Nutrition Essentials *for* Nursing Practice

SUSAN G. DUDEK, RD, CDN, BS

Former Nutrition Instructor, Dietetic Technology Program
Erie Community College
Williamsville, New York

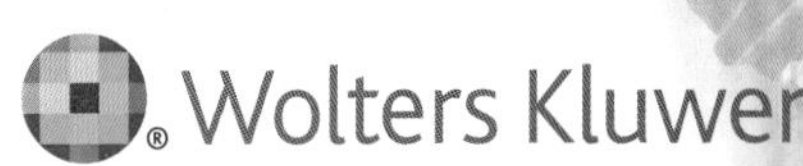

Philadelphia • Baltimore • New York • London
Buenos Aires • Hong Kong • Sydney • Tokyo

Vice President and Publisher: Julie K. Stegman
Acquisitions Editor: Jonathan Joyce
Manager, Nursing Education and Practice Content: Jamie Blum
Associate Development Editor: Rebecca J. Rist
Editorial Coordinator: Oliver Raj
Marketing Manager: Brittany Clements
Editorial Assistant: Molly Kennedy
Design Manager: Stephen Druding
Art Director, Illustration: Jennifer Clements
Senior Production Project Manager: Sadie Buckallew
Manufacturing Coordinator: Margie Orzech
Prepress Vendor: Lumina Datamatics

Ninth edition

9 8 7 6 5 4 3 2 1

Printed in China

Library of Congress Cataloging-in-Publication Data

Names: Dudek, Susan G., author.
Title: Nutrition essentials for nursing practice / Susan G. Dudek, RD, CDN, BS, Former Nutrition Instructor, Dietetic Technology Program, Erie Community College Williamsville, New York.
Description: Ninth edition. | Philadelphia, PA : Wolters Kluwer, [2022] | Includes bibliographical references and index.
Identifiers: LCCN 2021014575 | ISBN 9781975161125 (hardback) | ISBN 9781975161125
Subjects: LCSH: Diet therapy. | Nutrition. | Nursing. | BISAC: MEDICAL / Nursing / Nutrition
Classification: LCC RM216 .D8627 2022 | DDC 615.8/54--dc23
LC record available at https://lccn.loc.gov/2021014575

shop.lww.com

CCS0521

Dedicated to

All the people who on a personal or professional level made my initial dream of writing a book into a nine-edition-long reality. It has been a rewarding journey of teaching and learning, for which I am eternally grateful.

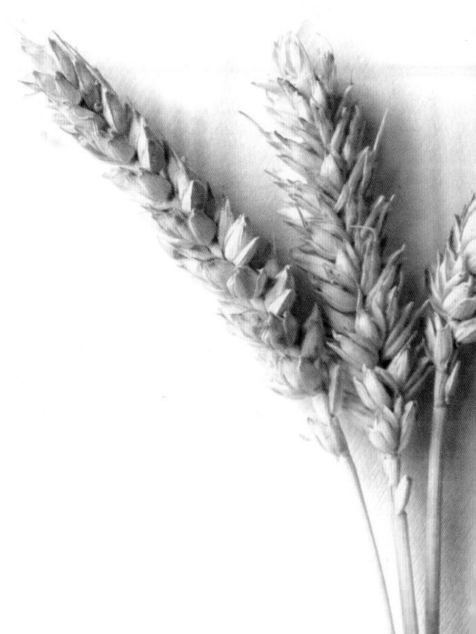

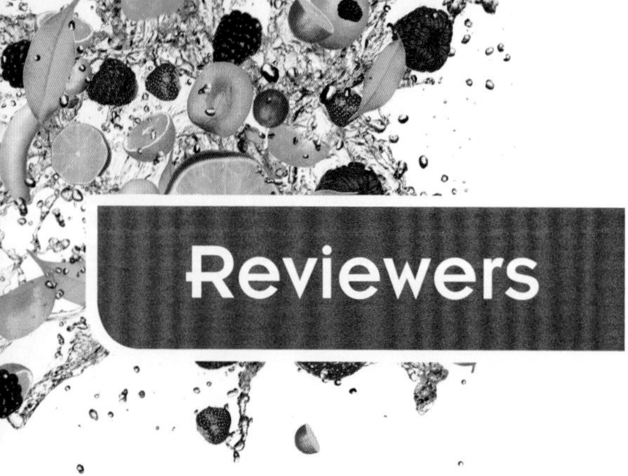

Reviewers

Claire Creamer, PhD, APRN-CPNP-PC
Associate Professor
Rhode Island College
Providence, Rhode Island

Claudia Kelley, PhD, RD, RN, CCS, CDE
Instructor
Los Angeles Mission College
Sylmar, California

Susan Kessler, RD, CDN, CHES
Senior Adjunct Professor
Adelphi University
Garden City, New York

Candace Pierce, DNP, RN, CNE
Assistant Professor
Troy University
Montgomery, Alabama

Colleen Tracy Snell, RN, MS
Faculty
Anoka-Ramsey Community College
Champlin, Minnesota

Stephanie R. Stewart, MSN, RN-BC
Associate Professor of Nursing
Missouri Western State University
St. Joseph, Missouri

Chantal Wolfe, MS, RDN, CSG, LDN, CLC
Pennsylvania College of Technology
Williamsport, Pennsylvania

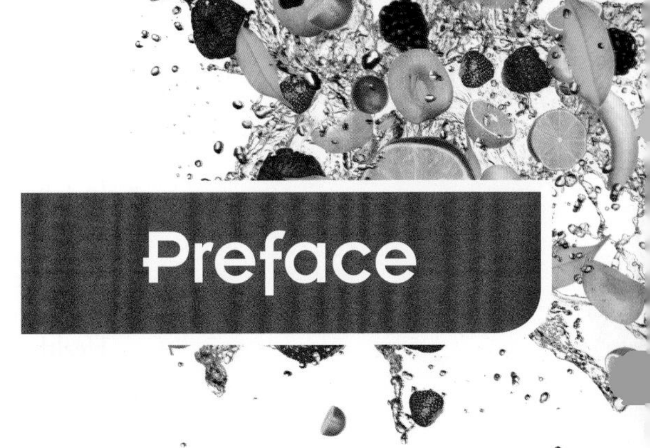

Preface

Like air and sleep, nutrition is a basic human need, essential for survival. From curing hunger to reducing the risk of chronic disease, nutrition is ever changing in response to technological advances and cultural shifts. Because nutrition at its most basic level is food—for the mind, body, and soul—it is a complex blend of science and art.

Although considered the realm of the dietitian, nutrition is a vital and integral component of nursing care across the life cycle and along the wellness–illness continuum. By virtue of their close contact with clients and families, nurses are often on the frontline in facilitating nutrition. Nutrition is woven into all steps of the nursing care process, from assessment and nursing analysis to implementation and evaluation. This textbook seeks to give student nurses an essential nutrition foundation to better serve themselves and their clients.

NEW TO THIS EDITION

This ninth edition of *Nutrition Essentials for Nursing Practice* has been reformatted to reflect the way students want to access information: quickly and concisely. To improve clarity and succinctness, bullet points are used where appropriate to present details. The depth of content is limited to what the nurse needs to know in an effort to avoid overwhelming the reader with unnecessary information. Some content has been reorganized to facilitate these changes.

- Content is updated throughout and reflects available evidence-based practice. In addition to the *Dietary Guidelines for Americans 2020–2025*, new guidelines or consensus reports included are those on nutrition therapy for adults with diabetes or prediabetes, guidelines on the primary prevention of cardiovascular disease, guidelines for the prevention and management of hypertension in adults, practice guidelines for obesity, and guidelines on nutrition in cancer care.
- The Table of Contents has been expanded to include a heading outline of each chapter.
- Concept Mastery Alerts clarify fundamental nursing concepts to improve the reader's understanding of potentially confusing topics, as identified by Misconception Alerts in Lippincott's Adaptive Learning Powered by prepU. Data from thousands of actual students using this program in courses across the United States identified common misconceptions that are clarified in this feature.
- Chapter 1 shifts from "Nutrition in Health and Health Care" to "Nutrition in Health." This chapter begins with recommended intake standards for nutrients and progresses to the relationship between nutrition and health, the importance of healthy eating, the concept of lifestyle medicine, and the future of nutrition research.
- The chapter entitled "Guidelines for Healthy Eating" is repositioned from Chapter 8 in the eighth edition to Chapter 2 in the ninth. This move improves the flow of content and provides the foundation for the chapters on nutrients that follow.
- Throughout the book, the focus on healthy eating patterns, such as the Mediterranean-style Eating Pattern and the DASH (Dietary Approaches to Stop Hypertension) diet, reflects the direction of nutrition guidelines and the widespread applicability of these patterns across the continuum of health and disease.

- In Chapter 9, "Food and Supplement Labeling," new content has been included on cannabidiol and labeling regulations regarding allergens, gluten, and country of origin.
- Adolescent pregnancy is moved from Chapter 13, "Nutrition for Infants, Children, and Adolescents," in the eighth edition to Chapter 12 in the ninth, "Healthy Eating for Healthy Babies."
- Healthy eating patterns promoted for healthy aging, namely the Mediterranean-Style Eating Pattern and the MIND diet, are added to Chapter 14, "Nutrition for Older Adults."
- The importance of consuming appropriate calories to attain and maintain healthy weight is emphasized throughout the units on health promotion and clinical practice (Chapters 9–24). This emphasis reflects the current prevalence of obesity and its significance as a major modifiable risk factor for chronic disease.
- Nursing analysis statements feature a nutrition problem, etiology of the problem, and the signs and symptoms of the problem. Because the priority in clinical nutrition is to prevent or treat malnutrition, risk of malnutrition is repeatedly cited as a nutrition problem throughout the unit on clinical nutrition.
- The Chapter Summary at the end of each chapter replaces the Key Concepts of the eighth edition. The straightforward outline format highlights the most salient information.

ORGANIZATION OF THE TEXT

The number of chapters has expanded from 22 to 24, by separating two large chapters into smaller chapters. "Consumer Issues" has been divided into "Food and Supplement Labeling" and "Consumer Interests and Concerns." A new separate chapter entitled "Enteral and Parenteral Nutrition" has been split from "Hospital Nutrition: Defining Nutrition Risk and Feeding Patients." These smaller chapters in the ninth edition are more cohesive and focused than their larger predecessors.

The chapters are organized into three units. Unit One is entitled "**Principles of Nutrition**." It flows from "Nutrition in Health" to "Guidelines for Healthy Eating" followed by chapters covering the six classes of nutrients—carbohydrates, protein, lipids, vitamins, water, and minerals. The health promotion section of each of these nutrient chapters explains why and how Americans are urged to shift their eating patterns to reduce the risk of chronic disease. The final chapter in this unit, "Energy Balance," explains how calorie needs are estimated, how body weight is evaluated, and strategies for balancing calorie intake with expenditure.

Unit Two, "**Nutrition in Health Promotion**," begins with Chapter 9, "Food and Supplement Labeling." Other chapters in this unit examine consumer interests, issues of food access, and cultural and religious influences on food and nutrition. The nutritional needs and concerns associated with the life cycle are presented in chapters devoted to pregnant and lactating women, infants, children and adolescents, and older adults.

Unit Three, "**Nutrition in Clinical Practice**," begins with "Hospital Nutrition: Defining-Nutrition Risk and Feeding Clients," which covers nutrition screening, nutrition in the nursing process, oral diets, and oral nutrition supplements. The chapter on enteral and parenteral nutrition follows. The unit continues with nutrition for obesity and eating disorders, critical illness, gastrointestinal disorders, diabetes, cardiovascular disorders, renal disorders, cancer, and HIV/AIDS. Pathophysiology is tightly focused as it pertains to nutrition.

FEATURES

This edition of *Nutrition Essentials for Nursing Practice* incorporates popular features to facilitate learning and engage students.

- **Unfolding Cases** present relevant nutrition information—in real-life scenarios—to provide an opportunity for students to apply theory to practice. Questions regarding the scenarios offer critical thinking opportunities for the student.
- **Key Terms** are defined in the margin for convenient reference.

- **Concept Mastery Alerts** clarify common misconceptions as identified by Lippincott's Adaptive Learning Powered by prepU.
- **Nursing Process** tables clearly present sample application of nutrition concepts in the context of the nursing process.
- **How Do You Respond?** helps students identify potential questions they may encounter and prepares them to think on their feet.
- **Review Case Study** along with the **Study Questions** challenge students to apply what they have learned.
- **Chapter Summaries** outlines the most important information from each chapter.

TEACHING AND LEARNING RESOURCES

To facilitate mastery of this textbook's content, a comprehensive teaching and learning package has been developed to assist faculty and students.

Lippincott® CoursePoint

Lippincott® CoursePoint is an integrated, digital curriculum solution for nursing education that provides a completely interactive and adaptive experience geared to help students understand, retain, and apply their course knowledge and be prepared for practice. The time-tested, easy-to-use, and trusted solution includes engaging learning tools, case studies, and in-depth reporting to meet students where they are in their learning, combined with the most trusted nursing education content on the market to help prepare students for practice. This easy-to-use digital learning solution of *Lippincott® CoursePoint*, combined with unmatched support, gives instructors and students everything they need for course and curriculum success!

Lippincott® CoursePoint includes the following:

- Engaging course content provides a variety of learning tools to engage students of all learning styles.
- Adaptive and personalized learning helps students learn the critical thinking and clinical judgment skills needed to help them become practice-ready nurses.
- Unparalleled reporting provides in-depth dashboards with several data points to track student progress and help identify strengths and weaknesses.
- Unmatched support includes training coaches, product trainers, and nursing education consultants to help educators and students implement CoursePoint with ease.

Resources for Instructors

Tools to assist you with teaching your course are available upon adoption of this textbook at https://thePoint.lww.com/Dudek9e.

- A **Test Generator** lets you put together exclusive new tests from a bank containing hundreds of questions to help you in assessing your students' understanding of the material. Test questions link to chapter learning objectives.
- **PowerPoint Presentations** provide an easy way for you to integrate the textbook with your students' classroom experience, either via slide shows or handouts. Multiple-choice and true/false questions are integrated into the presentations to promote class participation and allow you to use i-clicker technology.
- An **Image Bank** lets you use the photographs and illustrations from this textbook in your PowerPoint slides or as you see fit in your course.
- **Answers to Unfolding and Review Case Studies**
- **QSEN Map**

Resources for Students

An exciting set of free resources is available to help students review material and become even more familiar with vital concepts. Students can access all these resources at https://thePoint.lww.com/Dudek9e using the codes printed on the front of their textbooks.

- **Concepts in Action Animations** bring physiologic and pathophysiologic concepts to life.
- **Answers to Unfolding and Review Case Studies** from the text.
- **Learning Objectives** from the text.
- **Spanish–English Audio Glossary**.

I hope this textbook and teaching/learning resource package provide the impetus to embrace nutrition on both a personal and a professional level.

Susan G. Dudek, RD, CDN, BS

Acknowledgments

When I wrote the first edition of this book, I never imagined that the privilege would extend through nine editions. I am both humbled and thankful for the opportunity to do what I love—write, create, teach, and learn. It amazes me how much our understanding of nutrition evolves from one edition to the next. This project has been professionally rewarding, personally challenging, and rich with opportunities to grow.

- In large part, the success of this book rests with the dedicated and creative professionals at Wolters Kluwer. I especially thank **Jonathan Joyce**, Acquisitions Editor
- **Rebecca J. Rist**, Associate Development Editor
- **Oliver Raj**, Editorial Coordinator
- **Stephen Druding**, Design Manager
- **Jennifer Clements**, Art Director

I also appreciate the insightful comments and suggestions from **the reviewers of the eighth edition** that helped shape a new and improved edition.

And above all I thank **my husband, Joe**, who has been with me at every step of every edition with support, encouragement, and patience. Love you always.

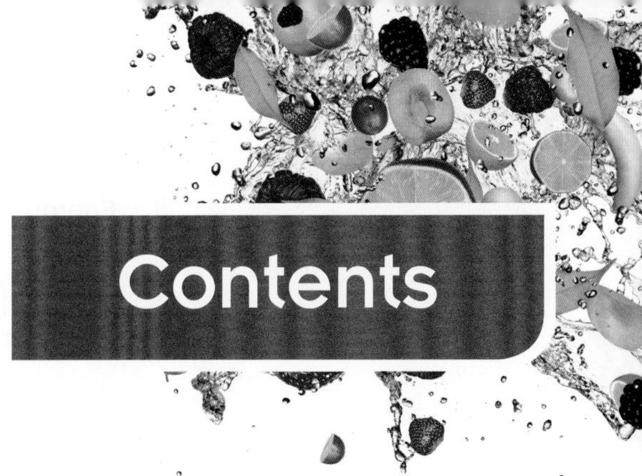

Contents

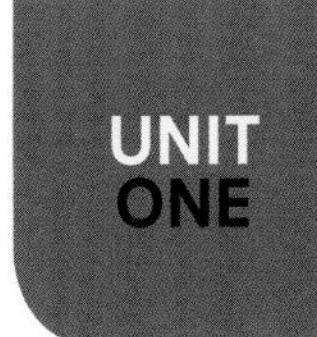

Nutrition Fundamentals 1

APPENDIX

UNIT
ONE

Nutrition Fundamentals

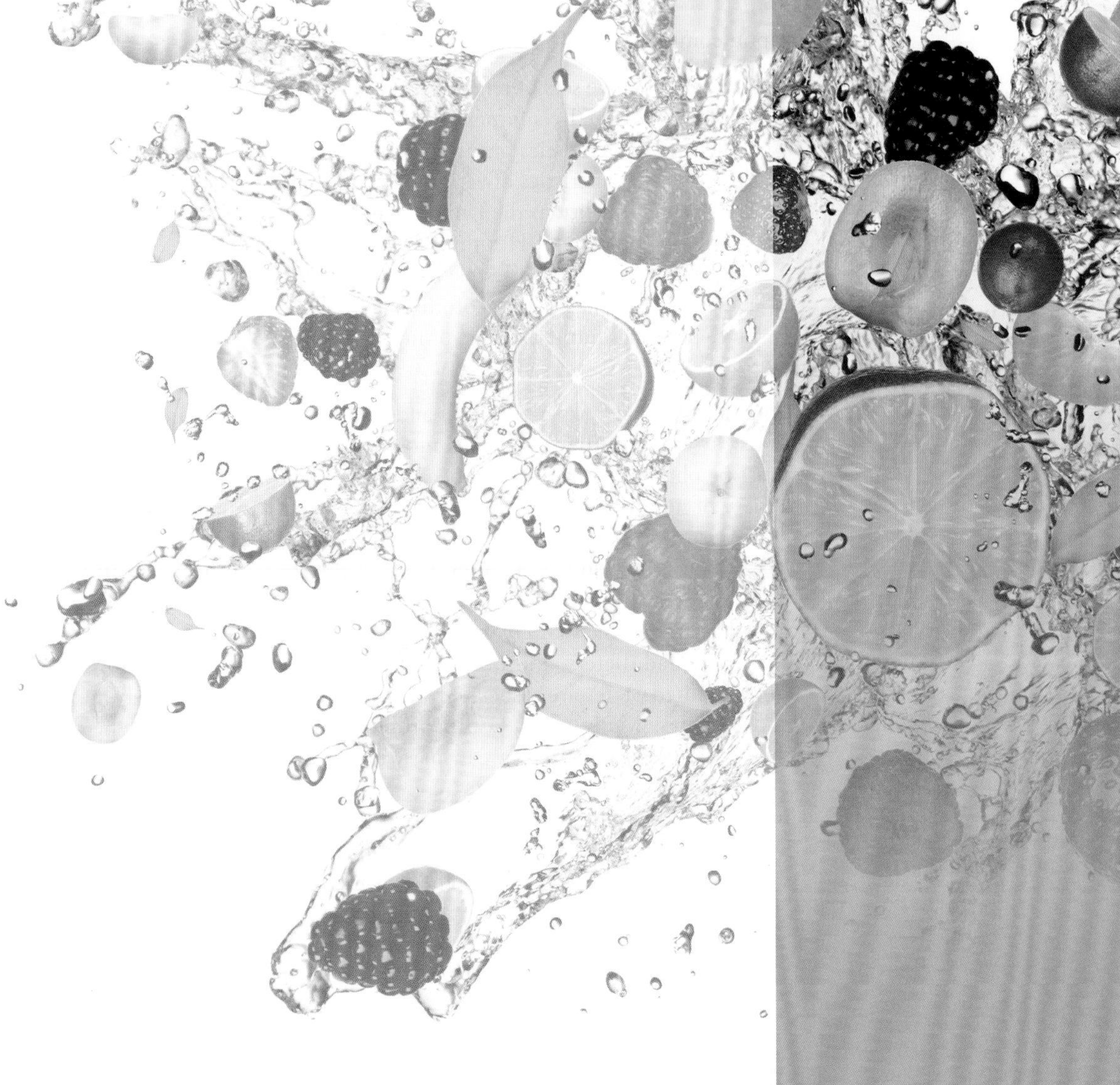

Chapter 1 Nutrition in Health

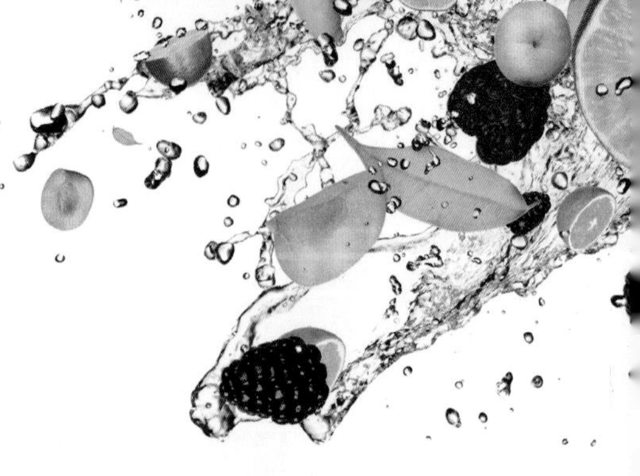

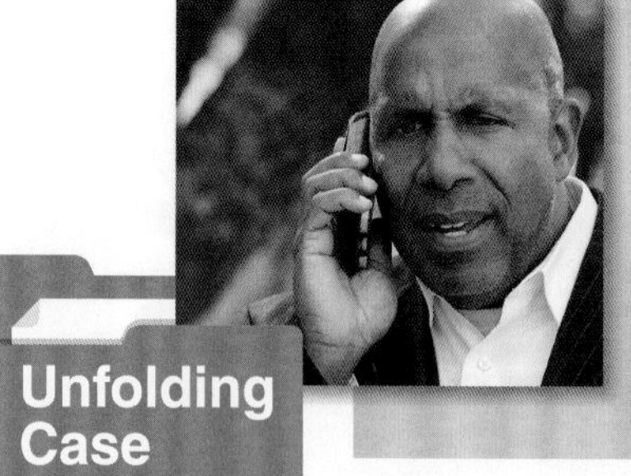

Unfolding Case

Tyrone Green

Tyrone is a 46-year-old national account executive who spends 4 out of 5 weekdays traveling on business. He was recently diagnosed with prediabetes and hypertension, which are two of the five diagnostic components of metabolic syndrome, which increases the risk of diabetes and cardiovascular disease. He blames his 25-pound weight gain on eating out while traveling.

Learning Objectives

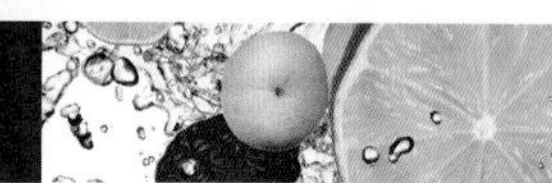

Upon completion of this chapter, you will be able to:

1 Describe the five sets of reference standards that make up the Dietary Reference Intakes.
2 Explain what the Recommended Dietary Allowances represent.
3 Describe characteristics of eating patterns associated with positive health outcomes.
4 Describe characteristics of eating patterns associated with detrimental health outcomes.
5 Discuss diet quality in the United States.
6 Define the purpose of Healthy People 2030.
7 Name four modifiable lifestyle risk factors for chronic disease.
8 Describe the characteristics of lifestyle medicine.
9 State potential future benefits of nutrigenomics.

Food is a complex mix of essential and nonessential components in various ratios and combinations. Essential nutrients, such as most vitamins, minerals, amino acids, fatty acids, and water, must be obtained through food because the body cannot make them. Plants provide fiber and a variety of nonnutrient compounds that have health-enhancing biological properties in the body. These beneficial nonnutrient compounds are known as *phytonutrients*.

When nutrition was a young science, the focus of healthy eating was to consume enough of all essential nutrients to avoid deficiency diseases. Today, nutrient deficiency diseases are generally rare in the United States except among specific population subgroups such as seniors, alcoholics, fad dieters, and hospitalized patients. In fact, several of the leading causes of death in the United States are associated with dietary excesses—namely, heart disease, cancer, stroke, and diabetes. Many other health problems, such as obesity, hypertension, and hypercholesterolemia, are related, at least in part, to dietary excesses. Although Americans in general are overconsuming some **nutrients** (e.g., saturated fat, sodium, sugar), other nutrients that are important for maintaining health (e.g., calcium and vitamin D) are being under-consumed. The current focus of nutrition is to reduce the risk of chronic diseases by improving overall dietary patterns. Lifestyle medicine is a medical specialty devoted to preventing and treating chronic disease through lifestyle changes.

Nutrients
chemical substances used by the body that are necessary for life and growth. Nutrient classes are carbohydrates, proteins, fats, vitamins, minerals, water.

This chapter begins with nutrient recommendations. The relationship between nutrition and health includes a discussion of characteristics of healthy and detrimental eating patterns, diet quality in the United States, Healthy People 2030, and the role of nutrition in chronic disease. Lifestyle medicine and nutritional genomics are presented.

DIETARY REFERENCE INTAKES

Dietary Reference Intakes (DRIs)
a set of five nutrient-based reference values used to plan and evaluate diets.

Dietary Reference Intakes (DRIs) are a collection of dietary reference standards that estimate nutrient intakes necessary to ensure that healthy populations meet nutrient needs to maintain health and prevent deficiency diseases (Institute of Medicine, 2006). For each essential nutrient, research studies were reviewed to help establish standards of adequacy and toxicity based on age and sex. Each reference value is viewed as an average daily intake over time, at least one week for most nutrients.

The four original DRI nutrient-based standards are the Recommended Dietary Allowances (RDAs), Estimated Average Requirement (EAR), Adequate Intake (AI), and Tolerable Upper Intake Level (UL). Each of these reference values has a specific purpose and represents a different level of intake (Fig. 1.1). Nutrients have either an RDA or an AI; not all nutrients have an established UL (Table 1.1). Additional reference sets that pertain to calories are Acceptable Macronutrient Distribution Ranges (AMDR) and the Estimated Energy Requirement (EER).

Chronic Disease Risk Reduction Intake (CDRR)
the level of intake associated with chronic disease risk. Recommendation specifies "reduce intake if above…" for sodium. For a nutrient that is inversely associated with disease risk, such as potassium, the recommendation would be to "increase intake if lower than…"

In 2019, the National Academies of Sciences, Engineering, and Medicine Food and Nutrition Board (formerly known as the Institute of Medicine, Food and Nutrition Board) created a new category of DRIs based on chronic disease risk, called the **Chronic Disease Risk Reduction Intakes (CDRR)** (National Academies of Sciences, Engineering, and Medicine, 2019). At this time, only sodium has a CDRR.

Since consumers eat *food* and not *nutrients*, nutrient recommendations are not suited to teaching people how to make healthy choices. Instead, nutrient recommendations are used by dietitians who plan and evaluate menus for specific populations such as senior citizens, schools, prisons, hospitals, assisted living communities, and military feeding programs. Nutrient recommendations are also used to assess the adequacy of an individual's intake by comparing estimated intake with estimated requirements. Keep in mind that obtaining a reliable estimate of a person's actual intake is difficult, due to reporting errors, flaws in estimating portion sizes, and day-to-day variation in food intake. Unless a person has participated in a nutrient requirement study, it is impossible to quantify exact nutrient requirements for an individual.

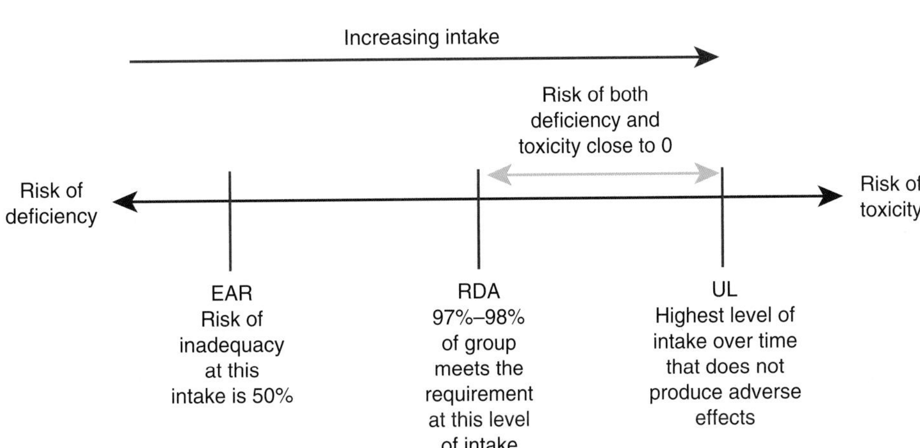

Figure 1.1 ▲ **Representation of Dietary Reference Intake along a continuum of intake.**

Table 1.1 Standards Applied to Each Nutrient for People Age 1 Year and Older

Nutrient	RDA	AI	UL[a]
Total water		✓	
Macronutrients			
Carbohydrate	✓		
Fiber		✓	
Linoleic acid		✓	
Alpha-linolenic acid		✓	
Protein	✓		
Fat-soluble vitamins			
Vitamin A	✓		✓
Vitamin D	✓		✓
Vitamin E	✓		✓
Vitamin K		✓	
Water-soluble vitamins			
Thiamin	✓		
Riboflavin	✓		
Niacin	✓		✓
Vitamin B_6	✓		✓
Folate	✓		✓
Vitamin B_{12}	✓		
Pantothenic acid		✓	
Biotin		✓	
Choline		✓	
Vitamin C	✓		
Elements			
Calcium	✓		✓
Chromium		✓	
Copper	✓		✓
Fluoride		✓	✓
Iodine	✓		✓
Iron	✓		✓
Magnesium	✓		✓
Manganese		✓	✓
Molybdenum	✓		✓
Phosphorus	✓		✓
Selenium	✓		✓
Zinc	✓		✓
Potassium		✓	
Sodium		✓	
Chloride		✓	

[a]A UL has also been established for boron and nickel, even though neither nutrient has an RDA or an AI.

Recommended Dietary Allowances

Recommended Dietary Allowances (RDAs)
the average daily dietary intake level sufficient to meet the nutrient requirement of 97% to 98% of healthy individuals in a particular life stage and gender group.

The **Recommended Dietary Allowances (RDAs)** represents the average daily recommended intake level that is sufficient to meet the nutrient requirements of 97% of healthy individuals by life stage and sex.

- RDAs exceed the requirements of almost all members of the group; therefore, intakes below the RDA cannot be assessed as inadequate.
- RDAs are set high enough to account for daily variations in intake.
- RDAs are used as a starting point when health professionals estimate the nutritional needs of people with health disorders and are individualized as needed.

Estimated Average Requirement

Estimated Average Requirement (EAR)
the nutrient intake estimated to meet the requirement of half of the healthy individuals in a specific group.

Estimated Average Requirement (EAR) values are used to determine RDA values; they are not used as a daily intake goal for individuals.

- The EAR of a nutrient is the average daily intake estimated to meet the nutrient needs of half of the healthy people in a life stage or gender group.
  - *Average* actually means *estimated median.*
  - Since it is an average, the EAR falls below the requirements of half of the specific group.
- The EAR is not based solely on the prevention of nutrient deficiencies:
  - it considers reducing the risk of chronic disease, and
  - accounts for the bioavailability of the nutrient—that is, how its absorption is affected by other food components.

Adequate Intake

Adequate Intake (AI)
an intake level thought to meet or exceed the requirement of almost all members of a specific group. An AI is set when there is insufficient data to define an RDA.

An **Adequate Intake (AI)** is set when an RDA cannot be determined due to lack of sufficient data on requirements.

- AI is a recommended average daily intake level that is expected to meet or exceed the needs of virtually all members of a specific group based on observed or experimentally determined estimates of nutrient intake by groups of healthy people.
- The primary purpose of the AI is to be a guide for an individual's nutrient intake.
- The difference between the RDA and the AI is that the RDA is expected to meet the needs of almost all healthy people whereas it is not known what percentage of people are covered with an AI.

Tolerable Upper Intake Level

Tolerable Upper Intake Level (UL)
the highest average daily intake level of a nutrient that probably poses no danger to most individuals in the group.

The **Tolerable Upper Intake Level (UL)** is the highest level of average daily nutrient intake that likely poses no risk of adverse health effects to almost all individuals in the general population.

- It is not intended to be a recommended level of intake: There is no benefit in consuming amounts greater than the RDA or AI.
- Not all nutrients have an established UL (Table 1.1).

Chronic Disease Risk Reduction Intake

Some essential nutrients are not only essential to life but are also linked to chronic disease risk, such as an excess of sodium. The category of CDRR was formed for the purpose of lowering chronic disease risk.

- The CDRR is based on evidence of the beneficial effect of lowering sodium intake on cardiovascular disease risk, hypertension risk, systolic blood pressure, and diastolic blood pressure (National Academies of Sciences, Engineering, and Medicine, 2019).
- The recommendation is written as "Reduce intake if above_____ mg/day."
- A CDRR for potassium was considered but not established due to lack of evidence that a low potassium intake increases the risk of chronic disease.

Acceptable Macronutrient Distribution Ranges

Acceptable Macronutrient Distribution Ranges (AMDRs)
an intake range for energy nutrients expressed as a percentage of total calories that is associated with a reduced risk of chronic disease.

The **Acceptable Macronutrient Distribution Ranges (AMDRs)** are broad ranges for each macronutrient expressed as a percentage of total calories consumed.

- These ranges are associated with reduced risk of chronic disease yet provide adequate amounts of essential nutrients.
- Over time, intakes above or below this range may increase the risk of chronic disease or deficiency, respectively.
- The AMDRs for adults are as follows:

	Percentage Total Calories Consumed
Carbohydrate	45–65
Protein	10–35
Fat	20–35
Essential fatty acids	
Linoleic acid (*n*-6)	5–10
Alpha-linolenic acid (*n*-3)	0.6–1.2

Estimated Energy Requirements

Estimated Energy Requirements (EERs)
level of calorie intake estimated to maintain weight in normal-weight individuals based on age, sex, height, weight, and activity.

The **Estimated Energy Requirements (EERs)** are the dietary calorie intake predicted to maintain weight in healthy, normal-weight individuals based on age, sex, weight, height, and level of physical activity.

- Exceeding EERs may produce weight gain.
- See Chapter 8 for more on determining energy needs.

FROM NUTRIENTS TO FOOD

Intake guidelines have often focused on nutrients more than food, such as limiting the total amount of fat consumed without consideration of the source of the fat. Such a narrow focus underestimates the complexity of food and the interactions between its components and ignores the possibility that many constituents of food and eating patterns may act synergistically to impact health (Jacobs & Orlich, 2014). For instance, populations that consume high amounts of fruit and vegetables were observed to have lower rates of epithelial cancers, so researchers speculated that beta carotene intake was protective; however, a study of giving large doses of supplemental beta carotene to people at high risk of lung cancer resulted in an increase in cancer and necessitated a premature halt to the study (Bjelakovic et al., 2007). This is a glaring example of how although certain food patterns may be associated with lower risk of disease, it is not known which components of a food, in what proportion, acting singularly or synergistically with other substances, are protective or detrimental to health. Thus, the health effects of foods may not be simply and accurately reduced to the effects of single nutrients (Jacobs & Orlich, 2014).

Focus on Total Diet

Researchers are increasingly focusing on the total diet—dietary patterns, nutrient density, and overall diet quality—to study the link between diet and health promotion/disease prevention (Millen, 2018).

Dietary Patterns

The 2020–2025 Dietary Guidelines for Americans (2020) defines *dietary patterns* as "the combination of foods and beverages that constitutes an individual's complete dietary intake over time. This may be a description of a customary way of eating or a description of a combination of foods recommended for consumption" (U.S. Department of Agriculture [USDA] and U.S. Department of Health and Human Services [USDHHS], 2020).

- Dietary patterns, commonly referred to as eating patterns, may be a better predictor of disease risk than specific nutrients or food (Wrobleski et al., 2018).
- A healthy eating pattern includes a variety of nutrient-dense foods across food groups that provide adequate amounts of nutrients within the appropriate calorie limits.

Healthy and detrimental eating patterns according to the 2020–2025 Dietary Guidelines for Americans (USDA & USDHHS, 2020) are as follows:

- Eating patterns associated with positive health outcomes are characterized by relatively high intakes of vegetables, fruits, legumes, whole grains, low- or nonfat dairy, lean meats and poultry, seafood, nuts, and unsaturated vegetable oils:
  - Examples of eating patterns consistently mentioned as healthy are plant-based eating patterns, the Mediterranean-Style Eating Pattern, and the Dietary Approaches to Stop Hypertension (DASH) diet.
  - Healthy eating patterns are presented in Chapters 2, 7, and 14 and are repeatedly referred to throughout Unit 3.
- Eating patterns associated with detrimental health outcomes are higher in the intake of red and processed meats, sugar-sweetened foods and beverages, and refined grains.

Nutrient Density

Nutrient density refers to foods and beverages that provide vitamins, minerals, and other beneficial substances relative to the number of calories with little or no added sugars, saturated fat, and sodium.

- Nutrient-dense foods include vegetables, fruits, whole grains, seafood, eggs, legumes, unsalted nuts and seeds, low-fat and fat-free dairy, and lean meats and poultry when prepared with no or little added sugars, saturated fat, and sodium.

Conversely, calorie density refers to the relative proportion of calories to nutrients in a food.

- Examples of calorie dense items include sugar-sweetened beverages, baked goods, full-fat fruited yogurt, and candy.
- Foods that are not in their most nutrient-dense form, such as whole milk compared to fat-free milk and fried chicken compared to baked chicken, have greater calorie density.

Overall Diet Quality

One way to measure diet quality is to use the **Healthy Eating Index-2015 (HEI-2015)**.

- The HEI-2015 uses a scoring tool to measure diet quality to assess how well a person's intake aligns with key dietary recommendations in the *Dietary Guidelines for Americans*—guidelines that are intended to help prevent diet-related chronic diseases, such as heart disease, type 2 diabetes, and cancer.
- There are 13 components that reflect different food groups and key recommendations (Table 1.2). The components are divided into two groupings:
  - The Adequacy group represents foods that are encouraged.
  - The Moderation group contains foods that should be limited.
- Most of the components are density-based (e.g., amounts per 1000 calories) and not absolute amounts.
- The HEI is revised with each new update of the *Dietary Guidelines* that occurs every 5 years. HEI-2020 has not yet been published.
- Evidence supports the validity and reliability of the HEI-2015 (Reedy et al., 2018).

Healthy Eating Index-2015 (HEI-2015)
a density-based (e.g., amounts per 1000 calories) measure of diet quality based on conformance with the *2015 Dietary Guidelines for Americans*. It is composed of food and nutrient characteristics that have established relationships with health outcomes. Previous versions were based on previous editions of the *Dietary Guidelines for Americans*.

Table 1.2 Components of the Healthy Eating Index-2015

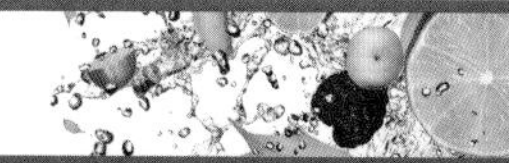

Component	Standard for Minimum Score of 0	Standard for Maximum Score
Adequacy: food components that are encouraged		
Total fruits	No fruit	≥0.8 c equivalents/1000 cal
Whole fruits	No whole fruit	≥0.4 c equivalents/1000 cal
Total vegetables	No vegetables	≥1.1 c equivalents/1000 cal
Greens and beans	No dark green vegetables or beans and peas	≥0.2 equivalents/1000 cal
Whole grains	No whole grains	≥1.5 oz equivalents/1000 cal
Dairy	No dairy	≥1.3 c equivalents/1000 cal
Total protein foods	No protein foods	≥2.5 oz equivalents/1000 cal
Seafood and plant proteins	No seafood or plant proteins	≥0.8 c equivalents/1000 cal
Fatty acids	Poly- + mono-unsaturated fatty acids/saturated fatty acids ≤1.2	Poly- + mono-unsaturated fatty acids/saturated fatty acids ≥2.5
Moderation: food components that should be consumed sparingly		
Refined grains	≥4.3 oz equivalents/1000 cal	≤1.8 oz equivalents/1000 cal
Sodium	≥2.0 g/1000 cal	≤1.1 g/1000 cal
Added sugars	≥26% of energy	≤6.5% of energy
Saturated fats	≥16% of energy	≤8% of energy

Source: United States Department of Agriculture, Food and Nutrition Service. (2019). *Healthy Eating Index (HEI)*. https://www.fns.usda.gov/resource/healthy-eating-index-hei#targetText=The%20Healthy%20Eating%20Index%20(HEI,the%20Dietary%20Guidelines%20for%20Americans.&targetText=The%20HEI%20uses%20a%20scoring,range%20from%200%20to%20100

Diet Quality in the United States

For Americans aged 2 and older, the average HEI-2015 score is 59 out of 100, indicating typical eating patterns consumed by Americans do not align with the *Dietary Guidelines for Americans* (USDA & USDHHS, 2020)

- Americans aged 60 and over have the highest diet quality with a score of 63
- Youth ages 14–18 have the lowest diet quality with a score of 51
- Americans fall short of nearly every component of diet quality measured (Wilson et al., 2016).

The term *poor* is often used to describe the typical American Eating Pattern, with poor referring to *quality*, not *inadequate quantity*, of food consumed. Compared to the Healthy U.S.-Style dietary pattern (USDA & USDHHS, 2020),

- 80% of Americans consume eating patterns that are low in vegetables, fruits, and dairy;
- more than 50% of the population is meeting or exceeding total grain and total protein foods recommendations but are not meeting the recommendations for the subgroups within each of these food groups (e.g., are not eating enough whole grains or seafood);
- average intakes of saturated fat, added sugars, and sodium exceed recommended amounts; and
- calorie intake in excess of need contributes to the high prevalence of overweight or obesity in adults (74%) and children (40%).

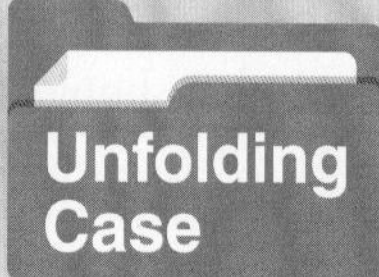

Think of Tyrone His typical intake while traveling is: two sandwiches containing eggs, cheese, and bacon for breakfast; a foot-long assorted deli meat submarine sandwich on white roll with a soft drink and bag of chips for lunch; and a dinner of steak, French fries, and salad. He snacks on candy, soft drinks, and granola bars in between meals.

How is Tyrone's intake of Adequacy components listed in the HIE-2015?

How is Tyrone's intake of Moderation components?

NUTRITION AND HEALTH

Across the lifespan, good nutrition supports all aspects of health: healthy pregnancy outcomes; normal growth, development, and aging; healthy body weight; lower risk of disease; and helping to treat acute and chronic disease (DiMaria-Ghalili et al., 2014). Nutrition is intimately entwined with health.

The World Health Organization (WHO, 1946) defines *health* as "a state of complete physical, mental, and social well-being, not merely the absence of disease or infirmity." In practice, health is defined subjectively and individually along a continuum that is influenced by an individual's perception of health. For instance, a recent survey found that although 53% of respondents ranked their health as very good or excellent, 61% of those respondents were overweight or obese (International Food Information Council Foundation, 2019). Likewise, older adults may consider themselves healthy despite having arthritis because they consider it a normal part of aging, not a chronic disease.

Healthy People 2030

Healthy People is a program under the jurisdiction of the U.S. Department of Health and Human Services (USDHHS) that focuses on improving the health and well-being of all Americans. Updated every 10 years since its inception, Healthy People sets public health goals and objectives and monitors the nation's progress toward meeting those objectives.

The newest edition, Healthy People 2030, has 355 core (measurable) objectives with 10-year targets. The objectives are organized into 5 categories: health conditions, healthy behaviors, populations, settings and systems, and social determinants of health. Box 1.1. lists core objectives

BOX 1.1 ***Healthy People 2030*** **Summary of Core Objectives for Nutrition and Healthy Eating and Overweight and Obesity**

Nutrition and Healthy Eating Objectives—General

- Reduce household food insecurity and hunger
- Eliminate very low food security in children
- Increase fruit consumption by people aged 2 years and over
- Increase vegetable consumption by people aged 2 years and older
- Increase consumption of dark green vegetables, red and orange vegetables, and beans and peas by people aged 2 years and over
- Increase whole grain consumption by people aged 2 years and over
- Reduce consumption of added sugars by people aged 2 years and over
- Reduce consumption of saturated fat by people aged 2 years and over
- Reduce consumption of sodium by people aged 2 years and over
- Increase calcium consumption by people aged 2 years and over
- Increase potassium consumption by people aged 2 years and over
- Increase vitamin D consumption by people aged 2 years and over
- Reduce iron deficiency in children aged 1 to 2 years

Adolescents

- Increase the proportion of students participating in the School Breakfast Program.

Heart Disease and Stroke

- Reduce the proportion of adults with high blood pressure
- Reduce cholesterol in adults

Infants

- Increase the proportion of infants who are breastfed exclusively through age 6 months
- Increase the proportion of infants who are breastfed at 1 year

Overweight and Obesity

- Reduce the proportion of adults with obesity
- Increase the proportion of health care visits by adults with obesity that include counseling on weight loss, nutrition, or physical activity

Women

- Increase the proportion of women of childbearing age who get enough folic acid
- Reduce iron deficiency in females aged 12 to 49 years

Overweight and Obesity Objectives

Overweight and Obesity—General

- Reduce the proportion of children and adolescents with obesity

(continued)

BOX 1.1 ***Healthy People 2030* Summary of Core Objectives for Nutrition and Healthy Eating and Overweight and Obesity (continued)**

Diabetes

- Reduce the proportion of adults who don't know they have prediabetes

Nutrition and Healthy Eating[a]

- Reduce the proportion of adults with obesity
- Increase the proportion of health care visits by adults with obesity that include counseling on weight loss, nutrition, or physical activity
- Reduce consumption of added sugars by people aged 2 years and over

Pregnancy and Childbirth

- Increase the proportion of women who had a healthy weight before pregnancy.

[a]These objectives appear under the broad topic of Nutrition and Healthy Eating and as a subtopic of Overweight and Obesity topics.
Source: U.S. Department of Health and Human Services. (2020, August 18). *Healthy People 2030. Building a healthier future for all.* https://health.gov/healthypeople/objectives-and-data/browse-objectives.

under the topics of Nutrition and Healthy Eating and Overweight and Obesity. Two additional categories of objectives differ from core objectives in that they lack either reliable baseline data (developmental objectives) or are not yet associated with evidence-based interventions (research objectives).

Chronic Disease

Changes in lifestyle over the last 50 years—an abundant, cheap food supply, increasing mechanization of daily life, sedentary occupations, and sedentary screen time—have been reflected in changes in disease patterns. Acute infectious diseases have been replaced by chronic diseases related to lifestyle as major causes of death. Preventable chronic disease is a major challenge to global health.

- Noncommunicable diseases account for 71% of all deaths worldwide (World Health Organization, 2018).
- In the United States, chronic diseases are responsible for 7 of the top 10 causes of death (Box 1.2) and are the leading causes of disability (CDC, 2019).
- Today, 60% of American adults have one or more diet-related chronic diseases (USDA & USDHHS, 2020), and 4 out of 10 adults have two or more chronic health conditions (Centers for Disease Control and Prevention [CDC], 2019). (See Table 1.3.)
- Children and adolescents also have chronic diseases, such as type 2 diabetes and hypertension.

BOX 1.2 **Ten Leading Causes of Death in the United States[a] (Data for 2018)**

1. Heart disease
2. Cancer
3. Accidents (unintentional injuries)
4. Chronic lower respiratory diseases
5. Cerebrovascular diseases
6. Alzheimer's disease
7. Diabetes mellitus
8. Influenza and pneumonia
9. Nephritis, nephrotic syndrome, and nephrosis
10. Suicide

[a]includes people of all origins, sex, age groups.
Source: Centers for Disease Control and Prevention. (2020, October 30). *Leading causes of death.* https://www.cdc.gov/nchs/fastats/leading-causes-of-death.htm.

Table 1.3 Facts about Nutrition-Related Health Conditions in the United States

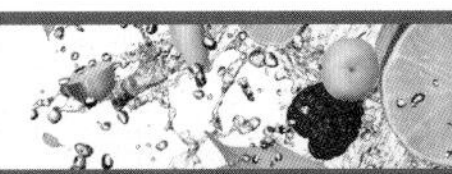

Health Conditions	Statistics
Overweight and obesity	• About 74% of adults are overweight or have obesity. • Adults ages 40–59 have the highest rate of obesity (43%) of any age group with adults 60 years and older having a 41% rate of obesity. • About 40% of children and adolescents are overweight or have obesity; the rate of obesity increases throughout childhood and teen years.
CVD and risk factors: • Coronary artery disease • Hypertension • High LDL and total blood cholesterol • Stroke	• Heart disease is the leading cause of death. • About 18.2 million adults have coronary artery disease, the most common type of heart disease. • Stroke is the 5th leading cause of death. • Hypertension, high LDL cholesterol, and high total cholesterol are major risk factors in heart disease and stroke. • Rates of hypertension and high total cholesterol are higher in adults with obesity than those who are at a healthy weight. • About 45% of adults have hypertension.[a] • More Black adults (54%) than White adults (46%) have hypertension. • More adults ages 60 and older (75%) than adults ages 40–59 (55%) have hypertension. • Nearly 4% of adolescents have hypertension.[b] • More than 11% of adults have high total cholesterol, ≥240 mg/dL. • More women (12%) than men (10%) have high total cholesterol, ≥240 mg/dL. • 7% of children and adolescents have high total cholesterol, ≥200 mg/dL.
Diabetes	• Almost 11% of Americans have type 1 or type 2 diabetes. • Almost 35% of American adults have prediabetes, and people 65 years and older have the highest rate (48%) compared to other age groups. • Almost 90% of adults with diabetes also are overweight or have obesity. • About 210,000 children and adolescents have diabetes, including 187,000 with type 1 diabetes. • About 6%–9% of pregnant women develop gestational diabetes.
Cancer[c] • Breast Cancer • Colorectal Cancer	• Colorectal cancer in men and breast cancer in women are among the most common types of cancer. • About 250,520 women will be diagnosed with breast cancer this year. • Close to 5% of men and women will be diagnosed with colorectal cancer at some point during their lifetime. • More than 1.3 million people are living with colorectal cancer. • The incidence and mortality rates are highest among those ages 65 and older for every cancer type.
Bone Health and Muscle Strength	• More women (17%) than men (5%) have osteoporosis. • 20% of older adults have reduced muscle strength. • Adults over 80 years, non-Hispanic Asians, and women are at the highest risk for reduced bone mass and muscle strength.

[a]For adults, hypertension is defined as systolic blood pressure (SBP) > 130 mm Hg and/or a diastolic blood pressure (DBP) > 90 mm Hg.
[b]For children, hypertension was defined using the 2017 American Academy of Pediatrics (AAP) Clinical Practice Guideline.
[c]The types of cancer included here are not a complete list of all diet- and physical activity–related cancers.
Source: USDA & USDHHS. (2020, December). *Dietary Guidelines for Americans*. https://www.dietaryguidelines.gov.

- Almost half of premature deaths in the United States are related to tobacco use, lack of physical activity, and poor diet (United Health Foundation, 2018).
- Box 1.3 features modifiable risk factors for chronic disease.

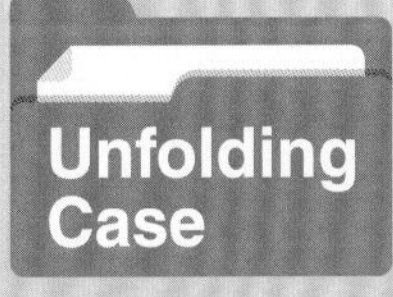

Consider Tyrone. From what we know about Tyrone, what modifiable risk factors for chronic disease does he have? What questions would you ask to further identify modifiable risk factors?

BOX 1.3 Modifiable Risk Factors for Chronic Disease

Poor Nutrition

- Fewer than 1 in 10 U.S. adults and adolescents eat enough fruit and vegetables.
- 6 in 10 young people and 5 in 10 adults consume a sugary drink on a given day.
- 9 out of 10 Americans aged 2 and older consume more than the recommended amount of sodium.
- U.S. diets are high in added sugars, sodium, and saturated fats.

Tobacco Use

- Tobacco use is the leading cause of preventable disease, disability, and death in the United States.
- About 34 million U.S. adults smoke cigarettes, and 58 million nonsmokers are exposed to secondhand smoke.
- Every day, about 2000 young people under age 18 smoke their first cigarette and >300 become daily cigarette smokers.
- Cigarette smoking causes >480,000 deaths annually, including 41,000 deaths from secondhand smoke. For every American who dies because of smoking, at least 30 are living with a serious smoking-related illness.
- Smoking causes cancer, heart disease, stroke, lung disease, type 2 diabetes, and other chronic health conditions.

Excessive Alcohol

- Excessive alcohol use is responsible for 88,000 deaths in the United States each year, including 1 in 10 total deaths among working-age adults.
- In 2010, excessive alcohol use cost the U.S. economy $249 billion, or $2.05 a drink.
- Binge drinking is responsible for over half the deaths related to excessive alcohol use.
- 9 in 10 adults who binge drink do not have an alcohol use disorder.

Physical Inactivity

- Only 1 in 4 U.S. adults and 1 in 5 high school students meet the recommended physical activity guidelines.
- About 31 million adults aged 50 or older are inactive, meaning that they get no physical activity beyond that of daily living.
- Low levels of physical activity can contribute to heart disease, type 2 diabetes, some kinds of cancer, and obesity.

Source: Centers for Disease Control and Prevention. (2019). National Center for Chronic Disease Prevention and Health Promotion. *About chronic diseases.* https://www.cdc.gov/chronicdisease/about/index.htm

Lifestyle Medicine

According to the American College of Lifestyle Medicine, "lifestyle medicine is the use of evidence-based lifestyle therapeutic approaches, such as a plant-predominant dietary lifestyle, regular physical activity, adequate sleep, stress management, avoiding use of risky substances, and pursuing other non-drug modalities to treat, reverse, and prevent chronic disease" (American College of Lifestyle Medicine [ACLM], 2019).

- Advocating for healthy lifestyles started when physicians began to see lifestyle as a critical tool in caring for patients but also healthy people (Yeh & Kong, 2013).
- The focus on food and lifestyle choices to prevent and treat chronic diseases, such as obesity, type 2 diabetes, cardiovascular disease, and many types of cancer, has become an increasingly popular medical paradigm (Retelny, 2017).
- Hippocrates' quote, "Let food be thy medicine and medicine be thy food," supports the present-day trend to view food as medicine based on the premise that good health depends on a healthy diet.
- Characteristics of lifestyle medicine differ from those of traditional medicine (Battersby et al., 2011):
  - Patients are an active partner in their own care and not a passive recipient.
  - Patients are required to make major changes.
  - Treatment is always long-term.
  - Medications are used as an adjunct to therapeutic lifestyle changes.

- Motivation and compliance are emphasized.
- The goal is primary, secondary, or tertiary prevention.
- Lifestyle medicine involves a multidisciplinary team approach that includes allied health professionals.
- The patient's home and community environment are assessed as contributing factors.

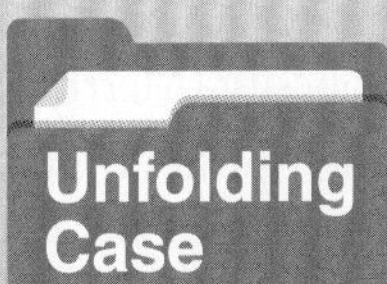

Remember Tyrone. Tyrone considers himself more interested in "natural" remedies than in conventional medicine. He asks you to explain lifestyle medicine and wants to know whether he is a good candidate. How would you respond?

Future Directions

Nutrition has the potential to help individuals live healthier, more productive lives and reduce the worldwide strain of chronic disease. The importance of nutrition as part of the solution to societal, environmental, and economic challenges facing the world has just begun to be fully recognized (Ohlhorst et al., 2013). Some of the questions driving nutrition research are featured in Box 1.4. New technology and scientific discoveries are deepening our understanding of how nutrients and eating patterns affect health and disease.

Database
a comprehensive collection of related information organized for convenient access.

Bioinformatics
an interdisciplinary field that uses computer science and information technology to develop and improve techniques that make it easier to acquire, store, organize, retrieve, and use complex biological data.

- Technology will enable researchers to expand and update nutrition **databases** to include more food items and substances in food previously not quantified, such as lycopene, resveratrol, and other phytonutrients, which will provide a more accurate and complete picture of food composition.
- **Bioinformatics** will enable researchers to make connections between intake and health that were not previously possible.
- **Nutrigenomics** has the potential to redefine the role of nutrition in health and disease risk in individuals.

BOX 1.4 Some Questions Driving Nutrition Research

- How do an individual's genes determine how the body handles specific nutrients?
- What role does a person's microbiota have in an individual's response to diet and food components? What is its role in disease prevention and progression?
- How does food intake affect a person's microbiota?
- How does an individual's genome affect responses to diet and food?
- How does diet during critical periods of development "program" long-term health and well-being? For instance, how does undernutrition during fetal life increase the risk of diabetes in adulthood?
- How can obesity be prevented? Can obesity be cured?
- How does nutrition influence the initiation of disease and its progression?
- What are the nutritional needs of aging adults?
- What are the biochemical and behavior bases for food choices? How can we most effectively measure, monitor, and evaluate dietary change?
- How can we get people to change their eating behaviors?

Source: Ohlhorst, S., Russell, R., Bier, D., Klurfeld, D., Li, Z., Mein, J., Milner, J., Ross, A., Stover, P., & Konopka, E. (2013). Nutrition research to affect food and a health life span. *American Journal of Clinical Nutrition, 98*, 620–625.

Nutrigenomics

Genomics
an area of genetics that studies the sequencing and analysis of an organism's genome.

Nutrigenomics
the study of the interaction between bioactive food components and genes and how that interaction impacts health and disease

Nutrigenomics is the study of the interaction between nutrients and other bioactive compounds with the human genome at the molecular level.

- Mapping the sequence of the human genome allows researchers to examine the relationship between a person's genetic makeup, response to diet, and health outcomes.
- Hundreds of links between genes, diet, and health outcomes have already been identified. Obesity is one area of particular interest. For instance,
  - It has been revealed that a variation in fat mass and an obesity-associated gene (FTO) is associated with susceptibility to obesity (Merritt et al., 2018).
  - Research findings suggest that a high protein intake may protect against the obesity effects of certain FTO genotypes (Merritt et al., 2018).
  - Further studies are needed to identify the mechanism of this gene–diet interaction, as well as explore the possibility of incorporating a high-protein diet in personalized weight loss plans.
- Nutrigenomics has the potential to produce major nutrition breakthroughs in the prevention of chronic disease and to identify new **biomarkers** that will more accurately assess a person's health and nutritional status. Additional benefits may include the following:
  - individualized dietary advice and customized dietary guidelines based on genetic background;
  - the development of healthier foods, such as functional foods, to provide specific health benefits based on genetic background beyond basic nutrition;
  - a reduction in health disparities that are related, at least in part, to the interaction between diet and genes;
  - reduced health care costs and improved quality of life (Singh & Sharma, 2019).
  - For instance, it is possible that certain components of food when matched with individual genotypes could take the place of more expensive drugs in the treatment of certain disorders.
- Genetic mutations only partially predict disease risk because most chronic diseases (e.g., cardiovascular disease, diabetes, and cancer) are multigenetic and multifactorial (Camp & Trujillo, 2014). For instance, tobacco use impacts the risk of chronic disease.
- It is not yet known whether knowledge gained from nutrigenomics will have practical application in the everyday life of consumers (Camp & Trujillo, 2014).

Biomarker
a measurable biological molecule found in blood, other body fluids, or tissues that is a sign of a normal or abnormal process or of a condition or disease.

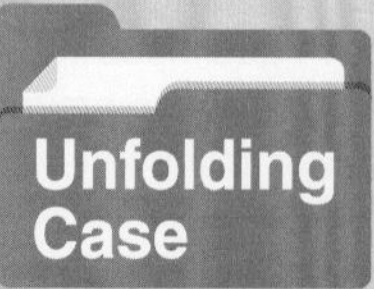

Recall Tyrone. He is admitted to the hospital for chest pain. Although screening did not find him to be at nutritional risk, he is counseled on the importance of eating healthier. He and his wife have many questions about how to implement a healthy eating pattern.

- Do you feel competent to reinforce the written and verbal instructions they've been given?
- How will you assure the patient that he can improve his eating pattern?
- What benefits could he realize with improved eating and exercise?

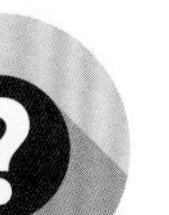

How Do You Respond?

Both of my parents had type 2 diabetes so I know I'm doomed. Why should I eat healthier to reduce my risk if it's in the genes? A healthy eating pattern and physical activity have been found to be effective in preventing or delaying the onset of diabetes among individuals with prediabetes, although eating healthier is not guaranteed to prevent type 2 diabetes. There are other potential health benefits to adopting a healthy eating pattern and increasing physical activity: improvements in weight status, blood pressure, low high-density lipoprotein cholesterol, and high triglyceride levels as well as possible reduced risk of certain cancers. There is not a downside to adopting healthier lifestyle behaviors, even though the benefits cannot be guaranteed.

REVIEW CASE STUDY

Kyla is 25 years old, overweight, and convinced a paleo diet will help her achieve her ideal weight. She eats only meat, fish, vegetables, nuts, and seeds. Fruit is acceptable to eat on a paleo diet, but Kyla avoids them because they are "high in sugar." She does not consume any dairy products, legumes, or grains in any form. She has lost weight but is concerned her diet may not be balanced or healthy for the long term.

- Using Table 1.2, what food components are missing from Kyla's diet?
- Is it possible for Kyla to eat too many calories despite the restrictiveness of her diet?
- Can a multivitamin adequately replace the nutrient and food components missing in Kyla's diet?
- When someone needs to lose weight for health benefits, is it okay to eat according to a less-than-healthy diet for the sake of weight loss, or should a healthy diet that provides all the adequate components always be the priority?
- There are no long-term clinical studies about the benefits and potential risks of the paleo diet. What would you say to Kyla about the efficacy and safety of her diet choice?

STUDY QUESTIONS

1 Recommended Dietary Allowances represent
  a. the average amount of a nutrient considered adequate to meet the needs of almost all healthy people.
  b. the minimum amount of a nutrient necessary to avoid deficiency disease.
  c. the optimal amount of a nutrient to prevent chronic disease.
  d. the highest amount of a nutrient that appears safe for most healthy people.

2 The typical American dietary pattern is
  a. low in refined grains.
  b. low in whole grains.
  c. high in fruit.
  d. high in dairy products.

3 Which statement is accurate regarding characteristics of a healthy eating pattern?
  a. The only healthy eating pattern is a vegetarian one.
  b. Healthy eating patterns eliminate foods that are high in saturated fat, added sugar, and sodium (fried foods, desserts, snack chips, etc.).
  c. Healthy eating patterns may reduce the risk of several chronic diseases: cardiovascular disease, type 2 diabetes, and certain cancers.
  d. Most young and middle-aged adults consume a healthy eating pattern.

4 Detrimental health outcomes are linked to excessive intakes of all of the following except
  a. Saturated fat.
  b. Carbohydrates.
  c. Added sugars.
  d. Sodium.

5 Which statement regarding the characteristics of lifestyle medicine is not true?
  a. Medications are not used in conjunction with lifestyle medicine.
  b. Patients are expected to be active participants in their care.
  c. Patients are required to make major lifestyle changes.
  d. Treatment is always long-term.

CHAPTER SUMMARY NUTRITION IN HEALTH

More than ever before, studies link dietary patterns, including nutrient density and diet quality, to health promotion and the prevention of disease.

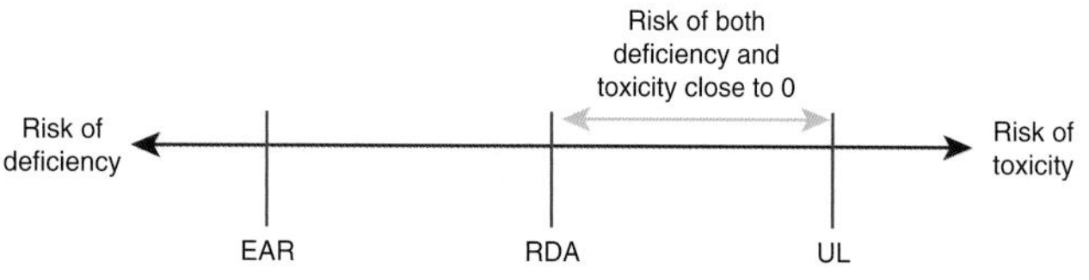

Dietary Reference Intakes

The DRIs are the set of accepted reference standards of estimated nutrient needs and intake recommendations for healthy people to maintain health and prevent deficiency diseases. The DRIs are primarily for professional use because they deal with nutrients, not food.

List of Dietary Reference Intakes

- **Recommended Dietary Allowances (RDAs):** amounts of nutrients considered adequate to meet the needs of almost all healthy people.
- **Adequate Intake (AI):** similar to RDA, but it is not known what percentage of people meet their nutritional needs by consuming the AI.
- **Tolerable Upper Intake Level (UL):** the highest intake of a nutrient over time that poses no risk.
- **Chronic Disease Risk and Reduction Intake (CDRR):** the level of a nutrient above or below which risk of chronic disease increases.
- **Acceptable Macronutrient Distribution Ranges (AMDRs):** the range of intake of each macronutrient, expressed as a percentage of total calories, associated with reduced risk of chronic disease.

From Nutrients to Food

The total diet approach to healthy eating encompasses eating patterns, nutrient density, and diet quality.

- **Dietary patterns:** the amount, proportions, variety, or combinations of different foods and beverages in diets, and the frequency with which they are usually eaten. Examples of healthy eating patterns are plant-based eating patterns, the Mediterranean-Style Eating Pattern, and the DASH diet.
- **Nutrient density:** the relative proportion of nutrients compared to calories in a food or serving
- **Overall diet quality:** the HEI-2015 is a numerical measure of diet quality based on food groups and key recommendations made in the *Dietary Guidelines for Americans*.

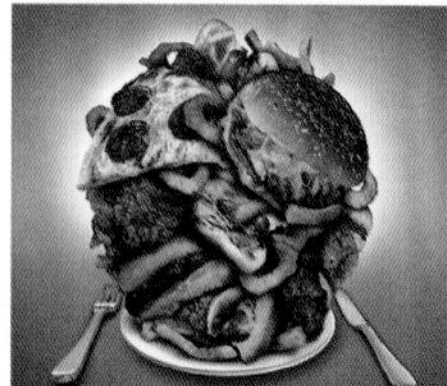

- **Diet quality in the United States:** the typical American Eating Pattern is low in fruits, vegetables, whole grains, dairy, and seafood and provides excessive saturated fat, added sugars, and sodium. An excessive intake of calories contributes to the high prevalence of overweight and obesity in children and adults.

Nutrition and Health

Nutrition plays a vital role in all aspects of health: growth, development, and health maintenance.

- Healthy People 2030 is a comprehensive blueprint for monitoring the nation's progress toward becoming healthier. Nutrition and Healthy Eating and Overweight and Obesity are among the topics with specific core objectives.
- Chronic disease is responsible for 7 of the top 10 causes of death in the United States. Modifiable risk factors for chronic disease include poor diet, tobacco use, excessive alcohol intake, and physical in activity.

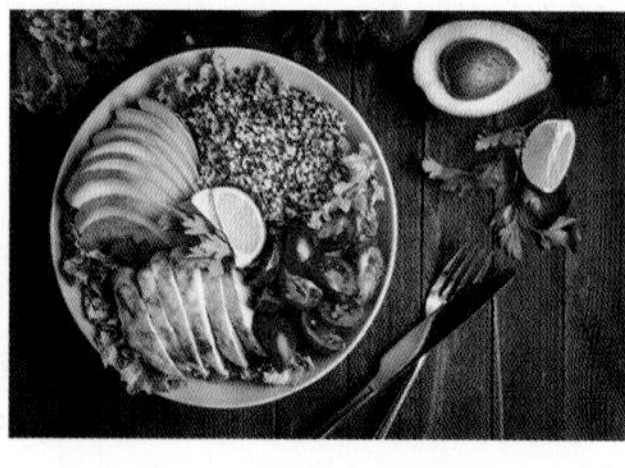

- Lifestyle medicine uses evidence-based lifestyle therapeutic approaches, such as a plant based eating pattern, regular physical activity, adequate sleep, stress management, avoiding the use of risky substances, and pursuing other non-drug modalities to treat, reverse, and prevent chronic disease.
- **Future directions:** new technology and scientific discoveries are deepening our understanding of how nutrients and eating patterns affect health and disease. Nutrigenomics studies the interaction between genes, diet, and health. It has the potential to revolutionize advances in individualized nutrition interventions.

Figure sources: *shutterstock.com/Lightspring and shutterstock.com/Elenadesign*

Student Resources on thePoint®
For additional learning materials, activate the code in the front of this book at https://thePoint.lww.com/activate

Websites

Dietary guidelines for Americans 2020–2025 at https://www.dietaryguidelines.gov/
Healthy Eating Index (HEI) at https://www.fns.usda.gov/resource/healthy-eating-index-hei
Healthy People 2030 at https://www.healthypeople.gov
United Health Foundation (a private, not-for-profit foundation dedicated to improving health and health care) at https://www.unitedhealthfoundation.org

References

American College of Lifestyle Medicine. (2019). *Mission/vision*. Available at https://www.lifestylemedicine.org/ACLM/About/Mission_Vision/ACLM/About/Mission_Vision.aspx?hkey=0c26bcd1-f424-416a-9055-2e3af80777f6

Battersby, M., Egger, G., & Litt, J. (2011). Introduction to lifestyle medicine. In: Egger, C., Binns, A., and Rossner, S., [eds]. *Lifestyle medicine: Managing diseases of lifestyle in the 21st century.* McGraw-Hill.

Bjelakovic, G., Nikolova, D., Gluud, L., Simonetti, R., & Gluud, C. (2007). Mortality in randomized trials of antioxidant supplements for primary and secondary prevention: Systematic review and meta-analysis. *JAMA, 297*(8), 842–857. https://doi.org/10.1001/jama.297.8.842

Camp, K., & Trujillo, E. (2014). Position of the Academy of Nutrition and Dietetics: Nutritional genomics. *Journal of the Academy of Nutrition and Dietetics, 114*(2), 299–312. https://doi.org/10.1016/j.jand.2013.12.001

Centers for Disease Control and Prevention. (2019). National Center for Chronic Disease Prevention and Health Promotion (NCCDPHP). *Chronic diseases in America*. https://www.cdc.gov/chronicdisease/resources/infographic/chronic-diseases.htm

DiMaria-Ghalili, R., Mirtallo, J., Tobin, B., Hark, L., Van Horn, L., & Palmer, C. (2014). Challenges and opportunities for nutrition education and training in the health care professions: Intraprofessional and interprofessional call to action. *American Journal of Clinical Nutrition, 99*(5), 1184S–1193S. https://doi.org/10.3945/ajcn.113.073536

Institute of Medicine. (2006). *Dietary reference intakes: The essential guide to nutrient requirements.* The National Academies Press. www.nap.edu

International Food Information Council Foundation. (2019). *2019 food & health survey*. https://foodinsight.org/wp-content/uploads/2019/05/IFIC-Foundation-2019-Food-and-Health-Report-FINAL.pdf

Jacobs, D., & Orlich, M. (2014). Diet pattern and longevity: Do simple rules suffice? A commentary. *American Journal of Clinical Nutrition, 100*(Suppl. 1), 313S–319S. https://doi.org/10.3945/ajcn.113.071340

Merritt, D., Jamnik, J., & El-Sohemy, A. (2018). FTO genotype, dietary protein intake, and body weight in a multiethnic population of young adults: A cross-sectional study. *Genes and Nutrition, 13*, 4. https://doi.org/10.1186/s12263-018-0593-7

Millen, B. (2018). Nutrition research advances and practice innovations. The future is very bright. *Journal of the Academy of Nutrition and Dietetics, 118*(9), 1587–1590. https://doi.org/10.1016/j.jand.2018.05.018

National Academies of Sciences, Engineering, and Medicine. (2019). *Consensus study report highlights. Dietary reference intakes for sodium and potassium.* https://www.nap.edu/resource/25353/030519DRISodiumPotassium.pdf

Ohlhorst, S., Russell, R., Bier, D., Klurfeld, D., Li, Z., Mein, J., Milner, J., Ross, A., Stover, P., & Konopka, E. (2013). Nutrition research to affect food and a healthy life span. *The Journal of Nutrition, 143*(8), 1349–1354. https://doi.org/10.3945/jn.113.180638

Reedy, J., Lerman, J., Krebs-Smith, S., Kirkpatrick, S., Pannucci, T., Wilson, M., Subar, A., Kahle, L., & Tooze, J. (2018). Evaluation of the healthy eating index-2015. *Journal of the Academy of Nutrition and Dietetics, 118*(9), 1622–1633. https://doi.org/10.1016/j.jand.2018.05.019

Retelny, V. (2017). Using food as lifestyle medicine. *Today's Dietitian, 19*, 36. https://www.todaysdietitian.com/newarchives/1217p36.shtml

Singh, R., & Sharma, L. (2019). Nutrigenomics: A combination of nutrition and genomics: A new concept. *International Journal of Physiology, Nutrition and Physical Education, 4*(1), 417–421. https://www.researchgate.net/profile/Richa_Singh25/publication/334603656_Nutrigenomics_A_combination_of_nutrition_and_genomics_A_new_concept/links/5d35596992851cd0467b4e9d/Nutrigenomics-A-combination-of-nutrition-and-genomics-A-new-concept.pdf

U.S. Department of Agriculture & U.S. Department of Health and Human Services. (2020). *Dietary guidelines for Americans, 2020–2025.* 9th ed. https://www.dietaryguidelines.gov

United Health Foundation. (2018). *America's health rankings. Annual report 2018.* https://assets.americashealthrankings.org/app/uploads/2018ahrannual_020419.pdf

United States Department of Agriculture, Food and Nutrition Service. (2019). *Healthy eating index (HEI).* https://www.fns.usda.gov/resource/healthy-eating-index-hei#targetText=The%20Healthy%20Eating%20Index%20(HEI,the%20Dietary%20Guidelines%20for%20Americans.&targetText=The%20HEI%20uses%20a%20scoring,range%20from%200%20to%20100

Wilson, M., Reedy, J., & Krebs-Smith, S. (2016). American diet quality: Where it is, where it is heading, and what it could be. *Journal of the Academy of Nutrition and Diet, 116*(2), 302–310. https://doi.org/10.1016/j.jand.2015.09.020

World Health Organization. (2018). *Noncommunicable diseases 2014.* Author. https://www.who.int/news-room/fact-sheets/detail/noncommunicable-diseases

World Health Organization. (1946). Preamble to the Constitution of the World Health Organization as adopted by the International Health Conference, New York, June 19–22, 1946; signed on July 22, 1946 by the representatives of 61 States (Official Records of the World Health Organization, no. 2, p. 100) and entered into force on April 7, 1948. http://whqlibdoc.who.int/hist/official_records/constitution.pdf

Wrobleski, M., Parker, E., Hurley, K., Oberlander, S., Merry, B., & Black, M. (2018). Comparison of the HEI and HEI-2010 diet quality measures in association with chronic disease risk among low-income African American urban youth in Baltimore, Maryland. *Journal of American College of Nutrition, 37*(3), 201–208. https://doi.org/10.1080/07315724.2017.1376297

Yeh, B. I., & Kong, I. D. (2013). The advent of lifestyle medicine. *Journal of Lifestyle Medicine, 3*(1), 1–8.

Chapter 2

Guidelines for Healthy Eating

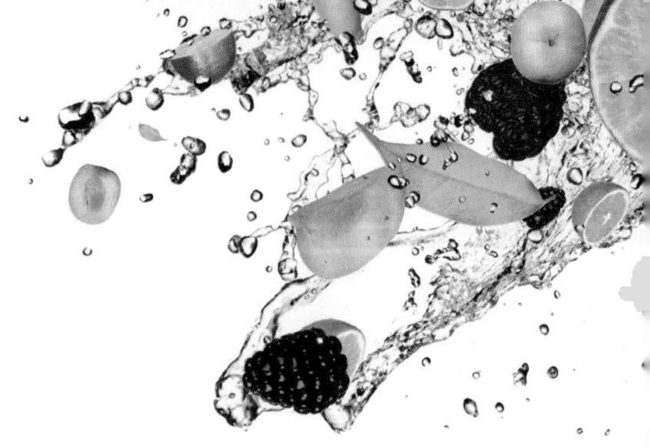

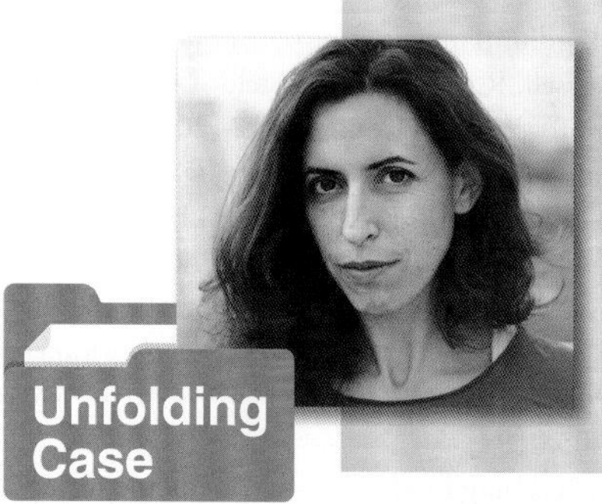

Unfolding Case

Aurea Espada

Aurea is 30 years old and has battled ulcerative colitis for more than 10 years. Medication helps keep her in remission, but she still has diarrhea that is sometimes bloody when she is stressed or eats too much fiber. She avoids fruits, vegetables, and whole grains to keep her gut calm. She worries that her diet lacks healthy foods and that it may place her at greater risk of chronic disease.

Learning Objectives

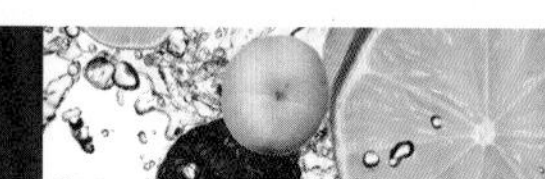

Upon completion of this chapter, you will be able to:

1 Discuss the four broad dietary guidelines and the key recommendations for each.
2 Explain how the Healthy U.S.-Style Eating Pattern differs from the typical American eating pattern.
3 List four underlying principles inherent in healthy eating.
4 Give examples of nutrient-dense foods.
5 Describe the MyPlate graphic.
6 List the nutritional attributes and potential health benefits associated with each of the MyPlate food groups.
7 Compare the nutrition recommendations from the American Heart Association, the American Cancer Society, and the American Institute for Cancer Research.

Healthy eating guidelines translate the science of nutrient needs into evidence-based public health recommendations for eating patterns to meet those needs. A healthy eating pattern provides adequate amounts of all essential nutrients, helps people attain and maintain a healthy body weight, promotes overall health, and reduces the risk of chronic disease. Following are the prominent characteristics of healthy eating patterns:

Variety in

- the color of fruits and vegetables
- the selections within each group
- methods of cooking

Balance

- inclusion of all food groups in reasonable proportions

Moderation

- limited amounts of saturated fat, added sugars, and sodium
- moderate amounts of alcohol and coffee, if adults so choose

Appropriate for the individual

- calorically, culturally, personally, and economically

No prohibition on any foods

This chapter discusses tools and resources for planning a healthy diet, including the *Dietary Guidelines for Americans*, MyPlate, and diet and lifestyle recommendations from leading health agencies. Guidelines and graphics from other countries are also introduced.

DIETARY GUIDELINES FOR AMERICANS

The *Dietary Guidelines for Americans* (DGA) have been published once every 5 years since 1980 jointly by the U.S. Department of Agriculture (USDA) and the U.S. Department of Health and Human Services (USDHHS). The report contains evidence-based advice on foods and beverages to consume to promote health, reduce the risk of chronic disease, and meet nutrient needs (USDA & USDHHS, 2020). The DGA are designed to meet the Recommended Dietary Allowances (RDA) and Adequate Intakes (AI) for essential nutrients while also staying within the Acceptable Macronutrient Distribution Ranges for carbohydrates, protein, and fat (USDA & USDHHS, 2020). The DGA serve as the basis of federal food, nutrition, and health policies and programs (USDA & USDHHS, 2020). They are intended to help all people shift to better food and beverage choices to achieve healthier eating patterns.

There are four broad guidelines with key recommendations for each (Box 2.1). Reflecting how the science of nutrition has evolved, the focus of the 2020–2025 DGA is

- to recognize the major public health problem caused by diet-related chronic diseases such as heart disease, type 2 diabetes, obesity, and some types of cancer,
- on dietary patterns, not individual nutrients or foods, and
- to provide guidance throughout the lifespan from infancy through older adulthood.

BOX 2.1 *Dietary Guidelines for Americans, 2020–2025*

The Guidelines

Make every bite count with the *Dietary Guidelines for Americans*. Here's how:

1. **Follow a healthy dietary pattern at every life stage.** At every life stage—infancy, toddlerhood, childhood, adolescence, adulthood, pregnancy, lactation, and older adulthood—it is never too early or too late to eat healthfully.
   - **For about the first 6 months of life,** exclusively feed infants human milk. Continue to feed infants human milk through at least the first year of life and longer if desired. Feed infants iron-fortified infant formula during the first year of life when human milk is unavailable. Provide infants with supplemental vitamin D beginning soon after birth.
   - **At about 6 months,** introduce infants to nutrient-dense complementary foods. Introduce infants to potentially allergenic foods along with other complementary foods. Encourage infant and toddlers to consume a variety of foods from all food groups. Include foods rich in iron and zinc, particularly for infants fed human milk.
   - **From 12 months through older adulthood,** follow a healthy dietary pattern across the lifespan to meet nutrient needs, help achieve a healthy body weight, and reduce the risk of chronic disease.
2. **Customize and enjoy nutrient-dense food and beverage choices to reflect personal preferences, cultural traditions, and budgetary considerations.** A healthy dietary pattern can benefit all individuals regardless of age, race, or ethnicity, or current health status. The *Dietary Guidelines* provides a framework intended to be customized to individual needs and preferences as well as the foodways of the diverse cultures in the United States.
3. **Focus on meeting food group needs with nutrient-dense foods and beverages, and stay within calorie limits.** An underlying premise of the *Dietary Guidelines* is that nutritional needs should be met primarily from foods and beverages—specifically, nutrient-dense foods and beverages. Nutrient-dense foods provide vitamins, minerals, and other health-promoting components and have no or little added sugars, saturated fat, and sodium. A healthy dietary pattern consists of nutrient-dense forms of foods and beverages

(continued)

BOX 2.1 Dietary Guidelines for Americans, 2020–2025 (continued)

across all food groups, in recommended amounts, and within calorie limits.

The core elements that make up a healthy dietary pattern include the following:

- **Vegetables of all types**—dark green; red and orange beans, peas, and lentils; starchy; and other vegetables
- **Fruits**, especially whole fruit
- **Grains**, at least half of which are whole grain
- **Dairy**, including fat-free or low-fat milk, yogurt, and cheese and/or lactose-free versions and fortified soy beverages and yogurt as alternatives
- **Protein foods,** including lean meats, poultry, and eggs; seafood; beans, peas, and lentils; and nuts, seeds, and soy products
- **Oils**, including vegetables oils and oils in food, such as seafood and nuts

4. **Limit foods and beverages higher in added sugars, saturated fat, and sodium and limit alcoholic beverages.** At every life stage, meeting food group recommendations—even with nutrient-dense choices—requires most of a person's daily calorie needs and sodium limits. A healthy dietary pattern doesn't have much room for extra added sugars, saturated fat, or sodium—or for alcoholic beverages. A small amount of added sugars, saturated fat, or sodium can be added to nutrient-dense foods and beverages to help meet food group recommendations, but foods and beverages high in these components should be limited. Limits are as follows:

- **Added sugars**—Less than 10% of calories per day starting at age 2. Avoid foods and beverages with added sugars for those younger than age 2.
- **Saturated fat**—Less than 10% of calories per day starting at age 2.
- **Sodium**—Less than 2300 mg/day—and even less for children younger than age 14.
- **Alcoholic beverages**—Adults of legal drinking age can choose not to drink or to drink in moderation by limiting intake to 2 drinks or less in a day for men and 1 drink or less in a day for women, when alcohol is consumed. Drinking less is better for health than drinking more. There are some adults who should not drink alcohol, such as women who are pregnant.

Source: U.S. Department of Agriculture & U.S. Department of Health and Human Services. (2020, December). *Dietary guidelines for Americans, 2020–2025.* https://www.dietaryguidelines.gov.

Recommended Eating Patterns

Three different healthy eating patterns are featured in the DGA to illustrate how the guidelines translate into types and amounts of foods. There are 12 different calorie levels within each style, ranging from 1000 to 3200 calories in 200-calorie increments. This wide range of calorie levels is intended to meet the needs of individuals across the lifespan. Each style lists recommended daily amounts of food within each food group for each calorie level. Patterns meet the standards for almost all nutrients while staying within limits for added sugars, saturated fat, and sodium. However, vitamin D, vitamin E, and choline may be marginal or below the RDA or AI standard for many or all age/sex groups (USDA & USDHHS, 2020). Table 2.1 compares each of the styles at 1600- and 2000-calorie levels. The styles are summarized in the following sections.

Healthy U.S.-Style Eating Pattern

The Healthy U.S.-Style Eating Pattern is based on the types and proportions of foods Americans typically consume in nutrient-dense forms and appropriate amounts.

- Because this pattern is designed as a healthier version of the typical American eating pattern, it is higher in fruits, vegetables, dairy, whole grains, and seafood than what the typical American consumes. It is also more restricted in the number of calories remaining for other uses, previously known as discretionary calories.
- It aligns closely with the Dietary Approaches to Stop Hypertension (DASH) diet (see Chapter 7).

Healthy Mediterranean-Style Eating Pattern

There is no single defined standard Mediterranean diet; this eating pattern is based on the food intakes of people who display positive health outcomes related to a Mediterranean-type diet. The traditional Mediterranean diet is higher in unsaturated fat and lower in saturated fat compared to the typical American diet.

Table 2.1 1600- and 2000-Calorie Patterns for Ages 2 and Older for the Healthy U.S.-Style Eating Pattern, the Healthy Mediterranean-Style Eating Pattern, and the Healthy Vegetarian Eating Pattern

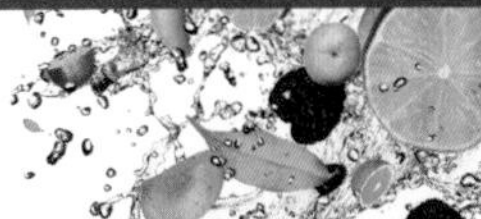

	Healthy U.S.-Style Eating Pattern		Healthy Mediterranean-Style Eating Pattern		Healthy Vegetarian Eating Pattern	
Calorie level of pattern	1600	2000	1600	2000	1600	2000
Food Group or Subgroup	**Daily Amount of Food from Each Group** (vegetable and protein foods subgroup amounts are per week)					
Vegetables (c-eq/day)	2	2½	2	2½	2	2½
	Vegetable subgroups in weekly amounts					
Dark green vegetables (c-eq/wk)	1½	1½	1½	1½	1½	1½
Red and orange vegetables (c-eq/wk)	4	5½	4	5½	4	5½
Beans, peas, lentils (c-eq/wk)	1	1½	1	1½	1	1½
Starchy vegetables (c-eq/wk)	4	5	4	5	4	5
Other vegetables (c-eq/wk)	3½	4	3½	4	3½	4
Fruits (cup eq/day)	1½	2	2	2½	1½	2
Grains (ounce eq/day)	5	6	5	6	5½	6½
Whole grains (oz-eq/d)	3	3	3	3	3	3½
Refined grains (oz-eq/d)	2	3	2	3	2½	3
Dairy (cup eq/day)	3	3	2	2	3	3
Protein foods (ounce eq/day)	5	5½	5½	6½	2½	3½
	Protein foods subgroups in weekly amounts					
Meats, poultry, eggs (ounce eq/week)	23	26	23	26	3 egg oz eq/week	3 egg oz eq/week
Seafood (ounce-eq/wk)	8	8	11	15	N/A	N/A
Nuts, seeds, soy products (ounce-eq/wk)	4	5	4	5	5 oz eq nuts and seeds/week 6 oz eq/week soy products	7 oz eq nuts and seeds/week 8 oz/eq/week soy products
Beans, peas, lentils (cup eq/week) (in addition to beans, peas, and lentils listed under vegetables)	N/A	N/A	N/A	N/A	4	6
Oils (grams/day)	22	27	22	27	22	27
Limit on calories for other uses, calories/day (% of total calories consumed)	100 (6%)	240 (12%)	120 (8%)	240 (12%)	150 (9%)	250 (13%)

Note. Food group amounts shown in cup equivalents (cup eq or c eq) or ounce equivalents (ounce eq or oz eq).
All foods are assumed to be in nutrient-dense form; lean or low fat; and prepared with minimal added sugars, refined starches (which are a source of calories but with few or no other nutrients), saturated fat, or sodium.
Source: U.S. Department of Agriculture & U.S. Department of Health and Human Services. (2020, December). *Dietary Guidelines for Americans, 2020–2025.* https://www.dietaryguidelines.gov/sites/default/files/2020-12/Dietary_Guidelines_for_Americans_2020-2025.pdf

Compared to the U.S.-Style Eating Pattern featured in the DGA, the Mediterranean-Style Eating Pattern

- provides slightly higher amounts of protein foods overall and significantly higher amounts of seafood/week.
- is higher in fruits.
- contains less dairy so the pattern is lower in calcium and vitamin D.

Healthy Vegetarian Eating Pattern

The Healthy Vegetarian Eating Pattern is a modified version of the Healthy U.S.-Style Eating Pattern and is similar to the eating patterns reported by self-identified vegetarians. Dairy and eggs are included because they are consumed by the majority of vegetarians studied. Compared to the Healthy U.S.-Style Eating Pattern, the Healthy Vegetarian Eating Pattern

- excludes meat, poultry, and seafood,
- lists the subgroups of protein foods as eggs; beans, peas, lentils; soy products; and nuts and seeds. The amount of beans, peas, and lentils recommended under protein foods is in addition to the amount recommended from the vegetable group,
- includes higher amounts of legumes, soy products, and nuts and seeds, and
- at some calorie levels, provides slightly higher amounts of whole grains and calories for other uses.

The Underlying Principles of Healthy Eating

Nutrient-Dense Foods
Nutrient-dense foods and beverages provide vitamins, minerals, and other beneficial substances relative to the number of calories with little or no added sugars, saturated fat, and sodium.

Certain underlying principles are inherent to healthy eating: Choose **nutrient-dense foods** and beverages; meet nutrient needs through food and beverages, not through supplements; use portion control to avoid exceeding calorie limits; and focus on variety to ensure nutritional adequacy.

Choose Nutrient Dense Foods and Beverages

At each calorie level, the amount of food recommended in each eating pattern is based on the assumption that all foods are chosen in their most nutrient-dense form. Figure 2.1 compares the calories in nutrient dense and non-nutrient-dense forms of various foods. Note that although whole milk is not made with added fat, it is not the leanest possible variety of milk; therefore, it is not as nutrient dense as fat-free milk. As such, eating patterns are based on the assumption that fat-free milk will be chosen.

- Eating nutrient-dense food, helps achieve nutrient requirements without exceeding calorie needs.
- The following foods and beverages are considered nutrient dense if they are prepared with little or no added solid fats, sugar, refined starches, or sodium: vegetables, fruits, whole grains, eggs, beans, peas, lentils, nuts, fat-free and low-fat dairy products, and lean proteins.
- If all food choices are nutrient dense, then a small number of calories will remain in the overall calorie limit of the eating pattern.
  - These calories are referred to "limit on calories for other uses."
  - If the limits for added sugars, saturated fat, and alcohol recommended by the DGA are not exceeded and the intake of carbohydrates, protein, and fat is within Acceptable Macronutrient Distribution Ranges, these calories can be used for
    - added sugars (e.g., a soft drink), added refined starches (e.g., white bread), solid fats (e.g., butter), or alcohol,
    - foods that are not the most nutrient-dense in a group, such as 2% milk instead of fat-free milk, and
    - eating more than the recommended amount of food in a food group (e.g., larger portion of seafood).

Meet Nutrient Needs through Foods and Beverages

People are urged to meet their nutrient needs through nutrient-dense foods and beverages, not through supplements, to the greatest extent possible.

- Foods and beverages provide complex mixtures of many nutrient and non-nutrient components that cannot be replicated in pill form, such as the wide variety of phytonutrients in fruits and vegetables that are not found in multivitamin supplements.

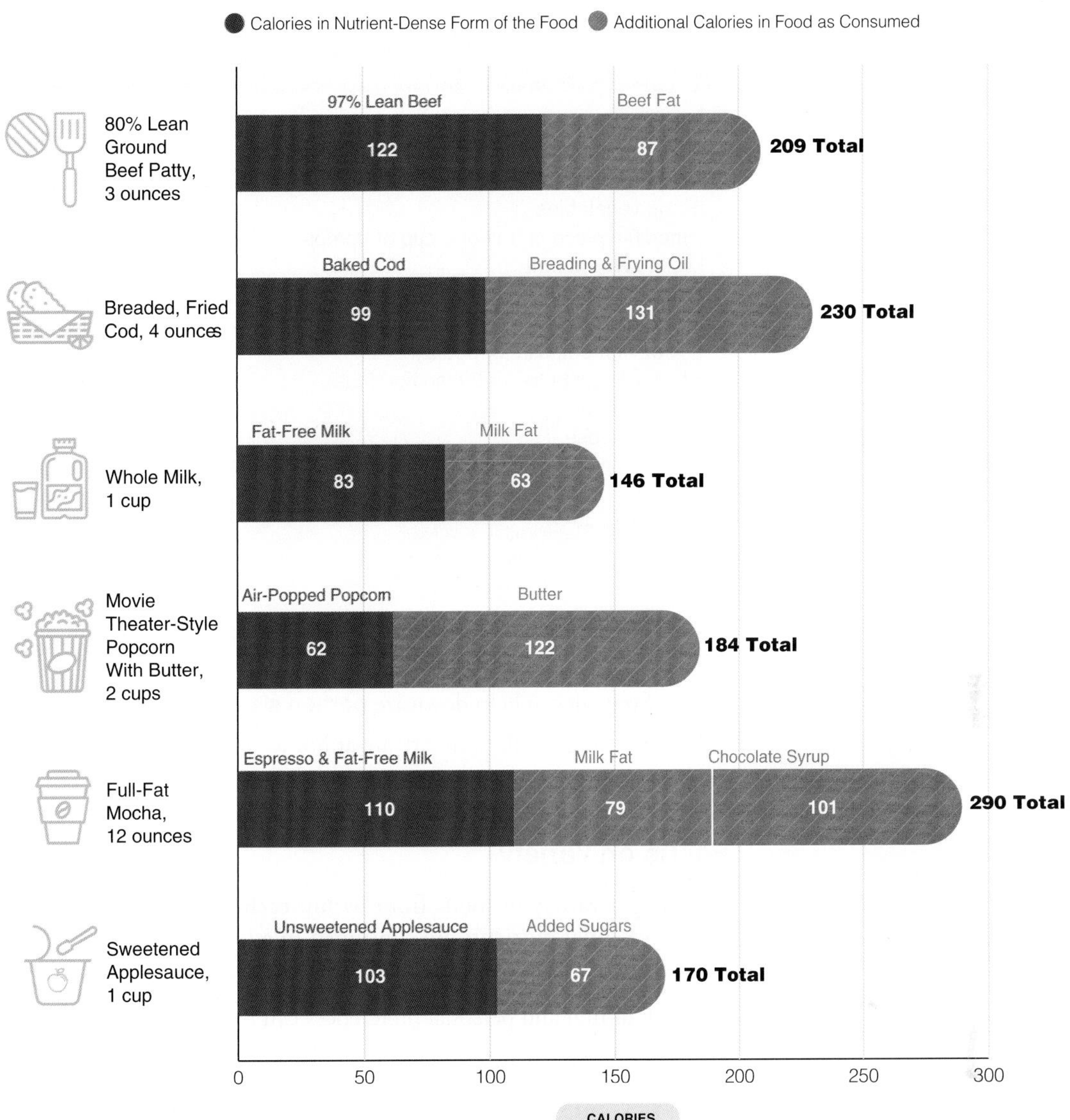

Figure 2.1 ▲ **Examples of calories in food choices that are nutrient dense and calories in nutrient-dense forms of these foods.** (*Source:* U.S. Department of Agriculture, Agricultural Research Service. [2019]. FoodData Central. fdc.nal.usda.gov).

- However, sometimes, fortified foods or supplements are necessary to meet certain nutrient needs, such as the use of calcium- and vitamin D–fortified orange juice by people who cannot or will not consume adequate amounts of dairy products.

Use Portion Control

Just as the quality of foods chosen influences total calorie intake, so does the quantity.

- Eating patterns specify daily or weekly amounts from each food group or subgroup, respectively, in "ounce-equivalents" or "cup-equivalents."
  - Total oils recommended per day are in grams.
  - Although these measures are more specific than the previously used term of *serving*, which consumers often confuse with portion, it is still a matter of estimating how much food is consumed.

BOX 2.2 Everyday Items to Help Estimate Recommended Serving Sizes

This Amount . . .	Looks Like . . .
1 cup raw vegetables	1 baseball
½ cup vegetables	1 computer mouse
1 medium piece of fruit or 1 cup of berries	1 tennis ball
½ cup canned fruit	1 computer mouse
1 cup dry cereal	1 baseball
½ cup cooked pasta	1 computer mouse
2–3 oz of meat, fish, or poultry	1 deck of cards
2 tbsp peanut butter or 2 tbsp hummus	1 pingpong ball
¼ cup of nuts	1 golf ball
1 oz of cheese	4 dice
1 teaspoon butter or oil	About the size of a penny

Source: Move, V.A. (n.d.). *Serving sizes*. Nutrition Handouts N21 version 5.0. https://www.move.va.gov/download/NewHandouts/Nutrition/N21_ServingSizes.pdf

Serving Size
the amount of food listed on the Nutrition Facts label that refers to the amount customarily consumed, for example, 1 cup of cooked spaghetti pasta.

Portion Size
the amount of food usually consumed at one time (e.g., 3 cups of spaghetti served as a restaurant entrée).

- Often, portion sizes exceed serving sizes; using common objects is an easy way to convey the concept of **serving sizes** (Box 2.2).
- Strategies to help downsize **portion sizes** include
  - using smaller dinnerware at home, and
  - using a tall slender glass instead of a short wide one.

Focus on Variety

Choosing a variety of foods from within each food group helps ensure that the more than 40 known essential nutrients are consumed in adequate amounts based on the rationale that some nutrients (e.g., iron, calcium, vitamin C, and vitamin A) are concentrated in a few foods.

- Cultural and personal preferences can be incorporated into healthy eating patterns.
- All foods, such as fresh, canned, dried, frozen, and 100% juices, can be included in healthy eating patterns when consumed in nutrient dense forms.
- Variety is promoted by dividing some groups into subgroups:
  - The vegetable group contains five subgroups with recommended cup-equivalents per week specified:
    - dark green
    - red and orange
    - legumes
    - starchy
    - other
  - Grains are divided into refined and whole grain categories.
    - At least half of all grains consumed should be whole grains.
    - Women of childbearing age who consume all their grains in the form of whole grains should be sure to choose some whole grains that are fortified with folic acid, such as some breakfast cereals.
  - There are three protein food subgroups for the Healthy U.S.-Style and Mediterranean-Style Eating Patterns:
    - meats, poultry, eggs
    - seafood
    - nuts, seeds, and soy products
  - The Healthy Vegetarian Eating Pattern also includes beans, peas, and lentils as a protein food subgroup.

MYPLATE

MyPlate is the graphic illustration of the DGA that was created to help consumers achieve healthy eating patterns. It features a place setting with one half of the dinner plate devoted to fruits and vegetables, one fourth to protein foods, and the one fourth to grains. Dairy is shown to accompany the plate (Fig. 2.2) (USDA, n.d.). MyPlate encompasses the same underlying principles as the DGA and promotes the following main points:

- Every bite counts—focus on variety, amount, and nutrition.
- Choose foods and beverages with less added sugars, saturated fat, and sodium.
- Small changes matter, and the benefits of healthy eating accumulate over time.

The serving sizes, nutritional attributes, and health benefits associated with each food group are listed in Table 2.2. Additional guidance on oils, added sugars, saturated fat, sodium, and alcohol are outlined in Table 2.3.

Fruit

Slightly less than one quarter of MyPlate is depicted as fruit.

- Generally, slightly fewer servings of fruit than vegetables are recommended per day in all the three styles of eating patterns.
- Fresh fruits provide more calories than vegetables and virtually all the calories in fruit are from natural sugars.
- Canned and frozen fruit with added sugar are higher in carbohydrates and calories.

Vegetables

Recommended amounts (based on age, sex, and level of physical activity) are specified for the total amount of vegetables per day and total amounts for each vegetable subgroup per week to be consumed.

- Vegetables are naturally low in calories; their calories come mostly from starch, with some incomplete protein.
- Vegetables are generally higher in vitamins and minerals than fruits.

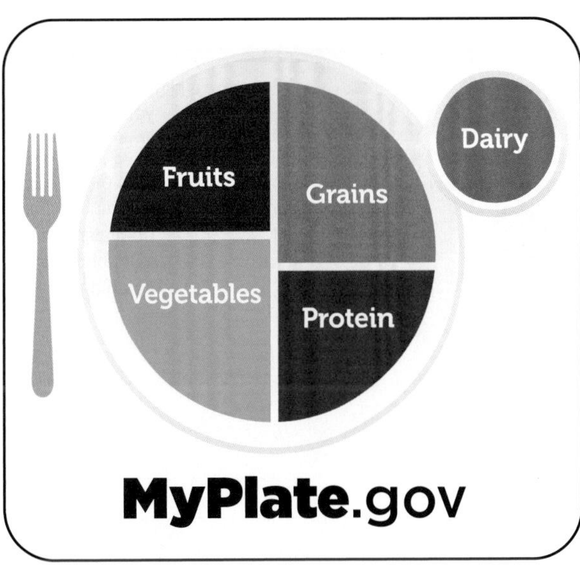

Figure 2.2 ▶ MyPlate graphic. (*Source:* MyPlate, U.S. Department of Agriculture. What's on your plate?. myplate.gov. MyPlate.gov is based on the *Dietary Guidelines for Americans, 2020–2025*)

Table 2.2 MyPlate Food Groups: Serving Sizes, Nutrition Attributes, Health Benefits

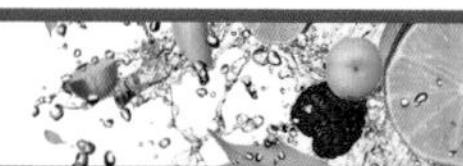

Food Group	What Counts as...	Nutritional Attributes as a Group	Health Benefits
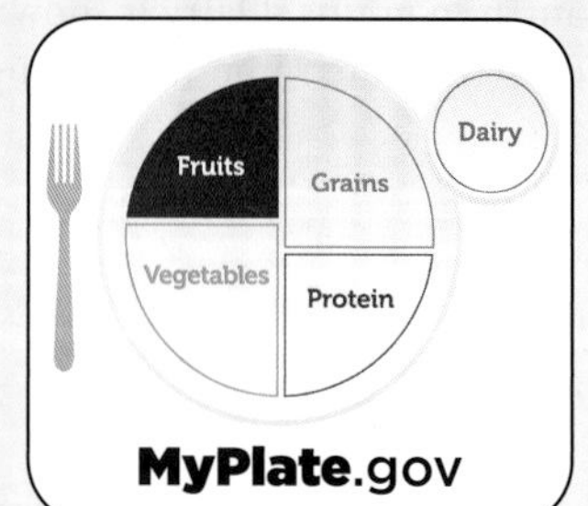	1 cup of fruit • 1 c fruit or 100% fruit juice • ½ c dried fruit	Most are low in fat, sodium, and calories All are cholesterol free Provide potassium, fiber, vitamin C, and folate Provide phytochemicals	May help lower calorie intake. Healthy eating patterns rich in fruits and vegetables may reduce the risk of heart disease (including heart attack and stroke) and certain types of cancer.
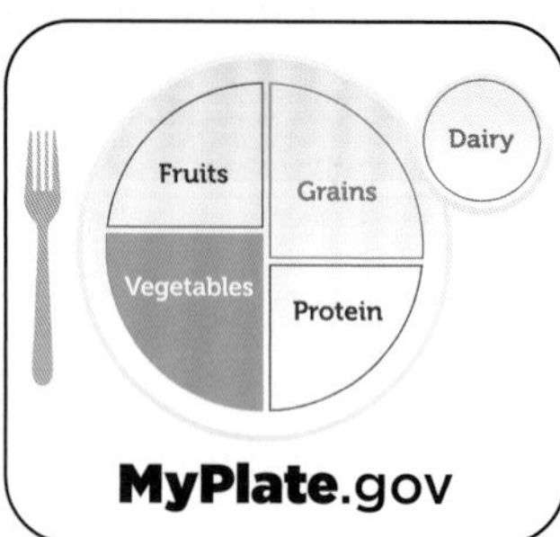	1 cup of vegetables • 1 c raw or cooked vegetables or vegetable juice • 2 cups raw leafy greens	Most are low in fat and calories All are cholesterol free Provide potassium, fiber, folate, vitamin A, and vitamin C	May help lower calorie intake. Healthy eating patterns rich in fruits and vegetables may reduce the risk of heart disease (including heart attack and stroke) and certain types of cancer.
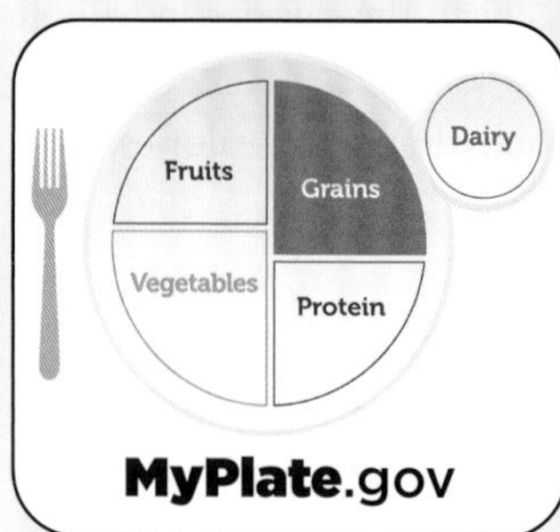	1 oz-equivalent • 1 slice of bread • 1 c of ready-to-eat cereal • ½ c cooked rice, cooked pasta, or cooked cereal	Whole grains provide fiber, thiamin, riboflavin, niacin, iron, magnesium, selenium, and phytonutrients. White (refined) flour is required to be enriched with thiamin, riboflavin, niacin, and iron and fortified with folic acid.	Eating whole grains within the context of a healthy eating pattern may reduce the risk of heart disease, prevent or alleviate constipation, and promote weight management. Folic acid–fortified grains help prevent neural tube defects when consumed before and during pregnancy.
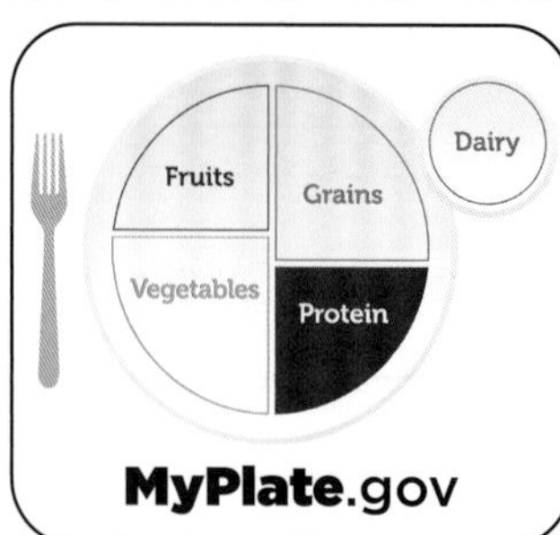	1 oz-equivalent of protein • 1 oz of meat, poultry, or fish • ¼ cup cooked beans • 1 egg • 1 tbsp peanut butter • ½ oz nuts or seeds • ¼ c cooked beans, peas, or lentils	Provide protein, B vitamins, vitamin E, iron, zinc, and magnesium. Seafood provides omega 3 fatty acids. Fatty meats, such as certain cuts of beef, pork, and lamb; regular ground beef, sausage, hot dogs, bacon, and certain luncheon meats should be limited because they are high in saturated fat. High cholesterol foods (e.g., egg yolk and organ meats) should be limited.	Health benefits associated with the protein group vary according to the selection: • Omega 3 fatty acids in seafood may help reduce the risk of heart disease. • Items high in saturated fats raise serum cholesterol levels and increase the risk of heart disease. • Nuts and seeds may reduce the risk of heart disease.
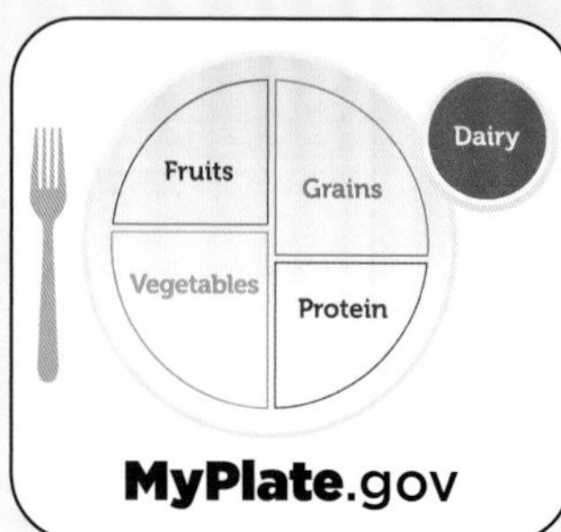	1 cup of dairy • 1 c milk, yogurt, or soy milk • 1.5 oz of natural cheese	Provide protein, calcium, phosphorus, vitamin A, vitamin D (if fortified), riboflavin, vitamin B_{12}, potassium, zinc, choline, magnesium, and selenium.	Calcium and vitamin D are important for bone health. Cultured dairy products provide probiotics that may regulate digestion or help maintain immune system functioning.

Table 2.3 MyPlate: Additional Key Topics and Points

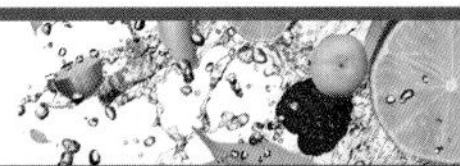

Key Topic	Key Points
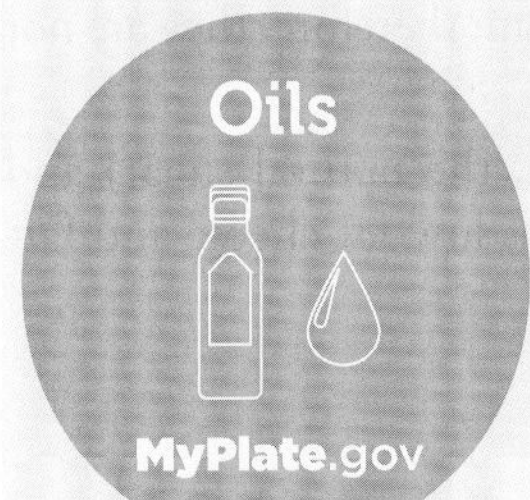	Use oils: They are not a food group but provide unsaturated fat and vitamin E. • Oils are derived from plants, such as olive oil, canola oil, and corn oil. • Three plant oils are high in saturated fat and should be limited: coconut oil, palm oil, and palm kernel oil. • Oil-containing foods include mayonnaise, salad dressings, soft margarine. • Using unsaturated fat in place of saturated fat can lower the risk of heart disease and increase high density lipoprotein (HDL) cholesterol.
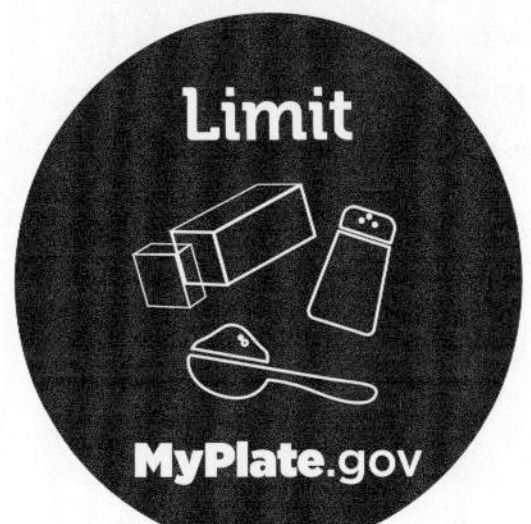	Added sugars: Syrups and sugars added to food or beverages during processing or preparation. • Children under the age of 2 should avoid all foods with added sugar • People aged 2 and older should limit added sugars Saturated fat: Fat that is solid at room temperature, such as butter, milk fat, and fat in and around meat. • Replace foods high in saturated fat with those higher in unsaturated fat, such as vegetable oils, fish, nuts, avocado. Sodium: Pervasive in the food supply as a seasoning and in preservatives. • People aged 14 and older should limit their sodium intake to 2300 mg/day. • Limiting sodium intake may lower the risk of hypertension and heart disease.
Alcohol	People who do not drink should not start drinking. Pregnant women and people with certain health conditions should not drink. Adults who choose to drink should do so in moderation: 1 drink or less for women and 2 drinks or less for men.

Source: U.S. Department of Agriculture. (n.d.) *More key topics.* https://www.myplate.gov/eat-healthy/more-key-topics

Grains

All foods made from wheat, rice, corn, barley, oats, or other grains are grain products.

- Grains are used primarily for flour, pasta, and breakfast cereals.
- Grains provide calories from starch and incomplete protein.
- Whole grains are made from the intact grain kernel: bran, endosperm, and germ.
- Refined grains contain only the endosperm; fiber, iron, phytochemicals, and many B vitamins are lost when the bran and germ are removed. Enrichment and fortification add back some of these nutrients to enriched grains.

Protein Foods

This group contains both animal (meat, poultry, seafood, eggs) and plant (nuts, seeds, beans, peas, lentils) protein sources.

- Calories come from protein and fat (animal proteins, nuts, seeds) and carbohydrate (beans, peas, lentils, and nuts).
- The fat and saturated fat content of meat and poultry choices vary with the specific selection; choices should be lean or low fat to help avoid excessive calorie and saturated fat intake.
- A variety of protein foods should be consumed to improve nutrient intake and health benefits, including at least 8 oz of seafood/week.

Dairy

The dairy group is comprised of dairy items that provide calcium: milk, yogurt, natural cheese, and fortified soy milk and yogurt.

- Items like butter, cream cheese, and cream have little or no calcium; therefore, they are not considered part of this group.
- Calories in dairy products come from carbohydrates (lactose, the natural sugar) and protein. Fat content varies: Low-fat and fat-free choices such as low-fat cheese and fat-free milk provide little to no calories from fat.

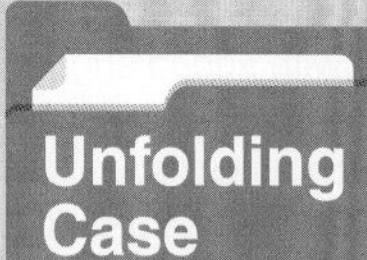

Recall Aurea. She may be able to achieve variety in fruits and vegetables. For instance, certain items in the vegetable subgroups of dark green (raw chopped spinach), red (tomato), orange (carrot juice), and other (zucchini) are low in fiber. However, Aurea may not be able to tolerate legumes or many whole grains. How do you respond to Aurea's frustration about having to adhere to a restrictive eating pattern?

MyPlate

The website MyPlate.gov provides a wealth of information under the headings of Eat Healthy, Life Stages, Resources, Professionals, and MyPlate Kitchen.

Users can obtain:

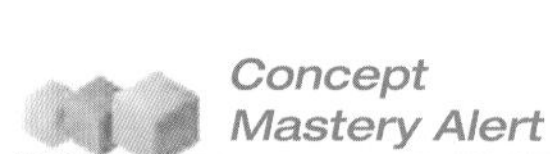

When providing an explanation of MyPlate, the nurse should note that it is a graphic of a place setting with a quarter of the plate devoted to grains and one half devoted to fruits and vegetables. MyPlate covers all aspects of the diet and reflects a philosophy that nutrient needs should be met through food as much as possible.

- details about each of the food groups, what counts as a cup or ounce equivalent for individual foods, and the nutritional value and health benefits of each group,
- a calorie-appropriate plan based on the individual's age, sex, height, weight, and activity level,
- age- and lifecycle-specific information and resources for women during pregnancy and lactation and older adults,
- activity ideas and mealtime tips for families,
- ideas for healthy eating on a budget,
- MyPlate videos and MyPlate app,
- MyPlate tools, such as quizzes,
- recipes, recipe videos, and recipe resources, and
- MyPlate graphics in multiple languages (Fig. 2.3).

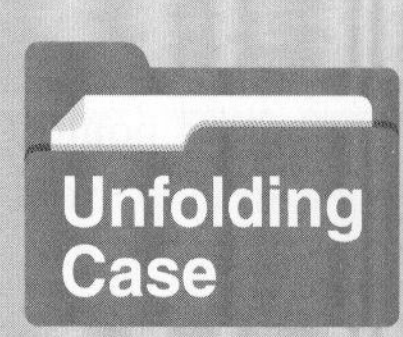

Think of Aurea. Aurea wants to add probiotics to her diet to see if they help. The American Gastroenterology Association's clinical practice guidelines for the management of mild to moderate ulcerative colitis do not make a recommendation regarding the use of probiotics due to insufficient evidence regarding their benefits (Ko et al., 2019). How would you respond to Aurea? What foods contain probiotics?

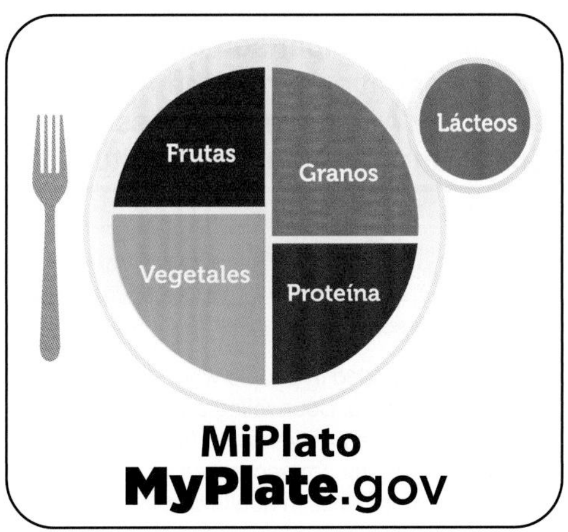

Figure 2.3 ▶ MyPlate graphic in Spanish. (*Source:* MyPlate, U.S. Department of Agriculture. What's on your plate?. myplate.gov. MyPlate.gov is based on the *Dietary Guidelines for Americans, 2020–2025*)

RECOMMENDATIONS FROM HEALTH AGENCIES

Many health agencies publish guidelines or recommendations for healthy eating, including the American College of Cardiology/American Heart Association (Arnett et al., 2019), the American Cancer Society (Kushi et al., 2012), and the American Institute for Cancer Research (World Cancer Research Fund & American Institute for Cancer Research, 2007) (Table 2.4). The recommendations of these agencies are similar to each other and to those of the DGA. Common themes are attaining or maintaining healthy weight, being physically active, choosing a nutrient-dense varied eating pattern, limiting certain foods and dietary components, and drinking alcohol in moderation, if at all.

EATING BEHAVIORS AMERICANS ARE TRYING TO IMPROVE

There is some evidence to indicate that people are at least trying to improve their eating patterns, although they fall short of current recommendations. The 2019 Food and Health Survey of the International Food Information Council (2019) shows that the top five ways in which people say their diets have changed over the past 10 years is

- limiting sugar intake,
- eating more fruits and vegetables,
- eating less carbohydrate,
- eating healthier protein sources, and
- eating better and healthier in general.

GUIDELINES AND GRAPHICS IN OTHER COUNTRIES

Cultural differences in symbolism and other cultural norms influence the shape of food guides in other countries. Similar to MyPlate, a circle or dinner plate with each section depicting relative proportion to the total diet is used in many countries, including Canada (Fig. 2.4), the United Kingdom, and Mexico. In the Republic of Korea, the back wheel of a bicycle is used to depict the food groups. China employs a pagoda shape to depict the food groups, while the Bahamas uses a more unique goatskin drum, divided into different food groups. Despite the differences in the shape of the graphics, guidelines generally contain several consistent concepts:

- Eat a variety of foods.
- Limit added sugar and salt.
- Be physically active.
- Attain and maintain healthy weight.

Table 2.4 A Summary Comparison of Nutrition and Physical Activity Recommendations from the American College of Cardiology/American Heart Association, the American Cancer Society, and the American Institute for Cancer Research

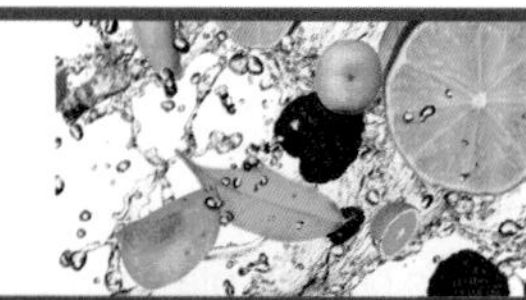

Criteria	American College of Cardiology/American Heart Association Guidelines on the Primary Prevention of Cardiovascular Disease[a]	American Cancer Society Guidelines on Nutrition and Physical Activity for Cancer Prevention[b]	American Institute for Cancer Research Recommendations for Cancer Prevention[c]
Weight status	Weight loss is recommended in people who are overweight or obese. Counseling and comprehensive lifestyle interventions, including calorie restriction, are recommended for achieving and maintaining weight loss in adults who are overweight or obese.	Be as lean as possible throughout life without being underweight. Avoid excess weight gain at all ages. Get regular physical activity and limit high calorie foods and drinks to help maintain healthy weight.	Keep weight within healthy range and avoid weight gain in adulthood.
Exercise and physical activity	Adults should engage in at least 150 minutes of moderate physical activity or 75 minutes of vigorous physical activity (or a combination of both) each week. Adults who are unable to meet the minimum physical activity recommendations can benefit from engaging in some moderate or vigorous activity even if less than the recommended amount. Decrease sedentary behaviors.	Aim for at least 150 minutes of moderate physical activity or 75 minutes of vigorous physical activity (or a combination of both) each week. Limit sedentary behaviors.	Aim for at least 150 minutes of moderate physical activity or 75 minutes of vigorous physical activity (or a combination of both) each week. Sit less.
Healthy diet	Emphasize the intake of • vegetables • fruits • legumes • nuts • whole grains • fish	Emphasize plant foods: • Eat at least 2½ cups of fruits and vegetables daily. • Choose whole grains in place of refined grains. • Choose food and beverages in amounts required to attain/maintain a healthy weight.	Eat a diet rich in • vegetables • fruits • whole grains • legumes
Limit certain foods and food components	Replace saturated fat with monounsaturated fatty acids (MUFA) and polyunsaturated fatty acids (PUFA). Reduce cholesterol and sodium intake. Minimize the intake of processed meats, refined carbohydrates, and sweetened beverages. Avoid trans fats.	Limit or avoid • red and processed meats • sugar-sweetened beverages • high processed foods and refined grain products	Limit fast foods and other processed foods high in fat, starches, or sugars. Limit • red meat and processed meat • sugar-sweetened drinks
Alcohol intake (for people who choose to drink)	Use in moderation to prevent or treat hypertension: no more than 1 drink/day for women and no more than 2 drinks/day for men	No more than 1 drink/day for women and no more than 2 drinks/day for men	No more than 1 drink/day for women and no more than 2 drinks/day for men
Other	Plant-based and Mediterranean diets are consistently associated with lower risk for all-cause mortality compared to standard diets in observational studies.	Plant-based eating patterns generally show the most health benefits.	Do not use supplements for cancer prevention. Mothers should breastfeed their babies if possible.

[a]Arnett, D. K., Blumenthal, R. S., Albert, M. A., Buroker, A. B., Goldberger, Z. D., Hahn, E. J., Himmelfarb, C. D., Khera, A., Lloyd-Jones, D., McEvoy, J. W., Michos, E. D., Miedema, M. D., Muñoz, D., Smith, S. C. Jr., Virani, S. S., Williams, K. A. Sr., Yeboah, J., & Ziaeian, B. (2019). 2019 ACC/AHA guideline on the primary prevention of cardiovascular disease: A report of the American College of Cardiology/American Heart Association Task Force on Clinical Practice Guidelines. *Circulation*, *140*, e596–e646. https://doi.org/10.1161/CIR.0000000000000678.
[b]Kushi, L., Doyle, C., McCullough, M., Rock, C. L., Demark-Wahnefried, W., Bandera, E. V., Gapstur, S., Patel, A., Andrews, K., Gansler, T., & American Cancer Society 2010 Nutrition and Physical Activity Guidelines Advisory Committee. (2012). American Cancer Society guidelines on nutrition and physical activity for cancer prevention: Reducing the risk of cancer with healthy food choices and physical activity. *CA: A Cancer Journal for Clinicians, 62*(1), 30–67. https://doi.org/10.3322/caac.20140.
[c]American Institute for Cancer Research. *10 Cancer Prevention Recommendations.* http://www.aicr.org/reduce-your-cancer-risk/recommendations-for-cancer-prevention

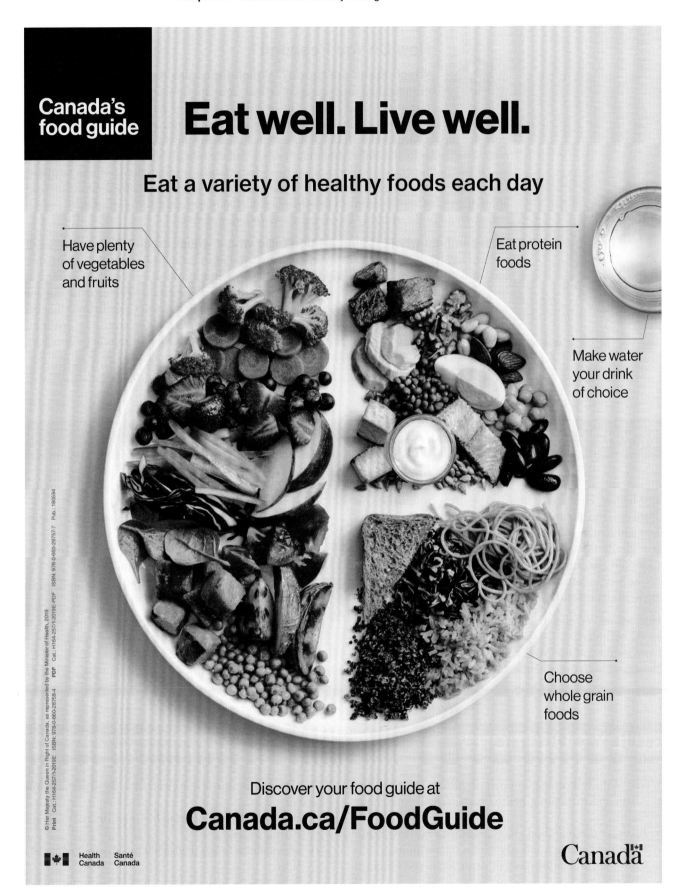

Figure 2.4 ▲ **Canada's food guide. Eat well. Live well.** (© Her Majesty the Queen in Right of Canada, as represented by the Minister of Health, 2019. Reprinted with permission)

How Do You Respond?

Which foods are "good?" Which foods are "bad"? Instead of thinking of individual foods as good or bad, consider how a food fits within the context of the total intake. For instance, broccoli is among the best plant foods available, yet if someone ate only broccoli all day long, it would not be "good" because broccoli does not supply adequate amounts of all essential nutrients for health. What matters is how often a particular food is eaten, the amount eaten, and the overall calorie and nutrient balance.

If most of a person's intake is of nutrient-dense foods, small amounts of less nutritious choices can fit into the eating pattern without wreaking havoc as long as total calorie intake is appropriate. The keys to fitting in less-than-healthy foods are to eat them *infrequently*, *in small amounts*, and *in the context of an otherwise healthy eating pattern*.

How can I eat whole grains if I don't like whole wheat bread? Just as there are no good or bad foods, there is no one particular food you must eat to be healthy or one particular food you must never eat to be healthy. White whole wheat bread or whole wheat versions of bagels, pita bread, or tortillas for sandwiches and wraps may be eaten. Whole grains like quinoa, brown rice, bulgur, or barley can be eaten as a side dish or as part of a grain bowl that can be a substitute for a sandwich. Whole grains can also be consumed as cereals (e.g., oatmeal, shredded wheat), as side dishes (e.g., quinoa, brown rice), as ingredients in other dishes (e.g., wild rice or sorghum added to soup), and even as snacks (e.g., popcorn).

REVIEW CASE STUDY

Andrew wants to eat healthier, so he went online to learn about MyPlate. He was overwhelmed by all the information on MyPlate.gov and became disenchanted by recommendations in cups and ounces—concepts that are unfamiliar to him. Andrew is clearly interested in changing his food habits, but he is stuck on the idea that he won't be able to make any changes unless he weighs and measures his food. He is wondering if eating healthier is worth the trouble.

- How would you encourage Andrew to approach the goal of eating healthier?
- How would you use MyPlate to help Andrew make better choices without overwhelming him?
- What would you tell him about weighing and measuring foods?
- How would you respond to these questions or statements from Andrew?
  - "I only like fruit juice and not whole fruits. Is it okay to consume all my fruit servings as juice?"
  - "I don't like fat-free milk. Can I drink 2% milk instead?"
  - "I noticed on my MyPlate plan that I should eat less than 2300 mg of sodium each day. I eat out a lot, so I don't have the option of calculating sodium intake from food labels for everything I eat."
  - "I like craft beers. Where does alcohol fit into MyPlate?"

STUDY QUESTIONS

1 Which of the following is not part of the four DGA?
   a. Attain and maintain a healthy body weight throughout life.
   b. Focus on meeting food group needs with nutrient-dense foods and beverages and stay within calorie limits.
   c. Customize and enjoy nutrient-dense foods and beverage choices.
   d. Follow a healthy dietary pattern at every life stage.

2 The DGA recommend that Americans do all of the following except
   a. limit saturated fat intake to less than 10% of total calories starting at age 2.
   b. limit sodium to less than 2300 mg/day for people 14 and older.
   c. limit total fat intake to less than 30% of calories beginning at age 2.
   d. limit added sugars to less than 10% of total calories beginning at age 2.

3 "Moderate" alcohol consumption is
  a. three to 4 drinks per week for women and 6 to 8 drinks per week for men.
  b. up to 1 drink per day for both men and women.
  c. up to 1 drink per day for women and up to 2 drinks per day for men.
  d. up to 2 drinks per day for women and up to 3 drinks per day for men.

4 The nurse knows that the client understands their instructions about grain equivalents when the client verbalizes that one grain equivalent is equal to
  a. one slice of bread.
  b. two cups of ready-to-eat cereal.
  c. one cup of cooked pasta.
  d. one cup of cooked rice.

5 A client states that there is no way they can eat all the vegetables recommended in their MyPlate plan. What is the nurse's best response?
  a. "If you can't eat all the vegetables, then make up for the difference by eating more fruit."
  b. "Be sure to take a daily multivitamin to provide the nutrients that may be missing from your diet."
  c. "Set a goal of eating larger quantities of the vegetable servings that you currently eat, and gradually increase the servings and variety as you become more skillful in adding vegetables to your diet."
  d. "No one can. The recommendations are only a guide. Just eat what you can."

6 The nurse knows that the client understands their instructions about estimating portion sizes when the client verbalizes that one cup of dry cereal looks like
  a. one baseball.
  b. one computer mouse.
  c. one ping-pong ball.
  d. one tennis ball.

7 Which of the following food items is not nutrient dense?
  a. Sweetened applesauce
  b. Whole wheat bread
  c. Plain shredded wheat
  d. Plain low-fat yogurt with fruit

8 Compared to a Healthy U.S.-Style Eating Pattern, a Mediterranean-Style Eating Pattern is generally
  a. higher in vegetables and whole grains.
  b. higher in seafood and lower in dairy.
  c. higher in oils and dairy.
  d. lower in protein foods and fruits.

CHAPTER SUMMARY GUIDELINES FOR HEALTHY EATING

Guidelines for healthy eating, put forth by the government and health organizations, are intended to help the public choose healthy eating patterns.

Dietary Guidelines for Americans

Revised every 5 years, the DGA provide evidence-based advice across the lifespan on food and beverages to consume to promote health, reduce the risk of chronic disease, and meet nutrient needs:

- Follow a healthy dietary pattern at every life stage.
- Customize and enjoy nutrient-dense food and beverage choices to reflect personal preferences, cultural traditions, and budgetary considerations.
- Focus on meeting food group needs with nutrient-dense foods and beverages, and stay within calorie limits.
- Limit foods and beverages higher in added sugars, saturated fat, and sodium, and limit alcoholic beverages.

The DGA feature healthy food patterns with three different eating pattern styles to illustrate how the guidelines and recommendations translate into food across 12 different calorie levels, from 1000 to 3200 calories:

- Healthy U.S.-Style Pattern
- Healthy Mediterranean-Style Pattern
- Healthy Vegetarian Pattern

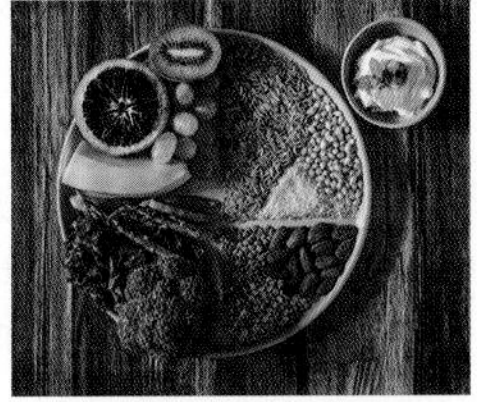

The underlying principles of healthy eating are to

- choose nutrient-dense foods and beverages,
- meet nutrient needs through foods and beverages not through supplements,
- use portion control, and
- focus on variety.

MyPlate

MyPlate is a graphic illustration of the DGA. It features a dinner plate with one half devoted to fruits and vegetables, one fourth to protein, and one fourth to grains. Dairy is alongside the plate.

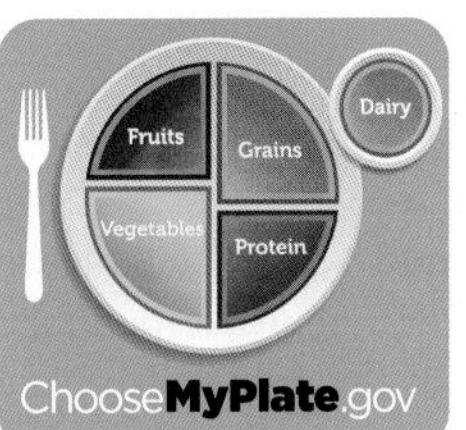

- Whole fruits that are fresh, frozen, canned, or dried are emphasized.
- The vegetable group is divided into subgroups with weekly recommended amounts specified for each group to ensure variety.
- At least half of grain servings should be whole grain.

(continued)

CHAPTER SUMMARY GUIDELINES FOR HEALTHY EATING (continued)

- Within the protein group, lean sources of meat and poultry are recommended, as are two weekly servings of seafood. Nuts, seeds, soy products, and legumes are healthy plant sources of protein with recommended amounts per week specified.
- The dairy group features low-fat or fat-free milk, yogurt, and soy milk.
- Additional points are to use oils and limit added sugars, saturated fat, sodium, and alcohol.

The website MyPlate.gov provides a myriad of online resources about healthy eating for all lifecycle stages.

Eating Behaviors Americans Are Trying to Improve

The typical American diet is far from ideal, yet many Americans surveyed say they are trying to

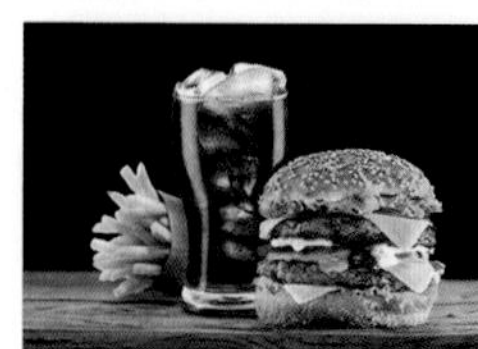

- limit sugar intake,
- eat more fruits and vegetables,
- eat less carbohydrate,
- eat healthier protein sources, and
- eat better and healthier in general.

Recommendations from Health Agencies

Many health agencies publish healthy eating recommendations or guidelines for the prevention of chronic disease. Recommendations made by the American Heart Association, the American Cancer Society, and the American Institute for Cancer Research are remarkably consistent:

- Attain and maintain a healthy weight.
- Be physically active.
- Eat a variety of foods, with an emphasis on fruits and vegetables, whole grains, and healthy proteins.
- Eat less saturated fat, sodium, and added sugars.
- Drink alcohol in moderation, if at all.

Guidelines and Graphics in Other Countries

Many countries use a circle or dinner plate to illustrate their dietary guidelines for healthy eating; however, there is still variety around the globe, such as a pagoda (China), bicycle wheel (Korea), and a goatskin drum (Bahamas). Global recurrent concepts are to

- be physically active,
- limit salt and added sugar,
- eat a variety of foods, and
- attain and maintain a healthy weight.

Figure sources: *shutterstock.com/P Kyriakos and shutterstock.com/Valentyn Volkov.*

Student Resources on thePoint®
For additional learning materials, activate the code in the front of this book at https://thePoint.lww.com/activate

Websites

American Cancer Society Guideline for Diet and Physical Activity for Cancer Prevention at http://www.cancer.org/healthy/eathealthygetactive/acsguidelinesonnutritionphysicalactivityforcancerprevention/index

The American Heart Association Diet and Lifestyle Recommendations at https://www.heart.org/en/healthy-living/healthy-eating/eat-smart/nutrition-basics/aha-diet-and-lifestyle-recommendations

American Institute for Cancer Research's cancer prevention recommendations at https://www.aicr.org/reduce-your-cancer-risk/recommendations-for-cancer-prevention/

Dietary Guidelines for Americans 2020–2025 at https://www.dietaryguidelines.gov/sites/default/files/2020-12/Dietary_Guidelines_for_Americans_2020-2025.pdf

Food and Agriculture Organization of the United Nations' food-based dietary guidelines at http://www.fao.org/nutrition/education/food-dietary-guidelines/regions/en/. Choose from the drop-down menu "Browse by countries" to select a particular country.

International Food Information Council's 2019 Food and Health Survey at https://foodinsight.org/2019-food-and-health-survey/

MyPlate at https://www.myplate.gov/

References

Arnett, D. K., Blumenthal, R. S., Albert, M. A., Buroker, A. B., Goldberger, Z. D., Hahn, E. J., Himmelfarb, C. D., Khera, A., Lloyd-Jones, D., McEvoy, J. W., Michos, E. D., Miedema, M. D., Muñoz, D., Smith, S. C. Jr., Virani, S. S., Williams, K. A. Sr., Yeboah, J., & Ziaeian, B. (2019). 2019 ACC/AHA guideline on the primary prevention of cardiovascular disease: A report of the American College of Cardiology/American Heart Association Task Force on Clinical Practice Guidelines. *Circulation, 140*, e596–e646. https://doi.org/10.1161/CIR.0000000000000678

International Food Information Council. (2019, May 22). *2019 food and health survey*. https://foodinsight.org/2019-food-and-health-survey/

Ko, C. W., Singh, S., Feuerstein, J. D., Falck-Ytter, C., Falck-Ytter, Y., Cross, R. K., & American Gastroenterological Association Institute Clinical Guidelines Committee. (2019). AGA clinical practice guidelines on the management of mild-to-moderate ulcerative colitis. *Gastroenterology, 156*(3), 748–764. https://doi.org/10.1053/j.gastro.2018.12.009

Kushi, L., Doyle, C., McCullough, M., Rock, C. L., Demark-Wahnefried, W., Bandera, E. V., Gapstur, S., Patel, A., Andrews, K.,

Gansler, T., & American Cancer Society 2010 Nutrition and Physical Activity Guidelines Advisory Committee. (2012). American Cancer Society guidelines on nutrition and physical activity for cancer prevention: Reducing the risk of cancer with healthy food choices and physical activity. *CA: A Cancer Journal for Clinicians, 62*(1), 30–67. https://doi.org/10.3322/caac.20140

U.S. Department of Agriculture. (n.d.). *MyPlate*. https://www.myplate.gov

U.S. Department of Agriculture & U.S. Department of Health and Human Services. (2020, December). *Dietary guidelines for Americans 2020–2025*. https://www.dietaryguidelines.gov/sites/default/files/2020-12/Dietary_Guidelines_for_Americans_2020-2025.pdf

World Cancer Research Fund & American Institute for Cancer Research. (2007). *Food, nutrition, physical activity, and the prevention of cancer: A global perspective*. American Institute for Cancer Research.

Chapter 3 Carbohydrates

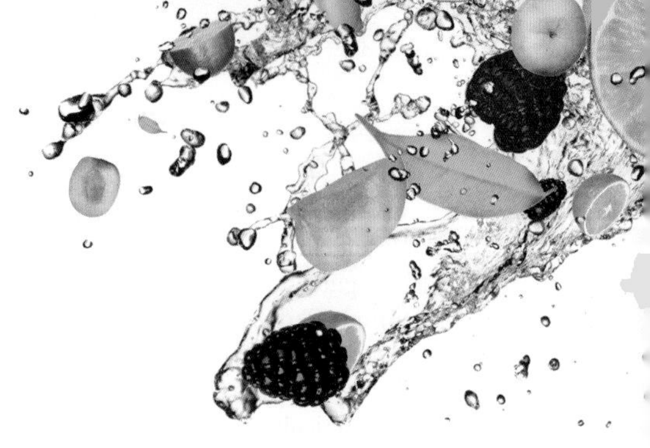

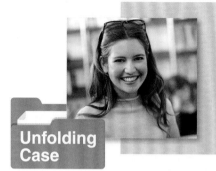

Krista Larson

Krista is a 24-year-old graduate student who complains of chronic constipation. She has used laxatives for years in an effort to control her weight, and eliminates as many carbohydrates from her diet as she can. She recently tried to stop using laxatives but is unable to have a bowel movement on her own.

Learning Objectives

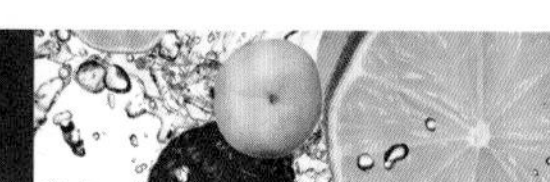

Upon completion of this chapter, you will be able to:

1 Explain how carbohydrates are classified.
2 Identify sources of carbohydrates.
3 Debate the usefulness of using glycemic load to make food choices.
4 Describe the functions of carbohydrates.
5 Modify a menu to replace low-fiber foods with higher-fiber foods.
6 Discuss the recommendations regarding carbohydrate intake in the Dietary Guidelines for Americans.
7 Suggest ways to increase whole grain intake.
8 Discuss the benefits and disadvantages of using sugar alternatives.

Carbohydrates (CHO)
a class of energy-yielding nutrients that contain only carbon, hydrogen, and oxygen, hence the common abbreviation of CHO.

Simple Sugars
a classification of carbohydrates that includes monosaccharides and disaccharides; commonly referred to as sugars.

Complex Carbohydrates
a group name for starch, glycogen, and fiber; composed of long chains of glucose molecules.

Starch
the storage form of glucose in plants.

Sugar and starch come to mind when people hear the word *carbs*, but carbohydrates are so much more than just table sugar and bread. Foods containing carbohydrates can be empty calories, nutritional powerhouses, or something in between. Globally, carbohydrates provide the majority of calories in almost all human diets.

This chapter describes what carbohydrates are, where they are found in the diet, and how they are handled in the body. Recommendations regarding intake and the role of carbohydrates in health are presented.

CARBOHYDRATE CLASSIFICATIONS

Carbohydrates (CHO) are composed of the elements carbon, hydrogen, and oxygen arranged into basic sugar molecules. They are classified as either **simple sugars** or **complex carbohydrates** (Fig. 3.1). Simple sugars contain only one (mono-) or two (di-) sugar (saccharide) molecules; they vary in sweetness and sources. Complex carbohydrates, of which **starch** is the most common, is made of long chains of many (poly) sugar (saccharide) molecules.

Figure 3.1 ▶ **Carbohydrate classifications.**

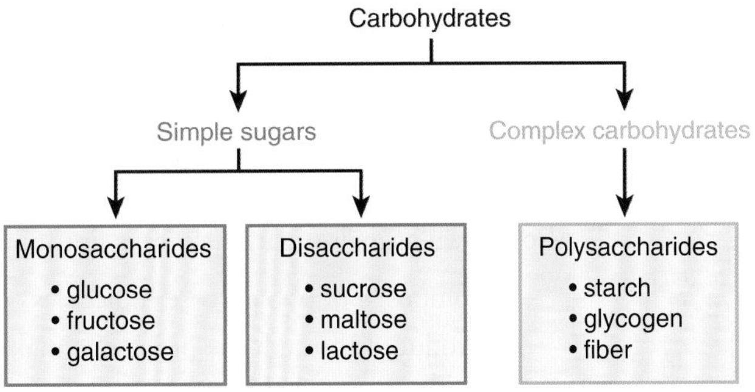

Monosaccharides

Monosaccharide
single (mono) molecules of sugar (saccharide); the most common monosaccharides in foods are hexoses that contain six carbon atoms.

Monosaccharides are the simplest form of carbohydrate. They cannot be digested into smaller molecules and thus are absorbed as they are. Hexoses, sugar molecules containing six carbon atoms, are the only monosaccharides that are abundant in food and nutritionally significant.

Glucose

Glucose, also known as dextrose, is the simple sugar of greatest distinction, which

- circulates through the blood to provide energy for body cells,
- is a component of all disaccharides, and is virtually the sole constituent of complex carbohydrates,
- is the sugar to which the body converts all other digestible carbohydrates, and
- is naturally found in fruit, vegetables, honey, corn syrup, and cornstarch.

Fructose

Fructose, also known as fruit sugar or levulose

- is the sweetest of all simple sugars,
- is naturally found in fruit, honey, and some vegetables, and
- comprises 42% to 55% of high-fructose corn syrup (HFCS).

Galactose

Galactose does not occur in appreciable amounts in foods. It is significant only as it combines with glucose to form lactose.

Disaccharides

Disaccharide
"double sugar" composed of two (di) monosaccharides (e.g., sucrose, maltose, lactose).

Disaccharides are double sugars made from one glucose molecule and one other monosaccharide.

Sucrose

Sucrose is the most familiar of all sugars and what comes to mind when the word *sugar* is used. It is

- composed of 50% glucose and 50% fructose,
- extracted from sugarcane and sugar beets and processed into its many forms, such as white, brown, powdered, turbinado, raw, and Baker's Special, and
- found naturally in maple syrup, bananas, dates, pineapple, peas, and sweet potato.

Lactose

Also known as milk sugar, lactose is the only animal source of carbohydrate in the diet, and

- is composed of 50% glucose and 50% galactose,
- is the least sweet of all sugars,

- enhances the absorption of calcium when consumed at the same time, and
- is often used by the pharmaceutical industry as filler in pills.

Maltose

Also known as malt sugar, maltose is not found freely in food. It is

- composed of two glucose molecules,
- produced through the process of malting (e.g., malted milk),
- used primarily as a flavoring and coloring agent in the manufacture of beer, and
- an intermediate in the digestion of starch.

Polysaccharides carbohydrates consisting of many (poly) sugar molecules.

Glycogen storage form of glucose in animals and humans.

Complex Carbohydrates

Complex carbohydrates, also known as **polysaccharides**, are composed of hundreds to thousands of glucose molecules linked together. Despite being made of sugar, polysaccharides do not taste sweet because their molecules are too large to fit on the tongue's taste bud receptors that sense sweetness. Starch, **glycogen**, and fiber are types of polysaccharides.

Starch

Plants synthesize glucose through the process of photosynthesis, and they use that glucose for energy. Glucose not used by the plant for immediate energy is stored in the form of starch in seeds, roots, or stems.

- Starch provides the majority of calories in grains, such as wheat, rice, corn, barley, millet, sorghum, oats, and rye. Other sources include legumes and starchy vegetables (e.g., potatoes, plantains, and parsnips).
- The majority of starch in grains comes from the endosperm, or the middle portion of the kernel, which is a component of both refined and whole grains.
- Cooking makes starch more digestible and slightly sweeter.

Glycogen

Glycogen is the animal (including human) version of starch. It is stored carbohydrate available for energy as needed. Humans have a limited supply of glycogen stored in the liver and muscles.

- There is virtually no dietary source of glycogen because any glycogen stored in animal tissue is quickly converted to lactic acid at the time of slaughter.
- The only exception is the miniscule amounts of glycogen in shellfish, such as scallops and oysters, which is why they taste slightly sweet compared to other fish.

Fiber

Fiber is a group name for non-digestible carbohydrates linked to an array of potential health benefits, including a lower risk of cardiovascular disease, stroke, hypertension, certain gastrointestinal conditions, obesity, type 2 diabetes, and some types of cancer (Box 3.1). Historically referred to as "roughage" or "bulk," fiber only occurs naturally in plants as a component of plant cell walls or intercellular structure. An estimated 85% of fiber in the U.S. food supply comes from grain products, vegetables, legumes, nuts, soy, and fruit (Dahl & Stewart, 2015). Table 3.1 lists the fiber content of selected fiber-rich foods. Almost all sources of fiber provide a mix of different types of fiber. No universal definition of fiber exists, and there are a number of ways it can be classified.

BOX 3.1 Potential Health Benefits Linked to Fiber

- A high fiber intake may improve serum lipid levels, lower blood pressure, and lower inflammatory marker levels, which may explain the link between fiber and lower risk of cardiovascular disease (CVD) (International Food Information Council, 2019).
- Observational data suggest a 15% to 30% lower risk in all-cause and CVD mortality, incidence of congenital heart disease, stroke incidence and mortality, type 2 diabetes, and colorectal cancer when comparing higher with lower intakes of dietary fiber (Reynolds et al., 2019).
- A high fiber intake is associated with a reduced risk of mortality from all cancers (Kim & Je, 2016).
- Observational studies show that populations with higher intakes of fiber often have lower body weight and that obese people tend to have lower intakes of fiber (Dahl & Stewart, 2015).
- Fiber promotes gastrointestinal health by increasing stool bulk to improve laxation (IFIC, 2019).
- A high fiber intake contributes to the maintenance of a healthy gut microbiota associated with increased diversity and functions, such as the production of short-chain fatty acids, which help maintain a functional immune system (Makki et al., 2018).

Table 3.1 Fiber Content of Fiber-rich Foods

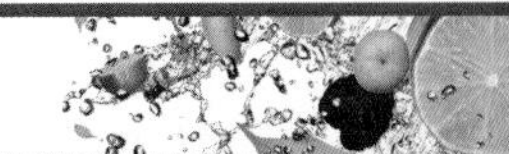

Food	Total Fiber (g)	Food	Total Fiber (g)
Fruit (1 medium, unless otherwise specified)		**Nuts (1 oz)**	
Apple with skin	4.0	Almonds	4.0
Banana	3.0	Cashews	1.0
Orange	4.0	Flaxseed	8.0
Pear	6.0	Pistachios	3.0
Strawberries (1 cup)	3.0	Walnuts	2.0
Raspberries (1 cup)	8.0	**Vegetables (½ cup cooked)**	
Grains (½ cup unless otherwise specified)		Broccoli	2.5
All-bran cereal	10.0	Brussels sprouts	3.0
Brown rice	2.0	Savoy cabbage	2.0
Bulgur	4.0	Collard greens	2.5
Oats (dry)	4.0	Mustard greens	2.5
Quinoa	2.5	Green peas	7.0
Whole wheat spaghetti, cooked	3.0	Edamame	3.0
Whole wheat bread (1 slice)	2.0	**Fiber Fortified Foods**	
Legumes (½ cup cooked)		Nature's Own Double Fiber Wheat Bread (1 slice)	5.0
Black	7.5	Bob's Red Mill Organic High Fiber Hot Cereal (1/3 c dry)	10.0
Kidney	8.0	Fiber One Yoplait Yogurt (4 oz)	5.0
Lentils	8.0		
Lima	7.0		
Navy	9.5		
White	9.5		

Source: Palmer, S. (2008). *The top fiber-rich foods list*. Today's Dietitian. https://www.todaysdietitian.com/newarchives/063008p28.shtml.

Soluble Fiber/Viscous Fiber
non-digestible carbohydrates that tend to form a thick, gel-like compound in the stomach that may then be fermented by bacteria in the colon.

Insoluble Fiber/ Non-Fermentable Fiber
non-digestible carbohydrates that cannot be broken down by bacteria in the colon but absorb water.

- Fiber has commonly been classified as either **soluble** or **insoluble**.
  - **Soluble fibers** dissolve in water to a gel-like substance (are **viscous**) and are easily digested (**fermentable**) by bacteria in the colon.
    - Sources include oatmeal, legumes, lentils, and citrus fruit.
    - Soluble fiber is credited with slowing gastric emptying time to promote a feeling of fullness, delaying and blunting the rise in postprandial serum glucose, and lowering serum cholesterol by promoting its excretion.
  - **Insoluble fibers** do not form gels, and they are not readily fermentable.
    - Insoluble fibers absorb water to add bulk to stools, and thereby promote laxation.
    - Whole grains, bran, and the skins and seeds of fruit and vegetables provide insoluble fiber.
  - The National Academy of Sciences recommends phasing out the terms *soluble* and *insoluble* and replacing them with terms that describe their physiochemical properties of viscosity and fermentability (Institute of Medicine, 2001). This means the term *soluble fiber* would be replaced by **viscous fiber** and *insoluble fiber* by **non-fermentable fiber**.
- Another way to classify fiber is by its source.
  - **Dietary fiber** is the intact and naturally occurring fiber in plants.
  - **Functional fiber** is fiber that has been isolated or extracted from plants and then added to food. For example, inulin is added to some yogurt.
  - **Total fiber** is the sum of dietary fiber and functional fiber.

Dietary Fiber
carbohydrates and lignin that are natural and intact components of plants that cannot be digested by human enzymes.

Functional Fiber
as proposed by the Food and Nutrition Board, functional fiber consists of extracted or isolated non-digestible carbohydrates that have beneficial physiologic effects in humans.

Total Fiber
total fiber = dietary fiber + functional fiber.

Recall Krista. Her restricted carbohydrate intake provides negligible fiber, because fiber occurs naturally only in plant sources of carbohydrates.

- What other nutrients may be lacking in her eating pattern due to her restricted intake of grains, fruit, vegetables, and legumes?
- What would you teach Krista about the role of carbohydrates and fiber in health?
- What does she need to know about increasing her fiber intake?

It is commonly assumed that fiber does not provide any calories because it is not truly digested by human enzymes and may actually trap macronutrients eaten at the same time, preventing them from being absorbed. Yet fibers that are soluble/viscous are fermented by bacteria in the colon to produce carbon dioxide, methane, hydrogen, and short-chain fatty acids, which serve as a source of energy (calories) for the mucosal lining of the colon. Although the exact energy value available to humans from the blend of fibers in food is unknown, it is estimated that the fermentation of fiber in the average human gut yields between 1.5 and 2.5 cal/g (Institute of Medicine, 2005).

Added Sugars
caloric sugars and syrups added to foods during processing or preparation, or consumed separately; do not include sugars naturally present in foods, such as fructose in fruit and lactose in milk.

SOURCES OF CARBOHYDRATES

Table 3.2 summarizes the amount of carbohydrate and fiber in servings of various foods. Americans consume approximately 50% of their total daily calorie intake in the form of carbohydrates, including starch from grains, legumes, and some vegetables; naturally occurring sugars in milk, fruit, and vegetables; and **added sugars** in items containing sugars and syrups added during processing, food preparation, or at the table (e.g., sugar in coffee).

Table 3.2 Sources of Carbohydrates: Average Amount of Carbohydrate and Fiber per Serving

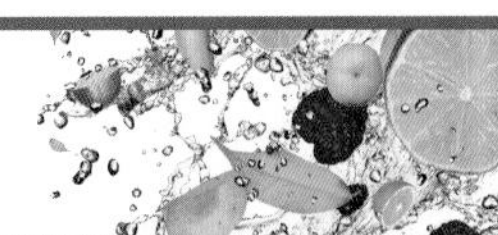

Fruit

Fresh, frozen, and dried fruit have about 15 g carbohydrate and about 2 g fiber per serving.

- 1 medium nectarine, peach, orange
- 1 large tangerine or pear
- ½ c unsweetened applesauce, fruit cocktail, sliced kiwi
- 1 c blackberries, raspberries, cubed papaya
- 2 tbsp dried fruit (raisins, blueberries, cranberries)

½ c fruit juice has 15 g carbohydrate and very little fiber.

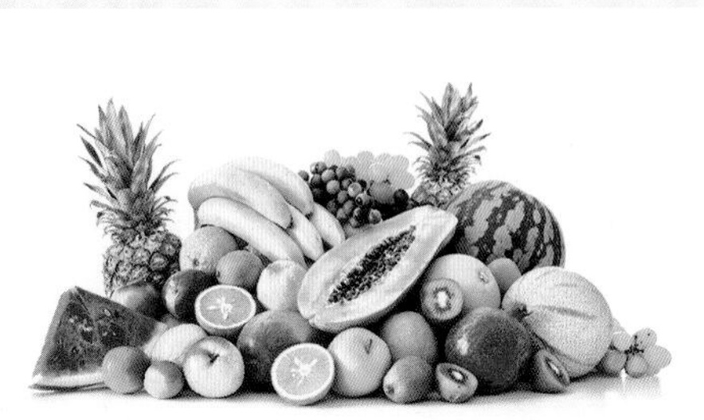

shutterstock.com/Alexander Raths

Vegetables

Non-starchy vegetables provide 5 g of carbohydrate and 2–3 g of fiber per serving.

- ½ c cooked broccoli, cabbage, carrots, cauliflower, eggplant, green beans, green peas, mushrooms, spinach, tomatoes
- 1 c of raw carrots, peppers

Starchy vegetables provide 15 g of carbohydrate and 2–4 g fiber per serving.

- ½ c cooked corn, yams, sweet potatoes, parsnips, green peas, succotash, potatoes
- 1 c cooked winter squash, french fries (oven baked)

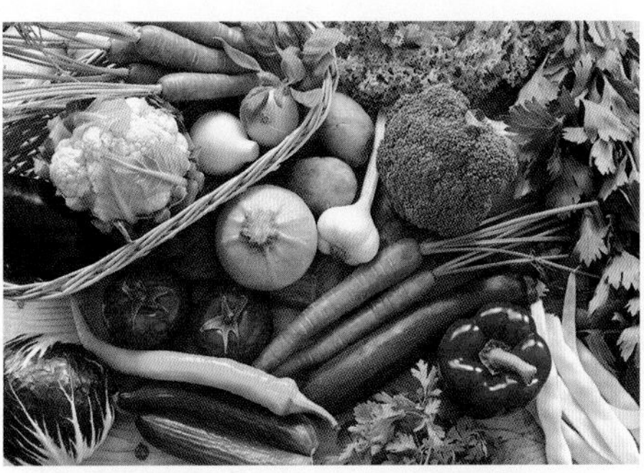

shutterstock.com/Ana Blazic Pavlovic

Grains

Grain products contain 15 g carbohydrate per serving.

Whole grains have 1–2 g fiber (or more). Refined grains have 0–1 g fiber per serving.

- 1 slice bread
- 1 oz ready-to-eat cereals
- ½ c cooked pasta, rice, oats, barley, bulgur, grits

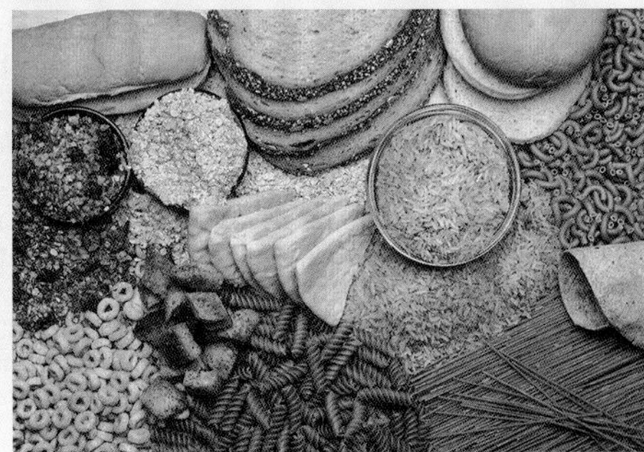

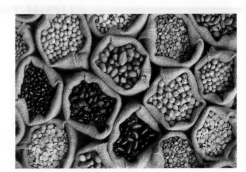

shutterstock.com/Stephen Cook Photography

Protein: Legumes

Legumes have 15 g carbohydrate and 5–8 g fiber per ½ c cooked or canned serving.

- ½ c black, garbanzo, kidney, lima, navy, pinto, white, black-eyed peas, lentils

shutterstock.com/Piyaset

Table 3.2 Sources of Carbohydrates: Average Amount of Carbohydrate and Fiber per Serving (continued)

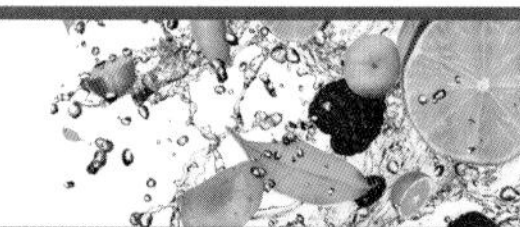

Dairy

Milk choices have about 12 g of carbohydrate per serving.
Milk choices do not naturally provide fiber although fiber-fortified yogurt is available.

- 1 c milk—fat-free, low-fat, 2%, or whole
- 2/3 c plain or Greek yogurt

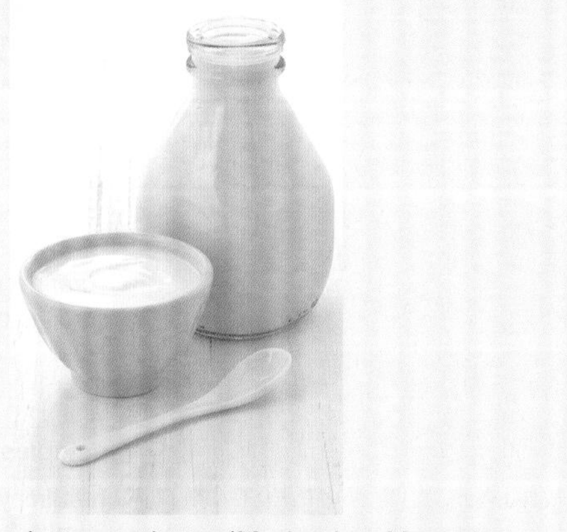

shutterstock.com/Modernista Magazine

Foods High in Added Sugar

Carbohydrate content varies considerably.
Fiber is generally negligible except for items made with fruit or whole grains.
Each of the following has about 15 g of carbohydrate:

- ½ c gelatin, regular or light ice cream
- 1 oz brownie, biscotti, milk or dark chocolate candy, 100 calorie pack cookies
- 1 tbsp sugar, jam, jelly, honey, pancake syrup

These foods provide about 30 g of carbohydrate:

- ½ c pudding, sorbet, sherbet
- 1 small frosted cupcake
- 2 tbsp chocolate syrup

Sweetened beverages vary in carbohydrate content[a]:

- 1 12 oz can of soft drink or Red Bull has approximately 40 g
- 16 oz of Starbucks Café Latte has 19 g
- 1 can of regular beer has 13 g
- 1 can of light beer has 6 g

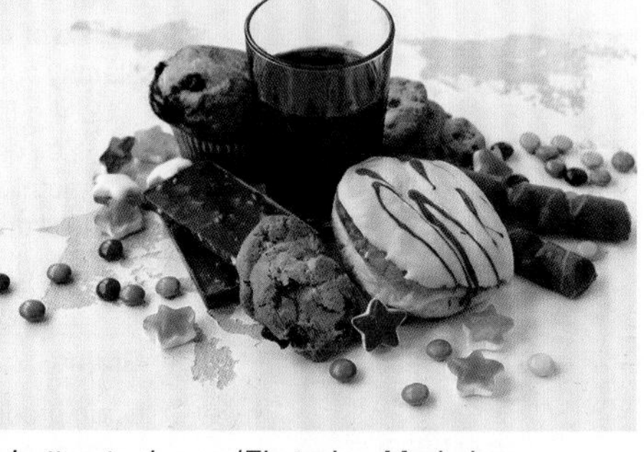

shutterstock.com/Ekaterina Markelova

[a]Based on product information.
Source: Academy of Nutrition and Dietetics and American Diabetes Association. (2019). *Choose your foods: Food lists for weight management.* Academy of Nutrition and Dietetics.

HOW THE BODY HANDLES CARBOHYDRATES

Digestion and Absorption

Carbohydrates are digested more quickly and completely than protein and fat. Normally, most starches and all sugars are digested within 1 to 4 hours after eating. Monosaccharides are the simplest form of carbohydrates and are the end product of disaccharide and polysaccharide digestion.

- Cooked starch begins to undergo digestion in the mouth by the action of salivary amylase, but the overall effect is small because food is not held in the mouth for very long (Fig. 3.2).
- The stomach churns and mixes its contents, but its acidic medium halts any residual effect of swallowed amylase.
- The principal site of carbohydrate digestion is the small intestine. Pancreatic amylase, secreted into the intestine by way of the pancreatic duct, reduces polysaccharides to shorter glucose chains and maltose.

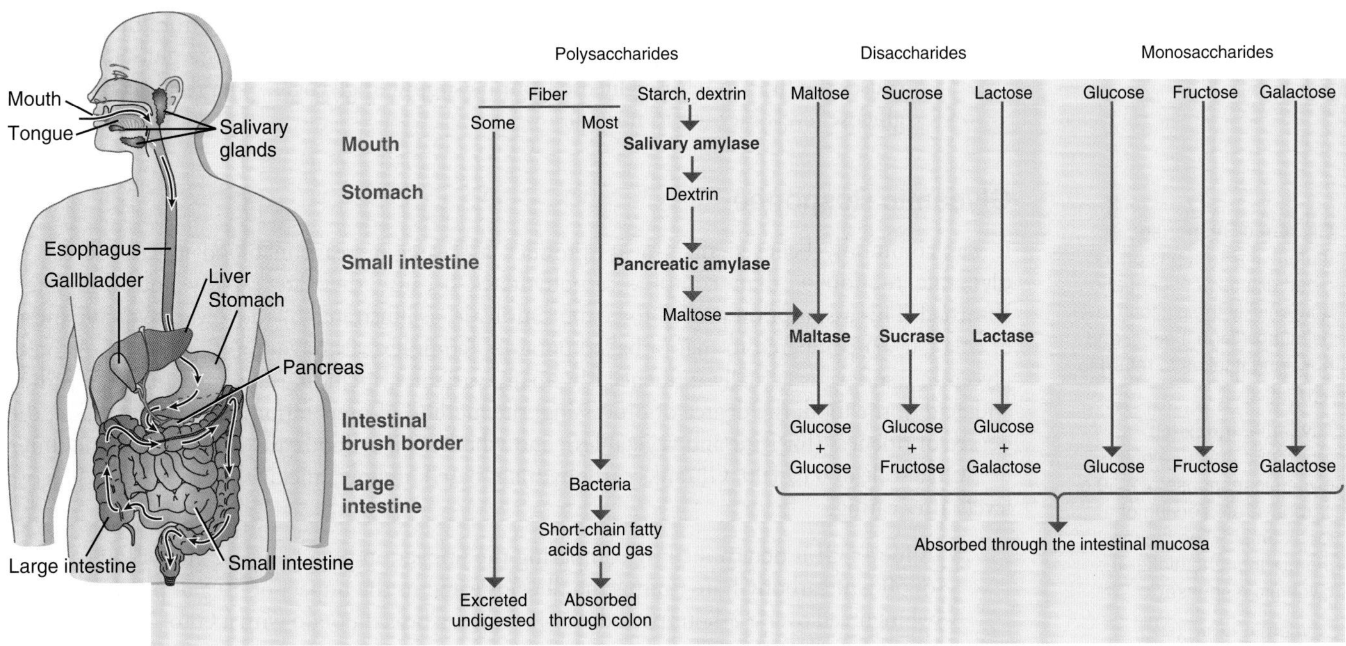

Figure 3.2 ▲ **Carbohydrate digestion.**

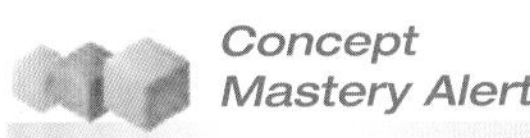
Concept Mastery Alert

Typically, two-thirds of the body's glycogen is stored in the muscle, where it is available only for use in the muscle, and the remaining one third is stored in the liver, where it is available for all body cells.

- Disaccharidase enzymes (maltase, sucrase, and lactase) within the brush border of the intestine split maltose, sucrose, and lactose, into monosaccharides.
- Monosaccharides, whether consumed as monosaccharides or resulting from the digestion of other carbohydrates, are absorbed through intestinal mucosa cells and travel to the liver via the portal vein.
- Small amounts of starch that have not been fully digested pass into the colon and are excreted in the stools.
- Fibers, which are non-digestible, advance to the large intestine.
    - Non-fermentable fibers attract water, which softens stools and promotes laxation.
    - Viscous fibers are fermented by gut microbiota, which yields water, methane, hydrogen, and short-chain fatty acids: These fatty acids are used by the colon for energy or are absorbed and metabolized by liver cells.

Metabolism

Fructose and galactose are converted to glucose in the liver. The liver releases glucose into the bloodstream, where its level is held fairly constant by hormones.

- A rise in blood glucose concentration after eating causes the pancreas to secrete insulin, which moves glucose out of the bloodstream and into the cells.
- Most cells take only as much glucose as they need for immediate energy needs.
    - Liver and muscle cells take up extra glucose molecules during times of plenty and join them together to form glycogen.
        - One-third of the body's total glycogen reserve is in the liver and can be released into circulation for all body cells to use
        - Two-thirds is in muscle, which is available only for use by muscles.
        - Unlike fat, glycogen storage is limited and may provide only enough calories for about a half-day of moderate activity.
- The movement of glucose out of the bloodstream and into cells eventually causes glucose levels to return to normal.

- Blood glucose concentration begins to drop as the body uses the energy from the last meal.
    - Even a slight fall in blood glucose stimulates the pancreas to release glucagon, which causes the liver to release glucose from its supply of glycogen. The result is that blood glucose levels increase to normal.

Glycemic Response
the effect a food has on the blood glucose concentration: how quickly the glucose level rises, how high it goes, and how long it takes to return to normal.

Glycemic Index (GI)
a numeric measure of the glycemic response of a 50 g carbohydrate serving of a food sample. The higher the number, the higher the glycemic response.

Glycemic Load (GL)
a formula that combines portion size and GI into one number to evaluate the impact on blood glucose levels.

Glycemic Response

It was commonly believed that sugars produce a greater increase in blood glucose levels, or **glycemic response**, than complex carbohydrates because they are rapidly and completely absorbed. This assumption proved to be too simplistic, as illustrated by the lower **glycemic index** of cola (sugar) compared to that of baked potatoes (complex carbohydrate) (Table 3.3). A food's glycemic response is actually influenced by many variables, including the amounts of fat, fiber, and acid in the food; the degree of processing; the method of preparation; the amount eaten; the degree of ripeness (for fruit and vegetables); and whether other foods are eaten at the same time.

On a scale of 0 to 100, GI ranks carbohydrates based on how quickly they raise blood glucose levels after eating.

- A food's GI is determined by comparing the impact on blood glucose after a food sample of 50 g of carbohydrate (minus the fiber) is eaten to the impact of 50 g of pure glucose or white bread over a 2-hour period: For instance, a boiled potato with a GI of 78 elicits 78% of the blood glucose response as an equivalent amount of pure glucose.
- The amount of carbohydrate contained in a typical portion of food also influences the glycemic response, so the concept of **glycemic load (GL)** was created; it combines portion size and GI into one value.

Table 3.3 Glycemic Index and Glycemic Load of Selected Foods, as Determined in People with Normal Glucose Tolerance

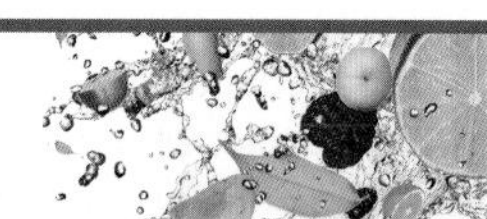

Item	Glycemic Index (Glucose = 100)	Glycemic Load/Serving
Pretzels (Canada)	83 ± 9	16
Puffed rice cakes, caramel flavored	82 ± 10	18
Corn flakes	77	19
Boiled white rice (Canada)	72 ± 9	30
Whole meal (whole wheat) bread (Canada)	72 ± 6	8
Clover honey	69 ± 8	15
Mars Bar	68 ± 12	27
Brown rice (Canada)	50 ± 8	24
Coca-Cola	63	16
Sweet corn, boiled	60	11
White spaghetti (Canada)	50 ± 8	24
V8 100% vegetable juice	43 ± 4	4
Whole milk	41 ± 2	5
Orange, raw (Canada)	40 ± 3	4
All-bran cereal	38	8
Chocolate cake with chocolate frosting	38 ± 3	20
Fat-free milk	32	4

Note. All items are U.S. formulations unless otherwise indicated.
Source: Atkinson, F., Foster-Powell, K., & Brand-Miller, J. (2008). International tables of glycemic index and glycemic load values: 2008. *Diabetes Care, 32*(12), 2281–2283. https://doi.org/10.2337/dc08-1239.

  - The carbohydrate content of a serving is multiplied by the food's GI, then divided by 100.
  - For example, the GI of beets is 64, but because they have only 13 g of carbohydrate per cup, the GL is only 8.3. ($13 \text{ g} \times 64 \div 100 = 8.3$)
  - In general, a GL > 20 is considered high, and 10 or less is considered low.
- In a practical sense, GL is not a reliable tool for choosing a healthy diet, and claims that a low-GI diet promotes significant weight loss or helps control appetite are unfounded.
  - Soft drinks, candy, sugars, and high-fat foods may have a low to moderate GI, but these foods are not nutritious and eating them does not promote weight loss.
- In addition, a food's actual impact on glucose levels is difficult to predict, due to the many factors influencing GL.
- GI may help people with diabetes fine-tune optimal meal planning (see Chapter 21), and athletes can use the GI to choose optimal fuels for before, during, and after exercise.

FUNCTIONS OF CARBOHYDRATES

Glucose metabolism is a dynamic state of balance between burning glucose for energy (*catabolism*) and using glucose to build other compounds (*anabolism*). This process is a continuous response to the supply of glucose from food and the demand for glucose for energy needs.

Glucose for Energy

The primary function of carbohydrates is to provide energy for cells.

- Glucose is burned more efficiently and more completely than either protein or fat, and it does not leave an end product that the body must excrete.
- Although muscles use a mixture of fat and glucose for energy, the brain is normally totally dependent on glucose for energy.
- All digestible carbohydrates—namely, simple sugars and complex carbohydrates—provide 4 cal/g. Depending on the extent to which fibers are fermented in the colon into short-chain fatty acids and metabolized, fibers provide 1.5 to 2.5 cal/g.

Protein Sparing

Consuming adequate carbohydrate to meet energy needs has the effect of "sparing protein" from being used for energy, leaving it available to do the special functions that only protein can perform, such as replenishing enzymes, hormones, antibodies, and blood cells. An adequate carbohydrate intake is especially important whenever protein needs are increased, such as for wound healing and during pregnancy and lactation.

Preventing Ketosis

Fat normally supplies about half of the body's energy requirement at rest. Yet, glucose fragments are needed to efficiently and completely burn fat for energy.

- Fat oxidation prematurely stops at the intermediate step of ketone-body formation without adequate glucose.
  - **Ketone bodies** are normally produced in small quantities.
  - They can be used by muscles and other tissues for energy.
- An increased production of ketone bodies and their accumulation in the bloodstream can cause nausea, fatigue, loss of appetite, and ketoacidosis.
  - Dehydration and sodium depletion may follow as the body tries to excrete ketones in the urine.

Ketone Bodies
intermediate, acidic compounds formed from the incomplete breakdown of fat when adequate glucose is not available.

Using Glucose to Make Other Compounds

After energy needs are met, excess glucose can be

- converted to other essential carbohydrates, such as ribose, a component of ribonucleic acid and deoxyribonucleic acid;
- broken down to provide a carbon stem that the body can use to make nonessential amino acids, if nitrogen and other necessary components are available.

Using Glucose to Make Fat

After energy needs are met, glycogen stores are saturated, and other specific compounds are made. Any glucose remaining at this point is converted by liver cells to triglycerides and stored in the body's fat tissue. The body does this by combining acetate molecules to form fatty acids, which then are combined with glycerol to make triglycerides. Although it sounds easy for excess carbohydrates to be converted to fat, it is not a primary pathway; the body prefers to make body fat from dietary fat, not from carbohydrates.

DIETARY REFERENCE INTAKES

Total Carbohydrate

The Recommended Dietary Allowance for total carbohydrate (starch, natural sugar, added sugar) is set at 130 g for both adults and children, based on the average *minimum* amount of glucose that is needed to fuel the brain and assuming total calorie intake is adequate (Institute of Medicine, 2005). Yet at this level, total calorie needs are not met unless protein and fat intakes exceed levels considered healthy.

- A more useful guideline for determining appropriate carbohydrate intake is the Acceptable Macronutrient Distribution Range (AMDR), which recommends carbohydrates provide 45% to 65% of total calories consumed (Institute of Medicine, 2005).
- As illustrated in Figure 3.3 the carbohydrate content using AMDR standards is significantly higher than the minimum of 130 g/day.
- Table 3.4 estimates the Carbohydrate Content of a 2000-calorie Healthy U.S.-Style Eating Pattern.

Table 3.4 Carbohydrate Content of the 2000-Calorie Healthy U.S.-Style Eating Pattern

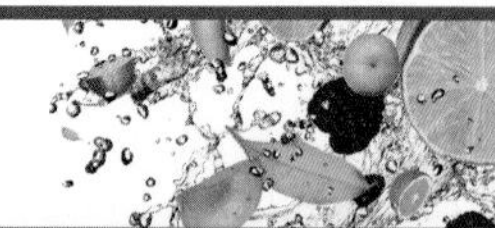

Food Group	Recommended Daily Amount	Average g Carbohydrate/Serving[a]	Estimated Total g Carbohydrate/Food Group
Vegetables[b]	2.5 c equivalent	5	25
Fruit	2 c equivalent	15	60
Grains	6 oz equivalent	15	90
Dairy	3 c equivalent	12	36
Protein foods	5.5 oz equivalents	0[c]	0
Oils	27 g	0	0
Total			211 g

Note. Healthy U.S.-Style Eating Pattern available at https://www.dietaryguidelines.gov/sites/default/files/2020-12/Dietary_Guidelines_for_Americans_2020-2025.pdf.

[a]Carbohydrate content based on: Academy of Nutrition and Dietetics and American Diabetes Association. (2019). *Choose your foods: Food lists for weight management.* Academy of Nutrition and Dietetics.

[b]Assuming all vegetables selected were non-starchy.

[c]Assuming no plant-based proteins were chosen.

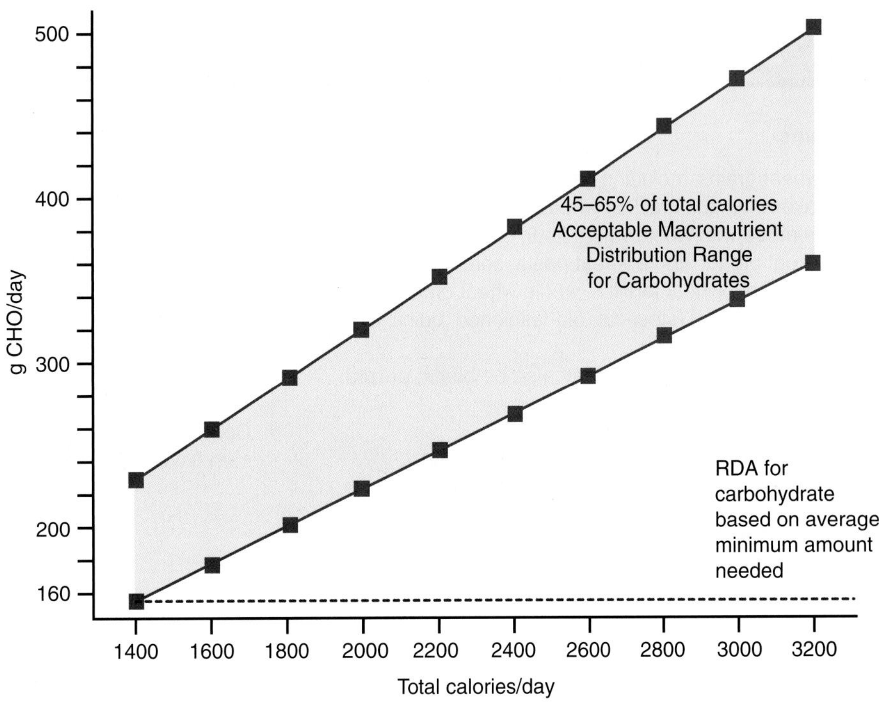

Figure 3.3 ▶ Amount of total carbohydrates appropriate at various caloric levels based on the Acceptable Macronutrient Distribution Range of 45% to 65% of total calories. The dotted line represents the Recommended Dietary Allowance for carbohydrate based on the average minimum amount needed.

Fiber

An Adequate Intake (AI) for total fiber is set at 14 g/1000 calories, or approximately 25 g/day for women and 38 g/day for men (Institute of Medicine, 2005). Fiber is not an essential nutrient that must be consumed through food in order to prevent a deficiency disease; the recommendation is based on intake levels that have been observed to protect against coronary heart disease based on epidemiologic and clinical data. Most Americans eat about half the amount of fiber recommended, most of which comes from vegetables (International Food Information Council [IFIC], 2019).

CARBOHYDRATES IN HEALTH PROMOTION

Refined Grains
consist of only the endosperm (middle part) of the grain and therefore do not contain the bran and germ portions.

Americans, on average, consume an appropriate percentage of their calories from carbohydrates but are urged to make healthier choices, namely, to use whole grains in place of **refined grains** (especially refined grains that are high in saturated fat, added sugars, or sodium) and to limit added sugars. For instance, the American College of Cardiology and the American Heart Association (AHA) recommend a healthy diet that emphasizes whole grains and minimizes the intake of refined carbohydrates and sugar-sweetened beverages (SSB) (Arnett et al., 2019).

Increase Whole Grains

Whole Grains
contain the entire grain, or seed, which is the endosperm, bran, and germ.

Americans are urged to eat **whole grains** for at least half of their total grain servings. Yet according to the *2020–2025 Dietary Guidelines for Americans*, 98% of Americans aged 1 and older consume less than the recommended amounts of whole grains (U.S. Department of Agriculture [USDA] & U.S. Department of Health and Human Services [USDHHS], 2020). Low intakes of whole grain (and also fruit and vegetables) negatively effects fiber intake. Fiber is identified as a shortfall nutrient in the typical American eating pattern and a dietary component of public health concern because underconsumption is associated with health concerns (USDA & USDHHS, 2020).

Grains are classified as "whole" or "refined," which means not whole (Box 3.2). Whole grains consist of the entire kernel of a grain bran, germ, and endosperm (Fig. 3.4). They may be eaten whole as a complete food (e.g., oatmeal, brown rice, popcorn) or milled into flour to be used as an ingredient in bread, cereal, pasta, and baked goods. Even when whole grains are

BOX 3.2 Sources of Whole and Not Whole Grains

Whole Grains

- Whole wheat grains, including varieties of spelt, emmer, farro, einkorn, bulgur, cracked wheat, and wheat berries
- Products made with whole wheat flour, such as 100% whole wheat bread, whole wheat pasta, shredded wheat, Wheaties, whole wheat tortillas, whole wheat crackers
- Whole oats, oatmeal (steel-cut, old-fashioned, quick, and instant), oat flour
- Brown rice. Whole grain rice may also be black, purple, or red
- Corn, popcorn, whole corn meal
- Whole-grain barley, whole rye, teff, triticale, millet, amaranth[a], buckwheat[a], sorghum[a], quinoa[a], wild rice[a]

Not Whole Grains (Missing one or more of the 3 components of a whole grain)

- Original Cream of Wheat, puffed wheat, refined ready-to-eat wheat cereals
- Products containing enriched white or wheat flour, even if "whole grain," "whole wheat," or "multigrain" are also listed, such as white, wheat, or multigrain breads, pasta, tortillas, and crackers
- Oat bran
- White rice, Rice Krispies, cream of rice, puffed rice, rice bran
- Cornstarch, grits, degerminated corn meal, white hominy, corn flakes

[a]Considered whole grains but are technically not cereals, but rather pseudocereals.

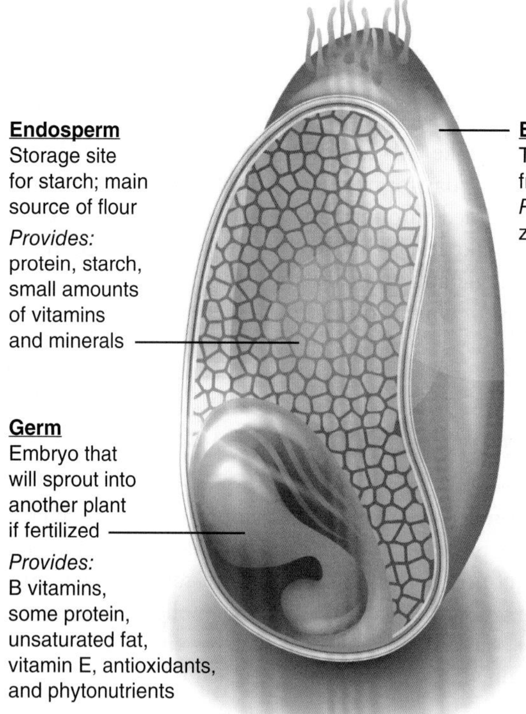
Endosperm
Storage site for starch; main source of flour
Provides: protein, starch, small amounts of vitamins and minerals
Germ
Embryo that will sprout into another plant if fertilized
Provides: B vitamins, some protein, unsaturated fat, vitamin E, antioxidants, and phytonutrients
Bran
Tough outer coating that protects rest of kernel from sunlight, pests, water, and disease.
Provides: fiber, antioxidants, B vitamins, iron, zinc, copper, magnesium, and phytonutrients

Figure 3.4 ▶ **Whole wheat. The components of the whole wheat kernel are the *bran*, the *germ*, and the *endosperm*.**

ground, cracked, or flaked, they must have the same proportion of the original three parts: bran, endosperm, and germ.

- Whole grains vary widely in their fiber content, providing slightly more than a half gram (e.g., brown rice) to around 3 g per serving (bulgur wheat).
- Whole grain cereals also vary in fiber content. Some bran cereals provide >10 g per serving, but they are not truly "whole" grain because they are only one part of the complete grain kernel.
- Although whole grains may be best known for their fiber content, the health benefits are probably due to the "whole package" of healthful components, including essential fatty acids, antioxidants, vitamins, minerals, and **phytonutrients**.

Phytonutrients are bioactive, nonnutrient plant compounds associated with a reduced risk of chronic diseases. Also known as phytochemicals.

- Just as there is not one "healthiest" vegetable, there is not one healthiest whole grain. Each whole grain (e.g., oats, quinoa, wheat, barley, rye) has a slightly different nutrient profile.
- People who choose whole grains for all of their grain choices are urged to choose some whole grains that are fortified with folic acid because the content of folic acid is naturally lower in whole grains than in fortified refined grains. This is especially true for women who are capable of becoming pregnant, because folic acid helps lower the risk of neural tube defects.

"Refined" grains are not whole because they are missing the bran and germ. They are rich in starch but have significantly lesser amounts of fiber, vitamin B_6, vitamin E, trace minerals, unsaturated fat, and most of the phytonutrients found in whole grains. Refined flour in the United States is **enriched** to add back some B vitamins (thiamin, riboflavin, and niacin) and iron to levels higher than found prior to processing. Enriched flour is also required to be **fortified** with folic acid, a mandate designed to reduce the risk of neural tube defects.

enriched
adding back certain nutrients (to specific levels) that were lost during processing.

Fortified
adding nutrients that are not naturally present in the food or were present in insignificant amounts.

- Other substances that are lost (other minerals, fiber, and phytonutrients) are not replaced by enrichment: For instance, fiber content is low—from 0 to 1 g per serving.
- Examples of refined grains include white flour, white bread, white rice, flour tortillas, and grits.
- Some refined grain products have added sugar such as: sweetened ready-to-eat cereals, muffins, and pancakes.

Identifying Whole Grains

At a quick glance, it is not always easy to distinguish between whole grain, "made with whole grain," and completely refined grains, especially with regard to bread and pasta.

- Labels that state a product is "100% whole wheat" or "100% whole grain" are whole grains.
  - "Whole wheat" or "whole (grain)" should be the first ingredient on the list or the second ingredient after water.
  - Enriched or refined flour should not appear on the ingredient list (Fig. 3.5).
- Breads, ready-to-eat cereals, and pastas labeled "made with whole grain" are not whole grains. They contain whole grains but also refined flour.
- Items containing "enriched flour" are refined.
  - Just seeing "wheat" on the label does not mean "whole wheat," such as in the case of breads identified as "honey wheat," "white wheat," or "made with 100% wheat flour."
  - With the exception of gluten-free breads, all bread contains wheat (e.g., rye bread contains rye and wheat flour) because it contains sufficient gluten to allow bread to rise.
- Tips for eating more whole grains appear in Box 3.3.

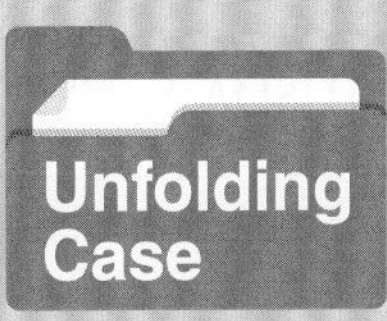

Think of Krista. She has increased her intake of grains, fruit, vegetables, and legumes but admits she doesn't like whole wheat bread or whole grains in any form.

- What other specific strategies should she try to increase her fiber intake?

Limit Added Sugars

Sugar has many functional roles in foods, including taste, physical properties, antimicrobial purposes, and chemical properties. Sugar adds flavor and interest. Few would question the value brown sugar adds to a bowl of hot oatmeal. Besides its sweet taste, sugar has important functions,

Figure 3.5 ▶

A comparison of ingredient lists to identify whole grains in bread.

A refined grain that contains only enriched wheat flour
White Bread
Ingredients
Unbromated Unbleached Enriched Wheat Flour (Flour, Niacin, Reduced Iron, Thiamin Mononitrate [Vitamin B1], Riboflavin [Vitamin B2], Folic Acid), Water, High-Fructose Corn Syrup, Yeast Soybean Oil, Nonfat Milk (adds a trivial amount of cholesterol). Contains 2% or less of th e following: Salt, Wheat Gluten...
Not a whole grain because it contains enriched wheat flour
White Bread made with Whole Grains
Ingredients
Water, Whole Wheat Flour, Enriched Wheat Flour (Unbleached Unbromated Flour, Malted Barley Flour, Niacin, Reduced Iron, Thiamin Mononitrate [Vitamin B1], Riboflavin [Vitamin B2], Folic Acid), Wheat Gluten, Honey. Contains 2% or less of the following: Sugar, Yeast, Soybean Oil...
A whole grain made from 2 types of whole wheat flour
100% Whole Wheat Bread
Ingredients
Stone Ground Whole Wheat Flour, Water, Whole Wheat Flour, Wheat Gluten, Honey. Contains 2% or less of the following: Soybean Oil, Sugar, Yeast...

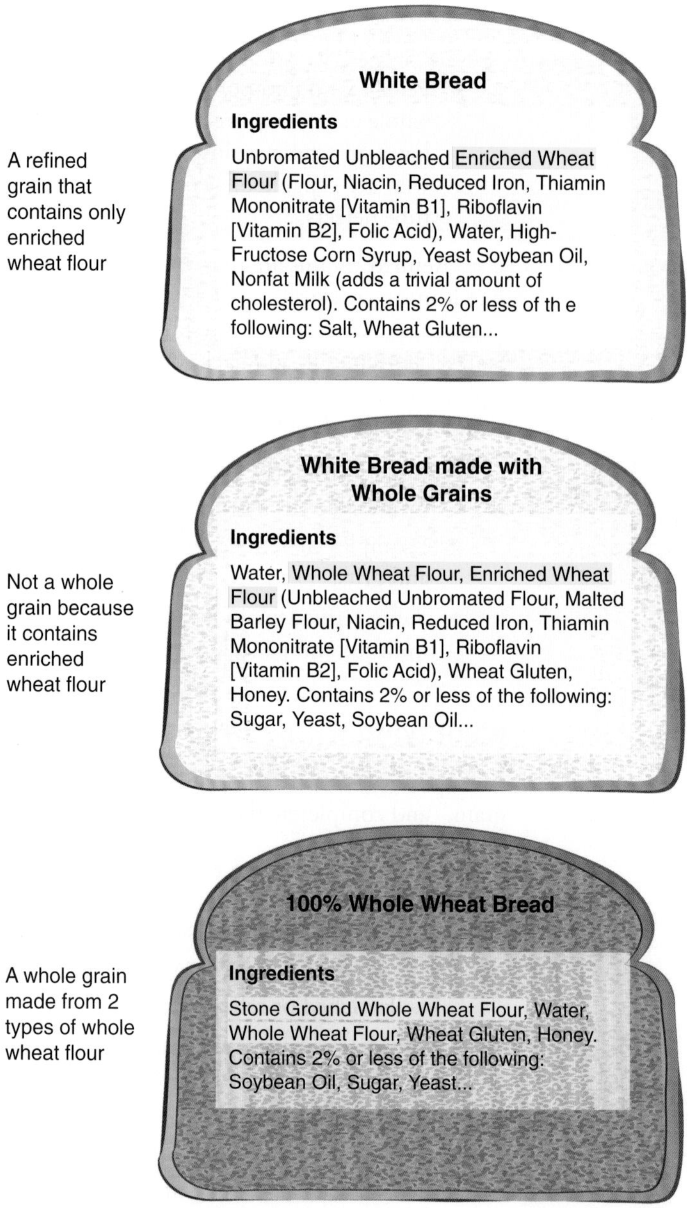

such as promoting tenderness in cakes, inhibiting the growth of mold in jams and jellies, and retaining moisture in cookies. However, added sugars are considered empty calories because they provide calories with few or no nutrients.

The *2020–2025 Dietary Guidelines for Americans* recommend added sugars be limited to <10% of total calories/day starting at age 2 (USDA & USDHHS, 2020). Foods and beverages with added sugars should be avoided for those younger than age 2. The rational for limiting added sugars is to help ensure an adequate intake of nutrients while keeping calorie intake at an appropriate level.

The average added sugar intake in the United States accounts for almost 270 calories or more than 13% of total calories per day (USDA & USDHHS, 2020). The biggest source of added sugars (24%) in the American population aged 1 and older is diet with SSB: soft drinks, fruit drinks, and sport and energy drinks (Fig. 3.6). A large body of evidence shows a strong link between SSB intake and weight gain (Malik et al., 2013) and risk of type 2 diabetes (Malik et al., 2010). SSB have also been linked to coronary heart disease (Malik & Hu, 2019). SSB are thought to promote weight gain because people do not compensate for their liquid calories by eating less at subsequent meals. Suggestions for limiting added sugar intake are in Box 3.4.

BOX 3.3 Tips for Increasing Whole Grain Intake

Substitute

- whole wheat bread or rolls for white bread or rolls
- brown rice for white rice
- whole wheat pasta or pasta that is part whole wheat, part white flour for white pasta
- whole wheat pita for white pita
- whole wheat tortillas for flour tortillas
- whole wheat English muffins for white English muffins
- whole grain for refined cereals
- whole wheat flour or oats for half of the white flour in pancakes, waffles, or muffins
- whole wheat bread or cracker crumbs for white crumbs as a coating or breading for meat, fish, and poultry
- whole corn meal for refined corn meal in corn cakes, corn bread, and corn muffins

Add

- barley, brown rice, or bulgur to soups, stews, bread stuffing, and casseroles
- handful of oats or whole grain cereal to yogurt

Snack on

- ready-to-eat whole grain cereal, such as shredded wheat or toasted oat cereal
- whole grain baked tortilla chips
- whole grain crackers
- popcorn

Decrease

- desserts and sweet snacks made with refined flour:
  - cakes, cookies, and pastries (which are also high in added sugars, solid fats, or both and a source of excess calories)

The AHA's recommendation to limit added sugar intake is even more restrictive based on a large body of evidence showing diets high in added sugars are linked to risk factors for cardiovascular disease, obesity, dyslipidemia, high blood pressure, and chronic inflammation (Johnson et al., 2009). As previously stated, a high intake of added sugars can displace nutrient-containing foods and contribute to excess calorie intake. The AHA recommends that added sugars should contribute no more than half of a person's daily discretional calorie allowance:

- For most American women, that is a maximum of 100 calories per day (25 g or 6 tsp).
- For most American men, the limit for added sugar intake is 150 calories per day (38 g or 9 tsp).

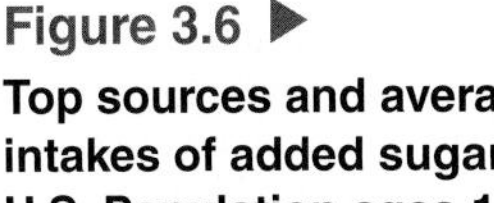

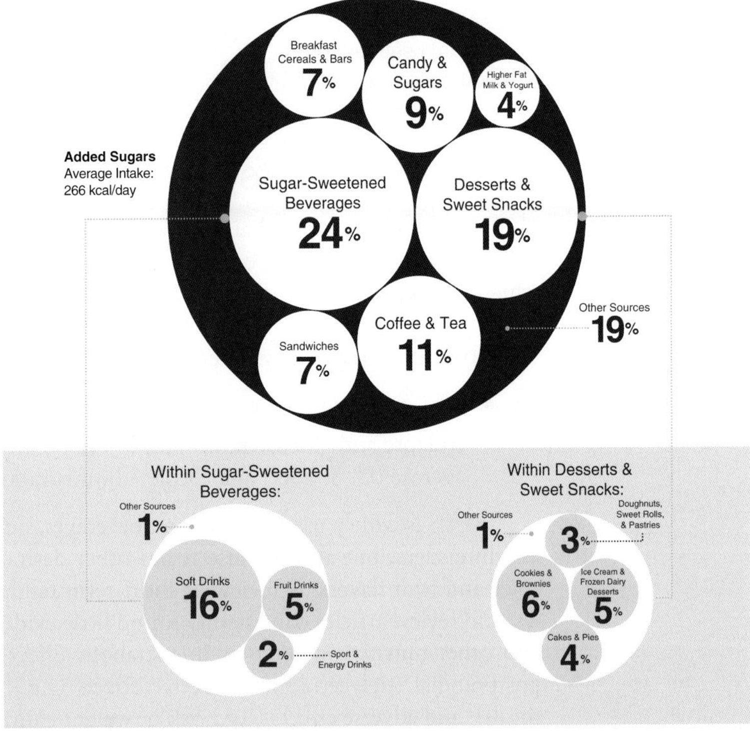

Figure 3.6 ▶
Top sources and average intakes of added sugars: U.S. Population ages 1 and older. (*Source:* U.S. Department of Agriculture & U.S. Department of Health and Human Services. (2020). *Dietary guidelines for Americans 2020–2025.* https://www.dietaryguidelines.gov/sites/default/files/2020-12/Dietary_Guidelines_for_Americans_2020-2025.pdf)

BOX 3.4 Ways to Limit Added Sugars

Cut Back On or Eliminate Sugar-Sweetened Beverages

- choose beverages with no added sugars: water or flavored water.
- consume SSB less often
- reduce portion size

Limit Sweetened Grain-based and Dairy-based Items

- smaller portions less often:
  - breakfast cereals and bars
  - sweetened yogurt
  - sweetened milks
  - candy
  - cookies
  - brownies
  - doughnuts
  - sweet rolls
  - pastries
  - cakes
  - ice cream
  - other frozen desserts
  - pudding

Rely on Natural Sugars in Fruit to Satisfy a "Sweet Tooth"

- Fruit also boosts vitamin, mineral, phytonutrient, and fiber intake

Read Labels

- "Nutrition Facts" labels (see Chapter 9) list the amount of total sugars and added sugars.
  - The Daily Value (DV) for added sugars is 50 g (10% of the calories the 2000 calorie standard used for DV). If total calories consumed are <2000, the percentage of the DV listed on the food label will underestimate the actual percent of calories from added sugar.
- Look for these sources of added sugar on the ingredient list:
  - agave sugar
  - brown sugar
  - cane juice
  - corn syrup
  - corn syrup solids
  - dextrose
  - fructose
  - glucose
  - HFCS
  - honey
  - invert sugar
  - lactose
  - maltose/malt sugar
  - maple syrup
  - molasses
  - nectars
  - raw sugar
  - sucrose
  - sugar
  - sugarcane juice
  - white granulated sugar

Consider Sugar Alternatives: Sugar Alcohols or Nonnutritive Sweeteners

- Products containing sugar alcohols (e.g., dietetic candy) are lower in calories from sugar but not necessarily lower in total calories.
  - Some sugar alcohols can cause diarrhea when eaten in large amounts.
- **Remember:** artificially sweetened low-calorie or calorie-free beverages can reduce calorie and added sugar intake, but their effectiveness as a long-term weight-loss strategy is not certain.
- The high-intensity sweeteners approved for use in the United States are safe for the general population when consumed under the intended conditions of use.

High-Fructose Corn Syrup

HFCS is an added sugar that generates a lot of controversy. It is a commercial sweetener made from enzymatically treated corn syrup. It is "high" in fructose compared to the corn syrup from which is it derived, which is essentially 100% glucose. HFCS is composed of glucose and either 42% or 55% fructose, making it similar in composition to sucrose, which is 50% glucose and 50% fructose. The primary differences between sucrose and the common forms of HFCS are that

- HFCS contains water;
- fructose and glucose molecules in HFCS are not joined by a chemical bond as they are in sucrose (U. S. Food and Drug Administration, 2018).

HFCS is widely used in food and beverages, not only because it provides the same sweetness as white sugar, but also because it has other desirable functional properties, such as enhancing spice and fruit flavors. A review of short-term randomized controlled trials, cross-sectional studies, and review articles consistently found little evidence that HFCS differs uniquely from sucrose and other nutritive sweeteners in metabolic effects (e.g., levels of circulating glucose, insulin, postprandial triglycerides), subjective effects (e.g., hunger, satiety, calorie intake at subsequent meals), and adverse effects (e.g., risk of weight gain) (Fitch & Keim, 2012).

Table 3.5 Polyols

Polyol	Relative Sweetness (Sucrose = 100)	Calories per Gram	Sources/Uses
Sorbitol	50%–70%	2.6	• made from corn syrup or glucose • used in sugar-free candies and chewing gums and sugar-free foods such as frozen desserts and baked goods
Mannitol	50%–70%	1.6	• extracted from seaweed or made from mannose • used as dusting powder on chewing gum, in chocolate-flavored coatings for ice cream and candy
Xylitol	100	2.4	• produced from birch bark and corn cob • used in chewing gum, hard candies, and foods for special dietary purposes
Maltitol	90	2.1	• made from maltose in corn syrup • used in sugarless hard candies, chewing gum, baked goods, ice cream
Lactitol	30%–40%	1.9	• derived from lactose • used in low-calorie, low-fat, and/or low-sugar foods such as ice cream, chocolate candy, baked goods, chewing gum
Isomalt	45%–65%	2.0	• made from sucrose • used in hard candies, toffee, chewing gum, baked goods, nutritional supplements
Hydrogenated starch hydrolysates	25%–50%	≤3.0	• produced from partial breakdown of corn, wheat, or potato starch • bulk sweetener in low-calorie foods: provides sweetness, texture, and bulk to a variety of sugarless items
Erythritol	60%–80%	0–0.2	• derived from glucose in corn or wheat starch • used as a bulk sweetener in reduced-calorie foods

Source: Grembecka, M. (2015). Sugar alcohols—their role in the modern world of sweeteners: A review. *European Food Research and Technology, 241*, 1. https://doi.org/10.1007/s00217-015-2437-7; Fitch, C., & Keim, K. S. (2012). Position of the Academy of Nutrition and Dietetics: Use of nutritive and non-nutritive sweeteners. *Journal of the Academy of Nutrition and Dietetics, 112*, 739–758.

Sugar Alternatives

One way to reduce sugar intake and not forsake sweetened foods is to consume sugar alternatives, such as **polyols** and **nonnutritive sweeteners (NNS)**, in place of regular sugar.

Polyols
sugar alcohols produced from the fermentation or hydrogenation of monosaccharides or disaccharides. Most originate from sucrose or glucose and maltose in starches.

Nonnutritive Sweeteners (NNS)
synthetically made sweeteners that provide minimal or no carbohydrate and calories. They are also known as artificial sweeteners.

Polyols

Polyols, or sugar alcohols, are used as sweeteners but are not true sugars or alcohols. They are derived from hydrogenated sugars and starches (Table 3.5).

- Although polyols occur naturally in some fruit, vegetables, and fermented foods (e.g., wine and soy sauce), the majority of polyols in the food supply are commercially synthesized.
- With the exception of xylitol, polyols are all less sweet than sucrose, so they are often combined with NNS in sugarless foods.
- Sugar alcohols are approved for use in a variety of products: candies, chewing gum, jams and jellies, baked goods, and frozen confections.
- Polyols are not sold as an ingredient for use at home.
- Foods containing polyols and no added sugars can be labeled as sugar-free.

Polyols offer some advantages to sugar.

- They are not fermented by mouth bacteria, and thus do not cause dental caries.
  - Since polyols are non-cariogenic, they are often used in items held in the mouth, such as chewing gum and breath mints.
- They are considered low-calorie sweeteners because they are incompletely absorbed.
  - Their calorie value generally ranges from 1.6 to 3.0 cal/g.
- They are generally slowly and incompletely absorbed and/or metabolized differently than true sugars, so they produce a smaller effect on blood glucose levels and insulin response, making them attractive to people with diabetes.

- Polyols that are not fully absorbed in the small intestine enter the large intestine where they function as a prebiotic.
    - They are fermented into short-chain fatty acids, which foster the growth of colonic bacteria.

The disadvantage of polyols is that, because they are incompletely digested and absorbed, they can lead to GI side effects such as diarrhea, abdominal pain, and gas. Therefore, it is recommended that sorbitol intake not exceed 50 g/day, and mannitol intake be limited to 20 g/day. Likewise, only limited amounts of xylitol are allowed in foods marketed for special diets (Brown, 2019). There is little research on the benefits of sugar alcohols for people with diabetes (Evert et al., 2019).

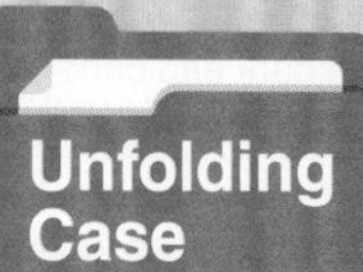

Consider Krista. She wondered if eating several pieces of dietetic chocolate candy sweetened with sugar alcohols every day would help prevent constipation. She was shocked to discover that five pieces of sugarless dark chocolate contains almost 200 calories, mostly from fat, and quickly ruled out candy as an option. She asks if she can chew several pieces of gum containing xylitol every day to improve laxation without consuming calories. How do you respond?

Nonnutritive Sweeteners

NNS are also known as intense sweeteners, artificial sweeteners, or sugar substitutes. They are hundreds to thousands of times sweeter than sugar and are virtually calorie-free because so little is needed. Sometimes combinations of NNS are used in a food to produce a synergistically sweeter taste, decrease the amount of sweetener needed, and minimize aftertaste. They have different functional properties, which influences how they are used in foods. Questions about their safety and efficacy are common.

Acceptable Daily Intake (ADI)
the estimated amount of a food additive that a person can safely consume every day over a lifetime without risk.

- NNS approved by the U.S. Food and Drug Administration (FDA) for use in the United States are featured in Table 3.6. When consumed at levels within the **Acceptable Daily Intake (ADI)**, all FDA-approved NNS are safe for use by the general public, including pregnant and lactating women.
    - Although it is difficult to determine the intake of food additives, including NNS, the FDA has determined that estimated daily intake would not exceed ADI limits even among high users (U.S. Food and Drug Administration, 2014).
- Evidence suggests that used judiciously, NNS *could* promote a decrease in added sugar intake and a decrease in calorie intake and potential loss of weight (Gardner et al., 2012).
    - These potential benefits can only be realized if there is not a compensatory increase in calories from other sources.
        - For instance, it has been proposed that NNS may lower awareness of calorie intake. Further research is needed.
- NNS appeal to people with diabetes because they do not raise blood glucose levels.
    - Again, there is not enough evidence to determine if sugar substitute use definitely leads to long-term decrease in body weight or cardiometabolic risk factors, including improved glycemic control (Evert et al., 2019).
    - Nutrition therapy for people with diabetes stresses replacing SSB with water as much as possible, and if NNS are used to lower calorie and carbohydrate intake, counseling should include how to avoid compensating by eating calories from other sources (Evert et al., 2019).

Dental Caries

Limiting added sugars is also one of the strategies to help reduce the risk of dental caries. Sugars—whether added or natural—and starches that stay on the teeth provide substrates oral bacteria feed on. This creates an acid that erodes tooth enamel. Although whole-grain crackers and orange juice are more nutritious than caramels and soft drinks, their potential damage to teeth is similar. The frequency of carbohydrate intake, the amount consumed, and the duration of time between eating and brushing teeth may be more important than whether or not they are "sticky sugars."

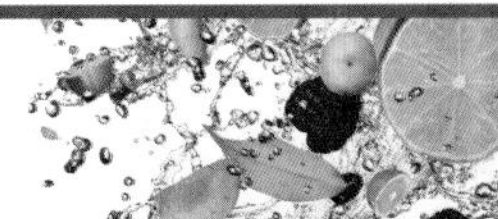

Table 3.6 Nonnutritive Sweeteners Approved for Use in the United States by the Food and Drug Administration

Sweetener	Times Sweeter than Sucrose	Taste Characteristics	Uses	Comments/ADI
Acesulfame Potassium (Sunette, Sweet One)	200	Bitter aftertaste like saccharin	Approved as a sweetener and flavor enhancer in foods (except in meat and poultry) • tabletop sweetener • dry beverage mixes • chewing gum	• Often mixed with other sweeteners to synergize the sweetness and minimize the aftertaste • Not digested; excreted unchanged in the urine • ADI: 15 mg/kg BW/day
Advantame	20,000	Clean, sugar-like taste	Approved as general sweetener and flavor enhancer (except in meat and poultry) under certain conditions of use: • baked goods • soft drinks • frozen desserts • chewing gum	• Chemically similar to aspartame • does not have to contain a warning about phenylalanine for people with PKU because only small amounts are needed due to its intense sweetness. • ADI: 32.8 mg/kg BW/day
Aspartame (NutraSweet, Equal, Sugar Twin)	200	Similar to sucrose; no aftertaste	Approved as a sweetener and flavor enhancer in foods • tabletop sweeteners • dry beverage mixes • chewing gum • beverages • confections • fruit spreads • toppings • fillings	• made from amino acids: aspartic acid and phenylalanine • people with PKU must avoid aspartame • degrades during heating so typically not used in baked goods • ADI: 50 mg/kg BW/day
Siraitia grosvenorri Swingle (Luo Han Guo) fruit extracts (SGFE) (Nectresse, Monk Fruit in the Raw, PureLo) (PureFruit)	100–250	Aftertaste at high levels	SGFE containing 25%, 45%, or 55% Mogroside V are approved as GRAS, so it is not officially considered a food additive and is exempt from legal requirement to prove safety Intended as • tabletop sweetener • food ingredient • a component of other sweetener blends	• ADI: not specified
Neotame (Newtame)	7000–13,000	Clean, sugar-like taste; enhances flavors of other ingredients	Approved as a sweetener and flavor enhancer in foods	• Like aspartame, neotame is made from aspartic acid and phenylalanine but it resists breakdown to these amino acids so a warning label is not required. • is heat stable, making it suitable for baked goods • has the potential to replace both sugar and HFCS • ADI: 0.3 mg/kg BW/day
Saccharin (Sweet Twin, Sweet'N Low)	200–700	Persistent aftertaste; bitter at high concentrations	Approved as a sweetener only in certain special dietary foods and as an additive used for certain technological purposes • soft drinks • assorted foods • tabletop sweetener	• potential (weak) carcinogen: the FDA has officially withdrawn its proposed ban, so a warning label is no longer required • ADI: 15 mg/kg BW/day
Stevia (glycosides purified from the leaves of *Stevia rebaudiana* (Truvia, PureVia, Enliten)	200–400	Sweet clean taste in usual amounts; some types may have bitter aftertaste	Refined stevia products are GRAS; whole leaf or crude extracts are not approved because of concerns about health effects Intended for use in • cereal • energy bars • beverages • tabletop sweetener	• ADI: 4 mg/kg BW

Table 3.6 Nonnutritive Sweeteners Approved for Use in the United States by the Food and Drug Administration (continued)

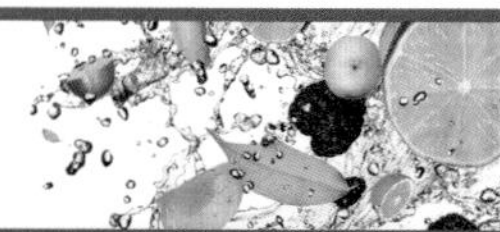

Sweetener	Times Sweeter than Sucrose	Taste Characteristics	Uses	Comments/ADI
Sucralose (Splenda)	600	Maintains flavor even at high temperatures	Approved as a sweetener in foods • soft drinks • baked goods • chewing gums • tabletop sweetener	• poorly absorbed; excreted unchanged in the feces • ADI: 5 mg/kg BW

Note. ADI = acceptable daily intake; BW = body weight; FDA = U.S. Food and Drug Administration; GRAS = generally recognized as safe; HFCS = high-fructose corn syrup; PKU = phenylketonuria.

Source: Brown, A. (2019). *Understanding food principles and preparation*. Cengage Learning; U. S. Food and Drug Administration. (2018, February 8). *Additional information about high-intensity sweeteners permitted for use in food in the United States*. https://www.fda.gov/food/food-additives-petitions/additional-information-about-high-intensity-sweeteners-permitted-use-food-united-states.

Anti-cavity strategies are

- eat a well-balanced diet—oral health is dependent on good nutrition;
- limit added sugars, especially SSB;
- limit in-between meal snacking, especially items that can remain on the surface of the teeth (e.g., candy, pretzels, and chips);
- avoid high-sugar items that stay in the mouth for a long time: hard candy, suckers, and cough drops;
- brush promptly after eating;
- chew gum sweetened with sugar alcohols (e.g., sorbitol, mannitol, and xylitol) or with NNS after eating. This may reduce the risk of cavities by stimulating production of saliva, which helps to rinse the teeth and neutralize plaque acids. Unlike sucrose and other nutritive sweeteners, sugar alcohols and NNS are not fermented by bacteria in the mouth, so they do not promote cavities
- use fluoridated toothpaste.

How Do You Respond?

Aren't carbohydrates fattening? At 4 cal/g, carbohydrates are no more fattening than protein and are less than half as fattening as fat at 9 cal/g. Whether or not a food is "fattening" has more to do with frequency of intake and total calories provided than whether the calories are in the form of carbohydrates, protein, or fat.

Is "white" whole wheat bread as nutritious as whole wheat? Whole "white" wheat flour is made from albino wheat that is white in color, not the characteristic brown color of whole wheat. It is a whole grain, so it is nutritionally comparable to whole wheat. Many people prefer not only its lighter color but also its milder flavor.

"Light" or "diet" breads are high in fiber. Can I use them in place of whole grain breads? "Light breads" usually have processed fiber from peas or other foods substituted for some starch. The result is a lower-calorie, higher-fiber bread that may help to prevent constipation but lacks the unique "package" of vitamins, minerals, and phytonutrients found in whole grains.

REVIEW CASE STUDY

Amanda is convinced that white flour and white sugar cause her to overeat, resulting in an extra 30 pounds of weight she is carrying around. To control her impulse to overeat, she has decided to eliminate all foods made with white flour and white sugar from her diet. Her total calorie needs are estimated to be 2000 per day. Yesterday, she ate the foods listed in the box. She asks if you think this is a healthy eating plan.

- What foods did she eat yesterday that contained carbohydrates? Estimate how many grams of carbohydrate she ate.
  - How does her intake compare with the amount of total carbohydrate recommended for someone needing 2000 cal/day?
  - Are all of the sources of carbohydrate she chose the "healthiest" in their food group?
    - What items is she consuming that contain added sugar?
- What sources of fiber did she consume? Estimate how many grams of fiber she ate.
  - How does her fiber intake compare with the AI amount recommended for women?
  - What would you tell her about her fiber intake?
- What would you tell her about her idea to forsake white flour and white sugar to manage her weight?
- What are the benefits and potential problems with her proposed diet?
- What suggestions would you make about her intake?

Breakfast: 2 scrambled eggs and 2 sausage links; 1 cup orange juice; tea with agave nectar
Snack: 2 oz of honey-roasted peanuts and a diet soft drink
Lunch: tossed salad with 1 hard cooked egg, 3 oz of sliced turkey, 2 oz of sliced cheese, 3 tbsp of honey mustard dressing; 1 can diet soft drink; 1 cup of diet gelatin
Snack: 2 oz of cheese curds and a diet soft drink
Dinner: 6 oz of fried chicken; 1 cup of white rice; ½ cup corn; ½ cup diet pudding with whipped cream; 1 can diet soft drink
Snack: 5 chicken wings with ¼ cup bleu cheese dressing

STUDY QUESTIONS

1 The nurse knows their explanation of glycemic index was effective when the client says?
   a. "Choosing foods that have a low GI is an effective way to eat healthier."
   b. "Low-GI foods promote weight loss because they do not stimulate the release of insulin."
   c. "GI could help me choose the best foods to eat before, during, and after training."
   d. "GI is a term used to describe the amount of refined sugar in a food."

2 Which of the following recommendations would be most effective for someone wanting to eat more fiber?
   a. Eat legumes more regularly.
   b. Eat raw vegetables in place of cooked vegetables.
   c. Use potatoes in place of white rice.
   d. Eat fruit for dessert in place of ice cream.

3 A client asks why sugar should be limited in the diet. What is the best response?
   a. "A high-sugar intake causes dental caries if you don't brush your teeth shortly after eating."
   b. "Sugar provides more calories per gram than starch, protein, or fat."
   c. "There is a direct correlation between sugar intake and increased hunger."
   d. "Foods high in sugar generally provide few nutrients other than calories and may make it hard to consume a diet that has enough of all the essential nutrients."

4 Compared to refined grains, whole grains have more
   a. Folic acid
   b. Vitamin A
   c. Vitamin C
   d. Phytonutrients

5 The nurse knows their instructions about choosing whole grains in place of refined grains are understood by the client when they verbalize that they will substitute
   a. Rice Krispies for puffed rice
   b. Bulgur for barley
   c. Shredded wheat cereal for puffed wheat cereal
   d. Quick oats for old-fashioned oats

6 Which might a client who has eaten too many dietetic candies sweetened with sorbitol experience?
   a. Diarrhea
   b. Heartburn
   c. Vomiting
   d. Low blood glucose

7 The client wants to eat fewer calories and lose weight by substituting regularly sweetened foods with those that are sweetened with sugar alternatives. Which would be the most effective at lowering calorie intake?
   a. Sugar-free cookies for regular cookies
   b. Sugar-free for regular chocolate candy
   c. Sugar-free soft drinks for regular soft drinks
   d. Sugar-free ice cream for regular ice cream

8 A client is on a low-calorie diet that recommends they test their urine for ketones to tell how well they are adhering to the guidelines of the diet. What does the presence of ketones signify about their intake?
   a. It is too low in carbohydrates.
   b. It is too high in fat.
   c. It is too high in carbohydrates.
   d. It is too high in protein.

CHAPTER SUMMARY CARBOHYDRATES

Carbohydrates are almost exclusively found in plants and provide the major source of energy in almost all human diets.

Carbohydrate Classifications

Monosaccharides are composed of one sugar molecule.

- Glucose (or dextrose) is a component of almost all carbohydrates, and is the sugar found in blood.
- Fructose, the sweetest of all natural sugars, is found in fruit, honey, and HFCS.

Disaccharides are composed of one glucose molecule and one other monosaccharide.

- Sucrose comes in many forms: table sugar, white sugar, brown sugar, granulated sugar, powdered sugar, raw sugar, and turbinado sugar.
- Lactose is the only animal source of carbohydrate. It is found in dairy products, and is the least sweet sugar.
- Maltose is an intermediate in starch digestion. It occurs in malted food products and is used to color beer.

Polysaccharides are made up of many glucose molecules. They do not taste sweet.

- Starch provides the majority of calories in grains. It is found in the endosperm portion of whole and refined grains.
- Fiber, the non-digestible part of plants, is commonly classified as either water soluble (or viscous and fermentable) or water insoluble (not viscous and not fermentable).

Sources of Carbohydrates

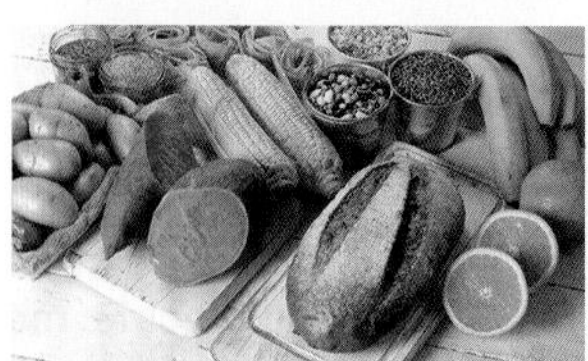

Natural sugars and starches are found in fruit, vegetables, grains, dairy, and legumes.

Added sugars are found in snacks and sweets, cereals, and sweetened yogurt. SSB are the biggest source of added sugars in the American diet.

How the Body Handles Carbohydrates

Digestion: The majority of carbohydrate digestion occurs in the small intestine. Disaccharides and starches are digested into monosaccharides. Fiber is not digested, but some types can be fermented by gut microbiota in the large intestine into water, gas, and short-chain fatty acids.

Absorption: Monosaccharides are absorbed through intestinal mucosal cells and transported to the liver through the portal vein.

Metabolism: In the liver, fructose and galactose are converted to glucose. The liver releases glucose into the bloodstream.

Glycemic response: The glycemic response is the effect a food has on the blood glucose concentration—how quickly the glucose level rises, how high it goes, and how long it takes to return to normal. It is hard to predict in practice.

Functions of Carbohydrates

- provide energy
- spare protein
- prevent ketosis
- produce specific body compounds: nonessential amino acids
- converts and stores remaining glucose as fat

Dietary Reference Intakes

The typical American diet provides an appropriate percentage of calories from carbohydrates but is too high in added sugars and low in fiber.

- Carbohydrates should provide 45% to 65% of total calories.
- Added sugars should contribute ≤10% of total calories.
- Women should consume approximately 25 g fiber per day and men about 38 g.

Carbohydrates in Health Promotion.

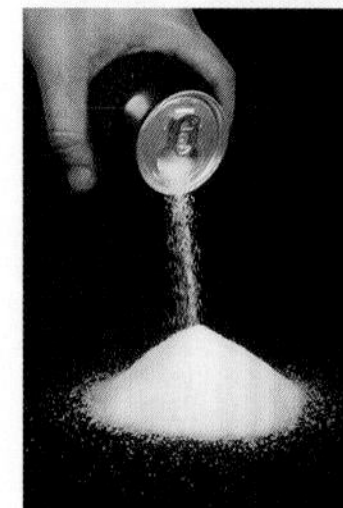

Americans are urged to make healthier carbohydrate choices:

- half or more of grain choices should be whole grain
- limit added sugars to <10% of calories/day starting at age 2. Added sugars in food and beverages should be avoided by those younger than age 2.

Sugar Alternatives

Polyols (sugar alcohols):

- provide fewer calories than sugar because they are incompletely digested and absorbed
- large amounts can cause osmotic diarrhea and cramping
- are not fermentable by mouth bacteria, so they do not contribute to tooth decay

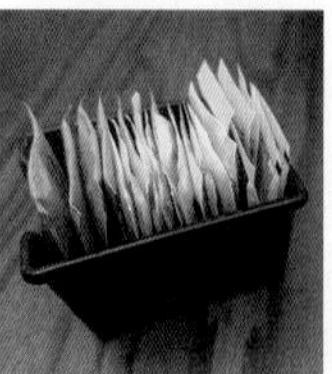

NNS (intense sweeteners, artificial sweeteners, or sugar substitutes):

- provide negligible or no calories
- are hundreds to thousands of times sweeter than sugar
- use is approved and regulated by the FDA
- it is unknown if their use helps people to reduce their calorie intake and better manage weight

Consuming a healthy diet that is limited in added sugars and in snacks that contain fermentable carbohydrates may help reduce the risk of dental caries.

Figure sources: *shutterstock.com/Tatjana Baibakova, shutterstock.com/Evan Lorne, and shutterstock.com/Mirror-Images*

Student Resources on thePoint®
For additional learning materials, activate the code in the front of this book at https://thePoint.lww.com/activate

Website

Learn about grains at https://wholegrainscouncil.org/

References

Academy of Nutrition and Dietetics & American Diabetes Association. (2019). *Choose your foods: Food lists for weight management.* American Diabetes Association & Academy of Nutrition and Dietetics.

Arnett, D. K., Blumenthal, R. S., Albert, M. A., Buroker A. B., Goldberger, Z. D., Hahn, E. J., Himmelfarb, C. D., Khera, A., Lloyd-Jones, D., McEvoy, J. W., Michos, E. D., Miedema, M. D., Muñoz, D., Smith, S. C. Jr., Virani, S. S., Williams, K. A. Sr., Yeboah, J., & Ziaeian, B. (2019). 2019 ACC/AHA guideline on the primary prevention of cardiovascular disease: A report of the American College of Cardiology/American Heart Association Task Force on Clinical Practice Guidelines. *Circulation, 140*, e596–e646. https://doi.org/10.1161/CIR.0000000000000678

Dahl, W., & Stewart, M. (2015). Position of the Academy of Nutrition and Dietetics: Health implications of dietary fiber. *Journal of the Academy of Nutrition and Dietetics, 115*(11), 1861–1870. https://doi: 10.1016/j.jand.2015.09.00

Evert, A., Dennison, M., Gardner, C., Garvey, W., Lau, K., MacLeod, J., Mitri, J., Pereira, R., Rawlings, K., Robinsion, S., Saslow, L., Uelmen, S., Urbanski, P., & Yancy, W. (2019). Nutrition therapy for adults with diabetes or prediabetes: A consensus report. *Diabetes Care, 42*(5), 731–754. https://doi.org/10.2337/dci19-0014

Fitch, C., & Keim, K. (2012). Position of the Academy of Nutrition and Dietetics: Use of nutritive and nonnutritive sweeteners. *Journal of the Academy of Nutrition and Dietetics, 112*(5), 739–758. https://doi.org/10.1016/j.jand.2012.03.009

Gardner, C., Wylie-Rosett, J., Gidding, S. S., Steffen, L. M., Johnson, R. K., Reader, D., Lichtenstein, A. H., American Heart Association Nutrition Committee of the Council on Nutrition, Physical Activity and Metabolism, Council on Arteriosclerosis, Thrombosis and Vascular Biology, Council on Cardiovascular Disease in the Young, & American Diabetes Association. (2012). Nonnutritive sweeteners: Current use and health perspectives—A scientific statement from the American Heart Association and the American Diabetes Association. *Diabetes Care, 35*(8), 1798–1808. https://doi.org/10.2337/dc12-9002

Institute of Medicine. (2001). *Dietary reference intakes: Proposed definition of dietary fiber.* The National Academies Press.

Institute of Medicine. (2005). *Dietary reference intakes for energy, carbohydrates, fiber, fat, fatty acids, cholesterol, protein, and amino acids (macronutrients).* The National Academies Press.

International Food Information Council Foundation. (2019). *Fiber.* https://foodinsight.org/wp-content/uploads/2019/07/IFIC-Foundation-Fiber-Fact-Sheet-for-HPs.pdf

Johnson, R., Appel, L., Brands, M., Brands, M., Howard, B., Lefevre, M., Lustig, R., Sacks, F., Steffen, L., Wylie-Rosett, J., & on behalf of the American Heart Association Committee of the Council on Nutrition, Physical Activity, and Metabolism and the Council on Epidemiology and Prevention. (2009). Dietary sugars intake and cardiovascular health: A scientific statement from the American Heart Association. *Circulation, 120*(11), 1011–1020. https://doi.org/10.1161/CIRCULATIONAHA.109.192627

Kim, Y., & Je, Y. (2016). Dietary fibre intake and mortality from cardiovascular disease and all cancers: A meta-analysis of prospective cohort studies. *Archives Cardiovascular Disease, 109*(1), 39–54. https://doi.org/10.1016/j.acvd.2015.09.005

Makki, K., Deehan, E., Walter, J., & Backhed, F. (2018). The impact of dietary fiber on gut microbiota in host health and disease. *Cell Host & Microbe, 23*(6), 705–715. https://doi.org/10.1016/j.chom.2018.05.012

Malik, V., & Hu, B. (2019). Sugar-sweetened beverages and cardiometabolic health: An update of the evidence. *Nutrients, 11*(8), 1840. https://doi.org/10.3390/nu11081840

Malik, V., Pan, A., Willett, W., & Hu, F. (2013). Sugar-sweetened beverages and weight gain in children and adults: A systematic review and meta-analysis. *American Journal of Clinical Nutrition, 98*(4), 1084–1102. https://doi.org/10.3945/ajcn.113.058362

Malik, V., Popkin, B., Bray, G., Despres, J.-P., Willett, W., & Hu, F. (2010). Sugar-sweetened beverages and risk of metabolic syndrome and type 2 diabetes: A meta-analysis. *Diabetes Care, 33*(11), 2477–2483. https://doi.org/10.2337/dc10-1079

Reynolds, A., Mann, J., Cummings, J., MDiet, N., MDiet, E., & Morenga, L. (2019). Carbohydrate quality and human health: A series of systematic reviews and meta-analyses. *Lancet, 393*(10170), 434–445. https://doi.org/10.1016/S0140-6736(18)31809-9

U.S. Department of Agriculture & U.S. Department of Health and Human Services. (2020). *Dietary guidelines for Americans 2020–2025.* https://www.dietaryguidelines.gov/sites/default/files/2020-12/Dietary_Guidelines_for_Americans_2020-2025.pdf

U. S. Food and Drug Administration. (2014). *High-intensity sweeteners.* https://www.fda.gov/food/food-additives-petitions/high-intensity-sweeteners

U. S. Food and Drug Administration. (2018). *High fructose corn syrup questions and answers.* https://www.fda.gov/food/food-additives-petitions/high-fructose-corn-syrup-questions-and-answers

Chapter 4 Protein

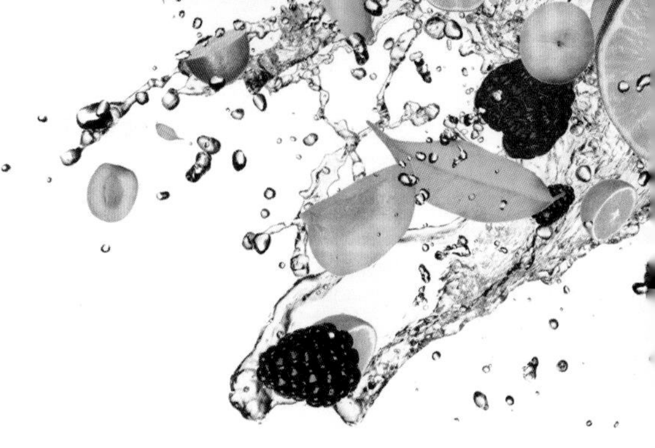

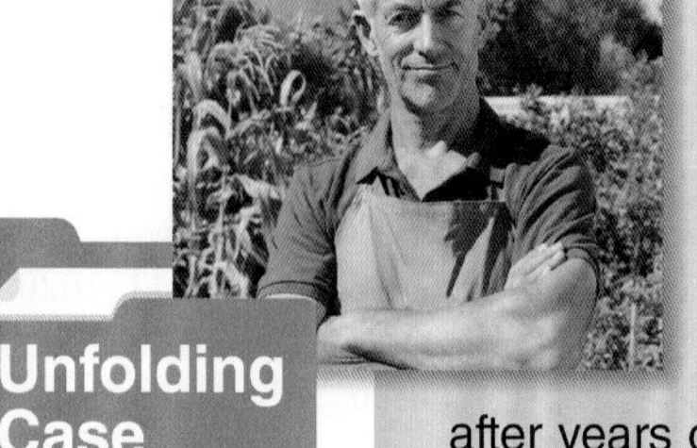

Unfolding Case

Robert Santos

Three years ago, Robert, a 50-year-old farmer, learned he has alpha-gal allergy. This allergy originates from a lone star tick bite that, in turn, causes a delayed anaphylactic reaction after eating meat. Robert must avoid beef, pork, lamb, rabbit, venison, and buffalo meats. Prior to the tick bite, his usual weight was 185 pounds (84 kg), which was within the healthy range for his height. However, after years of restricting the variety of protein foods he eats, Robert is now underweight and continues to lose weight. He does not like seafood and is tired of eating poultry.

Learning Objectives

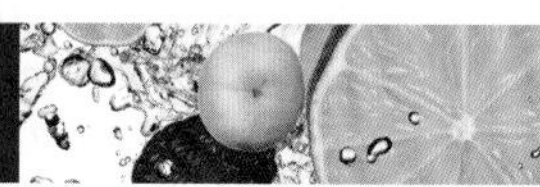

Upon completion of this chapter, you will be able to:

1 Explain the difference between essential and nonessential amino acids.
2 Discuss the functions of protein.
3 Give examples of conditions where people are in a positive nitrogen balance.
4 Name sources of complete and incomplete protein.
5 Calculate an individual's protein requirement.
6 Discuss how Americans should shift their protein food choices to improve their eating pattern.
7 Give examples of conditions that increase a person's protein requirement.
8 Name sources of lean protein foods.
9 Name sources of the nutrients that are most likely to be deficient in a vegetarian diet.
10 Describe nitrogen balance and how it is determined.

In Greek, *protein* means "to take first place," and truly life could not exist without protein. Protein is a component of every living cell: plant, animal, and microorganism. In adults, protein accounts for 20% of total weight. Dietary protein seems relatively immune to the controversy over optimal intake that surrounds both carbohydrates and fat.

This chapter discusses the composition of protein, its functions, and how it is handled in the body. Sources, Dietary Reference Intakes, and the role of protein in health promotion are presented.

PROTEIN COMPOSITION AND STRUCTURE

Proteins are composed of chains of amino acids that can be from several dozen to several hundred amino acids in length. Just as the 26 letters of the alphabet can be used to form an infinite number of words, so can amino acids be joined in different amounts, proportions, and sequences to form a great variety of proteins.

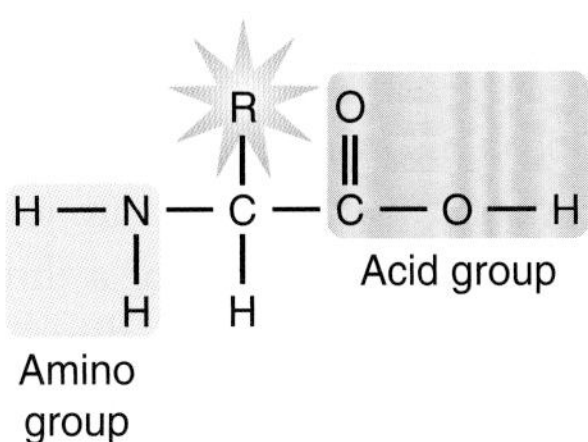

Figure 4.1 ▶ **Generic amino acid structure.**

Amino Acids

All amino acids have a carbon atom core with four bonding sites:

- one hydrogen atom
- one amino group (NH_2)
- one acid group (COOH) (see Fig. 4.1)
- one side group (R group)
  - contains atoms that give each amino acid its own distinct identity
  - some side groups contain
    - sulfur
    - some are acidic
    - some are basic
  - differences in side groups account for differences in amino acids:
    - size
    - shape
    - electrical charge

There are 20 common amino acids that make up proteins.

- Nine amino acids are classified as essential or indispensable.
  - They cannot be made by the body and so must be supplied through the diet (Box 4.1).
- Eleven amino acids are classified as nonessential or dispensable.
  - They can be made by cells, as needed, through the process of transamination.
- Some dispensable amino acids may become indispensable when metabolic need is great and endogenous synthesis is not adequate.
- Note that the terms *essential* and *nonessential* refer to whether the amino acid must be supplied by the diet, not to their relative importance: All 20 amino acids must be available for the body to make proteins.

BOX 4.1 Amino Acids

Essential (Indispensable)	Nonessential (Dispensable)	Conditionally[a] Essential (Indispensable)
Histidine	Alanine	Arginine
Isoleucine	Asparagine	Cysteine
Leucine	Aspartic acid	Glutamine
Lysine	Glutamic acid	Glycine
Methionine	Serine	Proline
Phenylalanine		Tyrosine
Threonine		
Tryptophan		
Valine		

[a]Under most normal conditions, the body can synthesize adequate amounts of these amino acids. A dietary source is necessary only when metabolic demands exceed endogenous synthesis.

Protein Structure

A protein's primary structure is determined by the types and amounts of amino acids and the unique sequence in which they are joined. Proteins also vary in shape. They may be straight, folded, coiled along one dimension, or a three-dimensional shape resembling a sphere. Larger proteins are created when two or more three-dimensional polypeptides combine. A protein's shape determines its function.

FUNCTIONS OF PROTEIN

Protein is the major structural and functional component of every living cell. Every tissue and fluid in the body contains some protein, except for bile and urine. In fact, the body may contain as many as 10,000 to 50,000 different proteins that vary in size, shape, and function.

Like carbohydrates, protein provides 4 cal/g. Protein is not the body's preferred fuel but is a source of energy when consumed in excess or when calorie intake from carbohydrates and fat is inadequate. Using protein for energy is a physiologic waste because amino acids used for energy are not available to be used for protein's specific functions (Box 4.2).

Intracellular within cells.

Interstitial between cells.

Edema the swelling of body tissues secondary to the accumulation of excessive fluid.

Denatured an irreversible process in which the structure of a protein is disrupted, leading to partial or complete loss of function.

Globular spherical.

Intravascular within blood vessels.

BOX 4.2 Functions of Protein

Body structure and framework

- >40% of protein in the body is found in each skeletal muscle and approximately 15% is found in the skin and the blood.
- Proteins also form tendons, membranes, organs, and bones.

Enzymes

- Enzymes are proteins that facilitate specific chemical reactions in the body without undergoing change themselves.
- Some enzymes (e.g., digestive enzymes) break down larger molecules into smaller ones.
- Other enzymes (e.g., enzymes involved in protein synthesis) combine molecules to form larger compounds.

Body secretions and fluids that are made from amino acids include

- Neurotransmitters such as serotonin and acetylcholine
- Antibodies
- Peptide hormones such as insulin, thyroxine, and epinephrine
- Breast milk
- Mucus
- Sperm
- Histamine

Fluid balance

- Proteins help to regulate fluid balance because they attract water, which creates osmotic pressure.
- Circulating proteins, such as albumin, maintain the proper balance of fluid among the **intravascular**, **intracellular**, and **interstitial** compartments of the body. A symptom of a low albumin level is **edema**.

Acid–base balance

- Because amino acids contain both an acid (COOH) and a base (NH_2), they can act as either acids or bases, depending on the pH of the surrounding fluid.
- The ability to buffer or neutralize excess acids and bases enables proteins to maintain normal blood pH, which protects body proteins from being **denatured**.

Transport molecules

- **Globular** proteins transport other substances through the blood. For instance, lipoproteins transport fats, cholesterol, and fat-soluble vitamins; hemoglobin transports oxygen; and albumin transports free fatty acids and many drugs.

Other compounds that contain amino acids

- Opsin, the light-sensitive visual pigment in the eye
- Thrombin, a protein necessary for normal blood clotting

Some amino acids have specific functions within the body

- Tryptophan is a precursor of the vitamin niacin, and is also a component of serotonin.
- Tyrosine is the precursor of melanin, the pigment that colors hair and skin, and is incorporated into the thyroid hormone.

HOW THE BODY HANDLES PROTEIN

Digestion and Absorption

Protein Digestibility
how well a protein is digested to make amino acids available for protein synthesis.

Protein digestibility varies among protein sources:

- 90% to 99% for animal proteins
- over 90% for soy and legumes
- 70% to 90% for other plant proteins

Chemical digestion of protein begins in the stomach. Hydrochloric acid denatures protein to make the peptide bonds more susceptible to the actions of enzymes (Fig. 4.2). Hydrochloric acid also converts pepsinogen to the active enzyme pepsin, which begins the process of breaking down proteins into smaller polypeptides and some amino acids.

The majority of protein digestion occurs in the small intestine.

- Pancreatic proteases reduce polypeptides to
  - shorter chains,
  - tripeptides,
  - dipeptides, and
  - amino acids.
- Enzymes trypsin and chymotrypsin break peptide bonds between specific amino acids.
- Carboxypeptidase breaks off amino acids from the acid end (carboxyl) of polypeptides and dipeptides.
- Enzymes located on the surface of the cells that line the small intestine complete the process of digestion:
  - Aminopeptidase splits amino acids from the amino ends of short peptides.
  - Dipeptidase reduces dipeptides to amino acids.

Amino acids, and sometimes a few dipeptides or larger peptides, are absorbed through the mucosa of the small intestine by active transport with the aid of vitamin B_6. Intestinal cells release amino acids into the bloodstream for transport to the liver via the portal vein.

Figure 4.2 ▶
Protein digestion.

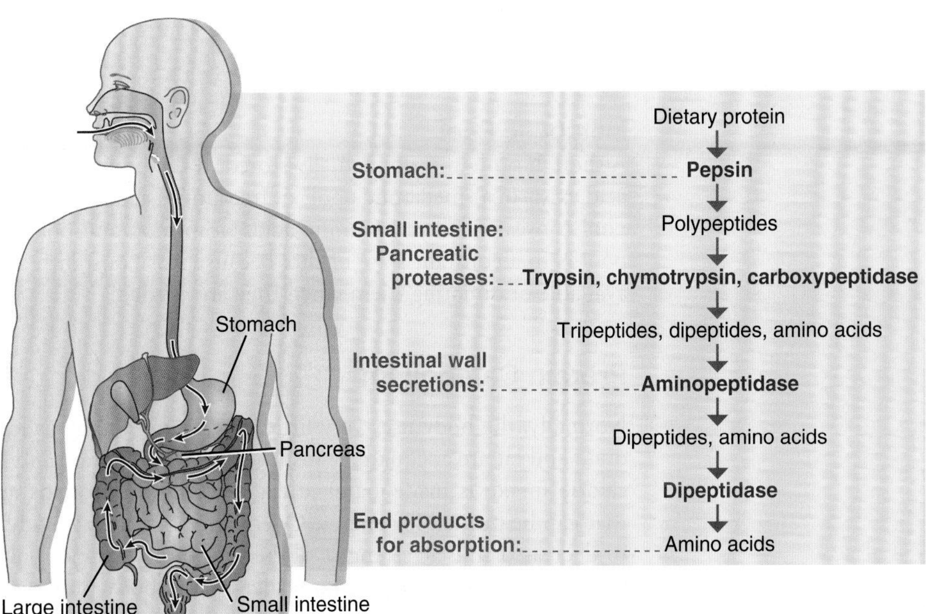

Metabolism

The liver acts as a clearing house for the amino acids it receives. It uses the amino acids it needs, releases those needed elsewhere, and handles the extra. The liver

- retains amino acids to make
  - liver cells
  - nonessential amino acids
  - plasma proteins such as heparin, prothrombin, and albumin
- regulates the release of amino acids into the bloodstream,
- removes excess amino acids from the circulation,
- synthesizes specific enzymes to degrade excess amino acids,
- removes the nitrogen from amino acids so that they can be burned for energy,
- converts certain amino acids to glucose, if necessary,
- forms urea from the nitrogenous wastes when protein and calories are excessively consumed, and
- converts protein to fatty acids that form triglycerides for storage in adipose tissue.

Protein Synthesis

Protein synthesis (anabolism) is a complicated but efficient process that quickly assembles amino acids provided through food or released from the breakdown of existing body proteins into proteins the body needs, such as those required for growth and development or lost through normal wear and tear. The body prioritizes muscle protein synthesis. Cells in the liver, heart, and diaphragm are replenished even during short-term periods of catabolism.

Part of what makes every individual unique are the minute differences in body proteins. These variations are caused by amino acid sequencing determined by genetics. Genetic codes created at conception hold the instructions for making all of the body's proteins. Cell function and life itself depend on the precise replication of these codes. Some important concepts related to protein synthesis are protein turnover and metabolic pool.

Protein Turnover

Protein turnover is a continuous process that occurs within each cell as proteins are broken down due to normal wear and tear, and replenished. Body proteins vary in their rate of turnover. For example, red blood cells are replaced every 60 to 90 days, gastrointestinal cells are replaced every 2 to 3 days, and enzymes used in the digestion of food are continuously replenished.

Metabolic Pool

Although protein is not actually stored in the body (glucose and fat are), a supply of each amino acid exists in a "metabolic pool" of free amino acids within cells and circulating in the blood. This pool consists of recycled amino acids from food and body proteins that have broken down. The pool is in a constant state of flux because it is constantly accepting amino acids as they become available or donating them when they are needed.

Protein Catabolism

Normally, the body uses very little protein for energy as long as intake and storage of carbohydrate and fat are adequate. If insufficient carbohydrate and fat are available for energy use (when calorie intake is inadequate), dietary and body proteins are sacrificed to provide amino acids that can be burned for energy. Over time, loss of lean body tissue occurs that, if severe, can lead to decreased muscle strength, altered immune function, altered organ function, and ultimately death. To "spare" protein—both dietary and body proteins—from being burned for calories, an adequate supply of energy from carbohydrate and fat is needed.

BOX 4.3 Calculating Nitrogen Balance

Mary is a 25-year-old woman who was admitted to the hospital with multiple fractures and traumatic injuries from a car accident. A nutritional intake study indicated a 24-hour protein intake of 64 g. A 24-hour UUN collection result was 19.8 g.

1. Determine nitrogen intake by dividing grams of protein intake by 6.25:

   64 g ÷ 6.25 = 10.24 g of nitrogen

2. Determine total nitrogen output by adding a coefficient of 4 to the UUN:

   19.8 g + 4 g = 23.8 g of nitrogen

3. Calculate nitrogen balance by subtracting nitrogen output from nitrogen intake:

   10.24 g − 23.8 g = −13.56 g in 24 hours

4. Interpret the results.

A negative number indicates that protein breakdown is exceeding protein synthesis. Mary is in a catabolic state.

Nitrogen Balance

Nitrogen balance reflects the state of balance between protein breakdown (catabolism) and protein synthesis (anabolism). It is determined by comparing nitrogen intake with nitrogen excretion over a specific period of time, usually 24 hours.

- Calculate total nitrogen intake for a 24-hour period:
  - Measure protein intake in grams over a 24-hour period.
  - Divide grams of protein consumed by 6.25 because protein is 16% nitrogen.
- Calculate nitrogen excretion in a 24-hour period:
  - Analyze a 24-hour urine sample for grams of urinary urea nitrogen (UUN).
  - Add a coefficient of 4 to account for the estimated daily nitrogen loss in feces, hair, nails, and skin.

Comparing grams of nitrogen excretion to grams of nitrogen intake will reveal the state of nitrogen balance, as illustrated in Box 4.3.

- A neutral nitrogen balance (or state of equilibrium) exists when nitrogen intake equals nitrogen excretion. This indicates that protein synthesis is occurring at the same rate as protein breakdown.
  - Healthy adults are in neutral nitrogen balance.
- Nitrogen balance is positive when protein synthesis exceeds protein breakdown.
  - This is the case during growth, pregnancy, or recovery from injury.
- A negative nitrogen balance indicates that protein catabolism is occurring at a faster rate than protein synthesis.
  - This occurs during starvation or the catabolic phase after injury.

SOURCES OF PROTEIN

Table 4.1 features protein sources and the average protein content per serving. The quality of dietary proteins differs based on their essential amino acid composition. Terms that refer to protein quality are *complete* and *incomplete*.

- Complete proteins provide all nine essential amino acids in adequate amounts and proportions needed by the body for protein synthesis.
  - All animal sources of protein—meat, poultry, seafood, eggs, milk—are complete proteins, with the exception of gelatin.

Table 4.1 Sources of Protein and Average Protein Content per Serving[a]

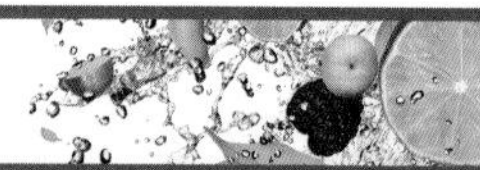

Vegetables

Non-starchy vegetables: 2 g of protein per serving

- ½ c cooked broccoli, cabbage, carrots, cauliflower, eggplant, green beans, green peas, mushrooms, spinach, tomatoes
- 1 c of raw carrots, peppers

Starchy vegetables: 3 g protein per serving

- ½ c cooked corn, yam, sweet potato, parsnips, green peas, succotash, potato
- 1 c cooked winter squash, french fries (oven baked)

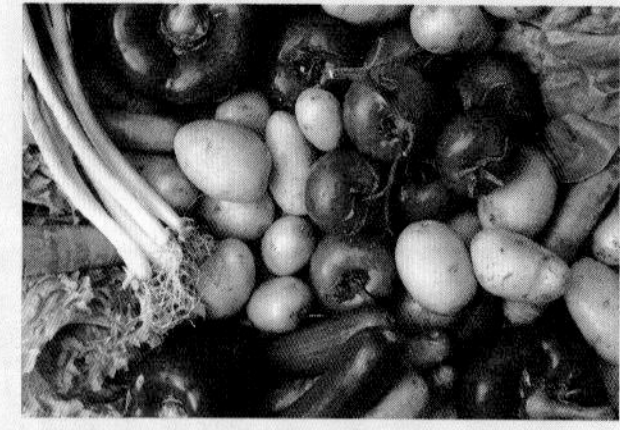

shutterstock.com/Gilles Lougassi

Grains

Grain products: 3 g protein per serving

- 1 slice bread
- 1 oz ready-to-eat cereals
- ½ c cooked pasta, rice, oats, barley, bulgur, grits

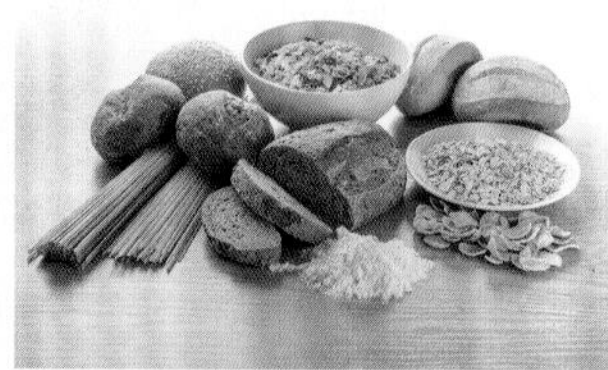

shutterstock.com/Billion Photos

Proteins

Both animal and plant proteins: approximately 7 g protein per serving

- 1 oz beef, pork, lamb, veal, poultry, seafood, deli meats
- 1 egg
- 1 oz cheese
- ½ c black, garbanzo, kidney, lima, navy, pinto, white, black-eyed peas, lentils
- ½ c tofu
- 1 tbsp nut "butters"
- 1 oz "beef" or "sausage" crumbles (meatless)
- ⅓ c hummus

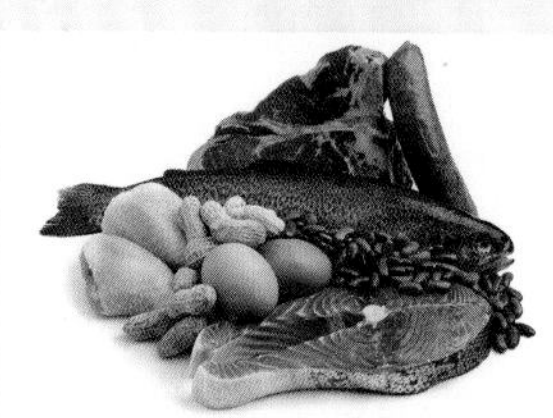

shutterstock.com/Hurst Photo

Dairy

Milk and yogurt choices: 8 g of protein per serving

- 1 c milk—fat-free, low-fat, 2%, or whole
- 6 oz yogurt

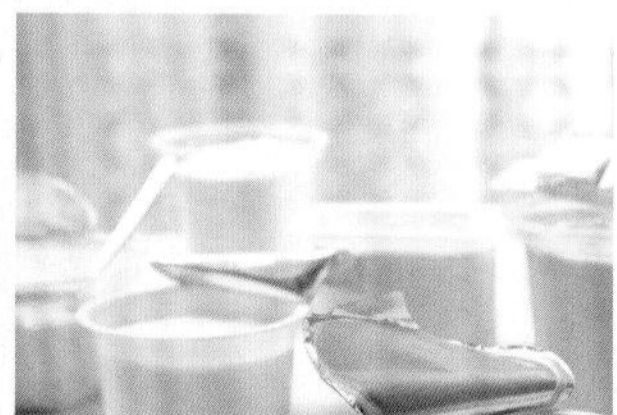

shutterstock.com/New Africa

[a] Based on American Diabetes Association, Academy of Nutrition and Dietetics. (2019). *Choose your foods: Food lists for diabetes*. American Diabetes Association & Academy of Nutrition.

- Incomplete proteins also provide all the essential amino acids, but one or more are present in insufficient quantities to support protein synthesis.
  - These amino acids are considered "limiting" in that they limit the process of protein synthesis. All plant proteins and gelatin are incomplete proteins.
- Different sources of incomplete proteins differ in their limiting amino acids.
  - For instance, grains are typically low in lysine and isoleucine. Legumes are low in methionine and cysteine.
- Two incomplete proteins that have different limiting amino acids are known as complementary proteins because together they form the equivalent of a complete protein.
  - Likewise, a complete protein combined with any incomplete protein is complementary.
  - Examples of foods that contain complementary proteins appear in Box 4.4.

BOX 4.4 Sources of Foods with Complementary Proteins

Two Incomplete Proteins	A Complete Protein Combined with an Incomplete Protein
Black beans and rice	Bread pudding
Bean tacos	Rice pudding
Pea soup with toast	Corn pudding
Lentils and rice curry	Cereal and milk
Falafel (ground chickpea patties) sandwich	Macaroni and cheese
Peanut butter sandwich	French toast
Pasta e fagioli (white beans and pasta soup)	Cheese sandwich
Hummus with crackers	Vegetable quiche
Tofu lasagna	Cheese enchilada

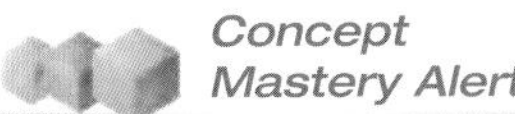

Two kinds of beans (e.g., black beans and kidney beans) do not create a complete, or complementary, protein because they have the same incomplete proteins. Consuming one of those kinds of beans with a different incomplete or complete protein (e.g., rice or cheese) would create a complete protein.

- It is not necessary to eat complementary proteins at the same meal; what is important is eating a variety of proteins over the course of a day and consuming adequate calories.
    - Protein quality is not important for most Americans because the amounts of protein and calories consumed over the course of a day are more than adequate. Quality becomes a crucial concern when protein needs are increased or protein intake is marginal.

DIETARY REFERENCE INTAKES

Protein has both a Recommended Dietary Allowance (RDA) and an Acceptable Macronutrient Distribution Range (AMDR).

Recommended Dietary Allowance and Mean U.S. Protein Intake

The RDA for protein for healthy adults age 19 years and older is 0.8 g/kg, and is derived from the absolute minimum requirement needed to maintain nitrogen balance, plus an additional factor to account for individual variations and the mixed quality of proteins typically consumed (National Research Council, 2005). The RDA is also based on the assumption that calorie intake is adequate.

- For reference, the RDA for an adult male weighing 154 pounds is 0.8 g/kg, which translates to 56 g protein/day.
- For reference, the RDA of an adult female weighing 127 pounds would need 46 g/day.
- To calculate a healthy adult's RDA for protein
    - determine weight in kilograms by dividing weight in pounds by 2.2.
    - multiply the weight in kilograms by 0.8 to determine total grams of protein needed per day.
- The RDA for protein is higher for people younger than 19 years (in grams per kilogram of body weight) and for pregnant or lactating women, to support growth and development (Table 4.2).
- A growing body of evidence suggests older adults may need more than the current RDA to help preserve muscle mass and function (Traylor et al., 2018).
- The RDA is intended for healthy people only.
    - Health impairments that require tissue repair increase a person's protein requirement (Box 4.5).
    - Conversely, protein restriction is appropriate for people with severe liver disease (because the liver metabolizes amino acids), and for those who are unable to adequately excrete nitrogenous wastes from protein metabolism, due to impaired kidney function.

Table 4.2 Recommended Dietary Allowance for Protein by Age and Life Stage

By Age	Gram Protein/kg Body Weight
For men and women:	
7–12 months	1.2
1–3 years	1.05
4–13 years	0.95
14–18 years	0.85
≥19 years	0.8
By life stage	
Pregnancy	1.1
Lactation	1.3

BOX 4.5 Conditions That Increase the Need for Protein

When Calorie Intake is Inadequate Resulting in Protein Being Used for Energy

- Very-low-calorie weight-loss diets
- Starvation
- PEM

When the Body Needs to Heal Itself

- Hypermetabolic conditions such as thermal injuries, sepsis, major infection, and major trauma
- Post-surgically
- Acute inflammation such as inflammatory bowel disease
- Skin breakdown
- Multiple fractures
- Hepatitis

When Excessive Protein Losses Need Replacement

- Long-term peritoneal or hemodialysis dialysis
- Protein-losing renal diseases
- Malabsorption syndromes such as protein-losing enteropathy and short bowel syndrome

When Periods of Normal Tissue Growth Occur

- Pregnancy
- Lactation
- Infancy through adolescence

According to the National Health and Nutrition Examination Survey 2015 to 2016 data, the mean protein intake for adult men and women age 20 years and older is 97 and 70 g, respectively. This amount is well above the RDA (U.S. Department of Agriculture, Agricultural Research Service, 2018a). It represents an average of 16% of total calories for both men and women age 20 and older (U.S. Department of Agriculture, Agricultural Research Service, 2018b). Table 4.3 estimates the protein content of a 2000-calorie Healthy U.S.-Style Eating Pattern.

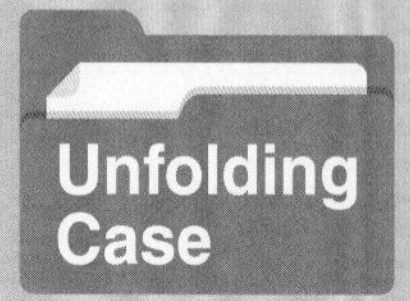

Think of Robert. What is Robert's RDA for protein at a healthy weight of 84 kg? His protein and calorie intakes are inadequate, as determined by food records and weight loss. He agrees to try in-between meal snacks. What snacks would you specifically suggest?

Acceptable Macronutrient Distribution Range

The AMDR for protein for adults is 10% to 35% of total calories (National Research Council, 2005). However, the AMDR is not a useful tool for assessing protein adequacy, because it is based on intake levels that are associated with a reduced risk of chronic disease while providing adequate intake

Table 4.3 Protein of the 2000-Calorie Healthy U.S.-Style Eating Pattern

Food Group	Recommended Daily Amount	Average g Protein/Serving[a]	Estimated Total g Protein
Vegetables	2.5 c eq	2 g/½ c	10
Fruits	2 c eq	0	0
Grains	6 oz eq	3 g/oz eq	18
Dairy	3 c eq	8 g/c eq	24
Protein Foods	5.5 oz eq	7 g/oz/eq	38.5
Oils	27 g	0	0
Total			90.5 g

Note. Healthy U.S.-Style Eating Pattern available at https://health.gov/dietaryguidelines/2015/guidelines/appendix-3/.
[a]Based on the American Diabetes Association, Academy of Nutrition and Dietetics. (2019). *Choose your foods: Food lists for weight management*. American Diabetes Association & Academy of Nutrition.

of essential nutrients. The AMDR ranges established for carbohydrate and fat are supported by evidence, but for protein, evidence is lacking. For instance, a Tolerable Upper Intake Limit has not been established for protein. The AMDR for protein was set, in part, to complement the ranges for carbohydrate and fat, and was not due to compelling evidence indicating a range based on risk of chronic disease.

Protein Deficiency

Protein deficiency usually occurs in conjunction with calorie deficiency. Protein–energy malnutrition (PEM), sometimes referred to as protein–energy undernutrition, is a calorie deficit due to a deficiency of all **macronutrients**—carbohydrates, protein, and fat. Accompanying deficiencies of **micronutrients** are common. It can occur simply from poor intake, or secondary to conditions or drugs that alter nutrient intake (e.g., anorexia nervosa), absorption (e.g., pancreatic insufficiency), utilization (e.g., cancer), or requirements (e.g., trauma).

- In developed countries, PEM is common among seniors, especially institutionalized seniors (Morely, 2018), hospitalized patients, and people with certain diseases.
- Children worldwide are most often affected by PEM. Globally, malnutrition affects almost half of the 5.6 million children who die before their fifth birthday each year (Black et al., 2013).
- **Marasmus** and **Kwashiorkor** are the two common forms of PEM in children (Table 4.4).

Macronutrients
nutrients required by the body in large amounts (gram quantities); namely, carbohydrate, protein, and fat.

Micronutrients
nutrients required by the body in small amounts (microgram or milligram quantities); namely, vitamins and minerals.

Marasmus
a type of PEM resulting from severe deficiency or impaired absorption of calories, protein, vitamins, and minerals.

Kwashiorkor
a type of PEM resulting from a deficiency of protein or infections.

Signs and Symptoms of Protein–energy Malnutrition

PEM affects all body organs and many body systems.

- Apathy and irritability are common.
- Work capacity is impaired.
- Temporary lactose deficiency can develop.
- Diarrhea is common and can be aggravated by a deficiency of lactase and other disaccharidases.
- Muscle and fat wasting are common.
- An impaired immune system increases the risk of infection.
- Infection in the intestinal tract impairs nutrient digestion and absorption.
- Wound healing is impaired. In senior patients, risk of hip fractures and pressure ulcers also increases.
- With acute or chronic severe PEM
  - cardiac output decreases, blood pressure falls, and respiratory rate decreases,
  - body temperature falls,
  - anemia occurs from a decreased production of hemoglobin,
  - diminished levels of serum albumin leads to edema,

Table 4.4 Comparison between Kwashiorkor and Marasmus

	Kwashiorkor	Marasmus
Intake	• More deficient in protein than calories • Tends to be confined to areas of the world where staple foods (e.g., yams, cassavas, green bananas) are low in protein and high in carbohydrates	• Inadequate calorie and protein intake
Cause	• Premature abandonment of breastfeeding • Acute illness or infections that cause loss of appetite while increasing nutrient requirements and losses. • Stressors in children in developing countries may be measles or gastroenteritis and often occurs during weaning • Less common than marasmus	• Severe prolonged starvation may occur in children from chronic or recurring infections with marginal food intake; in adults from developed countries, may occur secondary to chronic illness. • More common than Kwashiorkor
Onset	• Rapid, acute; may develop in a matter of weeks	• Slow, chronic; may take months or years to develop
Edema	• Characterized by peripheral edema due to low serum albumin	• Absent
Appearance	• May look plump due to ascites • Abdomen protrudes due to weakened abdominal muscles	• "Skin and bones" due to severe muscle loss and virtually no body fat
Weight loss	• Children present with poor weight gain or weight loss	• Severe
Other clinical symptoms that may be present	• Skin lesions; shedding skin • Hair loss, loss of hair color, easy pluckability • Enlarged fatty liver • Loss of appetite • Apathy and lethargy • Increased susceptibility to infections	• Dry, thin skin that easily wrinkles • Hair is sparse; easy pluckability • No fatty liver • Hypothermia • Increased susceptibility to infections

- jaundice and petechiae can develop, and
- liver, kidney, or heart failure may occur.

Treatment

Treatment is determined by the severity of PEM. Mild or moderate PEM can be treated with a balanced diet, preferably oral.

- Liquid supplements are useful if solid food intake is inadequate.
- Lactose is restricted if diarrhea persists.
- Multivitamin supplements are given.

In severe PEM or chronic starvation, the following apply:

- Nutrition therapy begins with correcting fluid and electrolyte imbalances to help raise the blood pressure and increase the heart rate.
- Infections are treated.
- In children with diarrhea, feeding may be delayed for 24 to 48 hours to avoid worsening diarrhea.
  - It is usually not necessary to delay feeding in adults.
- Oral or enteral feedings (e.g., nasogastric tube feedings) begin with small amounts to avoid overwhelming the absorptive capacity of the small intestine (Morley, 2018).
- Intake progresses as tolerated.
- Multivitamin supplements at about twice the RDA are given until recovery is complete.

Protein Excess

There are no proven risks from eating an excess of protein. A Tolerable Upper Intake Level has not been established, but this does not mean that there is no potential for adverse effects from a high protein intake from food or supplements (National Research Council, 2005). Data are limited on the adverse effects of high levels of amino acid intake from supplements, so caution is advised in taking any single amino acid in amounts significantly higher than what is found in food (National Research Council, 2005).

PROTEIN IN HEALTH PROMOTION

The *Dietary Guidelines for Americans (DGA) 2020–2025* urge people to consume a healthy eating pattern that includes a variety of protein foods in nutrient-dense forms. This means meat and poultry should be consumed fresh, frozen, or canned forms instead of processed products and that choices be lean or low fat (Box 4.6) (U.S. Department of Agriculture [USDA] & U.S. Department of Health and Human Services [USDHHS] , 2020). This advice is consistent with guidelines from other health agencies.

- The American College of Cardiology/American Heart Association recommendations for the primary prevention of cardiovascular disease suggests that adults consume lean vegetable or animal protein and fish, and minimize the intake of red and processed meats (Arnett et al., 2019).
- The American Cancer Society recommends limiting processed meat and red meat (Kushi et al., 2012).
- The American Institute for Cancer Research advises consumers to limit consumption of red meats (e.g., beef, pork, and lamb) to moderate amounts and to eat little, if any, processed meat, such as: ham, bacon, salami, hot dogs, and sausages. (American Institute for Cancer Research, 2020).

Protein Food Group

Dietary Reference Intakes for protein refer to protein (the nutrient); protein foods (the group) refer to a set of foods that provide significant protein as well as fat and/or carbohydrates and micronutrients. Subgroups within the protein food group include: meats, poultry, eggs; seafood; nuts, seeds, and soy products; and beans, peas, and lentils.

Intake of Protein Foods

While Americans eat enough of the nutrient protein and come close to the target amounts for the protein food group, many people do not meet recommendations for specific protein subgroups (USDA & USDHHS, 2020):

- Approximately 75% of Americans meet or exceed the recommendation for meats, poultry, and eggs.

BOX 4.6 Lean Animal and Plant Protein Choices

Animal

- Beef: USDA Choice or Select grades trimmed of fat: 90% or higher lean ground beef, roast (chuck, round, rump, sirloin), steak (cubed, flank, porterhouse, T-bone), tenderloin
- Beef jerky
- Lean pork choices: pork loin, tenderloin, center loin, ham, and Canadian bacon
- Skinless poultry: chicken, Cornish hen, turkey, well-drained domestic duck or goose; lean ground turkey or chicken
- Veal: culet without breading, loin chop, roast
- Any of the following processed items in varieties that provide 3 g of fat or less per oz: sausage, hot dogs, deli meat, cheese
- Fish: fresh or frozen; canned salmon, sardines, tuna (in water or oil, drained)
- Shellfish: clams, oysters, crab, lobster, scallops, shrimp
- Game: buffalo, ostrich, rabbit, venison
- Egg substitutes or egg whites
- Goat: chop, leg, loin
- Organ meats: heart, kidney, liver

Plant

- Beans, peas, and lentils
- Edamame
- Light tofu
- Meatless crumbles, soy-based bacon strips, meatless burger, meatless chicken tenders, meatless hotdog, meatless deli slices

Source: American Diabetes Association, Academy of Nutrition and Dietetics. (2019). *Choose your food: Food lists for weight management.* American Diabetes Association & Academy of Nutrition.

- Almost 90% do not meet the recommendation for seafood.
- More than 50% do not meet the recommendation for nuts, seeds, and soy products.
- 48% of protein foods consumed are eaten as part of a mixed dish, such as sandwiches, burgers, and tacos. The protein in mixed dishes may have higher amounts of saturated fat than protein foods consumed as a separate food (e.g., a chicken breast or fillet of fish) and mixed dishes may have other ingredients that are not in nutrient-dense form.

Seafood

Seafood is known for providing the omega-3 fatty acids eicosapentaenoic acid (EPA) and docosahexaenoic acid (DHA) yet it contains an array of other nutrients including protein, selenium, iron, zinc, iodine, vitamin B12, and vitamin D. Healthy eating patterns that include a focus on fish are recommended to lower atherosclerotic cardiovascular disease (Arnet et al., 2019). It is not completely known whether health benefits are solely due to fish oil intake or if other nutrients contribute to its benefits (Gribble et al., 2016).

The healthy U.S. style eating patterns intended for adults (total daily calorie intake from 1600 to 3200) recommend Americans consume at least eight ounces of seafood/week (USDA & USDHHS, 2020). A variety of seafood is recommended to limit exposure to **methylmercury**, which is present in varying amounts in nearly all fish.

Methylmercury
Mercury, a neurotoxin, is a heavy metal that occurs naturally in the environment and is released into the air through industrial pollution. It changes to methylmercury when it falls from the air into the water. As a fat-soluble element, it accumulates in the fat tissue of large predatory fish. Pregnant and lactating women and children younger than age 8 years are vulnerable to the toxic effects of mercury because it can damage the developing brain and spinal cord.

- Most fish have minute amounts of methylmercury that are not harmful to humans; large predatory fish with long lifespans have more.
- Evidence suggests the benefits of consuming moderate amounts of fish on cardiovascular health very likely outweigh the risk of any potential harm related to mercury exposure (Rimm et al., 2018).
- Still, to minimize potential risk from methylmercury, it is recommended that people choose seafood that is high in EPA and DHA and lower in methylmercury: salmon, anchovies, herring, shad, sardines, Pacific oysters, and Atlantic and Pacific mackerel (Fig. 4.3).
- People who eat more than the recommended 8 oz of seafood per week are encouraged to choose a mix of seafood that is relatively low in methylmercury.
- Because fish provides vital nutrients for developing fetuses and infants, especially omega-3 fatty acids, pregnant and lactating women are urged to eat 8 to 12 oz of a variety of seafood per week, from choices that are lower in mercury a week (FDA & Environmental Protection Agency [EPA], 2019). See Chapter 12 for additional recommendations regarding seafood intake during pregnancy.

Vegetarian Diets

A healthy vegetarian-style eating pattern is one of three eating patterns featured in the *Dietary Guidelines for Americans 2020-2025* (USDA & USDHHS 2020). The health benefits of a plant-based diet may come from eating less of certain substances (such as saturated fat), eating more of others (such as fiber, antioxidants, and phytonutrients), or a combination of the two. Plant-based foods are also low in calorie density.

Vegetarianism is a general term assigned to plant-based eating patterns that restrict animal foods (e.g., meat, poultry, seafood, dairy, and eggs) and products made with them.

- Restrictions range from total elimination of all animal products to simply excluding one or more types of animal proteins (Box 4.7).
- Each defined category of vegetarianism has different characteristics, and individuals differ in how strictly they adhere to the eating pattern. For instance, some vegans do not eat refried beans that contain lard because lard is an animal product, but other vegans do not avoid animal products so conscientiously.
- Nationally, 3.3% of American adults describe themselves as vegetarians and about half of the vegetarians are also vegan (Vegetarian Resource Group, 2016).

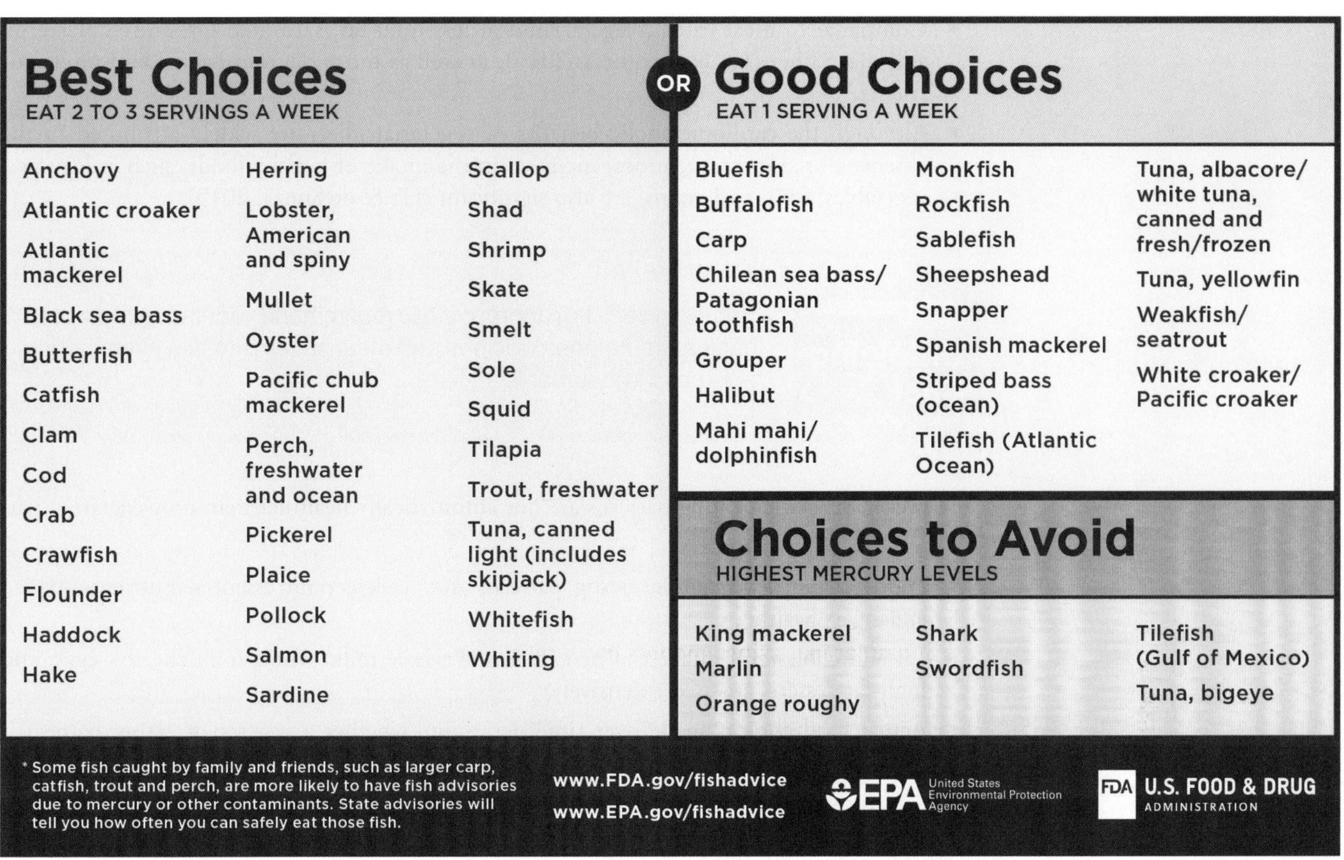
Best Choices
EAT 2 TO 3 SERVINGS A WEEK
OR
Good Choices
EAT 1 SERVING A WEEK
Anchovy
Atlantic croaker
Atlantic mackerel
Black sea bass
Butterfish
Catfish
Clam
Cod
Crab
Crawfish
Flounder
Haddock
Hake
Herring
Lobster, American and spiny
Mullet
Oyster
Pacific chub mackerel
Perch, freshwater and ocean
Pickerel
Plaice
Pollock
Salmon
Sardine
Scallop
Shad
Shrimp
Skate
Smelt
Sole
Squid
Tilapia
Trout, freshwater
Tuna, canned light (includes skipjack)
Whitefish
Whiting
Bluefish
Buffalofish
Carp
Chilean sea bass/ Patagonian toothfish
Grouper
Halibut
Mahi mahi/ dolphinfish
Monkfish
Rockfish
Sablefish
Sheepshead
Snapper
Spanish mackerel
Striped bass (ocean)
Tilefish (Atlantic Ocean)
Tuna, albacore/ white tuna, canned and fresh/frozen
Tuna, yellowfin
Weakfish/ seatrout
White croaker/ Pacific croaker
Choices to Avoid
HIGHEST MERCURY LEVELS
King mackerel
Marlin
Orange roughy
Shark
Swordfish
Tilefish (Gulf of Mexico)
Tuna, bigeye
* Some fish caught by family and friends, such as larger carp, catfish, trout and perch, are more likely to have fish advisories due to mercury or other contaminants. State advisories will tell you how often you can safely eat those fish.
www.FDA.gov/fishadvice
www.EPA.gov/fishadvice
EPA United States Environmental Protection Agency
FDA U.S. FOOD & DRUG ADMINISTRATION

Figure 4.3 ▲ **Recommended fish choices based on mercury content.** (*Source:* United States Food and Drug Administration. (2019). *Advice about eating Fish.* https://www.fda.gov/food/consumers/advice-about-eating-fish)

- Properly planned vegan, lacto-vegetarian, and lacto-ovo vegetarian eating patterns are healthful and are nutritionally adequate during all phases of the life cycle, including pregnancy, lactation, infancy, childhood, and adolescence, older adulthood, and for athletes (Melina et al., 2016).
- Vegetarian diets improve several modifiable risk factors for heart disease, including abdominal obesity, blood pressure, serum lipids, and blood glucose as well as lowered C-reactive protein (Melina et al., 2016).
- Vegetarian eating patterns can provide health benefits in the prevention and treatment of certain health conditions: ischemic heart disease, type 2 diabetes, and certain cancers.

BOX 4.7 Types of Vegetarian Diets

The basis of all vegetarian diets is the exclusion of meat, fish, and poultry. Additional traits vary with the type of vegetarian diet.

- **Vegan:** also excludes eggs, dairy products, and may exclude honey
- **Raw vegan:** a strictly uncooked food eating pattern based on fruit, vegetables, nuts, seeds, legumes, and sprouted grains. Uncooked food ranges from 75% to 100% of total food consumed.
- **Lacto-ovo vegetarian:** includes dairy products and eggs.
- **Lacto-vegetarian**: excludes eggs but includes dairy products.
- **Ovo-vegetarian**: excludes dairy products but includes eggs.
- Other eating patterns that restrict the types of protein consumed are loosely defined.
  - **Pesco-vegetarian:** excludes all animal products except fish
  - **Semi-vegetarian:** does not eat red meat
  - **Flexitarian:** eats chicken and fish, occasionally eats red meat

- Compared to meat eaters, vegetarians eat less total fat, saturated fat, and cholesterol, and more fiber (Ha & de Souza, 2015), as well as more micronutrients and phytonutrients.
- Although the cardiometabolic benefits of vegetarian diets are widely attributed to the absence of red meat, reciprocal increases in the intake of healthy foods, such as legumes, vegetables, fruit, and grains, are also significant (Ha & de Souza, 2015).

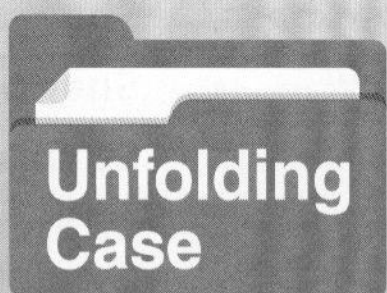

Recall Robert. Is it appropriate to recommend vegetarian resources that feature nonmeat recipes and meal patterns to him even though he is not a vegetarian?

However, vegetarian eating patterns are not automatically healthier than nonvegetarian patterns.

- Poorly planned vegetarian eating patterns may lack certain essential nutrients, which endangers health.
- Fat and cholesterol intake can be excessive if whole milk, whole-milk cheeses, eggs, and high-fat desserts are used extensively.
- Actual food choices made over time determine whether a vegetarian eating pattern is healthy or detrimental to health.
- Tips for vegetarians appear in Box 4.8.

Nutrients of Concern

The concerns that vegetarian eating patterns are deficient in total protein or provide poor overall protein quality are unfounded.

- Most vegetarian eating patterns, even vegan ones, meet or exceed the RDA for protein. Box 4.9 illustrates how a vegan menu can exceed the RDA for the average adult.
- Eating a variety of plant proteins and adequate calories ensures that the supply of essential amino acids is adequate.
- Iron, zinc, calcium, vitamin D, omega-3 fatty acids, and iodine are nutrients of concern, not because they cannot be obtained in sufficient quantities from plants, but because they may not be adequately consumed, depending on an individual's food choices.
- Vitamin B_{12} is of concern because it does not occur naturally in plants. Table 4.5 lists vegetarian sources of these nutrients of concern.

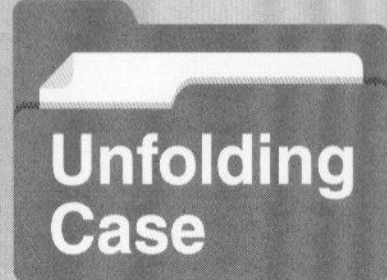

Think of Robert. Robert's intake of heme iron is low because he does not eat red meat.

What other nutrients may he consume in inadequate amounts? Would he benefit from a multivitamin with minerals?

Protein for Muscle Building

High-protein diets and protein supplements are popular among athletes based on the rationale that muscle is protein tissue; thus eating more protein makes more muscle. Building muscle is not simply a matter of increasing protein intake, even though protein recommendations for athletes are higher than for nonathletes. Both resistance training and an adequate overall intake are necessary to increase muscle mass.

BOX 4.8 Tips for Following a Vegetarian Diet

- *Eat a variety of foods that provide protein, including whole grains, vegetables, legumes, nuts, seeds, and, if desired, dairy products and eggs.*
  - Consider meatless versions of familiar favorites, such as vegetable pizza, vegetable lasagna, vegetable stir-fry, vegetable lo mein, and vegetable kabobs.
- *Experiment with meat substitutes made from vegetables.*
  - For variety, try soy sausage patties or links, veggie burgers, quinoa chili, or scrambled tofu.
- *Include legumes.*
  - Try vegetarian chili, three-bean salad, navy bean soup, hummus, lentil stew, bean burritos, or black bean burgers.
- *Substitute soy milk in place of cow's milk*
  - such as in french toast, rice pudding, and smoothies.
- *Experiment with tofu*
  - such as in place of eggs (e.g., scrambled "eggs") or ricotta cheese (e.g., lasagna).
- *Include nuts.*
  - Snack on unsalted nuts, or add to salads or main dishes.
- *Eat enough calories.*
  - Adequate calories are necessary to avoid using amino acids for energy, which could lead to a shortage of amino acids for protein synthesis.
- *Consume a rich source of vitamin C at every meal.*
  - Eating a good source of vitamin C at every meal helps to maximize iron absorption from plants.
  - Try citrus fruits and juices, tomatoes, kiwi, red and green peppers, broccoli, brussels sprouts, cantaloupe, and strawberries.
- *Include foods that supply plant omega-3 fat*
  - such as flaxseeds, tofu, chia seeds, walnuts, and canola and soybean oils.
- *Don't go overboard on high-fat cheese as a meat substitute.*
  - Full-fat cheese has more saturated fat and calories than many meats.
- *Experiment with ethnic cuisines.*
  - Many Asian, Middle Eastern, and Indian restaurants offer a variety of meatless dishes.
- *Choose vitamin B_{12}-fortified foods, or take a vitamin B_{12} supplement daily.*
- *Supplement nutrients that are lacking from food.*
  - See Table 4.5 for sources of other nutrients of concern.

BOX 4.9 Protein Content of a Sample Vegan Menu

Food Item	g Protein*
Breakfast	
1 cup oatmeal	6
With 2 tbsp walnuts	1
1 cup soymilk	8
Banana	
Lunch	
Black bean burger	10
On whole wheat bun	6
Condiments as desired	
Side salad with dressing	2
Fresh orange	
Dinner	
4 oz tofu	12
Stir fried with 1½ cup vegetables	6
Served over 1 cup brown rice	4
Fresh watermelon	
Snack	
1 cup soy yogurt	10
With 2 tbsp almonds	2
Total grams protein/day	67

*Estimates based on averages listed in Table 4.1.

Note. The RDA for reference man is 56 g/day and for reference woman 46 g/day.

Table 4.5 Sources of Nutrients of Concern in Vegan Eating Patterns

Nutrient	Vegetarian Sources	Comments
Iron	Iron-fortified bread and cereals Baked potato with skin Kidney beans, black-eyed peas, chickpeas, and lentils Cooked soybeans Tofu, tahini Veggie "meats" Dried apricots, prunes, and raisins Cooking in a cast iron pan, especially with acidic foods such as tomatoes	Vegetarians generally consume as much or more iron than meat eaters but their iron stores are lower (Melina et al., 2016). It is recommended that vegetarians consume good sources of iron such as iron-fortified breads and cereals, legumes, lentils, and raisins, with a source of vitamin C because vitamin C enhances the bioavailability of iron from plants.
Zinc	Whole grains Legumes Zinc-fortified cereals Soybean products Seeds Nuts	Compared to meat eaters, adult vegetarians consume similar or somewhat lower amounts of zinc and have serum levels that are lower but within normal range (Melina et al., 2016) Overt zinc deficiency is not evident in American vegetarians.
Calcium	Bok choy Broccoli Chinese/Napa cabbage Collard greens Kale Turnip greens Calcium-fortified orange juice Calcium-set tofu Calcium-fortified plant milks, breakfast cereals	Calcium recommendations are met or exceeded by lacto-ovo vegetarians. Calcium intake among vegans varies widely and may be less than recommended (Melina et al., 2016) Beet greens, spinach, and Swiss chard are also high in calcium, but their oxalate content greatly impairs calcium absorption, so they are not considered good sources. Calcium supplements are recommended for people who do not meet their calcium requirement through food.
Vitamin D	Sunlight Fortified milk Fortified ready-to-eat cereals Fortified fruit juices Fortified soy milk Fortified nondairy milk products	Supplements may be necessary depending on the quality of sunlight exposure and adequacy of vitamin D–fortified food choices.
Omega-3 fatty acids	Fortified foods, such as breakfast cereals, soy milk, and yogurt Sources of alpha-linolenic acid are the following: Ground flaxseed and flaxseed oil Chia seeds Walnuts and walnut oil Canola oil Soybean oil	Diets that exclude fish do not contain a direct source of omega-3 fatty acids EPA and DHA. The body can convert small amounts of alpha-linolenic acid into DHA and EPA. Adequate DHA and EPA is especially important during pregnancy, infancy, and in seniors. Low-dose microalgae-based DHA supplements are available
Vitamin B_{12}	Fortified soy milk, breakfast cereals, and veggie burgers	Vitamin B_{12} is naturally present only in foods derived from animals Seaweed, algae, spirulina, tempeh, miso, beer, and other fermented foods cannot be relied up as adequate or practical sources of B_{12} (Melina et al., 2016) Vegans must regularly consume B_{12}-fortified foods or supplements containing B_{12} to avoid deficiency. Supplemental vitamin B_{12} through food or pills is recommended for all people over the age of 50 years regardless of the type of diet they consume because absorption decreases with age. Vitamin B_{12} deficiency during pregnancy and lactation may lead to severe developmental problems in the fetus and infant.
Iodine	Iodized salt Sea vegetables	Vegans who do not consume iodized salt or sea vegetables may be at risk for iodine deficiency (Melina et al., 2016) Sea salt, kosher salt, and salt-based seasonings are generally not iodized, nor is iodized salt used in processed foods. Vegan women of childbearing age should consume a iodine supplement of 150 mcg/day (Melina et al., 2016)

Resistance training, also called weight or strength training, is exercise that causes muscle to contract against an external force for the purpose of increasing strength, tone, mass, or endurance. Resistance training causes microscopic tears in muscle tissue (catabolism), which the body quickly repairs to regenerate and strengthen muscle (anabolism). Although an adequate protein is important, so is an adequate intake of overall calories—energy to fuel the activity as well as repair the tissue.

- Athletes need to consume adequate calories timed to meet energy needs during high-intensity and/or long-duration training (Thomas et al., 2016).
- Recommendations for protein intake typically range from 1.2 to 2.0 g protein/kg/day (Thomas et al., 2016). This amount of protein can generally be met through food alone, without the need for protein or amino acid supplements.
- An even distribution of protein intake after exercise and throughout the day may optimize muscle protein synthesis (Thomas et al., 2016).
- Vitamin and mineral supplements are unnecessary for athletes who consume adequate calories from a variety of nutrient-dense foods (Thomas et al., 2016).
- The use of sports supplements is a personal choice, and is controversial (Thomas et al., 2016).
    - Safety and efficacy are concerns. Athletes may take inappropriately large doses or problematic combinations of products. Aids should be used only after careful consideration of potential benefits and risk (Thomas et al., 2016).

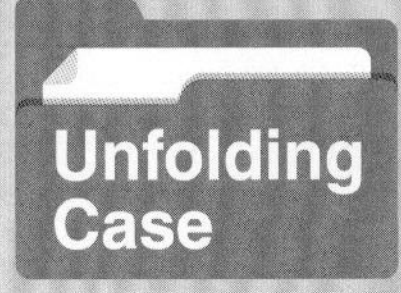

Consider Robert. Robert wants to know if whey protein powder or amino acid supplements would be beneficial. How would you respond?

How Do You Respond?

Is ground turkey a low-fat alternative to ground beef? Not necessarily. Ground turkey may contain skin, dark meat, and fat, which makes it a higher-fat product than 95% lean ground beef. Ground turkey breast and chicken breast are both made only from white meat and are lower in fat (approximately 3 g/3 oz cooked) than all varieties of ground beef (5.5–15 g fat/3 oz cooked).

Are amino acid supplements a good idea to boost protein intake or sports performance? Amino acid supplements often provide only one or few particular amino acids, unlike the natural array of amino acids found in food. An imbalance of amino acids is not beneficial: an excess of one amino acid can interfere with the absorption of other amino acids, and cause them to become the limiting amino acid for protein synthesis. An abnormally high serum concentration of an amino acid raises the possibility of toxicity. Caution is advised in using any single amino acid at levels other than what is supplied by food.

REVIEW CASE STUDY

Emily does not eat meat, eggs, or milk for ethical reasons, although she will still eat baked goods that may contain milk or eggs. Over the last 6 months, she has gained 15 pounds. Emily admits that she expected to see weight loss instead of gain.

She needs 2000 cal/day according to MyPlate, and a typical daily intake for Emily is shown on the right.

- What kind of vegetarian is Emily? What sources of protein is she consuming? Is she consuming enough protein?
  - How does her daily intake compare to MyPlate recommendations for a 2000-calorie diet? What suggestions would you make to her to improve the quality of her diet?
- Is Emily at risk of any nutrient deficiencies?
  - If so, what would you recommend she do to ensure nutritional adequacy?
- What would you tell Emily about her weight gain? What food would you recommend limiting to promote weight loss? What could she substitute for those foods?

Breakfast: a glazed donut and a smoothie made with soy milk, tofu, and fresh fruit
Snack: potato chips and soda
Lunch: peanut butter sandwich, soy yogurt, oatmeal cookies, and a soft drink
Snack: candy bar
Dinner: stir-fried vegetables over rice, bread w/margarine, glass of soy milk, apple pie
Snack: buttered popcorn

STUDY QUESTIONS

1 What is the RDA for protein for a healthy adult who weighs 165 pounds?
a. 40 g
b. 60 g
c. 75 g
d. 132 g

2 The client asks what foods are rich in protein and are less expensive than meat. Which foods would the nurse recommend they eat more of?
a. Breads and cereals
b. Fish and shellfish
c. Fruit and vegetables
d. Beans, peas, and lentils

3 Which of the following is a lean source of protein?
a. Eggs
b. Turkey breast without skin
c. 80% lean ground beef
d. Prime beef rib roast

4 Which statement indicates the client understands vegetarian diets?
a. "Vegetarian diets are not adequate during pregnancy and lactation."
b. "Vegetarians may need to take a vitamin B_{12} supplement and other nutrients, depending on their actual food selection."
c. "Vegetarian diets are always healthier than nonvegetarian diets."
d. "Vegetarians usually do not consume enough protein."

5 A client who is in a positive nitrogen balance is most likely to be
a. Pregnant.
b. Starving.
c. A healthy adult.
d. Losing weight.

6 What should the nurse tell a client who likes fish but refuses to eat it because of fear of mercury poisoning?
a. "You are justified to be concerned. To be safe, use fish oil supplements instead."
b. "You can eat as much fish as you want because most fish are not contaminated with even small amounts of mercury."
c. "The benefits of eating 8 oz/week of a variety of fish outweigh any potential risks from mercury."
d. "As a compromise, eat 4 oz of fish per week instead of 8 oz."

7 The nurse knows that instructions have been effective when the client verbalizes that a source of complete, high-quality protein is found in
a. Peanut butter
b. Black-eyed peas
c. Corn
d. Cottage cheese

8 To move toward healthier eating patterns, Americans should
a. Eat more seafood
b. Eat more total protein
c. Eat more mixed protein dishes, such as sandwiches, in place of eating protein as a separate food
d. Replace seafood with poultry

CHAPTER SUMMARY PROTEIN

Protein is a component of every living cell. It provides the structure and framework of the body. Amino acids are components of enzymes, hormones, neurotransmitters, and antibodies. Proteins play a role in fluid balance and acid–base balance, and are used to transport substances through the blood. Protein provides 4 cal/g.

Protein Composition and Structure

Amino acids are the building blocks of protein.

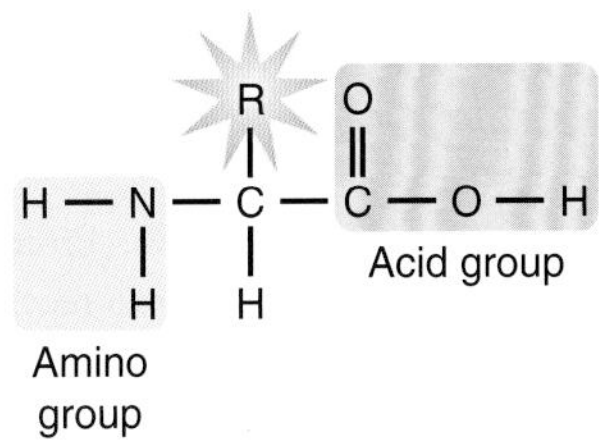

- They are composed of carbon, hydrogen, oxygen, and nitrogen atoms.
- Amino acids are joined in different amounts, proportions, and sequences to form the thousands of different proteins in the body.
- Nine are essential and must be supplied through the diet.
- The remaining 11 are considered nonessential only because they can be made if nitrogen is available.

Functions of Protein

Amino acids or proteins are involved in or components of

- body structure and framework: muscle, skin, blood, tendons, organs, and bones,
- enzymes,
- other body secretions and fluids: neurotransmitters, antibodies, and peptide fluid balance,
- acid–base balance,
- transport molecules,
- fueling the body (protein provides 4 cal/g).

How the Body Handles Protein

- The small intestine is the principal site of protein digestion.
- Amino acids and some dipeptides are absorbed through the portal bloodstream.
- Amino acids consumed in excess are burned for energy or converted to fat and stored.
- Healthy adults are in nitrogen balance, which means that protein synthesis is occurring at the same rate as protein breakdown.

Sources of Protein

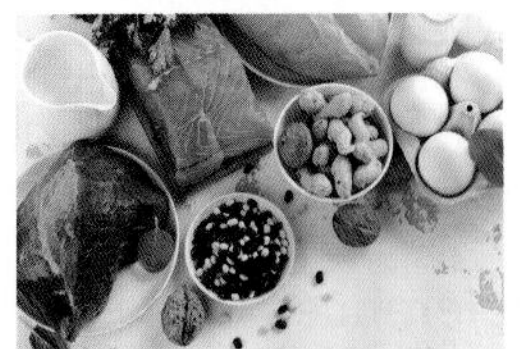

Complete proteins contain all essential amino acids in adequate amounts and proportions to support protein synthesis:

- meat, poultry, seafood, eggs
- milk, yogurt, cheese

Incomplete proteins contain insufficient quantities of one or more essential amino acids:

- grains and products made with grains
- legumes and lentils
- nuts and seeds
- vegetables
- gelatin

Dietary Reference Intakes

- The RDA for protein is 0.8 g/kg/day for adults.
- Protein should provide 10% to 35% of total calories consumed.
- Protein need is higher during growth, pregnancy, lactation, recovery from injury, or when calorie intake is inadequate.
- Protein is restricted in certain liver and kidney diseases.
- Protein deficiency is rare in the United States except among hospitalized patients and certain others.

Protein in Health Promotion

- Americans eat enough protein foods but are urged to make more nutrient dense selections, such as avoiding fatty and processed meats.
- Americans are urged to eat 8 oz or more/week of a variety of seafood that is low in methylmercury.
- Vegetarian diets exclude animal products. Most vegetarian diets meet or exceed the RDA for protein. Pure vegans who do not have reliable sources of vitamin B_{12} and vitamin D need supplements.
- Resistance exercise helps build muscle mass. Adequate calories and protein are necessary. The use of sports food and supplements should be carefully considered.

Figure sources: *shutterstock.com/Ekaterina Markelova and shutterstock.com/Elena Veselova*

Student Resources on thePoint®
For additional learning materials, activate the code in the front of this book at https://thePoint.lww.com/activate

Websites

Soyfoods Association of North America at www.soyfoods.org
Vegan Health at www.veganhealth.org
The Vegan Society at www.vegansociety.com
Vegetarian Nutrition Dietetic Practice Group's at www.vegetariannutrition.net
Vegetarian Resource Group at www.vrg.org
Vegetarian-Nutrition Info at https://vegetarian-nutrition.info/
VegWeb at www.vegweb.com

References

American Institute for Cancer Research. (2020). *Cancer prevention recommendations.* https://www.aicr.org/reduce-your-cancer-risk/recommendations-for-cancer-prevention/index.html

Arnett, D. K., Blumenthal, R. S., Albert, M. A., Buroker, A. B., Goldberger, Z. D., Hahn, E. J., Himmelfarb, C. D., Khera, A., Lloyd-Jones, D., McEvoy, J. W., Michos, E. D., Miedema, M. D., Muñoz, D., Smith, S. C. Jr., Virani, S. S., Williams, K. A., Sr., Yeboah, J., & Ziaeian, B. (2019). ACC/AHA guideline on the primary prevention of cardiovascular disease: A report of the American College of Cardiology/American Heart Association Task Force on Clinical Practice Guidelines. *Journal of American College of Cardiology, 74*, e177–e232. https://doi.org/10.1016/j.jacc.2019.03.010

Gribble, M., Karimi, R., Feingold, B., Nyland, J., O'Hara, T., Gladyshev, M., & Chen, C. Y. (2016). Mercury, selenium and fish oils in marine food webs and implications for human health. *Journal of the Marine Biological Association of the United Kingdom, 96*(1), 43–59. https://doi.org/10.1017/S0025315415001356

Ha, V., & de Souza, R. (2015). "Fleshing out" the benefits of adopting a vegetarian diet. *Journal of the American Heart Association, 4*, e002654. https://doi.org/10.1161/JAHA.115.002654

Kushi, L., Doyle, C., McCullough, M., Rock, C. L., Demark-Wahnefried, W., Bandera, E. V., Gapstur, S., Patel, A. V., Andrews, K., Gansler, T., & American Cancer Society 2010 Nutrition and Physical Activity Guidelines Advisory Committee. (2012). American Cancer Society Guidelines on nutrition and physical activity for cancer prevention: Reducing the risk of cancer with healthy food choices and physical activity. *CA: A Cancer Journal for Clinicians, 62*, 30–67. https://doi.org/10.3322/caac.20140

Melina, V., Craig, W., & Levin, S. (2016). Position of the Academy of Nutrition and Dietetics: Vegetarian diets. *Journal of the Academy of Nutrition and Dietetics, 116*, 1970–1980. https://doi.org/10.1016/j.jand.2016.09.025

Morley, J. (2018). *Protein-energy undernutrition.* Merck Manual Professional Version. https://www.merckmanuals.com/professional/nutritional-disorders/undernutrition/protein-energy-undernutrition-PEM?query=Undernutrition

National Research Council. (2005). *Dietary reference intakes for energy, carbohydrate, fiber, fat, fatty acids, cholesterol, protein, and amino acids (macronutrients).* The National Academies Press.

Thomas, D., Erdman, K., & Burke, L. M. (2016). Position of the Academy of Nutrition and Dietetics, Dietitians of Canada, and the American College of Sports Medicine: Nutrition and athletic performance. *Journal of the Academy of Nutrition and Dietetics, 116*, 501–528. https://doi.org/10.1016/j.jand.2015.12.006

Traylor, D., Gorissen, S., & Phillips, S. (2018). Perspective: Protein requirements and optimal intakes in aging: Are we ready to recommend more than the Recommended Daily Allowance. *Advances in Nutrition, 9*, 171–182. https://doi.org/10.1093/advances/nmy003

U.S. Department of Agriculture, Agricultural Research Service. (2018a). Nutrient intakes from food and beverages: Mean amounts consumed per individual, by gender and age. What we eat in America, NHANES 2015–2016. www.ars.usda.gov/nea/bhnrc/fsrg

U.S. Department of Agriculture, Agricultural Research Service. (2018b). Energy intakes: Percentages of energy from protein, carbohydrate, fat, and alcohol, by gender and age. What we eat in America, NHANES 2015–2016. www.ars.usda.gov/nea/bhnrc/fsrg

U.S. Department of Agriculture & U.S. Department of Health and Human Services. (2020). *Dietary guidelines for Americans 2020–2025.* https://www.dietaryguidelines.gov/sites/default/files/2020-12/Dietary_Guidelines_for_Americans_2020-2025.pdf

Vegetarian Resource Group. (2016). *How many adults in the United States are vegetarian and vegan? How many adults eat vegetarian and vegan meals when eating out?* https://www.vrg.org/nutshell/Polls/2016_adults_veg.htm

Chapter 5

Lipids

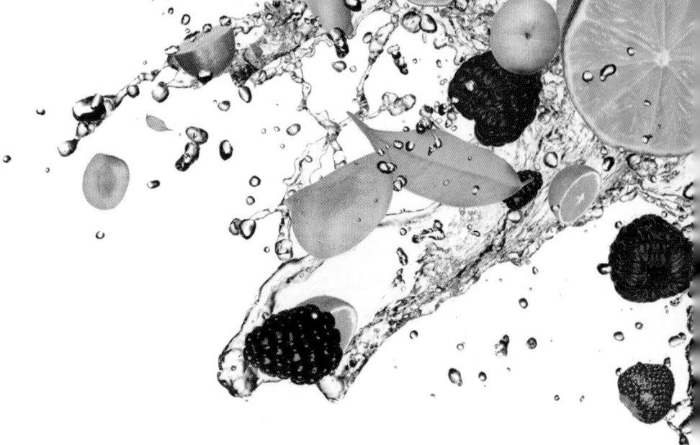

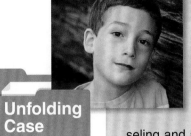

Unfolding Case

Dylan Masters

Dylan is a 5-year-old boy who has up to 20 seizures a day due to epilepsy. He is a candidate for a ketogenic diet because antiseizure medications have failed to control his seizures. Although there are several different levels of the diet, it is characterized as a high-fat, adequate-protein, very-low-carbohydrate diet. Dylan's classic ketogenic diet will provide 1200 calories, 120 g of fat, 18 g of protein, and 12 g of carbohydrate. The family has undergone extensive counseling and agreed to try the diet for at least 12 weeks; they understand the risks and that all foods must be carefully prepared and weighed on a gram scale. Dylan will be under close medical and nutritional supervision and will start the diet in the hospital, where he will be closely monitored by a neurologist and registered dietitian. Lab work will be used to identify metabolic abnormalities and evaluate serum nutrient levels.

Learning Objectives

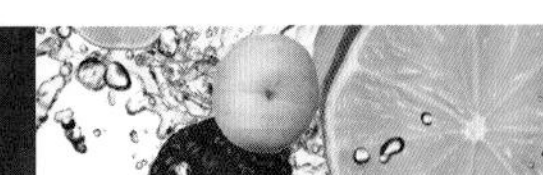

Upon completion of this chapter, you will be able to:

1 List sources of saturated, monounsaturated, and polyunsaturated fatty acids and discuss how they impact health.
2 List sources of dietary cholesterol.
3 Name sources of synthetic trans fats.
4 Explain the functions of fat in the body.
5 Discuss the digestion and absorption of fat.
6 Give examples of foods that provide omega-3 fatty acids.
7 Discuss strategies for making healthier food choices based on fat.

Fat has many vital functions in food and improves the overall palatability of the diet. It absorbs the flavors and aromas of ingredients to improve overall taste. It adds juiciness to meats and mouthfeel to milk. Fat is the ingredient that makes cakes tender, ice cream creamy, and pie crusts flaky. Nothing can duplicate the unique properties of fats in foods.

However, the amount and quality of fat in the typical American diet has been the subject of study and debate for decades. "Avoid too much fat" appeared in the first edition of the *Dietary Guidelines for Americans* published in 1980 (the 1980 DGA can be found with a quick Google search). Since then, studies have shown that the relationship between fat and health is far more complex than that statement implies. Current recommendations put forth by many American and international health and government agencies recommend emphasizing or limiting specific sources of fat rather than addressing total fat intake.

Sterols
one of three main classes of lipids, which include cholesterol, bile acids, sex hormones, the adrenocortical hormones, and vitamin D.

Lipids
a group of water-insoluble, energy-yielding organic compounds composed of carbon, hydrogen, and oxygen atoms.

There are three classes of **lipids**, which are referred to as *fat* throughout the rest of this chapter and book: triglycerides (fats and oils), which account for 98% of the fat in food; phospholipids (e.g., lecithin); and sterols (e.g., cholesterol). This chapter describes the classes of fats, their dietary sources, and how they are handled in the body. The functions of fat and recommendations regarding intake are presented.

TRIGLYCERIDES

Triglycerides
a class of lipids composed of a glycerol molecule as its backbone with three fatty acids attached.

Fatty Acids
organic compounds composed of a chain of carbon atoms to which hydrogen atoms are attached. An acid group (COOH) is attached at one end, and a methyl group (CH_3) at the other end.

Glycerol
a three-carbon atom chain that serves as the backbone of triglycerides.

Chemically, **triglycerides** are made of the same elements as carbohydrates—namely, carbon, hydrogen, and oxygen. There are proportionately more carbon and hydrogen atoms to oxygen atoms, so triglycerides yield more calories per gram than carbohydrates. Structurally, triglycerides are composed of a three-carbon atom glycerol backbone with three fatty acids attached (Fig. 5.1). An individual triglyceride molecule may contain one, two, or three different types of fatty acids.

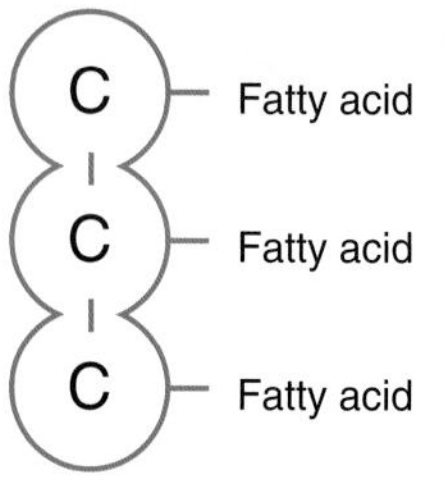

Figure 5.1 ▲
Generic triglyceride molecule.

Fatty Acids

Fatty acids are basically chains of carbon atoms with hydrogen atoms attached (Fig. 5.2). At one end of the chain is a methyl group (CH_3), and at the other end is an acid group (COOH).

- Fatty acids attach to **glycerol** molecules in various ratios and combinations to form a variety of triglycerides within a single food fat.
- The types and proportions of fatty acids present influence the sensory and functional properties of the food fat. For instance, butter tastes and acts differently from corn oil, which tastes and acts differently from lard.

Fatty Acid Chain Length

Fatty acids vary in the length of their carbon chain. Almost all naturally occurring fatty acids have an even number of carbon atoms in their chain, generally between 4 and 24.

- Long-chain fatty acids (containing more than 12 carbon atoms) predominate in meat, fish, and vegetable oils and are the most common length fatty acid in the diet.
- Smaller amounts of medium-chain (8–12 carbon atoms) and short-chain (up to 6 carbon atoms) fatty acids are found primarily in dairy products.

Figure 5.2 ▶
Fatty acid configurations.

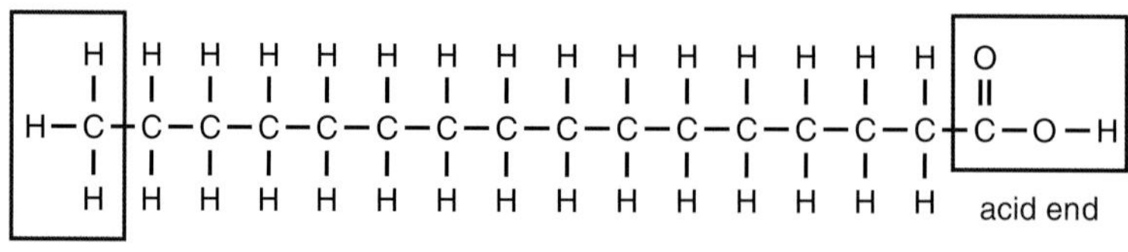

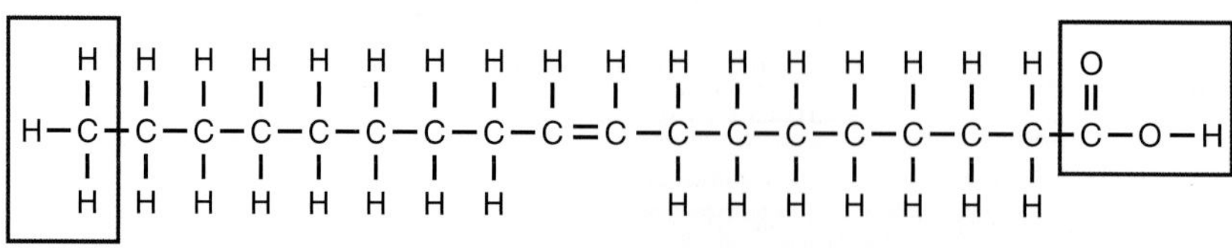

Oleic acid: 18 carbon *n*-9, monounsaturated fatty acid

Fatty Acid Saturation

Saturated Fatty Acids (SFAs) fatty acids in which all the carbon atoms are bonded to as many hydrogen atoms as they can hold, so no double bonds exist between carbon atoms.

Fatty acid saturation refers to the types of bonds between carbon atoms. Based on degree of saturation, fatty acids differ in their function, major sources, and impact on health (Table 5.1).

- When all the carbon atoms have four single bonds, the fatty acid is "saturated" with hydrogen atoms.
    - **Saturated fatty acids** are straight-line molecules that can pack tightly together; thus, they are solid at room temperature and referred to as "solid fat."

Table 5.1 Types of Fatty Acids, Their Functions, Sources, and Impact on Health

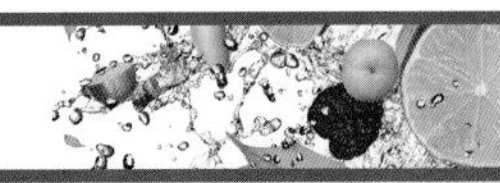

Types of Fatty Acids and Functions	Common Food Sources	Impact on Health
Saturated fatty acids (SFA) Functions: • Provide structure to cell membranes • Facilitate normal function of proteins	• Animal fats—beef, pork, poultry, veal, egg yolks, dairy products (the fat in milk does not appear as a solid due to the process of homogenization). • The only vegetable oils that are saturated are palm oil, palm kernel oil, and coconut oil. • Products containing palm, palm kernel, or coconut oils or any oil that is fully hydrogenated • The body makes more than enough saturated fats to meet its need	• As a category, saturated fat is associated with a higher risk of total and cause-specific death (Arnett et al., 2019). Although not all saturated fatty acids may negatively impact health, "good" and "bad" saturated fatty acids share the same food sources, so foods high in saturated fat should be limited. • Reducing saturated fat intake by replacing it with unsaturated fats, particularly PUFA, lowers the incidence of cardiovascular disease (CVD) in adults and reduces serum total and low-density cholesterol in all adults and some children (Dietary Guidelines Advisory Committee, 2020).
Monounsaturated fatty acids (MUFA) Functions: • Key components of membrane lipids, especially nervous tissue myelin	• Olives, olive oil, canola oil, avocado, peanut oil, and most nuts. • Meat fat contains moderate amounts of monounsaturated fats, providing approximately 50% of MUFAs in a typical American eating pattern (National Research Council, 2005).	• When substituted for saturated fatty acids, plant sources of MUFA but not animal sources may lower mortality risk (Guasch-Ferre et al., 2019).
Polyunsaturated fatty acids (PUFA) ***n*-3 fatty acids:** Components of phospholipids that form the structures of cell membranes		
Alpha linolenic acid (ALA) Function: • Precursor of EPA and DHA	• Soybean, flaxseed, and canola oils. • Other sources include walnuts and chia and hemp seeds. • Grass-fed cows produce beef with ALA but in very low amounts.	• May provide modest protection against CVD although the evidence is not as strong as the association of fish oils and CVD (Rajaram, 2014).
Eicosapentaenoic acid (EPA) and docosahexaenoic acid (DHA) Functions: • EPA is precursor for *n*-3 eicosanoids. • Eicosanoids made from *n*-3 tend to have anti-inflammatory, antiarrhythmic, and anticlotting effects. • DHA is a structural component of red blood cell membranes and is abundant in retinal tissue, neuron cells, the liver, and testes.	• Fatty fish, especially salmon, anchovy, sardines, tuna, herring, and mackerel. • Food products fortified with EPA and/or DHA are available, such as soy milks, cooking oils, margarine-like spreads, breakfast cereals, baked goods, infant formulas, and baby food and juices.	• *n*-3 fatty acids are best known for their heart health benefits, which are attributed to their antiinflammatory, anticlotting, and anti-arrhythmic effects. • Evidence supports recommendations to consume seafood, especially species that are higher in *n*-3 fatty acids, 1–2 times per week for cardiovascular benefits, including lower risk of cardiac death, coronary heart disease, and ischemic stroke, especially when seafood replaces the intake of less healthy foods (Rimm et al., 2018).
***n*-6 fatty acids** Functions: • LA is a precursor of arachidonic acid and other *n*-6 fatty acids • Components of membrane lipids • Play a role in cell signaling pathways • Play a role in maintaining normal skin cell function • Precursor of eicosanoids, including prostaglandins • Involved in regulation of genes for proteins that regulate fatty acid synthesis	• Linolenic acid: Soybean ("vegetable oil"), corn oil, safflower oil, poultry, nuts, seeds • Arachidonic acid: Found in small amounts in meat, poultry, and eggs	• Epidemiologic evidence shows an inverse relationship between *n*-6 fatty acid intake and CVD, coronary artery disease (CAD), diabetes, and CVD mortality and generally supports lower cardiometabolic disease risk with higher intakes of *n*-6 PUFA (Maki et al., 2018).

Unsaturated Fatty Acids fatty acids that are not completely saturated with hydrogen atoms, so one or more double bonds form between the carbon atoms.

- An "unsaturated" fatty acid does not have all the hydrogen atoms it can potentially hold; therefore, one (monounsaturated) or more (polyunsaturated) double bonds form between carbon atoms in the chain.
  - Because of the double bond, **unsaturated fatty acids** are physically kinked and unable to pack together tightly; they are liquid at room temperature and are referred to as "oils."

Further Unsaturated Fatty Acid Classification Based on the First Double Bond

Unsaturated fatty acids can be classified according to the location of their double bonds along the carbon chain. The most common method of identifying the bond is to count the number of carbon atoms from the methyl (CH_3) end, as denoted by the term *n* or *omega*.

Omega-3 (*n*-3) Fatty Acid an unsaturated fatty acid the endmost double bond of which occurs three carbon atoms from the methyl end of its carbon chain.

Polyunsaturated Fatty Acids (PUFA) fatty acids that have two or more double bonds between carbon atoms.

Fish Oils a common term for the long-chain, polyunsaturated omega-3 fatty acids EPA and DHA found in the fat of fish, primarily in cold-water fish.

Omega-6 (*n*-6) Fatty Acid an unsaturated fatty acid the endmost double bond of which occurs six carbon atoms from the methyl end of its carbon chain.

Monounsaturated Fatty Acids (MUFA) fatty acids that have only one double bond between two carbon atoms.

Essential Fatty Acids fatty acids that cannot be synthesized in the body and thus must be consumed through food.

- **Omega-3 fatty acids (*n*-3)** are **polyunsaturated fatty acids (PUFA)** with the first double-bond three carbons from the methyl end. Several *n*-3 fatty acids exist, but the majority of research focuses on three: alpha-linolenic acid (ALA) found in certain plants and the two "**fish oils**" eicosapentaenoic acid (EPA) and docosahexaenoic acid (DHA).
- **Omega-6 fatty acids (*n*-6)** are PUFA that have the first double-bond 6 carbons from the methyl end. The two major *n*-6 fatty acids are linoleic acid (LA) and arachidonic acid (ARA).
- Omega-9 (*n*-9) fatty acids are **monounsaturated fatty acids (MUFA)** with the only double-bond 9 carbon atoms from the methyl end.

Essential Fatty Acids

The location of the first double bond is significant because it determines if the fatty acid is essential. *Essential* does not refer to importance but rather to whether it must be consumed through food because it cannot be synthesized in the body.

- The body is unable to synthesize fatty acids with double bonds closer than *n*-9, so one *n*-6 fatty acid (LA) and one *n*-3 fatty acid (ALA) are deemed essential.
  - Although the body cannot make **essential fatty acids**, it does store them, making cases of deficiencies of either *n*-3 or *n*-6 fatty acids virtually nonexistent in the United States.
- MUFAs are *n*-9 fatty acids and thus are not essential.
- Saturated fatty acids do have double bonds, so none are essential.

Linoleic Acid (*n*-6)

LA accounts for 80% to 90% of total dietary PUFA intake (Micha et al., 2014).

- The richest source of LA in the typical American diet is soybean oil (often labeled as vegetable oil) because it used extensively in processed foods.
- The body can make other *n*-6 fatty acids, such as ARA, from LA. However, if a deficiency of LA develops, ARA becomes "conditionally essential" because the body is unable to synthesize it without a supply of LA.

Alpha-Linolenic Acid (*n*-3 from plants)

ALA is the most prominent *n*-3 fatty acid in most Western diets because average seafood intake (source of EPA and DHA) is low.

- The richest sources of ALA are soybean and canola oils.
- Humans can convert ALA into the *n*-3 fatty acids EPA and DHA to only a very limited extent, so the only practical way to increase the levels of these fatty acids in the body is to

Figure 5.3 ▶
Trans and cis fatty acid configurations.

Trans-position: H on opposite sides of double bond

Cis-position: H on same side of double bond

Cis Fats
unsaturated fatty acids whose hydrogen atoms occur on the same side of the double bond.

Trans Fats
unsaturated fatty acids that have at least one double bond the hydrogen atoms of which are on the opposite sides of the double bond; *trans* means "across" in Latin.

Hydrogenation
a process of adding hydrogen atoms to unsaturated vegetable oils (usually corn, soybean, cottonseed, safflower, or canola oil), which reduces the number of double bonds; the number of saturated and monounsaturated bonds increases as the number of polyunsaturated bonds decreases.

Rancidity
the chemical change that occurs when fats are oxidized, which causes an offensive taste and smell and the loss of fat-soluble vitamins A and E.

Low-Density Lipoprotein (LDL) Cholesterol
the major class of atherogenic lipoproteins that carry cholesterol from the liver to the tissues.

Generally Recognized as Safe (GRAS)
compounds exempt from the definition of "food additive" because they are GRAS, based on "a reasonable certainty of no harm from a product under the intended conditions of use."

Partial or Light Hydrogenation
some, but not all, unsaturated fatty acids are converted to saturated fatty acids. Some of the unsaturated fatty acids are changed from a cis to a trans configuration.

consume seafood or take *n*-3 fatty acid supplements (National Institutes of Health, Office of Dietary Supplements, 2019).

Trans Fatty Acids

The term *trans* refers to the placement of the hydrogen atoms in relation to double carbon bonds. Almost all double bonds in nature exist in the **cis** position; **trans** bonds are rare in nature (Fig. 5.3).

- Only small amounts of trans fats occur naturally in some animal foods, such as beef, lamb, and dairy products.
- Synthetic sources of trans fats were once widespread in the food supply from partially hydrogenated oils (e.g., stick margarine and shortening) and processed foods containing them (e.g., crackers, doughnuts, frozen french fries).
  - The process of **hydrogenation** of oils extends stability (e.g., longer shelf life because fewer double bonds lower the risk of **rancidity**) and functionality (e.g., crispier french fries, creamier frosting), so partially hydrogenated oils permeated the food supply.
  - It eventually became evident that synthetic trans fats are detrimental to health, because they increase **low-density lipoprotein (LDL)**–cholesterol and increase the risk of CVD.
  - Based on extensive research and public input, the U.S. Food & Drug Administration (FDA) withdrew partially hydrogenated oils status as **Generally Recognized as Safe (GRAS)** (Food & Drug Administration [FDA], 2018).
- In place of **partial or light** hydrogenated fats, food manufacturers are using palm oil, fully hydrogenated palm oil, or a blend of oils. The result is that trans fatty acids are eliminated, but saturated fat content increases.
- Trans fatty acid content is listed on the Nutrition Facts label. There is no %Daily Value, because it is recommended that trans fat intake be as close to zero as possible.

Food Fats

All food fats contain a mixture of saturated, monounsaturated, and PUFA (Fig. 5.4). When used to characterize fat in food, *unsaturated* and *saturated* are not absolute terms; rather, they are relative descriptions that indicate which kinds of fatty acids are present in the largest proportion. For instance, olive oil is classified as monounsaturated fat, because 73% of its fatty acids are MUFA. Of its remaining fatty acids, 10% are PUFA and 14% are saturated.

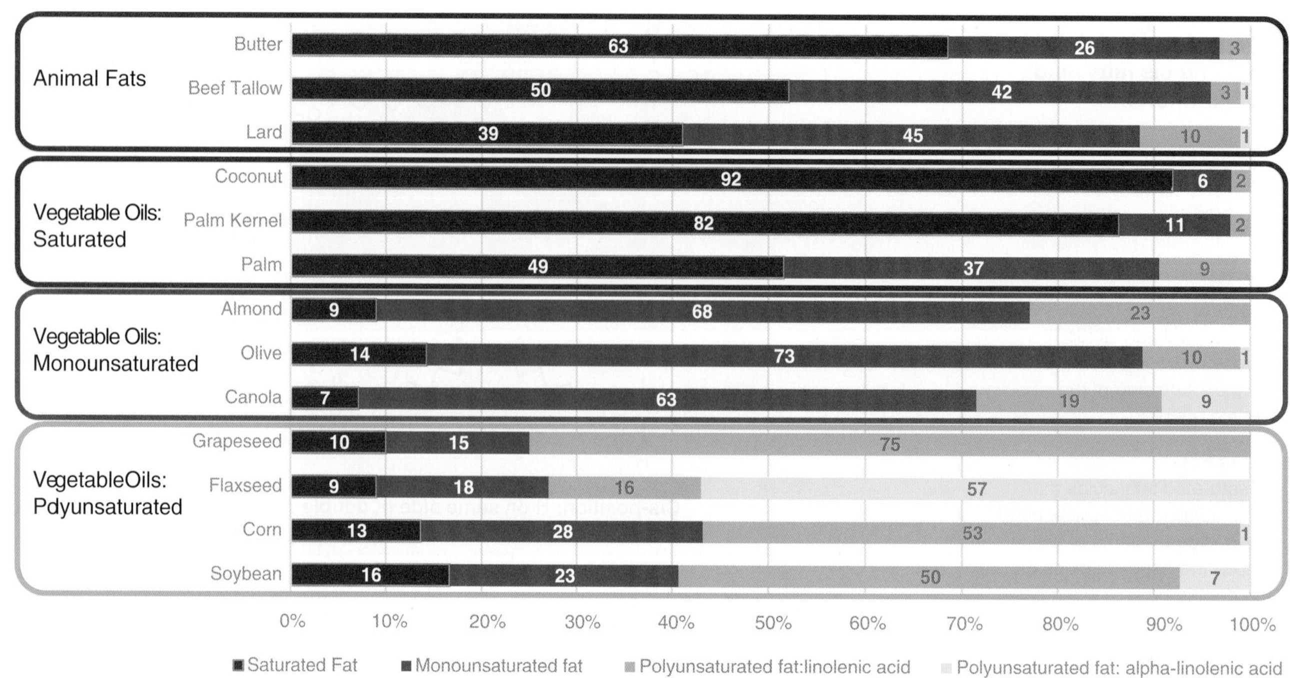

Figure 5.4 ▲ Fatty acid profile of selected animal fats and vegetable oils. (*Source:* Maki, K., Eren, F., Cassens, M., Dicklin, M. R., & Davisdon, M. H. [2018]. n-6 polyunsaturated fatty acids and cardiometabolic health: Current evidence, controversies, and research gaps. *Advances in Nutrition, 9*, 688–700. https://doi.org/10.1093/advances/nmy038; Garavaglia, J., Markowski, M., Oliveira, A., & Marcadenti, A. [2016]. Grapeseed oil compounds: Biological and chemical actions for health. *Nutrition and Metabolic Insights, 9*, 59–64; Flax Council of Canada (n.d.). A focus on fatty acids. https://flaxcouncil.ca/resources/nutrition/general-nutrition-information/a-focus-on-fatty-acids.)

Note. Expressed as percentages. Numbers may not total 100 due to the presence of other fatty acids, such as naturally present trans fatty acids in butter.

OTHER LIPIDS

Phospholipids and cholesterol are two other types of lipids.

Phospholipids

Phospholipids
a group of compound lipids that is similar to triglycerides in that they contain a glycerol molecule and two fatty acids. In place of the third fatty acid, phospholipids have a phosphate group and a molecule of choline or another nitrogen-containing compound.

Emulsifier
a stabilizing compound that helps to keep both parts of an emulsion (oil and water mixture) from separating.

Like triglycerides, **phospholipids** have a glycerol backbone with fatty acids attached. What makes them different from triglycerides is that a phosphate group replaces one of the fatty acids. Although phospholipids occur naturally in almost all foods, they make up a very small percentage of total fat intake.

- Phospholipids are both fat soluble (because of the fatty acids) and water soluble (because of the phosphate group), which is a unique feature that enables them to act as **emulsifiers**.
- As emulsifiers, they surround fats and keep them suspended in blood and other body fluids.
- As a component of all cell membranes, phospholipids provide structure and help to transport fat-soluble substances across cell membranes.
- Phospholipids are also precursors of prostaglandins.
- Lecithin is the best-known phospholipid.

Cholesterol

Cholesterol is a sterol, a waxy substance whose carbon, hydrogen, and oxygen molecules are arranged in a ring.

- Cholesterol is found in all cell membranes and in myelin. Brain and nerve cells are especially rich in cholesterol.
- The body makes cholesterol from acetyl-coenzyme A (acetyl-CoA), which can originate from carbohydrates, protein, fat, or alcohol. Eating an excess of calories, regardless of the source, can increase cholesterol synthesis.
- All body cells are capable of making enough cholesterol to meet their needs, so cholesterol is not an essential nutrient. In fact, daily endogenous cholesterol synthesis is approximately two to three times more than average cholesterol intake.
- Although cholesterol is made from acetyl-CoA, the body cannot break down cholesterol into CoA molecules to yield energy, so cholesterol does not provide calories.
- The body synthesizes bile acids, steroid hormones, and vitamin D from cholesterol.
- Dietary cholesterol is found exclusively in animals, with organ meats and egg yolks the richest sources. Meats, shrimp, lobster, and full-fat dairy products provide moderate amounts.
- The cholesterol in food is just cholesterol; descriptions of "good" and "bad" cholesterol refer to the lipoprotein packages that move cholesterol through the blood (see Chapter 22). You cannot eat more "good" cholesterol, but you can make lifestyle changes, such as quitting smoking, exercising, and losing weight if overweight, that increase the amount of "good" cholesterol in the blood.

FUNCTIONS OF FAT IN THE BODY

The primary function of fat is to fuel the body. At rest, fat provides about 60% of the body's calorie needs. All fat—whether saturated, unsaturated, cis, or trans—provides 9 cal/g, which is more than double the amount of calories as an equivalent amount of either carbohydrate or protein. Although fat is an important energy source, it cannot meet all of the body's energy needs, because certain cells, such as brain cells and cells of the central nervous system, normally rely solely on glucose for energy.

Fat has other important functions in the body. Fat deposits insulate and cushion internal organs to protect them from mechanical injury. Fat under the skin helps to regulate body temperature by serving as a layer of insulation against the cold. And dietary fat facilitates the absorption of the fat-soluble vitamins A, D, E, and K when consumed at the same meal. Table 5.1 lists the functions of fatty acids by type.

HOW THE BODY HANDLES FAT

Digestion and Absorption

A minimal amount of chemical digestion of fat occurs in the mouth and stomach through the action of lingual lipase and gastric lipases, respectively (Fig. 5.5).

- Fat entering the duodenum stimulates the release of the hormone cholecystokinin, which, in turn, stimulates the gallbladder to release bile.
- Bile, an emulsifier produced in the liver from bile salts, cholesterol, phospholipids, bilirubin, and electrolytes, prepares fat for digestion by suspending the hydrophobic molecules in the watery intestinal fluid. Emulsified fat particles have enlarged surface areas on which digestive enzymes can work.
- Most fat digestion occurs in the small intestine. Pancreatic lipase, the most important and powerful lipase, splits off one fatty acid at a time from the triglyceride molecule, working from the outside in until two free fatty acids and a **monoglyceride** remain.
- Usually, the process stops at this point, but sometimes, digestion continues and the monoglyceride splits into a free fatty acid and a glyceride molecule.

Monoglyceride
a glyceride molecule with only one fatty acid attached.

Figure 5.5 ▶ **Fat digestion.**

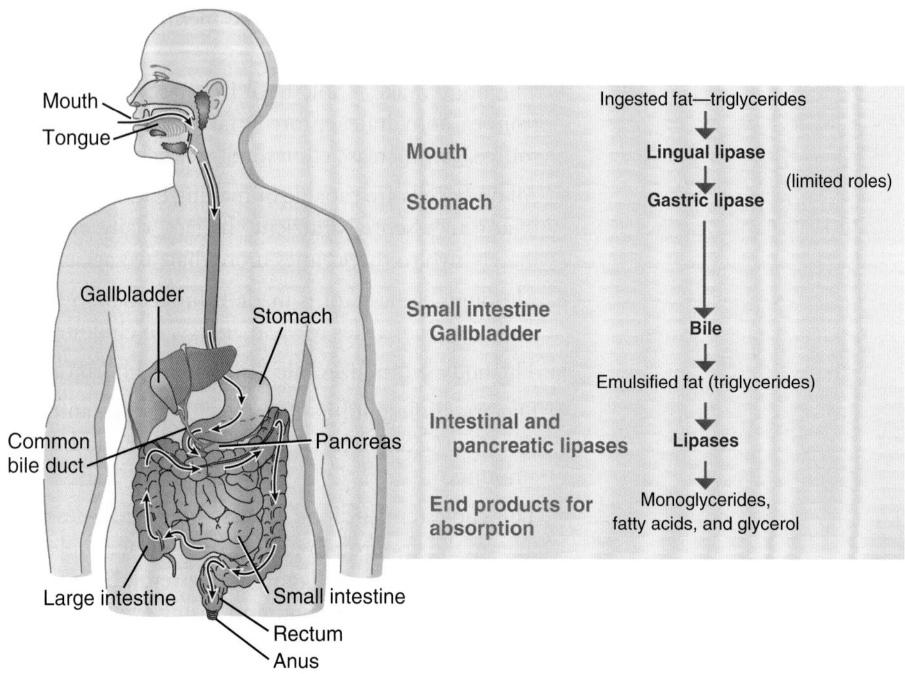

- The end products of digestion—mostly monoglycerides with free fatty acids and little glycerol—are absorbed into intestinal cells. It is normal for a small amount of fat (4–5 g) to escape digestion and be excreted in the feces.
- The digestion of phospholipids is similar, with the end products being two free fatty acids and a phospholipid fragment.
- Cholesterol does not undergo digestion; it is absorbed as is.

Absorption

- About 95% of consumed fat is absorbed, mostly in the duodenum and jejunum.
- Small fat particles, such as short- and medium-chain fatty acids and glycerol, are absorbed directly through the mucosal cells into capillaries. They bind with albumin and are transported to the liver via the portal vein.
- The absorption of larger fat particles—namely, monoglycerides and long-chain fatty acids—is more complex. Although they are insoluble in water, monoglycerides and long-chain fatty acids dissolve into **micelles**, which deliver fat to the intestinal cells. Once inside the intestinal cells, the monoglycerides and long-chain fatty acids combine to form triglycerides. The reformed triglycerides, along with phospholipids and cholesterol, become encased in protein to form **chylomicrons** and enter circulation via the lymphatic system.
- Once in the bloodstream, lipoprotein particles circulate, delivering dietary lipids to various organs for oxidation, metabolism, or to store in adipose tissue.
- Their job done, most of the released bile salts are reabsorbed in the terminal ileum, transported back to the liver, and recycled (enterohepatic circulation). Some bile salts become bound to fiber in the intestine and are excreted in the feces.

Micelles
fat particles encircled by bile salts to facilitate their diffusion into intestinal cells.

Chylomicrons
lipoproteins that transport absorbed lipids from intestinal cells through the lymph and eventually into the bloodstream.

Fat Catabolism

Whether from the most recent meal or from storage, triglycerides that are needed for energy are split into glycerol and fatty acids by lipoprotein lipase, and are released into the bloodstream to be picked up by cells.

- The catabolism of fatty acids increases when carbohydrate intake is inadequate (e.g., while on a very-low-calorie or low-carbohydrate diet) or unavailable (e.g., in the case of uncontrolled diabetes). Without adequate glucose, the breakdown of fatty acids is incomplete, and ketones are formed. Eventually, ketosis and acidosis may result.
- Since fatty acids break down into two-carbon molecules, not three-carbon molecules, they cannot be reassembled to make glucose. Only the glycerol component of triglycerides can be used to make glucose, making fat an inefficient choice of fuel for glucose-dependent brain cells, nerve cells, and red blood cells. Fortunately, most body cells can use fatty acids for energy.

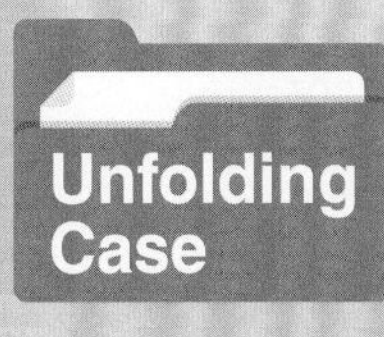

Recall Dylan. It is well known that starvation causes a decrease in seizure activity, although the mechanism of action is not known. Starvation causes acidosis, ketosis, dehydration, and hypoglycemia. The ketogenic diet provides calories and carbohydrate at levels that mimic a starved state in which the primary fuel is fat. Dylan's blood work confirms a low pH related to ketoacids. What does that finding indicate in terms of dietary compliance?

Fat Anabolism

Most newly absorbed fatty acids recombine with glycerol to form triglycerides that end up stored in adipose tissue. Fat stored in adipose cells represents the body's largest and most efficient energy reserve; most other body cells are able to store only minute amounts of fat.

- Unlike glycogen, which can be stored only in limited amounts and is accompanied by water, adipose cells have a virtually limitless capacity to store fat, and carry very little additional weight as intracellular water.
- Fat reserves can last up to 2 months in people of normal weight.
- Each pound of body fat provides 3500 calories.

SOURCES OF FAT

Food categories that provide naturally occurring fat are protein foods, dairy, and oils (Table 5.2). Vegetables and grains naturally provide little or no fat; however, some items within each group may have added fat, such as fried or creamed vegetables and granola cereals and biscuits. Fruit is naturally fat free, with the exception of avocado, coconut, and olives. Within all calorie levels of MyPlate meal patterns and across all food groups, the amount of food recommended is based on the assumption that all foods chosen are in their most nutrient-dense form: vegetables, fruits, whole grains, seafood, eggs, beans, peas, lentils, unsalted nuts and seeds, fat-free and low-fat dairy products, and lean meats and poultry—all prepared with no or little saturated fat.

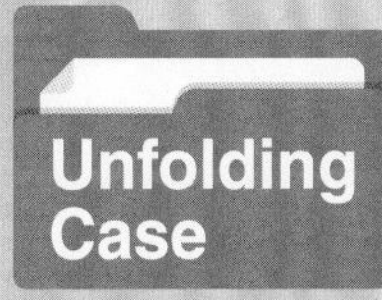

Think of Dylan. A typical ketogenic meal consists mostly of fats (e.g., 5 tbsp heavy whipping cream) with approximately an ounce of protein (e.g., chicken) and a small amount of carbohydrate (e.g., <½ cup green beans). What serving suggestions would you make to help make the high-fat diet more palatable?

Table 5.2 Sources of Fat: Average Fat Content per Serving

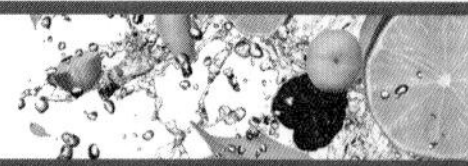

Protein

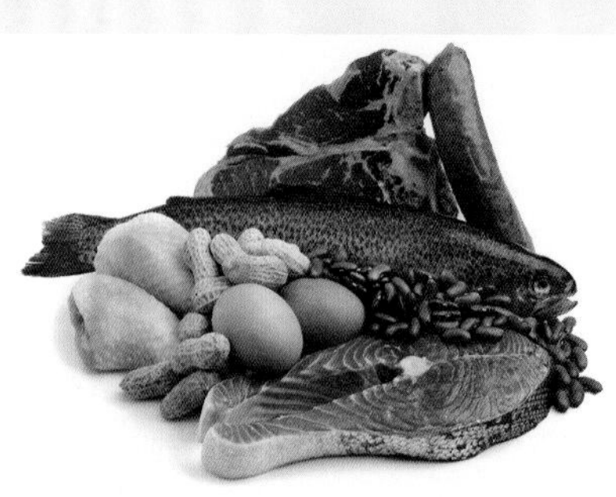

Lean proteins provide 2 g fat per oz

- Lean cuts of beef, pork veal, ham
- Skinless poultry
- Ninety percent lean or higher ground beef, chicken, or turkey
- Fish and shellfish
- Game: buffalo, ostrich, rabbit, venison
- Organ meats: heart, kidney, liver
- Veal: cutlet, loin chop, roast
- Egg substitutes, egg whites
- Processed deli meats with 3 g or fat or less per oz

Medium-fat proteins provide 5 g fat per oz

- Beef trimmed of visible fat, 85% or lower lean ground beef, USDA Prime cuts of beef
- Cheeses with 4–7 g fat/oz, such as feta and mozzarella
- Egg
- Fried fish
- Poultry with skin; fried chicken

High-fat proteins provide 8 g fat per choice

- 1 oz regular cheese
- 2 slices pork bacon or 3 slices turkey bacon
- Turkey or chicken hot dogs
- 1 oz of certain processed deli meats, such as bologna, hard salami, pastrami
- 1 oz certain sausages, such as bratwurst, chorizo, Italian, Knockwurst, Polish, smoked, summer

Plant-based proteins vary in fat content from very little in legumes to 8 g in a tablespoon of nut spreads such as peanut butter, almond butter, and soy nut butter

Milk, yogurt, and milk substitutes

Milk, yogurt, and milk substitute choices vary in fat content

- 0–3 g fat in fat-free or low-fat (1% fat) choices: 1 cup milk, 2/3 cup plain yogurt, or 1 cup light soy milk
- 5 g fat in 2% choices: 1 cup milk, 2/3 cup plain yogurt, 1 cup regular-fat plain soy milk, 1 cup flavored coconut milk
- 8 g fat in whole-milk choices: 1 cup milk or 1 cup plain yogurt

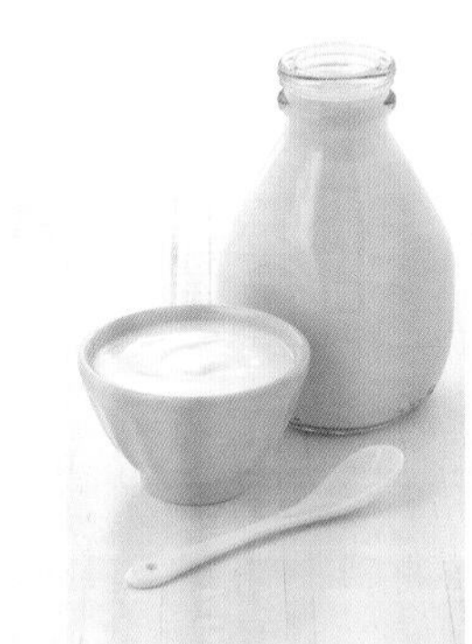

Oils and fats

1 serving provides 5 g fat

- 1 tsp oil, such as canola, olive, corn, soybean, flaxseed, or coconut
- 1 tsp solid fat, such as stick or tub margarine, stick butter, regular mayonnaise, lard, or shortening
- 1 tbsp salad dressing, such as regular Italian
- 6 almonds or cashews
- 2 tbsp avocado
- 1 tbsp pumpkin, sesame, or sunflower seeds
- 2 tbsp half and half, whipped cream, or regular sour cream

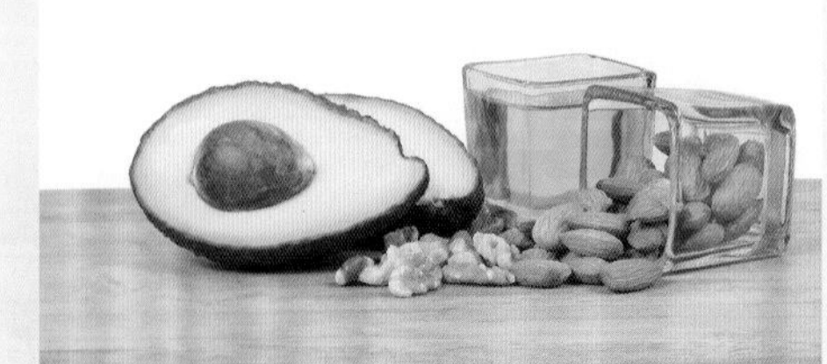

Note. Based on American Diabetes Association, Academy of Nutrition and Dietetics. (2019). *Choose your foods. Food lists for diabetes*. American Diabetes Association & Academy of Nutrition.

Source: shutterstock.com/Hurst Photo; shutterstock.com/Modernista Magazine; shutterstock.com/Photo Art Lucas

Adequate Intake (AI)
an intake level thought to meet or exceed the requirement of almost all members of a life stage and gender group; AI is set when there are insufficient data to define an RDA.

Recommended Dietary Allowance (RDA)
the average daily dietary intake level sufficient to meet the nutrient requirements of 97% to 98% of healthy people in a particular life stage and gender group.

DIETARY REFERENCE INTAKES

Fats that the body can synthesize—namely, saturated fatty acids, MUFAs, and cholesterol—do not need to be consumed through food. Trans fats provide no known health benefits, and so they are not essential. Neither an **Adequate Intake (AI)** nor a **Recommended Dietary Allowance (RDA)** exists for any of these fats. Box 5.1 outlines the DRI for adults for total fat and specific types of fat.

Total Fat Recommendation and Average Intake

An **Acceptable Macronutrient Distribution Range (AMDR)** for total fat intake is estimated to be 20% to 35% of the total calories for adults (Fig. 5.6). There is insufficient data to define a level of total fat intake at which the risk of deficiency or prevention of chronic disease occurs, so there is not an AI or RDA for total fat (National Research Council, 2005).

BOX 5.1 Dietary Reference Intakes for Adults for Total Fat and Specific Types of Fat

Total Fat

- AMDR 20% to 35% of total calories
- No RDA, AI, or **Tolerable Upper Intake Level (UL)**

Saturated Fatty Acids, Cholesterol, and Trans Fat

- No RDA or AI because a dietary source is not required
- No UL because any incremental increase in intake increases the risk of coronary heart disease

Monounsaturated Fatty Acids

- No RDA or AI because a dietary source is not required
- Evidence is insufficient to set a UL

Alpha-Linolenic Acid (*n*-3 Fatty Acid)

- AMDR 0.6% to 1.2% of total calories
- AI: 1.1 g/day for women; 1.6 g/day for men
- Evidence insufficient to set a UL

Linoleic Acid (*n*-6 Fatty Acid)

- AMDR 5% to 10% of total calories
- AI: 11 to 12 g/day for women; 14 to 17 g/day for men
- Evidence insufficient to set a UL

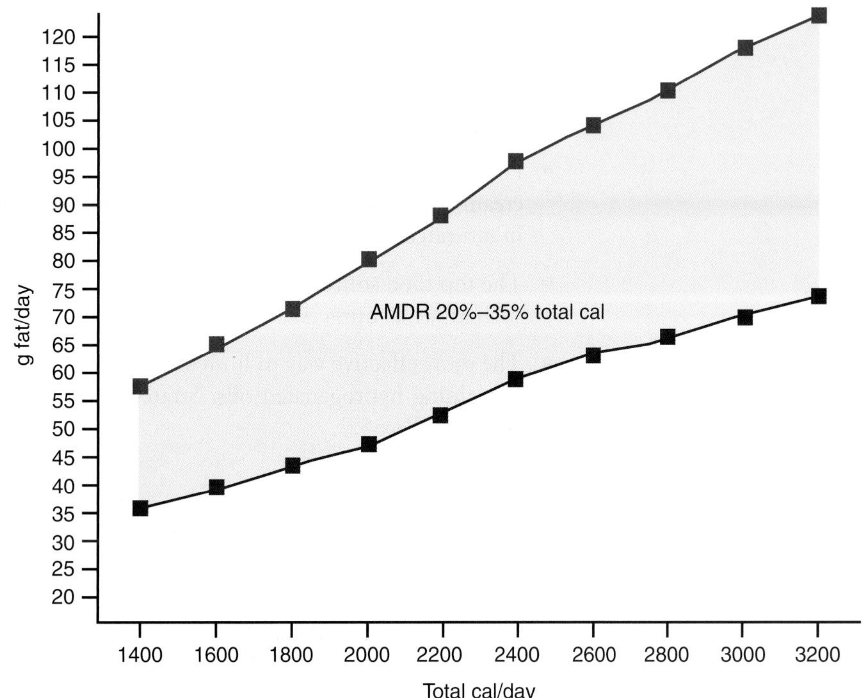

Figure 5.6 ▶ **Amount of total fat appropriate at various calorie levels based on AMDR of 20% to 35% of total calories.**

Acceptable Macronutrient Distribution Range (AMDR)
an intake range as a percentage of total calories for energy nutrients.

Tolerable Upper Intake Level (UL)
the highest average daily intake level of a nutrient likely to pose no danger to most individuals in the group.

Unlike carbohydrate and protein, Americans consume more than the AMDR for fat. The National Health and Nutrition Examination Survey 2015 to 2016 data show that 36% of total calories consumed by males and females age 20 and older come from fat, with 12% of total calorie intake from saturated fat (USDA & Agricultural Research Service [ARS], 2018). As total fat intake increases, the amount of saturated fat increases; therefore, limiting total fat intake to 35% of total calories or less may help limit saturated fat intake.

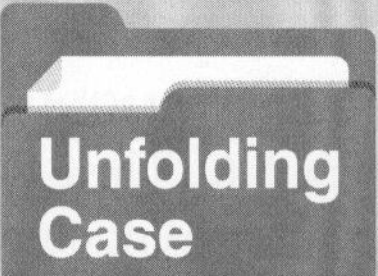

Consider Dylan. His 1200 calorie eating pattern provides 18 g of protein, 12 g of carbohydrate, and 120 g of fat.

- What are the percentages of calories from protein, carbohydrate, and fat?
- How do these percentages compare to the AMDR for each of these macronutrients?
- What nutrients are deficient in the diet due to the severe restriction on carbohydrates?

FAT IN HEALTH PROMOTION

In general, health is "promoted" when total fat intake and the types of fat consumed are appropriate based on calorie needs. Exactly what "appropriate" is in terms of individual fatty acids is not entirely clear. Dietary advice on fat intake generally centers specifically on saturated fat content and broadly on healthy eating patterns.

Limit Saturated Fat

The *Dietary Guidelines for Americans 2020–2025* recommend limiting saturated fat intake to less than 10% of total calories for all people age 2 and older and replacing saturated fat with unsaturated fats, particularly polyunsaturated fats (U.S. Department of Agriculture [USDA] & U.S. Department of Health and Human Services [USDHHS], 2020). Making this shift lowers the incidence of CVD in adults and reduces serum total and low-density cholesterol in all adults and some children (Dietary Guidelines Advisory Committee, 2020).

- Even with nutrient-dense food choices, approximately 5% of the calories in the Healthy U.S.-Style Eating Pattern comes from saturated fat present in lean meat, poultry, eggs, nuts, seeds, grains, and oils, leaving little room for higher saturated fat choices (USDA & USDHHS, 2020).
- Foods highest in saturated fat include fatty meats; full-fat milk, yogurt, cheese, and ice cream; and butter. The tropical oils coconut oil, palm kernel oil, and palm oil are also high in saturated fat.
- The top food sources of saturated fat among Americans ages 1 and older are sand wiches, such as tacos, burgers, and chicken sandwiches (Fig. 5.7).
- The most effective way to limit saturated fats is to eat less animal fats and processed foods containing hydrogenated oils. Strategies for making healthier food choices based on fat appear in Box 5.2.

Healthy Eating Patterns

With the exception of quantifying limits on saturated fat, most intake recommendations from leading health organizations emphasize healthy eating patterns and types of food rather than specific types of fat. For instance, the American College of Cardiology/American Heart Association guidelines to reduce the risk of atherosclerotic cardiovascular disease (ASCVD) recommend an eating pattern that emphasizes vegetables, fruits, legumes, nuts, whole grains,

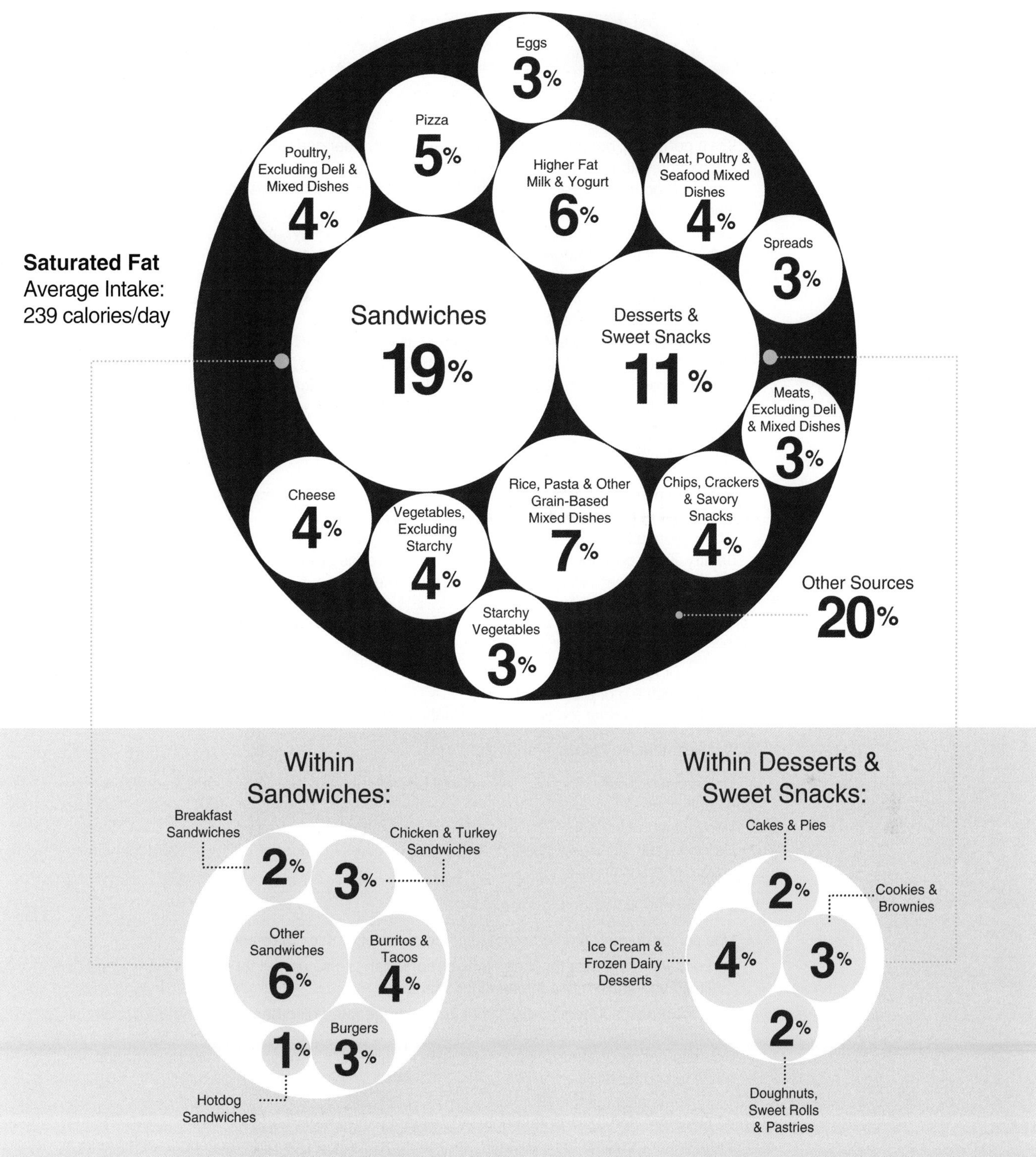

Figure 5.7 ▲ **Top sources and average intakes of saturated fat: U.S. population ages 1 and older.** (*Source:* U.S. Department of Agriculture, U.S. Department of Health and Human Services. [2020]. *Dietary Guidelines for Americans 2020–2025.* https://www.dietaryguidelines.gov; Data Source: What We Eat in America, NHANES, 2013–2016, ages 1 and older, 2 days intake data, weighted).

BOX 5.2 Strategies for Making Healthier Food Choices Regarding Fat

Make better protein choices

- Keep portion sizes of protein to the amount recommended for your appropriate calorie level. 5½ oz-equivalents are recommended per day for a 2000-calorie eating pattern. Limit the intake of red meat (beef, pork, veal, lamb) to 3 to 4 times per week or 12 to 18 oz total per week.
- Minimize processed meat intake: bacon (regular and turkey), hot dogs, corned beef, pepperoni, salami, beef jerky, bologna, canned meats, etc.
- Eat 8 oz of fish per week; best choices regarding mercury content include salmon, sardines, herring, freshwater trout, and Atlantic mackerel (see Fig. 4.3 for more choices). If you eat more than 8 oz of fish per week, choose a variety of seafood.
- Choose lean cuts of meat that are labeled as "round," "loin," or "sirloin."
- "Select" grades of beef have less fat marbled through than "Choice" grades.
- Choose ground beef that is at least 90% lean. This is indicated on the label.
- Trim all visible fat from meat before cooking and drain fat after cooking.
- Remove poultry skin.
- Bake, broil, grill, stew, or roast meats, poultry, and seafood. Avoid frying and breading meat or poultry.
- Eat more plant-based meals: bean burritos, black beans and rice, meatless chili, vegetable stir-fry with tofu, and lentil soup.
- Choose unsalted nuts or seeds as a snack, on salads, or in main dishes to replace meat or poultry. Keep portions small because nuts and seeds are high in calories.
- Replace deli meats with leftover chicken or turkey; use canned tuna or salmon, hummus, or nut butters for sandwiches.

Choose low-fat or fat-free dairy items.

- fat-free or low-fat milk and yogurt
- cheese with 3 g or less per serving
- sherbet, reduced-fat ice cream, and nonfat ice cream

Limit solid fats used in food preparation.

- Use nonstick spray, olive oil, or canola oil in place of margarine or butter to sauté foods and "butter" pans.
- Use imitation butter spray to season vegetables and hot-air popcorn.
- Use oils—especially soybean, canola, corn, or olive—instead of butter or shortening for cooking and baking.

Use oils as a healthier option to solid fat.

- Use soft margarine (liquid or tub) in place of butter or stick margarine.
  - Look for margarine that contains no more than 2 g saturated fat per tablespoon and has liquid vegetable oil as the first ingredient.
- Look for processed foods made with non-hydrogenated oil other than coconut oil, palm oil, or palm kernel oil.
- Eat nuts and nut butters that are rich in unsaturated fats: peanuts, walnuts, almonds, hazelnuts, pecans
  - Walnuts also contain ALA.
  - Cashews and macadamia nuts are higher in saturated fats.
- Sprinkle ground flaxseed, chia seeds, or hemp seed (1–2 tbsp/day) over cereal or yogurt.
  - Use ground flaxseed as a fat substitute in many recipes: 3 tbsp of ground flaxseed can replace 1 tbsp of fat or oil.

Replace fatty foods with fruit and vegetables.

- Eat fruit for dessert instead of baked goods or full-fat ice cream.
- Snack on raw vegetables or fresh fruit instead of snack chips.

Consider the following foods as "treats" to be used only on occasion and in small portions.

BOX 5.2 Strategies for Making Healthier Food Choices Regarding Fat (continued)

- Baked goods: cakes, cookies, pies, doughnuts, muffins, etc.
- candy
- Full-fat dairy: whole milk, sour cream, cheese, and ice cream
- pizza and fast food
- Fatty meats: ribs, Prime rib, fried chicken, etc.
- Processed meats: bacon (regular and turkey), hot dogs, corned beef, pepperoni, salami, beef jerky, bologna, canned meats, etc.

and fish to decrease ASCVD risk factors (Arnett et al., 2019). Additional fat-related intake recommendations state that

- replacing saturated fat with monounsaturated and polyunsaturated fats can help lower ASCVD risk (see Box 5.2)
- reducing cholesterol intake can be beneficial to decrease ASCVD risk, and
- within the context of a healthy eating pattern, it is reasonable to minimize the intake of processed meats (e.g., sausage, hot dogs, salami, cured bacon, salted and cured meats, and canned meats) and avoid the intake of trans fats (e.g., foods containing partially hydrogenated oils).

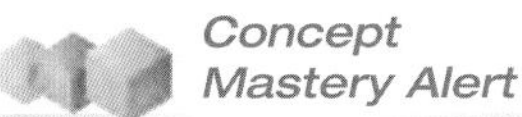

When providing instruction about what constitutes a "good" fat, nurses should emphasize soybean oil, flaxseed, walnuts, and salmon. Whole wheat bread for sandwiches is a healthy choice, but processed meat (like bologna) should be limited in the diet.

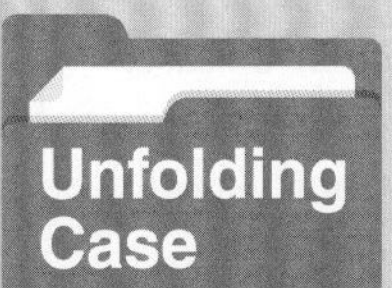

Recall Dylan. The most common adverse side effect of the ketogenic diet is constipation related to the very low carbohydrate intake. Children are closely monitored for other potential side effects, such as kidney stones, hyperlipidemias, dyslipidemias, hypoglycemia, pancreatitis, and cardiomyopathy. How do the potential risks of the diet compare to the risk of uncontrolled seizures, severe adverse side effects from medication, or the possible option of brain surgery?

How Do You Respond?

Is coconut oil healthy? Coconut oil is being touted as a healthy fat that helps promote weight loss, control diabetes, and reverse Alzheimer's disease (Gordon, 2019). Unfortunately, studies showing weight loss benefits were small and not well designed. Likewise, studies on its beneficial effects in managing diabetes were done on animals and may not be applicable to humans, and as of yet, there is no scientific evidence supporting the value of coconut oil in the treatment of Alzheimer's. Eighty-two percent of the fatty acids in coconut oil are saturated, and saturated fats may raise cholesterol and increase the risk for CVD, so coconut oil intake should be limited.

What is flaxseed? Flaxseed is derived from the flax plant and is the same plant used to make linen. It is a nutritional powerhouse that provides essential fatty acids, fiber, and lignans. Specifically, 57% of its fat is from ALA, the essential *n*-3 fatty acid that is only found in plants. The fiber in flaxseed is predominately soluble, which helps to lower cholesterol levels and improves glucose levels in people with diabetes. Flaxseed contains 100 to 800 times more lignans than other grains. Lignans are a group of plant estrogens, and they may help to reduce the risk of breast and prostate cancers. Although flaxseed oil and flaxseed oil pills provide the benefits of ALA, they lack the fiber found in the whole grain, and the lignan content is variable. Humans are unable to digest the tough outer coating, so flaxseeds must be eaten ground, not whole. They are prone to rancidity because they are high in polyunsaturated fat. Ground flaxseed should be refrigerated and used within a few weeks.

REVIEW CASE STUDY

Michael is a 40-year-old man who lost about 25 pounds 10 years ago by reducing his fat intake. He has slowly regained the weight and now wants to go back to a low-fat diet to manage his weight. (A sample of his usual intake is in the box on the right.)

- What foods and beverages did Michael eat that contain fat?
  - What sources of saturated fat did he eat? What sources of unsaturated fat? What sources of *n*-3 fats? What sources of cholesterol?
  - What specific suggestions would you make for him to eat less fat and/or improve the type of fat he eats?
- What would you tell Michael about cutting fat intake to lose weight?
  - What would you suggest he do to "eat healthier"?

Breakfast: 3 cups of coffee with sugar and nondairy creamer
On the way to work: A bagel with low-fat cream cheese and jelly
Snack before lunch: Low-fat coffee cake, more coffee with sugar and nondairy creamer
Lunch: Usually a burger, a large order of french fries, and a diet soda from the fast-food restaurant near his office
Snack before dinner: A glass of wine with cheese and crackers
Dinner: Meat, potato, and vegetable; often double portions of meat; a salad with Italian dressing; bread and butter; sherbet for dessert
Snack: A bowl of cornflakes with 2% milk and sugar

STUDY QUESTIONS

1 The client asks if the cholesterol in shrimp is the "good" or "bad" type. What is the nurse's best response?
a. "All cholesterol is bad cholesterol."
b. "Bad and good refer to how cholesterol is packaged for transport through the blood. The cholesterol in food is unpackaged and neither bad nor good."
c. "Good cholesterol is found in plants, and bad cholesterol is found in animal sources."
d. "Shrimp has good cholesterol because it is low in saturated fat; foods high in cholesterol and saturated fat are a source of bad cholesterol."

2 When developing a teaching plan for a client who needs to limit saturated fat, which of the following foods would the nurse suggest the client limit?
a. Seafood and poultry
b. Nuts and seeds
c. Olive oil and canola oil
d. Prime cuts of red meat and whole milk

3 What is the primary function of fat?
a. Facilitate protein metabolism
b. Provide energy
c. Promote the absorption of fat-soluble vitamins
d. Facilitate carbohydrate metabolism

4 The nurse knows that instructions have been effective when the client verbalizes that an ingredient that provides synthetic trans fats is
a. Fully hydrogenated oil
b. Partially hydrogenated oil
c. Palm oil
d. Palm kernel oil

5 A client asks why lowering saturated fat intake is necessary for lowering serum cholesterol levels. What is the nurse's best response?
a. "Replacing saturated fats with unsaturated fats helps lower LDL (the 'bad' cholesterol) and the risk of cardiovascular disease."
b. "Sources of saturated fat also provide monounsaturated fat, and both should be limited to control blood cholesterol levels."
c. "Saturated fat is high in calories, and excess calories from any source increase the risk of high blood cholesterol levels."
d. "Saturated fats make blood more likely to clot, increasing the risk of heart attack."

6 Which of the following is the best source of polyunsaturated fats?
a. Soybean oil
b. Corn oil
c. Vegetable oil
d. Olive oil

7 Which statement indicates the client understands how to choose low-fat foods from MyPlate?
a. "All items within a food group have approximately the same amount of fat so my fat intake isn't affected by the specific foods I choose from any group."
b. "You don't have to consciously select low-fat items because the calories for other uses allowance will account for higher-fat choices."
c. "All fats are bad fats. It is best to eliminate as much fat from your diet as possible."
d. "Within each food group, the foods lowest in fat should be chosen most often."

8 Which of the following is the top source of saturated fat intake among Americans?
a. Desserts and sweet snacks
b. Pizza
c. Sandwiches
d. Chips, crackers, and savory snacks

CHAPTER SUMMARY LIPIDS

Ninety-eight percent of lipids consumed in the diet are triglycerides, which are composed of one glyceride molecule and three fatty acids. Phospholipids and sterols are the other two types of dietary lipids.

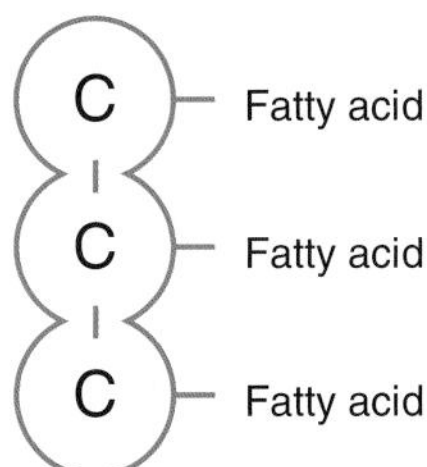

Fatty Acids

Saturation refers to each carbon atom in the fatty-acid chain having four single bonds.

- Saturated fatty acids have four single bonds and are "saturated" with hydrogen.
  - They are "solid" fats—solid at room temperature.
- Monounsaturated fatty acids have one double bond between carbon atoms; polyunsaturated fatty acids have more than one double bond.
- They are liquid at room temperature and are considered "oils."

Double bond position is identified by counting the number of carbon atoms from the methyl (CH_3) end, as denoted by the term *n* or *omega*.

- Monounsaturated fats (*n*-9) can be made by the body, so they are not essential in the diet (like saturated fats).
- One *n*-3 and one *n*-6 PUFA are deemed essential because they cannot be made in the body.

Artificial trans fatty acids are created from the partial hydrogenation of oils.

- They have no function in the body and their impact on health is negative, so they are no longer considered GRAS and are being removed from the food supply.

All food fats are a mixture of saturated and unsaturated fatty acids. Sources of fat are classified according to the type of fatty acid present to the largest degree.

Other Lipids

- Phospholipids occur naturally in almost all foods but in very small amounts. They are similar in structure to triglycerides but have only two fatty acids plus a phosphate group.
  - They act as emulsifiers to keep fat (e.g., cholesterol) suspended in water (e.g., blood)
- Cholesterol is a sterol found in all animal tissues. It does not supply calories. The body makes cholesterol from an excess of calories from any source, so it is not an essential nutrient. "Good" cholesterol and "bad" cholesterol refer to how it is packaged in the blood, not its dietary sources.

Functions of Fat in the Body

The primary function of fat is to supply energy. It provides 9 cal/g. Fat also insulates and cushions internal organs, helps regulate body temperature, and facilitates the absorption of fat-soluble vitamins. Individual fatty acids have other specific functions.

How the Body Handles Fat

Fat digestion occurs mostly in the small intestine.

- Short- and medium-chain fatty acids and glycerol are absorbed through mucosal cells into capillaries leading to the portal vein.
- Larger fat molecules—namely, cholesterol, phospholipids, and reformed triglycerides made from monoglycerides and long-chain fatty acids—are absorbed in chylomicrons and transported through the lymph system.
- Not all body cells can use fat for energy. The complete oxidation of fatty acids requires adequate glucose.
  - Ketones are formed when catabolism is incomplete.
- Fat consumed in excess of need is stored in adipose tissue.

Sources of Fat

Fat is naturally found in protein foods, dairy, and the category of oils. Grains and vegetables may have fat added during preparation. Fruits are considered fat free with the exception of olive, avocado, and coconut.

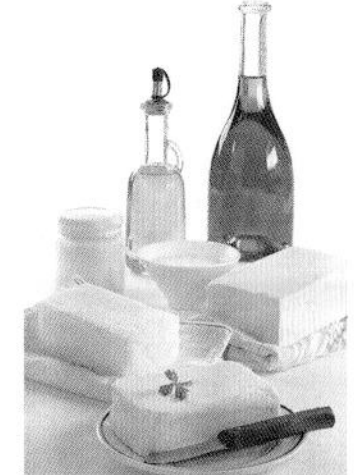

Dietary Reference Intakes

- The AMDR for total fat intake is 20% to 35% of total calorie intake.
  - Americans exceed this on average.

(continued)

CHAPTER SUMMARY LIPIDS (continued)

- AI are established for ALA (*n*-3 fatty acid) and LA (*n*-6).
- Dietary reference intakes do not exist for total fat, saturated fat, monounsaturated fat, cholesterol, and trans fatty acids.

Fat in Health Promotion

Americans are urged to consume an eating pattern that emphasizes the intake of vegetables, fruits, legumes, nuts, whole grains, and fish to lower the risk of heart disease. Other fat-related recommendations are to

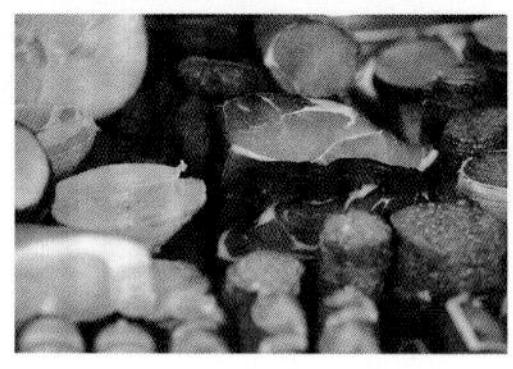

- replace saturated fat with polyunsaturated and monounsaturated fats,
- reduce cholesterol intake,
- minimize the intake of processed meats, and
- avoid trans fats.

Figure sources: *shutterstock.com/JPC-PROD and shuterstock.com/stockfour*

Student Resources on thePoint®
For additional learning materials, activate the code in the front of this book at https://thePoint.lww.com/activate

Websites

American Heart Association at www.heart.org
Calorie Control Council's glossary of fat replacers at www.caloriecontrol.org/articles-and-video/feature-articles/glossary-of-fat-replacers
Dietary Guidelines for Americans, 2020–2025 at www.dietaryguidelines.gov
Institute of Shortening and Edible Oils at www.iseo.org
International Food Information Council at www.foodinsight.org
National Heart, Lung, and Blood Institute at www.nhlbi.nih.gov

References

Arnett, D. K., Blumenthal, R. S., Albert, M. A., Buroker A. B., Goldberger, Z. D., Hahn, E. J., Himmelfarb, C. D., Khera, A., Lloyd-Jones, D., McEvoy, J. W., Michos, E. D., Miedema, M. D., Muñoz, D., Smith, S. C. Jr., Virani, S. S., Williams, K. A. Sr., Yeboah, J., & Ziaeian, B. (2019). 2019 ACC/AHA guideline on the primary prevention of cardiovascular disease: A report of the American College of Cardiology/American Heart Association Task Force on Clinical Practice Guidelines. *Circulation, 140*, e596–e646. https://doi.org/10.1161/CIR.0000000000000678

Dietary Guidelines Advisory Committee. (2020). Scientific report of the 2020 Dietary Guidelines Advisory Committee: Advisory Report to the Secretary of Agriculture and the Secretary of Health and Human Services. U.S. Department of Agriculture, Agricultural Research Service, Washington, DC. https://www.dietaryguidelines.gov/2020-advisory-committee-report

Gorden, B. (2019). *The facts about coconut oil.* https://www.eatright.org/food/nutrition/nutrition-facts-and-food-labels/the-facts-about-coconut-oil

Guasch-Ferre, M., Zong, G., Wilett, W., Zock, P. L., Wanders, A. J., Hu, F. B., & Sun, Q. (2019). Associations of monounsaturated fatty acids from plant and animal source with total and cause-specific mortality in two U.S. prospective cohort studies. *Circulation Research, 124*, 1266–1275. https://doi.org/10.1161/CIRCRESAHA.118.313996

Micha, R., Khatibzadeh, S., Shi, P., Fahimi, S., Lim, S., Andrews, K. G., Engell, R. E., Powles, J., Ezzati, M., & Mozaffarian, D. (2014). Global, regional, and national consumption levels of dietary fats and oils in 1990 and 2010: A systematic analysis including 266 country-specific nutrition surveys. *British Medical Journal, 348*, g2272. https://doi.org/10.1136/bmj.g2272

National Institutes of Health, Office of Dietary Supplements. (2019). *Omega-3 fatty acids: Fact sheet for professionals.* https://ods.od.nih.gov/factsheets/Omega3FattyAcids-HealthProfessional/

National Research Council. (2005). *Dietary reference intakes for energy, carbohydrate, fiber, fat, fatty acids, cholesterol, protein, and amino acids (macronutrients).* The National Academies Press.

Rajaram, S. (2014). Health benefits of plant-derived alpha-linolenic acid. *American Journal of Clinical Nutrition, 100*(suppl 1), 443S–448S. https://doi.org/10.3945/ajcn.113.071514

Rimm, E., Appel, L., Chiuve, S., Djoussé, L., Engler, M. B., Kris-Etherton, P. M., Mozaffarian, D., Siscovick, D. S., Lichtenstein, A. H. and On behalf of the American Heart Association Nutrition Committee of the Council on Lifestyle and Cardiometabolic Health; Council on Epidemiology and Prevention; Council on Cardiovascular Disease in the Young; Council on Cardiovascular and Stroke Nursing; and Council on Clinical Cardiology. (2018). Seafood long-chain n-3 polyunsaturated fatty acid and cardiovascular disease: A science advisory from the American Heart Association. *Circulation, 138*, e35–e47. https://doi.org/10.1161/CIR.0000000000000574

U.S. Department of Agriculture, Agricultural Research Service. (2018). *Percentages of energy from protein, carbohydrate, fat, and alcohol, by gender and age, in the United States, 2015–2016.* https://www.ars.usda.gov/ARSUserFiles/80400530/pdf/1516/Table_5_EIN_GEN_15.pdf

U.S. Department of Agriculture & U.S. Department of Health and Human Services. (2020, December). *Dietary guidelines for Americans 2020–2025.* www.dietaryguidelines.gov

U.S. Food & Drug Administration. (2018). *Final determination regarding partially hydrogenated oils (removing trans fat).* https://www.fda.gov/food/food-additives-petitions/final-determination-regarding-partially-hydrogenated-oils-removing-trans-fat

U.S. Food & Drug Administration. (2019). *Advice about eating fish: For women who are or might become pregnant, breastfeeding mothers, and young children.* https://www.fda.gov/food/consumers/advice-about-eating-fish

Chapter 6 Vitamins

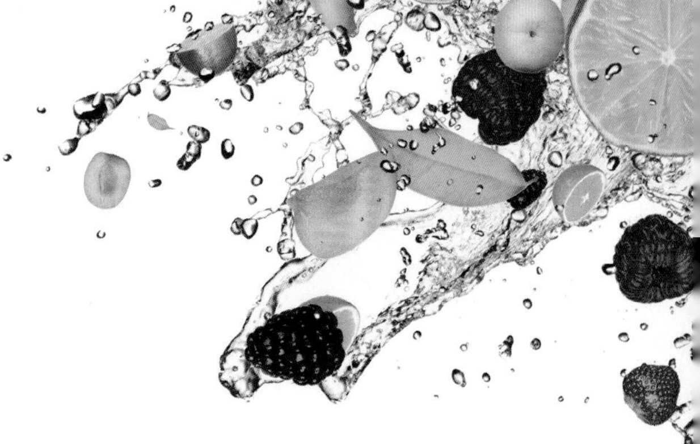

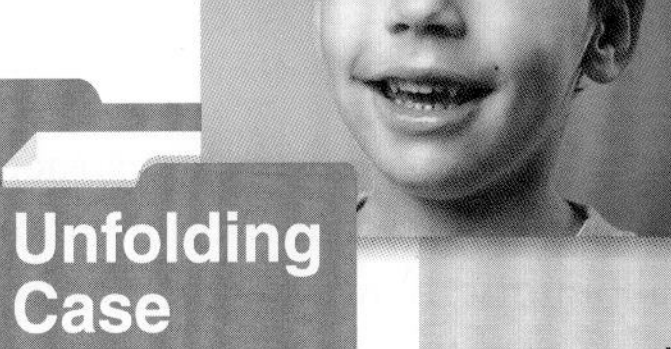

Unfolding Case

Marcus Skinner

Marcus is a 4-year-old boy with autism spectrum disorder who has communication impairments and social difficulties and exhibits repetitive behavior. His treatment includes medical nutrition therapy, speech-language therapy, occupational therapy, and physical therapy. Marcus does not eat a well-balanced eating pattern for several reasons: A feature of his compulsive behavior is that he only accepts a limited variety of foods, he is unable to eat when overstimulated at mealtime, and he has poor fine motor coordination that impairs his ability to feed himself. He is on a gluten-free/casein-free diet because these peptides are believed to cause a variety of effects in the neurotransmitter systems of the brain. Eliminating all foods containing gluten (foods containing wheat, barley, oats, and rye) and casein (the major protein in milk and other dairy products and used as an additive in other foods such as soy products) is theorized to improve social and cognitive behaviors and speech in some children with autism, although there is a lack of scientific evidence of benefit.

Learning Objectives

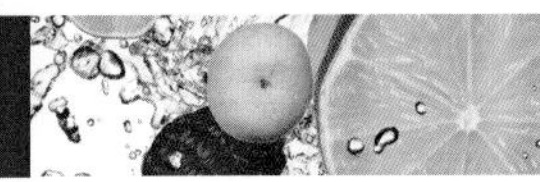

Upon completion of this chapter, you will be able to:

1. Compare and contrast fat- and water-soluble vitamins.
2. Describe general functions and uses of vitamins.
3. Judge when vitamin supplements may be necessary.
4. Give examples of food sources for individual vitamins.
5. Discuss how Americans can shift their food choices to improve their intake of shortfall vitamins.
6. Identify characteristics to look for when choosing a vitamin supplement.

In 1913, thiamin was discovered as the first vitamin, the "vital amine" necessary to prevent the deficiency disease beriberi. Today, 13 vitamins have been identified as important for human nutrition; vitamin deficiency diseases are generally rare in the United States, and vitamin research focuses on whether consuming various vitamins above the minimum basic requirement can reduce the risk of heart disease, cancer, vision disorders, cognitive decline in seniors, and other chronic diseases.

This chapter describes vitamins and their uses. Generalizations about fat- and water-soluble vitamins are presented. The unique features of each vitamin are covered individually, and criteria for selecting a vitamin supplement are discussed.

UNDERSTANDING VITAMINS

Vitamins are organic compounds made of carbon, hydrogen, oxygen, and sometimes nitrogen or other elements. They differ in their chemistry, biochemistry, function, and availability in foods. Vitamins facilitate biochemical reactions within cells to help regulate body processes such as growth and metabolism. They are essential to life. Unlike the organic compounds covered previously in this unit (carbohydrates, protein, and fat), vitamins

- are individual molecules, not long chains of molecules linked together,
- do not provide energy but are needed for the metabolism of energy, and
- are needed in microgram or milligram quantities (not gram quantities), so they are called **micronutrients**.

Micronutrients
nutrients that are needed in very small amounts.

Chemical Substances

Vitamins are extremely complex chemical substances that differ widely in their structures. Because vitamins are defined chemically, the body cannot distinguish between natural vitamins extracted from food and synthetic vitamins produced in a laboratory. However, the absorption rates of natural and synthetic vitamins sometimes differ because of different chemical forms of the same vitamin (e.g., synthetic folic acid is better absorbed than natural folate in foods) or because the synthetic vitamins are "free," not "bound" to other components in food (e.g., synthetic vitamin B_{12} is not bound to small peptides as natural vitamin B_{12} is).

Susceptible to Destruction

As organic substances, vitamins in food are susceptible to destruction and subsequent loss of function. Individual vitamins differ in their vulnerability to heat, light, **oxidation**, acid, and alkalis:

- Thiamin is heat sensitive and is easily destroyed by high temperatures and long cooking times.
- Riboflavin is resistant to heat, acid, and oxidation but is quickly destroyed by light. That is why riboflavin-rich milk is sold in opaque, not transparent, containers.
- From 50% to 90% of folate in foods may be lost during preparation, processing, and storage.
- Vitamin C is destroyed by heat, air, and alkalis.

Oxidation
a chemical reaction in which a substance combines with oxygen; oxidation reactions involve the loss of electrons in an atom.

Multiple Forms

Many vitamins exist in more than one active form. Different forms perform different functions in the body. For instance, vitamin A exists as retinol (important for reproduction), retinal (needed for vision), and retinoic acid (acts as a hormone to regulate growth). Some vitamins have **provitamins**, an inactive form found in food that the body converts to the active form. Beta carotene is a provitamin of vitamin A. Dietary Reference Intakes (DRIs) take into account the biologic activity of vitamins as they exist in different forms.

Provitamins
precursors of vitamins.

Essentiality

Vitamins are essential in the diet because the body cannot make them with a few exceptions. The body can make vitamin A, vitamin D, and niacin if the appropriate precursors are available. Microorganisms in the gastrointestinal (GI) tract synthesize vitamin K and vitamin B_{12} but not in amounts sufficient to meet the body's needs.

Coenzymes

Many **enzymes** cannot function without a **coenzyme**, and many coenzymes are vitamins. All B vitamins work as coenzymes to facilitate thousands of chemical conversions. Thiamin, riboflavin, niacin, and biotin participate in enzymatic reactions that extract energy from glucose, amino

Enzymes
proteins produced by cells that catalyze chemical reactions within the body without undergoing change themselves.

Coenzymes
organic molecules that activate an enzyme.

acids, and fat. Folacin facilitates both amino acid metabolism and nucleic acid synthesis. Protein synthesis and cell division are impaired without adequate folacin. An adequate and continuous supply of B vitamins in every cell is vital for normal metabolism.

Antioxidants

Free Radicals
highly unstable, highly reactive molecular fragments with one or more unpaired electrons.

Antioxidants
substances that donate electrons to free radicals to prevent oxidation.

Free radicals are produced continuously in cells as they burn oxygen during normal metabolism. Ultraviolet radiation, air pollution, ozone, the metabolism of food, and smoking can also generate free radicals in the body. The problem with free radicals is that they oxidize body cells and deoxyribonucleic acid (DNA) in their quest to become stable by gaining an electron. These structurally and functionally damaged oxidized cells are believed to contribute to aging and various health problems such as cancer, heart disease, and cataracts. Polyunsaturated fatty acids (PUFAs) in cell membranes are particularly vulnerable to damage by free radicals.

Antioxidants protect body cells from being oxidized (destroyed) by free radicals by undergoing oxidation themselves, which renders free radicals harmless.

- Vitamins and other substances in fruits, vegetables, and other plant-based food provide dozens, if not hundreds, of antioxidants.
- Vitamins that function as major antioxidants are vitamin C, vitamin E, folate, and the provitamin beta carotene.
- Each has a slightly different role, so one cannot completely substitute for another.
  - For instance, water-soluble vitamin C works within cells to disable free radicals, and fat-soluble vitamin E functions within fat tissue.
- Whether high doses of individual antioxidants offer the same health benefits as the package of substances found in food sources is an area of ongoing research.

Food Additives
substances added intentionally or unintentionally to food that affect its character.

Enrich
to add nutrients back that were lost during processing; for example, white flour is enriched with certain B vitamins lost when the bran and germ layers are removed.

Megadoses
amounts at least 10 times greater than the Recommended Dietary Allowance (RDA).

Food Additives

Some vitamins are used as **food additives** in certain foods to boost their nutritional content: vitamin C–enriched fruit drinks, vitamin D–fortified milk, and **enriched** flour. Other foods have certain vitamins added to them to help preserve quality: vitamin C is added to frozen fish to help prevent rancidity and to luncheon meats to stabilize the red color. Vitamin E helps slow rancidity in vegetable oils, and beta carotene adds color to margarine.

Medications

In **megadoses**, vitamins function like drugs, not nutrients. Large doses of niacin are used to lower cholesterol, low-density lipoprotein (LDL) cholesterol, and triglycerides in people with hyperlipidemia who do not respond to diet and exercise. Tretinoin (retinoic acid, a form of vitamin A) is used as a topical treatment for acne vulgaris. Gram quantities of vitamin C promote healing in patients with impaired bone and wound healing.

VITAMIN CLASSIFICATIONS BASED ON SOLUBILITY

Vitamins are classified according to their solubility. Vitamins A, D, E, and K are fat soluble. Vitamin C and the B vitamins (thiamin, riboflavin, niacin, folate, B_6, B_{12}, biotin, and pantothenic acid) are water soluble. Solubility determines vitamin absorption, transportation, storage, and excretion (Table 6.1).

Fat-Soluble Vitamins

Table 6.2 highlights recommended intakes, sources, functions, deficiency symptoms, and toxicity symptoms of each fat-soluble vitamin. Additional features of individual fat-soluble vitamins follow.

Table 6.1 Group Characteristics of Fat-Soluble and Water-Soluble Vitamins

Characteristic	Fat-Soluble Vitamins	Water-Soluble Vitamins
Sources	The fat and oil portion of foods	The watery portion of foods
Absorption	With fat encased in chylomicrons that enter the lymphatic system before circulating in the bloodstream Conditions that impair fat absorption increase the risk of fat-soluble vitamin deficiencies	Directly into the bloodstream
Transportation through the blood	Attach to protein carriers because fat is not soluble in watery blood	Move freely through the watery environment of blood and within cells
When consumed in excess of need	Are stored—primarily in the liver and adipose tissue	Are excreted in the urine, although some tissues may hold limited amounts of certain vitamins
Safety of consuming high intakes through supplements	Can be toxic; this applies primarily to vitamins A and D; large doses of vitamins E and K are considered relatively nontoxic	Are generally considered nontoxic, although side effects can occur from consuming very large doses of vitamin B_6 over a prolonged period
Frequency of intake	Generally do not have to be consumed daily because the body can retrieve them from storage as needed	Generally must be consumed daily because there is no reserve in storage

Table 6.2 Summary of Fat-Soluble Vitamins

Vitamin and Sources	Functions	Deficiency/Toxicity Signs and Symptoms
Vitamin A Adult RDA: Men: 900 mcg Women: 700 mcg • Retinol: beef, liver, milk, butter, cheese, cream, egg yolk, fortified milk, margarine, and ready-to-eat cereals • Beta carotene: "greens" (turnip, dandelion, beet, collard, mustard), spinach, kale, broccoli, carrots, peaches, pumpkin, red peppers, sweet potatoes, winter squash, mango, apricots, cantaloupe	The formation of visual purple, which enables the eye to adapt to dim light Normal growth and development of bones and teeth The formation and maintenance of mucosal epithelium to maintain healthy functioning of skin and membranes, hair, gums, and various glands Important role in immune function	**Deficiency** Slow recovery of vision after flashes of bright light at night is the first ocular symptom, which can progress to xerophthalmia and blindness Bone growth ceases; bone shape changes; enamel-forming cells in the teeth malfunction; teeth crack and tend to decay Skin becomes dry, scaly, rough, and cracked; keratinization or hyperkeratosis develops; mucous membrane cells flatten and harden: eyes become dry (xerosis); irreversible drying and hardening of the cornea can result in blindness Decreased saliva secretion → difficulty chewing, swallowing → anorexia Decreased mucous secretion of the stomach and intestines → impaired digestion and absorption → diarrhea, increased excretion of nutrients Impaired immune system functioning → increased susceptibility to respiratory, urinary tract, and vaginal infections increases **Toxicity** Headaches, vomiting, double vision, hair loss, bone abnormalities, liver damage, which may be reversible or fatal Can cause birth defects during pregnancy
Vitamin D Adult RDA: Up to age 70 years: 600 IU/day 70 years and older: 800 IU/day UL: 4000 IU/day Sunlight on the skin • Fatty fish (salmon, tuna, sardines, swordfish), cod liver oil, egg yolks, beef liver; fortified foods: milk (dairy and nondairy), ready-to-eat cereals, orange juice, and infant formula	Maintains serum calcium concentrations by the following: Stimulating GI absorption Stimulating the release of calcium from the bones Stimulating calcium absorption from the kidneys Other roles include cell growth, neuromuscular and immune function, and reducing inflammation	**Deficiency** Rickets (in infants and children) Retarded bone growth Bone malformations (bowed legs) Enlargement of ends of long bones (knock-knees) Deformities of the ribs (bowed with beads or knobs) Delayed closing of the fontanel → rapid enlargement of the head Decreased serum calcium and/or phosphorus Malformed teeth; decayed teeth

Table 6.2 Summary of Fat-Soluble Vitamins (continued)

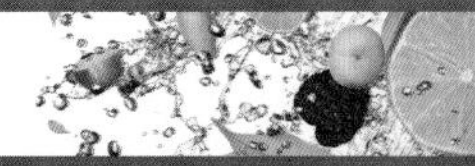

Vitamin and Sources	Functions	Deficiency/Toxicity Signs and Symptoms
	Most tissues and cells have vitamin D receptors (e.g., in the skin, pancreas, colon, kidney, parathyroid and pituitary glands, ovaries, and lymphocytes), which suggests vitamin D has many diverse roles	Protrusion of the abdomen related to relaxation of the abdominal muscles Increased secretion of parathyroid hormone Osteomalacia (in adults) Softening of the bones → deformities, pain, and easy fracture Decreased serum calcium and/or phosphorus, increased alkaline phosphatase Involuntary muscle twitching and spasms **Toxicity** Kidney stones, irreversible kidney damage, muscle and bone weakness, excessive bleeding, loss of appetite, headache, excessive thirst, calcification of soft tissues (blood vessels, kidneys, heart, lungs), death
Vitamin E Adult RDA: 15 mg • Vegetable oils, margarine, salad dressing, other foods made with vegetable oil, nuts, seeds, wheat germ, dark-green vegetables, whole grains, fortified cereals	Acts as an antioxidant to protect vitamin A and polyunsaturated fatty acids from being destroyed Protects cell membranes Also involved in inhibiting cell division, enhancing immune system functioning, regulating gene expression, inhibiting platelet aggregation, and promoting blood vessel dilation	**Deficiency** Increased red blood cell hemolysis In infants, anemia, edema, and skin lesions **Toxicity** Relatively nontoxic High doses enhance action of anticoagulant medications
Vitamin K Adult Adequate Intake (AI): Men: 120 mcg Women: 90 mcg Menaquinone: meat, dairy products, eggs; synthesized by intestinal microbiota Phylloquinone: brussels sprouts, broccoli, cauliflower, Swiss chard, spinach, loose leaf lettuce, carrots, green beans, asparagus	Coenzyme for reactions involved in blood clotting and bone metabolism	**Deficiency** Hemorrhaging **Toxicity** No symptoms have been observed from excessive intake of vitamin K.

Vitamin A

Two forms of vitamin A are available in the diet:

- Preformed vitamin A
  - It exists as an alcohol (retinol), aldehyde (retinaldehyde), or acid (retinoic acid).
  - It is found only in animal sources such as liver, whole milk, and fish.
    - Low-fat milk, skim milk, margarine, and ready-to-eat cereals are **fortified** with vitamin A.
- Provitamin A carotenoids
  - Beta carotene, alpha carotene, and cryptoxanthin can be converted to retinol.
  - Other **carotenoids** (e.g., lycopene, lutein, and zeaxanthin) do not have vitamin A activity.

The body can store up to a year supply of vitamin A, 90% of which is in the liver. It may take 1 to 2 years for deficiency symptoms to appear because they do not develop until body stores are exhausted.

- Vitamin A deficiency is rare in the United States. Premature infants, infants with malabsorption disorders, and people with cystic fibrosis are the groups most at risk.

Fortified
to fortify is to add nutrients to a food that were either not originally present or were present in insignificant amounts; for instance, many brands of orange juice are fortified with vitamin D.

Carotenoids
natural plant pigments found in deep-yellow and orange fruits and vegetables and most dark-green leafy vegetables. Well-known carotenoids that cannot be converted to vitamin A in the body are zeaxanthin, lutein, and lycopene.

- In sub-Saharan Africa and South Asia, vitamin A deficiency affects approximately one third of children living in low- and middle-income settings (Stevens et al., 2015), causing a range of vision problems, including permanent blindness.
  - Vitamin A deficiency is also linked to an increased risk of mortality from measles and diarrhea in children.

Preformed Vitamin A
the active form of vitamin A.

Only **preformed vitamin A**, the form found in animal foods, fortified foods, and supplements, is toxic in high doses.

- Chronic excessive vitamin A intake can cause central nervous system changes, bone and skin changes, and liver abnormalities that range from reversible to fatal.
- Toxicity is usually caused by consuming too much vitamin A from supplements.
- At high doses during pregnancy (three to four times the recommended intake), vitamin A is teratogenic.
  - Supplementation is not recommended during the first trimester of pregnancy unless there is specific evidence of vitamin A deficiency.

Beta carotene is nontoxic because the body makes vitamin A from it only as needed and the conversion is not rapid enough to cause hypervitaminosis A.

- Carotene is stored primarily in adipose tissue and may accumulate under the skin to the extent that it causes the skin color to turn yellowish orange, a harmless and reversible condition known as carotenodermia.
- The Tolerable Upper Intake Level (UL) for vitamin A does not apply to vitamin A derived from carotenoids.

Beta carotene is a major antioxidant in the body, which prompted researchers to study whether it can prevent heart disease and cancer. A landmark trial designed to test whether beta carotene supplements could decrease cancer incidence in people at high risk was prematurely halted when results showed a surprising increase in lung cancer incidence and deaths in smokers and male asbestos workers (Omenn et al., 1996; The Alpha Tocopherol, Beta Carotene Cancer Prevention Study Group, 1994).

Vitamin D

Essential Nutrient
A nutrient that must be supplied by the diet because it is not synthesized in the body. Essentiality does not refer to importance but to the need for a dietary source.

Vitamin D is unique in that the body has the potential to make all it needs if exposure to ultraviolet rays from sunlight is optimal and liver and kidney functions are normal. Because vitamin D can be endogenously synthesized, it is not an **essential nutrient** in the diet.

- Vitamin D also known as calciferol, exists in two forms:
  - Vitamin D_3 or cholecalciferol, which is derived from animal foods in the diet and synthesis in the skin
  - Vitamin D_2 or ergocalciferol, which is found in plant foods in the diet
- Vitamin D naturally occurs in very few foods; fortified foods are the major dietary source (Box 6.1).
- Vitamin D from sunlight or food is inert and requires two hydroxylation reactions to become active.
  - The first reaction occurs in the liver where vitamin D is converted to 25-hydroxyvitamin D [25(OH)D], also known as calcidiol.
  - The second reaction occurs primarily in the kidney where 25(OH)D is converted to the biologically active form of vitamin D, $1,25(OH)_2D$, also known as calcitriol. This conversion is tightly regulated by parathyroid hormone in response to serum calcium and phosphorus levels.
- Because vitamin D is synthesized in one part of the body (skin) and stimulates functional activity elsewhere (e.g., GI tract, bones, and kidneys), it is actually a prohormone.

The RDA for vitamin D is based on the assumption of minimal or no sun exposure.

BOX 6.1 Vitamin D Content of Selected Items

	IUs of Vitamin D
1 tbsp cod liver oil	1360
3 oz swordfish	566
3 oz Atlantic salmon	447
3 oz canned tuna in water, drained	154
1 cup fortified orange juice	137
1 cup nonfat, reduced fat, and whole milk fortified with vitamin D	115–124
1 tbsp fortified margarine	60
1 large egg yolk	41

Source: USDA National Nutrient Database for Standard Reference Release 28. https://ods.od.nih.gov/pubs/usdandb/VitaminD-Content.pdf

- The basis for determining the RDA for vitamin D is its cause-and-effect relationship with bone health only.
  - The Institute of Medicine (IOM) maintains that evidence linking vitamin D with extra-skeletal outcomes (e.g., cancer, cardiovascular disease, diabetes, and autoimmune disorders) is inconsistent, inconclusive, and insufficient to use in determining vitamin D requirements (Food and Nutrition Board, Institute of Medicine [IOM], 2011).
- The current UL for vitamin D is set at 4000 IU/day for ages 9 years and older.
  - Factors considered in determining the UL included hypercalcemia, hypercalciuria, and vascular and soft-tissue calcification.
- Vitamin D toxicity from overexposure to the sun does not occur because the body limits the amount it produces.

Although it is possible for the body to make all the vitamin D it needs, a dietary source is considered necessary because few people meet those conditions.

- Cloud cover, time of day, dark skin pigmentation, air pollution, and the use of sunscreen are the factors that affect ultraviolet (UV) radiation exposure and vitamin D synthesis in the skin (Food and Nutrition Board, IOM, 2011).
- Season also impacts vitamin D synthesis.
  - During the winter months, people living in latitudes above 37° do not receive enough UVB radiation, preventing most or all endogenous synthesis of previtamin D (Fig. 6.1).
- Although it is difficult to determine how much sun exposure is adequate, some experts suggest 5 to 30 minutes of sun exposure between 10 a.m. and 3 p.m. at least twice a week to the face, arms, legs, or back without sunscreen is sufficient (Holick, 2007).

Overt deficiency of vitamin D causes poor calcium absorption, leading to a calcium deficit in the blood, which the body corrects by releasing calcium from bone.

- The result is **rickets** in children, a condition characterized by abnormal bone shape and structure.
- In adults, vitamin D deficiency can result in **osteomalacia**, a softening of the bones.

Rickets
vitamin D deficiency disease in children; most prominently characterized by bowed legs.

Osteomalacia
adult rickets characterized by inadequate bone mineralization due to the lack of vitamin D.

Food fortification, particularly milk, has virtually eradicated these two deficiency diseases in the United States (Pfotenhauer & Shubrook, 2017). However, many Americans may have inadequate serum concentrations of vitamin D.

Because the major source of vitamin D for children and adults is sunlight exposure, the major cause of vitamin D inadequacy or deficiency is inadequate sun exposure (Nair & Maseeh, 2012).

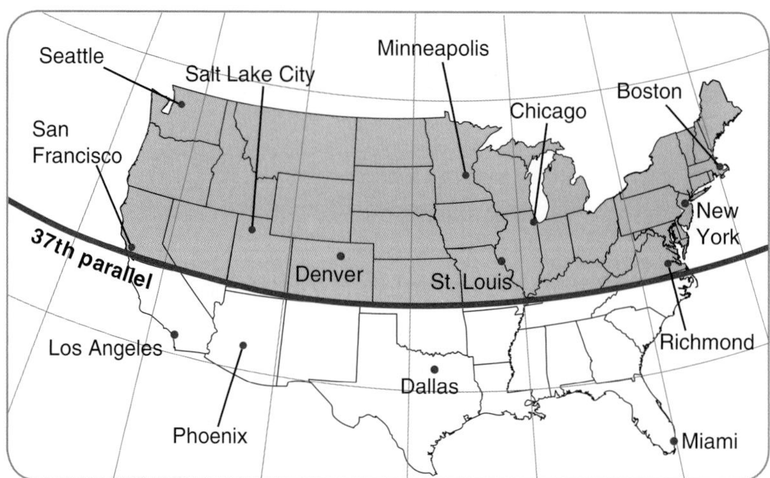

Figure 6.1 ▲ Americans living north of 37° latitude (shaded area) are at great risk for vitamin D deficiency because of low or absent UVB sunlight from late October to late April. (*Source:* Wickham, R. [2012]. Cholecalciferol and cancer: Is it a Big D3-eal? *Journal of the Advanced Practitioner in Oncology, 3*(4), 249–257. https://doi.org/10.6004/jadpro.2012.3.4.6)

- Senior persons are particularly at risk for vitamin D deficiency because of various factors: inadequate intake, limited sun exposure, reduced skin thickness, and impaired activation by the liver and kidneys.
- Other groups at risk of vitamin D deficiency include breastfed infants who do not receive vitamin D supplements, people with fat malabsorption or inflammatory bowel conditions, and people who are obese or have had gastric bypass surgery (National Institutes of Health, Office of Dietary Supplements, 2019a).
- Certain medications, such as anticonvulsants, glucocorticoids, and highly active antiretroviral therapy can interfere with vitamin D metabolism.

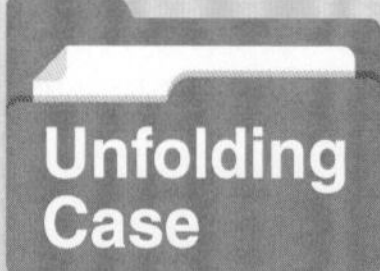

Recall Marcus. His gluten-free/casein-free diet restricts many types of grain and milk products, and some children following this diet have developed amino acid deficiencies, which is essentially a form of protein malnutrition. Marcus has difficulty chewing meat, which further limits his intake of protein. What foods can provide protein within the context of his dietary restrictions? Which vitamins may he be under consuming given his restricted intake of grains, milk, and meats? Will vitamin supplements compensate for the lack of variety in his intake?

Vitamin E

Vitamin E is a group name that describes a group of at least eight structurally related, naturally occurring compounds.

- Alpha tocopherol is considered the most biologically active form of vitamin E, although other forms also have important roles in maintaining health.
- As a group, vitamin E functions as the primary fat-soluble antioxidant in the body, protecting PUFAs and other lipid molecules, such as LDL cholesterol, from oxidative damage. By doing so, it helps to maintain the integrity of PUFA-rich cell membranes, protects red blood cells against hemolysis, and protects vitamin A from oxidation.

The need for vitamin E increases as the intake of PUFA increases.

- Fortunately, vitamin E and PUFA share many of the same food sources, particularly nuts, seeds, fortified cereals, vegetable oils, and products made from oil such as margarine, salad dressings, and other prepared foods.

- Not all oils are rich in alpha tocopherol, the active form of vitamin E.
    - Sunflower oil, canola oil, and olive oil all have higher amounts of the active form of vitamin E than does soybean oil, the most commonly used oil in food processing.

It is noteworthy that deficiency symptoms have never been reported in healthy people eating a low–vitamin E diet. Mean intake in the United States is somewhat less than recommended (U.S. Department of Agriculture [USDA], Agricultural Research Service [ARS], 2018).

- Total fat intake, thus vitamin E intake, may be underreported.
- It is difficult to estimate the amount of fat used in food preparation (e.g., frying).
- Vitamin E content cannot be determined when the ingredient list of a food states "may contain one or more of the following oils" because vitamin E content differs among oils.

Vitamin E deficiency is rare and more likely to occur secondary to fat malabsorption syndromes, such as cystic fibrosis and short bowel syndrome, than from an inadequate intake.

- Premature infants who have not benefited from the transfer of vitamin E from mother to fetus in the last weeks of pregnancy are at risk for red blood cell hemolysis.
    - The breaking of their red blood cell membranes is caused by oxidation; vitamin E corrects red blood cell hemolysis by preventing oxidation.
- Prolonged vitamin E deficiency symptoms include peripheral neuropathy, ataxia, and impaired vision and speech.

Large amounts of vitamin E are relatively nontoxic as evidenced by a UL that is 66 times higher than the RDA.

- Excessive vitamin E can interfere with vitamin K action (blood clotting) by decreasing platelet aggregation.
- Large doses may also potentiate the effects of blood-thinning drugs, increasing the risk of hemorrhage.

Vitamin K

Vitamin K occurs naturally in two forms. Phylloquinone is found in plants, and menaquinones, the animal form, is found in modest amounts in meat, dairy products, and eggs. It is the form of vitamin K synthesized in the intestinal tract by microbiota. It is not known how much vitamin K produced by microbiota are absorbed. A UL has not been set because no adverse effects are associated with vitamin K intake from food or supplements. Vitamin K is a coenzyme essential for the synthesis of prothrombin and at least 6 of the other 13 proteins needed for normal blood clotting.

- Without adequate vitamin K, life is threatened.
    - Even a small wound can cause someone deficient in vitamin K to bleed to death.
- Vitamin K also activates at least three proteins involved in building and maintaining bone.

Newborns are prone to vitamin K deficiency for a few reasons.

- Vitamin K transport across the placenta is low.
- Breast milk is low in vitamin K.
- Newborns have sterile GI tracts that cannot synthesize vitamin K.
- To prevent hemorrhagic disease, a single intramuscular dose of vitamin K is given prophylactically at birth.

Clinically significant vitamin K deficiency is defined as vitamin K–responsive hypoprothrombinemia and is characterized by an increase in prothrombin time.

- Vitamin K deficiency does not occur from inadequate intake but may occur secondary to malabsorption syndromes.
- The use of certain medications that interfere with vitamin K metabolism or synthesis, such as anticoagulants and antibiotics, can cause vitamin K deficiency.

- Anticoagulants, such as warfarin (Coumadin), interfere with hepatic synthesis of vitamin K–dependent clotting factors.
  - People who take warfarin do not need to avoid vitamin K, but they should try to maintain a consistent intake so that the effect on coagulation time is as constant and as predictable as possible.
- Antibiotics kill the intestinal bacteria that synthesize vitamin K.

Water-Soluble Vitamins

Table 6.1 summarizes the group characteristics of water-soluble vitamins. Table 6.3 highlights sources, functions, deficiency symptoms, and toxicity symptoms of each water-soluble vitamin. Additional features of individual water-soluble vitamins are summarized in the following sections.

Table 6.3 Summary of Water-Soluble Vitamins

Vitamin and Sources	Functions	Deficiency/Toxicity Signs and Symptoms
Thiamin (vitamin B_1) Adult RDA Men: 1.2 mg Women: 1.1 mg • Whole grain and enriched breads and cereals, liver, nuts, wheat germ, pork, dried peas and beans	Coenzyme in energy metabolism Promotes normal appetite and nervous system functioning	**Deficiency** Beriberi Mental confusion, decrease in short-term memory Fatigue, apathy Peripheral paralysis Muscle weakness and wasting Painful calf muscles Anorexia, weight loss Edema Enlarged heart Cardiac and renal complications can be fatal **Toxicity** No toxicity symptoms reported
Riboflavin (vitamin B_2) Adult RDA Men: 1.3 mg Women: 1.1 mg • Milk and other dairy products; whole-grain and enriched breads and cereals; liver, eggs, meat, spinach	Coenzyme in energy metabolism Aids in the conversion of tryptophan into niacin	**Deficiency** Dermatitis Cheilosis Glossitis Photophobia Reddening of the cornea **Toxicity** No toxicity symptoms reported
Niacin (vitamin B_3) Adult RDA Men: 16 mg Women: 14 mg • All protein foods, whole grain and enriched breads and cereals	Coenzyme in energy metabolism Promotes normal nervous system functioning	**Deficiency** Pellagra: 4 Ds Dermatitis (bilateral and symmetrical) and glossitis Diarrhea Dementia, irritability, mental confusion → psychosis Death, if untreated **Toxicity** (from supplements/drugs) Flushing, liver damage, gastric ulcers, low blood pressure, diarrhea, nausea, vomiting
Vitamin B_6 Adult RDA Men: 1.3–1.7 mg Women: 1.3–1.5 mg • Fish, beef liver and other organ meats, potatoes, other starchy vegetables, non-citrus fruits, fortified cereals, beef, and poultry	Coenzyme in >100 enzyme reactions, mostly concerned with protein metabolism Involved in the metabolism of carbohydrates and lipids Plays a role in gluconeogenesis, immune system functioning, hemoglobin formation, and the synthesis of neurotransmitters	**Deficiency** Microcytic anemia, dermatitis, cheilosis, glossitis, abnormal brain wave pattern, convulsions, depression and confusion, weakened immune system functioning **Toxicity** Depression, fatigue, irritability, headaches; sensory neuropathy characteristic
Folate Adult RDA: 400 mcg • Liver, okra, spinach, asparagus, dried peas and beans, seeds, orange juice; breads, cereals, and other grains are fortified with folic acid	Coenzyme in DNA synthesis; therefore, vital for new cell synthesis and the transmission of inherited characteristics Coenzyme in homocysteine metabolism	**Deficiency** Glossitis, diarrhea, macrocytic anemia, depression, mental confusion, fainting, fatigue **Toxicity** Too much can mask vitamin B_{12} deficiency

Table 6.3 Summary of Water-Soluble Vitamins (continued)

Vitamin and Sources	Functions	Deficiency/Toxicity Signs and Symptoms
Vitamin B_{12} Adult RDA: 2.4 mcg • Animal products: meat, fish, poultry, shellfish, milk, dairy products, eggs • Some fortified foods	Coenzyme in the synthesis of new cells Activates folate Maintains myelin sheath around nerve cells Helps metabolize some fatty acids and amino acids Coenzyme in homocysteine metabolism	**Deficiency** GI changes: glossitis, anorexia, indigestion, recurring diarrhea or constipation, and weight loss Macrocytic anemia: pallor, dyspnea, weakness, fatigue, and palpitations Neurologic changes: paresthesia of the hands and feet, decreased sense of position, poor muscle coordination, poor memory, irritability, depression, paranoia, delirium, and hallucinations **Toxicity** No toxicity symptoms reported
Pantothenic acid Adult AI: 5 mg • Widespread in foods • Meat, poultry, fish, whole-grain cereals, and dried peas and beans are among best sources	Part of coenzyme A used in energy metabolism	**Deficiency** Rare; general failure of all body systems **Toxicity** No toxicity symptoms reported, although large doses may cause diarrhea
Biotin Adult AI: 30 mcg • Widespread in foods • Eggs, liver, milk, and dark-green vegetables are among best choices • Synthesized by GI flora	Coenzyme in energy metabolism, fatty acid synthesis, amino acid metabolism, and glycogen formation	**Deficiency** Rare; anorexia, fatigue, depression, dry skin, heart abnormalities **Toxicity** No toxicity symptoms reported
Choline Adult AI Men: 550 mg Women: 425 mg • Widespread: milk, liver, beef, beans, eggs, peanuts, cruciferous vegetables (broccoli, brussels sprouts, cauliflower) • Processed foods with added lecithin (an emulsifier): salad dressings, gravies, margarine	Important for structural integrity of cell membranes Necessary for acetylcholine (a neurotransmitter) formation Plays a role in modulating gene expression, cell membrane signaling, lipid transport and metabolism, and early brain development	**Deficiency** Muscle damage, liver damage, and nonalcoholic fatty liver disease **Toxicity** Extremely high intakes may cause fishy body odor, sweating, salivation, hypotension, and hepatoxicity
Vitamin C Adult RDA Men: 90 mg Women: 75 mg • Citrus fruits and juices, red and green peppers, broccoli, cauliflower, brussels sprouts, cantaloupe, kiwifruit, mustard greens, strawberries, tomatoes	Synthesis of collagen, the most abundant protein in fibrous tissues, such as connective tissue, cartilage, bone matrix, tooth dentin, skin, and tendon. Antioxidant that protects vitamin A, vitamin E, PUFA, and iron from destruction Promotes iron absorption Involved in the metabolism of certain amino acids Thyroxin synthesis Immune system functioning	**Deficiency** Scurvy, characterized by the following: Hemorrhaging that begins with pinpoint hemorrhages under the skin and progresses to massive internal bleeding Muscle degeneration Skin changes Delayed wound healing: reopening of old wounds Softening of the bones → malformations, pain, easy fractures Soft, loose teeth Anemia Increased susceptibility to infection Hysteria and depression **Toxicity** Diarrhea, mild GI upset

Thiamin

Thiamin (vitamin B_1) is a coenzyme in the metabolism of carbohydrates and branched-chain amino acids. In addition to its role in energy metabolism, thiamin is important in nervous system functioning.

- In the United States and other developed countries, the use of enriched breads and cereals has virtually eliminated the thiamin deficiency disease known as beriberi.

- Today, thiamin deficiency is usually seen only in alcoholics with limited food consumption.
  - Chronic alcohol abuse impairs thiamin intake, absorption, and metabolism. Edema occurs in wet beriberi, and muscle wasting is prominent in dry beriberi. Cardiac and renal complications can be fatal.

Riboflavin

Riboflavin (vitamin B_2) is an integral component of the coenzymes flavin adenine dinucleotide and flavin mononucleotide that function to release energy from nutrients in all body cells.

Homocysteine
an amino acid correlated with increased risk of heart disease.

Methionine
an essential amino acid.

- Flavin coenzymes are also involved in the formation of some vitamins and their coenzymes and in the conversion of **homocysteine** to **methionine**.
- Riboflavin is unique among water-soluble vitamins in that milk and dairy products contribute the most riboflavin to the diet.
- Biochemical signs of an inadequate riboflavin status can appear after only a few days of a poor intake.
- Seniors and teens are at greatest risk for riboflavin deficiency.
- Riboflavin deficiency interferes with iron handling and contributes to anemia when iron intake is low.
- Certain diseases, such as cancer, heart disease, and diabetes, precipitate or exacerbate riboflavin deficiency.

Niacin

Niacin Equivalents (NEs)
the amount of niacin available to the body, including that made from tryptophan.

Niacin (vitamin B_3) exists as nicotinic acid and nicotinamide. A unique feature of niacin is that the body can make it from the amino acid tryptophan. Because of this additional source of niacin, niacin requirements are stated in **niacin equivalents (NEs)**. Niacin is part of the coenzymes nicotinamide adenine dinucleotide and nicotinamide adenine dinucleotide phosphate (NADP), which are involved in energy transfer reactions in the metabolism of glucose, fat, and alcohol in all body cells.

- Reduced NADP is used in the synthesis of fatty acids, cholesterol, and steroid hormones.

Pellagra, the disorder caused by severe niacin deficiency, was common in the southern United States before grain products were enriched with niacin in the early 20th century.

- Today, pellagra is rare in the United States and usually is seen only in alcoholics.
- Once widespread in areas that rely on corn as a staple, such as parts of Africa and Asia, pellagra is now mostly seen only in populations during food emergencies.
- Niacin deficiency may be treated with niacin, tryptophan, or both.

Because a deficiency of niacin rarely occurs alone, treatment is most effective when other B-complex vitamins are also given, especially thiamin and riboflavin. Large doses of niacin in the form of nicotinic acid (1000–2000 mg/day) are used therapeutically to lower total LDL cholesterol, lower triglycerides, and raise high-density lipoprotein cholesterol.

- Flushing is a common side effect caused by vasodilation.
- Large doses may cause liver damage and gout and should be used only with a doctor's supervision.
- The UL of 35 mg of NE does not apply for clinical applications using niacin as a drug.

Vitamin B_6

Vitamin B_6 and pyridoxine are group names for six related compounds that include pyridoxine, pyridoxal, and pyridoxamine. All forms can be converted to the active form, pyridoxal phosphate, which is involved in nearly 100 enzymatic reactions, mostly involving protein metabolism.

- Unlike other B vitamins, vitamin B_6 is stored extensively in muscle tissue.

- A combination of vitamin B_6 and doxylamine succinate (an antihistamine) in a delayed-release combination pill is associated with a 70% reduction in nausea and vomiting in pregnancy (Niebyl, 2010).
  - A randomized, placebo-controlled clinical trial showed that it is safe (not a teratogen) and effective as an antiemetic for mild to moderate nausea and vomiting during pregnancy (Nuangchamnong & Niebyl, 2014).

Deficiencies of vitamin B_6 are uncommon but are usually accompanied by deficiencies of other B vitamins, such a folic acid and vitamin B_{12}.

- People at risk of vitamin B_6 deficiency include those with impaired renal function, autoimmune diseases, and malabsorption disorders such as celiac disease.
- Vitamin B_6 deficiency also occurs in people with alcohol dependency (because the metabolism of alcohol promotes the destruction and excretion of vitamin B_6) and those on certain drug therapies such as isoniazid, the antituberculosis drug that acts as a vitamin B_6 antagonist.

No adverse effects have been reported with high intakes of vitamin B_6 from food.

- High intake of supplemental vitamin B_6 (1–6 g oral/day for 12–40 months) can cause severe and progressive sensory neuropathy characterized by ataxia (Kulkantrakorn, 2014).
  - The severity of symptoms is dose dependent.
  - Symptoms usually disappear if supplements are discontinued as soon as symptoms appear (National Institutes of Health, Office of Dietary Supplements, 2019b).

Folate

Folate is the generic term for this B vitamin that includes both synthetic folic acid found in vitamin supplements and fortified foods and naturally occurring folate in foods such as green leafy vegetables, legumes, seeds, liver, and orange juice.

- Dietary folate equivalents, used in establishing folate requirement, are based on the assumption that natural food folate is approximately only half as available to the body as synthetic folic acid.
- A large number of factors influence the bioavailability of natural folates, and different plant and animal sources of folate may have varied levels of bioavailability (Saini et al., 2016).

Much like the enterohepatic circulation of bile, folate is recycled through the intestinal tract. A healthy GI tract is essential to maintain folate balance.

- When GI integrity is impaired, as in malabsorption syndromes, failure to reabsorb folate quickly leads to folate deficiency.
- GI cells are particularly susceptible to folate deficiency because they are rapidly dividing cells that depend on folate for new cell synthesis. Without the formation of new cells, GI function declines and widespread malabsorption of nutrients occurs.

Folate deficiency impairs DNA synthesis and cell division and results in macrocytic anemia and other clinical symptoms.

- It is prevalent in all parts of the world. In developing countries, folate deficiency commonly is caused by parasitic infections that alter GI integrity.
- In the United States, alcoholics are at highest risk of folate deficiency because of alcohol's toxic effect on the GI tract.
- The groups at risk because of poor intake include seniors, fad dieters, and people of low socioeconomic status.
- New tissue growth increases folate requirements, so infants, adolescents, and pregnant women may have difficulty consuming adequate amounts.

Studies show that an adequate intake of folate before conception and during the first trimester of pregnancy reduces the risk of neural tube defects (e.g., spina bifida) in infants (Medical Research Council Vitamin Study Research Group, 1991).

- This discovery prompted the U.S. Public Health Service to recommend that all women of childbearing age who are capable of becoming pregnant consume 400 mcg of synthetic folic acid from fortified food and/or supplements in addition to folate from a varied diet (U.S. Preventive Services Task Force, 2017).
- Folic acid fortification of enriched bread and grain products is mandatory in the United States. These products have become an important source of folic acid because grains are so widely consumed in the United States.

The UL for folic acid is 1000 mg/day from fortified food or supplements, exclusive of food folate.

- Large amounts of folic acid may mask vitamin B_{12} deficiency by correcting the megaloblastic anemia. However, it does not correct the neurologic abnormalities, which if left untreated, may be irreversible.

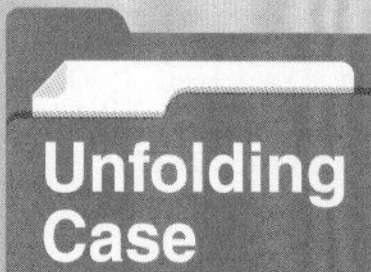

Recall Marcus. He has a restricted diet and accepts only a limited variety of foods, so he may be under- or overconsuming certain nutrients. His parents give him a multivitamin with minerals, plus additional supplements of vitamin D, vitamin C, and calcium. What questions would you ask about the supplements he is taking? Should Marcus's parents keep a food diary so that his total vitamin intake from food and supplements can be estimated?

Vitamin B_{12}

Vitamin B_{12} (cobalamin) has several interesting features.

- First, vitamin B_{12} has an interdependent relationship with folate: Each vitamin must have the other to be activated.
- Because it activates folate, vitamin B_{12} is involved in DNA synthesis and maturation of red blood cells.
- Like folate, vitamin B_{12} functions as a coenzyme in homocysteine metabolism.
- Unlike folate, vitamin B_{12} has important roles in maintaining the myelin sheath around nerves.
    - For this reason, large doses of folic acid cannot halt the progressive neurologic impairments that only vitamin B_{12} can treat, although they can alleviate the anemia caused by vitamin B_{12} deficiency.
        - Nervous system damage may be irreversible without early treatment with vitamin B_{12}.

Vitamin B_{12} also holds the distinction of being the only water-soluble vitamin that does not occur naturally in plants.

- Fermented soy products and algae may be enriched with vitamin B_{12}, but it is in an inactive, unavailable form.
- Some ready-to-eat cereals are fortified with vitamin B_{12}.
- All animal foods contain vitamin B_{12}.

Another unique feature of vitamin B_{12} is that it requires an intrinsic factor (IF), a glycoprotein secreted in the stomach, to be absorbed from the terminal ileum.

- But before it can bind to the IF, natural vitamin B_{12} must first be separated from the small peptides to which it is bound in food sources. Separation is accomplished by pepsin and gastric acid.

- Conversely, synthetic vitamin B_{12} found in enriched foods and supplements does not require this separation step because it is in free form.

Vitamin B_{12} deficiency symptoms may take 5–10 years or longer to develop because the liver can store relatively large amounts of B_{12} and the body recycles B_{12} by reabsorbing it. Vitamin B_{12} deficiency can be caused by the following:

- Dietary deficiencies, especially in vegans who consume no animal products.
  - Although once thought to be rare, studies show relatively high vitamin B_{12} deficiency prevalence among vegetarians (Pawlak et al., 2014).
    - Vegans who do not consume vitamin B_{12} supplements are especially at high risk.
  - A dietary deficiency is preventable with regular consumption of oral supplements or vitamin B_{12}–fortified foods.
- Pernicious anemia is an autoimmune gastritis in which destruction of parietal cells leads to achlorhydria and failure to produce IF.
  - Even when intake is adequate, vitamin B_{12} deficiency occurs from severe vitamin B_{12} malabsorption.
- Conditions that impair the integrity of the stomach (e.g., total or partial gastrectomy, gastric bypass or other bariatric surgery) or bowel (e.g., ileal resection, inflammatory bowel disease) and Supplementation via injections, nasal gels, and sprays are available. Large oral doses have also been found to be an effective treatment (Chan et al., 2016).
  - These conditions can cause severe deficiency related to vitamin B_{12} malabsorption.
- Protein-bound vitamin B_{12} malabsorption is a milder form of atrophic gastritis in which low gastric acid secretion impairs the freeing of protein-bound vitamin B_{12} in foods.
  - It is frequently attributed to aging and affects up to 20% of older adults (Lewerin et al., 2008).
  - It may also occur secondary to the use of medications that suppress gastric acid secretion.
    - This mild form of malabsorption can be treated with large doses of oral supplements.
  - As a preventive measure, the National Academy of Sciences Food and Nutrition Board recommends that people older than age 50 years obtain most of their requirement from fortified foods or supplements (Food and Nutrition Board, IOM, 1998).

Other B Vitamins

Pantothenic acid is part of coenzyme A (CoA), the coenzyme involved in the formation of acetyl-CoA and in the tricarboxylic acid (TCA) cycle.

- Pantothenic acid participates in >100 different metabolic reactions.
- It is assumed that the average American diet provides adequate amounts of pantothenic acid.

As a coenzyme, biotin is involved in the TCA cycle, gluconeogenesis, fatty acid synthesis, and chemical reactions that add or remove carbon dioxide from other compounds.

- Significant amounts of biotin are synthesized by GI flora, but it is not known how much is available for absorption.
- It is assumed that the average American diet provides adequate amounts of biotin.

Choline

Choline is an essential nutrient commonly categorized with the B vitamins.

- Choline is required for the structural integrity of cell membranes.
- Although essential to life, few data exist on the effects of inadequate dietary intake in healthy people (Food and Nutrition Board, IOM, 1998).
- It is possible that the requirement for choline can be met by endogenous synthesis at some stages of the life cycle.

Vitamin C

Vitamin C (ascorbic acid) may be the most famous vitamin. Its long history dates back more than 250 years when it was determined that something in citrus fruits prevents scurvy, a disease that killed as many as two thirds of sailors on long journeys. Years later, British sailors acquired the nickname "Limeys" because of Great Britain's policy to prevent scurvy by providing limes to all sailors. It wasn't until 1932 that the anti-scurvy agent was identified as vitamin C. Acute vitamin C deficiency leads to scurvy.

- Overt deficiency symptoms occur only if vitamin C intake is approximately ≤10 mg/day for many weeks.
- Even though scurvy is deadly, it can be cured within a matter of days with moderate doses of vitamin C.
- Severe vitamin C deficiency is rare in developed nations but can occur in people who do not eat enough fruits and vegetables.
    - It is estimated that 90% of vitamin C in the typical diet comes from fruits and vegetables.
- The groups most at risk of vitamin C inadequacy include smokers who need more vitamin C because smoking increases oxidative stress and metabolic turnover of vitamin C (Food and Nutrition Board, IOM, 2000).
    - Smokers are advised to increase their intake by 35 mg/day.
- The other groups at risk of inadequate intake are people with severe malabsorption and those with end-stage renal disease on chronic hemodialysis.

There is no clear and convincing evidence that large doses of vitamin C prevent colds in the general population; however, in five trials, vitamin C decreased the risk of colds in people under physical stress (e.g., marathon runners or soldiers in subarctic environments) by 50% (Hemilä & Chalker, 2013). Efficacy is difficult to measure because it may be influenced by how much, how often, and how long supplements are used and by which outcome it is measured, such as frequency of colds, length of cold, and severity of symptoms.

VITAMINS IN HEALTH PROMOTION

A premise of the *Dietary Guidelines for Americans, 2020–2025* is that nutrient needs should be met primarily from nutrient-dense foods and beverages, not from supplements (U.S. Department of Agriculture [USDA], U.S. Department of Health and Human Services [USDHHS], 2020). Vitamins are found in all MyPlate food groups; however, items within each group vary in type and amount of vitamins they provide. For instance, kiwifruit is high in vitamin C (83 mg/½ cup) whereas pears are not (3 mg/½ cup). Eating a variety of nutrient-dense items within each group helps ensure nutritional adequacy.

Shortfall Vitamins

Concept Mastery Alert

Folate is found in fruits, vegetables, and protein foods and is beneficial to everyone, especially pregnant clients. Folic acid is found in fortified grains.

Based on data from National Health and Nutrition Examination Survey 2015 to 2016, the mean intake of vitamin A, vitamin D, vitamin E, vitamin C, and choline among both men and women age 20 and older is less than the Dietary References Intakes (USDA, ARS, 2018). Vitamin D is among the dietary components of public health concern for the general population because low intakes are associated with health concerns (USDA, USDHHS, 2020). Figure 6.2 illustrates mean intake of these shortfall vitamins expressed as a percentage of DRIs for each vitamin. The majority of the U.S. population has low intakes of key food groups or certain subgroups that provide these specific vitamins.

- Vitamin A: orange fruits and vegetables, dark-green vegetables, and fortified dairy products.
- Vitamin D: fortified dairy products and seafood.

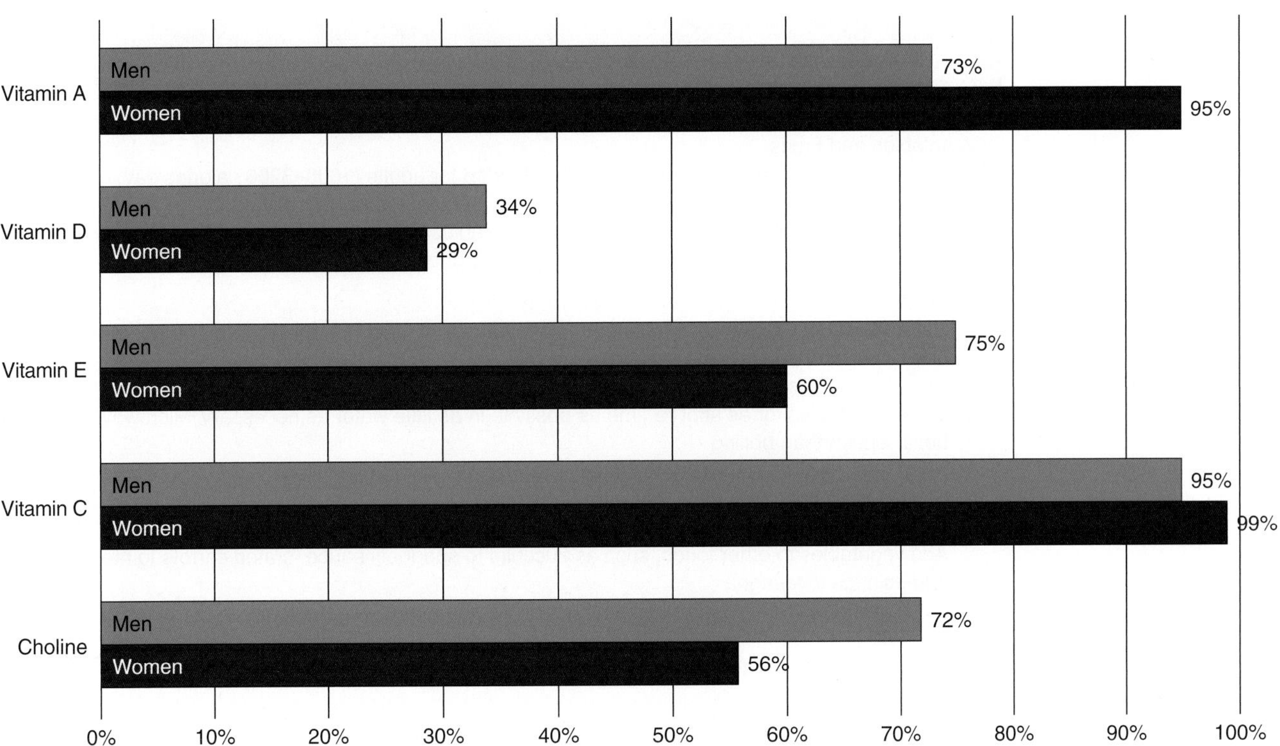

Figure 6.2 ▲ Mean intake of shortfall vitamins as a percentage of the Recommended Dietary Allowance in adult men and women. (Data from the USDA, ARS. [2018]. *Nutrient intakes from food and beverages: Mean amounts consumed per individual, by gender and age, What We Eat in America, NHANES 2015–2016.* www.ars.usda.gov/nea/bhnrc/fsrg)

- Vitamin E: oils, whole grains, and dark-green vegetables.
- Vitamin C: fruits and vegetables.
- Choline: dairy products, certain vegetables

Vitamin-Rich Eating Patterns

Healthy eating patterns recommended by leading health agencies encourage plant-based diets that emphasize fruits, vegetables, beans, peas, lentils, nuts, whole grains, seafood, and other lean proteins—all in nutrient-dense forms. Even further, they promote limiting foods that are nutrient poor, such as sugar-sweetened beverages and processed meats. Strategies that will help Americans increase their intake of shortfall nutrients and improve intake overall are as follows:

- Consume more vegetables from all subgroups, concentrating on variety. Box 6.2 provides tips for boosting fruit and vegetable intake.
- Consume more fruit.
- Consume more whole grains in place of refined grains. Whole grains provide more vitamin E than refined grains as well as phytonutrients and antioxidants.
- Consume more nonfat and low-fat dairy products, especially those fortified with vitamins A and D.
- Include a greater variety of nutrient-dense items within the protein foods group, such as more seafood (e.g., provides vitamin D) and nuts and seeds (e.g., provide vitamin E).
- Replace solid fats with oils, which will improve vitamin E intake.

BOX 6.2 Tips for Boosting Fruit and Vegetable Intake

Vegetables and Fruits

- Intake recommendations among patterns intended for adults (1600–3200 calories/day) range from 1½ to 2½ c of fruit per day and from 2 to 4 c of vegetables per day.
- Fill half the dinner plate with vegetables or vegetables and fruit.
- Buy a new fruit or vegetable when you go grocery shopping.

Vegetables

- Eat a variety of vegetables in different colors. Aim for at least one green, one orange, one red, one citrus, and one legume serving every day.
- Store vegetables correctly to preserve vitamin content. Keep most in the refrigerator.
- Cook vegetables for as short a time as possible in as little water as necessary. Microwaving is a better option than boiling.
- Keep fresh vegetables on the top shelf of the refrigerator in plain view.
- Start at least one meal each day with a fresh salad.
- Eat raw vegetables for snacks.
- Add vegetables to other foods, such as zucchini to spaghetti sauce, grated carrots to meat loaf, and spinach to lasagna.
- Eat occasional meatless entrees such as pasta primavera, vegetable stir fry, or black beans and rice.
- Order a vegetable when you eat out.

Fruit

- Leave a bowl of fruit on the center of your table.
- Snack on fruit. Add fruit to salads.
- Use fruit as a side dish.
- Eat fruit for dessert.

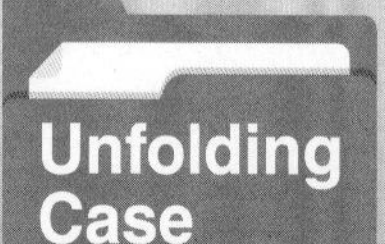

Consider Marcus. One of his food obsessions is a fortified gluten-free cereal. It is fortified with 100% of the Daily Value (DV) for many vitamins—but those DVs are based on adult requirements, not recommendations for children. Marcus eats a few servings of this cereal daily, so he is getting much larger amounts of certain vitamins and minerals than is required. If the percentage of the DV is not valid due to his age, how can his vitamin intake from the cereal be determined? Would you encourage Marcus's parents to find a nonfortified gluten-free cereal? Would you recommend they discontinue his vitamin and mineral supplements?

Phytonutrients: Technically Not Vitamins but Health Enhancing

Phytonutrients
bioactive, nonnutrient plant compounds associated with a reduced risk of chronic diseases.

Phytonutrients, also known as phytochemicals, are literally plant ("phyto" in Greek) chemicals. They are a broad, diverse, and bioactive class of nonnutritive compounds that function like the immune system of plants to protect them against viruses, bacteria, and fungi. In foods, phytonutrients impart color, taste, aroma, and other characteristics. When eaten in the "package" of fruit, vegetables, whole grains, or nuts, these chemicals work together with nutrients and fiber to promote health by acting as antioxidants, detoxifying enzymes, stimulating the immune system, regulating hormones, or inactivating bacteria and viruses. More than 25,000 phytochemicals have been identified; often, their actions in the body are complementary and overlapping.

BOX 6.3 Examples of Phytonutrients and Their Connection to Health

Lycopene in tomatoes and tomato products may reduce the risk of prostate cancer.
Lignans in flaxseed and whole grains may reduce the risk of certain kinds of cancer.
Genistein in soybeans may decrease the risk of breast and uterine cancer.
Isothiocyanates in cruciferous vegetables (broccoli, cabbage, kale, etc.) may induce detoxification of carcinogens.
Lutein in dark-green leafy vegetables may reduce the risk of age-related eye diseases.
Resveratrol in red wine and red grape juice may lower the risk of heart disease by improving blood flow to the heart and preventing blood clots.
Catechins in green tea may help prevent DNA damage by neutralizing free radicals.

Phytonutrients are hypothesized to be a large part of the reason why eating patterns high in plants, namely, fruits and vegetables; whole grains; legumes; nuts; and tea are associated with lower risk of chronic disease, such as heart disease, cancer, and diabetes. Box 6.3 lists examples for phytonutrients and their connection to health.

- At this time, researchers simply do not know all the components in plants, how they function, which ones are beneficial, which ones are potentially harmful, and the ideal combination and concentration of these chemicals to be able to create a pill to substitute for a varied diet rich in plants.
- More than likely, it is the total package and balance of nutrients and nonnutritive substances that make fruits and vegetables so healthy.
- Until science catches up to nature, the best advice is to eat a diet rich in a variety of plants.

Vitamin Supplements

Multivitamin and mineral (MVM) supplements are the most commonly used dietary supplements among American adults in the United States (Marra & Bailey, 2018). Depending on the definition of MVM, an estimated one third of American adults use MVM and among adults age 60 and older the percentage rises to 40 (Kantor et al., 2016). Supplement use is associated with several sociodemographic variables (Kantor et al., 2016):

- Supplement use increases with age.
- Women are more likely than men to use supplements.
- Use is highest among non-Hispanic white adults.
- Supplement use is highest among the most highly educated.
- Supplement users most often report their health status as excellent.
- "Improve overall health," "maintain health," "supplement the diet," and "prevent health problems" are the most commonly cited motivations for general supplement use (Baily et al., 2012).

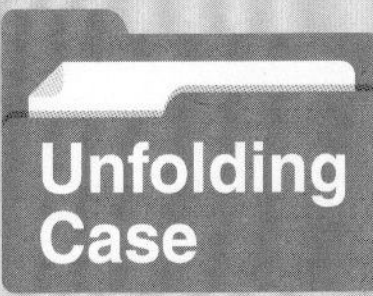

Think of Marcus. As with healthy adults, studies of children with autism taking supplements show that the children most likely to take supplements were less likely to need them. This may reflect heightened awareness of nutrition by some families in regard to both food and supplements. Is too much better than too little?

The shortfall nutrients identified above, namely vitamins A, C, D, E, and choline, indicate that a high prevalence of inadequate intakes relative to the DRIs exists across the population and that underconsumption has been linked to adverse health outcomes (Marra& Bailey, 2018). Many Americans do not eat the amount and types of foods necessary to meet recommended nutrient intakes. MVM supplements can bridge the gap in meeting those nutrient needs.

Although MVM can help Americans consume an adequate intake of nutrients, they are not a guarantee of good health.

- Consuming nutrients in supplement form increases the risk of exceeding the UL of some nutrients.
- Supplements have not been shown effective at reducing the risk of chronic diseases in generally healthy people (Huang et al., 2007). Table 6.4 summarizes studies that examined the role of vitamin supplements in chronic disease.

The U.S. Preventative Services Task Force position on the use of multivitamins is that current evidence is insufficient to assess the balance of benefits and risks for the prevention of cardiovascular disease or cancer (U.S. Preventive Services Task Force, 2014). Specially formulated supplements containing carotenes, vitamin E, and vitamin C have been found to reduce the risk of developing advanced age-related macular degeneration (AMD) among people at high risk (see Table 6.4). In general, groups that may benefit from a multivitamin supplement include the following:

- Dieters who consume fewer than 1200 cal/day.
  - Even with optimal food choices, it may not be possible to consume adequate amounts of all nutrients on a low-calorie diet.
- Vegans, who eat no animal products, need supplemental vitamin B_{12} because it is found naturally only in animal products.
  - Vegetarians may also need vitamin D if sunlight exposure is inadequate because the only plant sources of vitamin D are some fortified margarines, mushrooms exposed to UV light, and some fortified cereals.
- People with poor appetite or illness or those who intentionally eliminated one or more food groups from their diet on a regular basis.
- Older adults. Risk factors in this population include limited food budget, impaired chewing and swallowing, social isolation, physical limitations that make shopping or cooking difficult, or a decreased sense of taste leading to poor appetite.
  - It is recommended that people 50 and over consume 2.4 mcg/day of vitamin B_{12} through supplements or fortified food.
- Women of childbearing age who may become pregnant. The U.S. Preventive Services Task Force recommends all women who are capable of becoming pregnant take a daily supplement containing 400 to 800 mcg of folic acid for the prevention of neural tube defects (U.S. Preventive Services Task Force, 2017).
- Alcohol-dependent people because alcohol alters vitamin intake, absorption, metabolism, and excretion; the nutrients most profoundly affected are thiamin, riboflavin, niacin, folic acid, and pantothenic acid.
- People who are food insecure, meaning they may not always have sufficient money or other resources for food for all household members.
- People with chronic illness or chronic use of a medication that impairs nutrient absorption or increases nutrient metabolism or excretion.

Choosing a Supplement

Although there is little scientific evidence to suggest that vitamin supplements can benefit the average person, there is also little evidence of harm from low-dose multivitamin or MVM supplements.

- Vitamins work best together and in balanced proportions, so a multivitamin that provides no more than 100% of the DV is usually better than single-vitamin supplements that tend to provide doses much greater than the RDA.
- Pills are not a substitute for healthy food: "supplement" means "add to," not "replace."
  - MVM supplements are limited in what they contain. They do not provide all the health-enhancing compounds found in foods, such as phytonutrients and fiber.

Table 6.4 What Studies Reveal about Vitamin Supplements and Chronic Disease Prevention

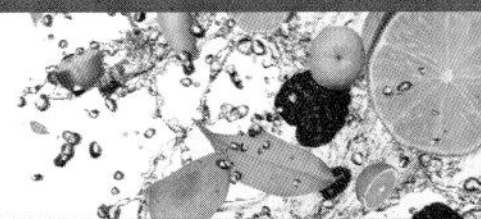

Vitamins	Chronic Disease	What Research Reveals
Beta carotene	Heart disease and cancer	A landmark trial designed to test whether beta-carotene supplements could decrease cancer incidence in people at high risk was prematurely halted when results showed a surprising increase in lung cancer incidence and deaths in smokers and male asbestos workers (Omenn et al., 1996; The Alpha-Tocopherol, Beta-Carotene Cancer Prevention Study Group, 1994). The U.S. Preventive Services Task Force recommends against beta-carotene supplements for the prevention of cardiovascular disease or cancer (Moyer, 2014).
Carotenes, Vitamin E, Vitamin C	Age-related macular degeneration	The Age-Related Eye Disease Study found that participants at high risk of developing advanced AMD reduced their risk of developing advanced AMD by 25% by taking a daily supplement containing beta carotene, vitamin E, vitamin C, and zinc for 5 years (Age-Related Eye Disease Study Research Group, 2001).
Vitamin D	Autoimmune diseases such as multiple sclerosis (hypertension, cardiovascular diseases, metabolic syndrome, type 2 diabetes, several types of cancer, cognitive decline, depression, and respiratory diseases)	A large review of observation and randomized controlled trials of vitamin D was used to examine vitamin D and 137 outcomes, including skeletal, cancer, cardiovascular, autoimmune, infections, metabolic, and other diseases (Theodoratou et al., 2014). • No highly convincing evidence was found of a clear role of vitamin D with any outcome. • There was some evidence for some outcomes (e.g., decreased risk of colorectal cancer, cardiovascular disease prevalence, hypertension, high body mass index, type 2 diabetes), but researchers concluded more evidence is needed. • Probable associations were found with a few selected outcomes, such as birth weight, dental cavities in children, and parathyroid hormone concentrations in people on dialysis. Likewise, a 5-year-old nationwide, randomized, placebo-controlled trial of vitamin D among healthy American adults showed that high-dose vitamin D did not reduce the incidence of cancer or major cardiovascular events (Manson et al., 2019).
Vitamin E	Cancer	Most randomized trials find that vitamin E is not beneficial with regard to total or site-specific cancers (Wang et al., 2014). A study in the post-trial follow-up to the Selenium and Vitamin E Cancer Prevention Trial (SELECT) found that vitamin E supplementation significantly *increased* the risk of prostate cancer in healthy men (Klein et al., 2011). The U.S. Preventive Services Task Force recommends against vitamin E supplements for the prevention of cardiovascular disease or cancer (Moyer, 2014).
Vitamin B_6, folic acid, and B_{12}	Cardiovascular disease	Large clinical trials have failed to show that supplemental B vitamins lower the risk of cardiovascular events, even though they lower homocysteine levels (National Institutes of Health, Office of Dietary Supplements, 2019b). To date, there is little evidence to support the use of B_6 alone or in combination with folic acid and B_{12}, to lower the risk or severity of cardiovascular disease and stroke.
Vitamin B_6	Cancer	The few clinical trials completed to date do not show that vitamin B_6 supplementation helps prevent cancer or lowers its mortality risk (National Institutes of Health, Office of Dietary Supplements, 2019b).
	Cognitive decline	More evidence is needed to determine if vitamin B_6 supplementation helps prevent or treat cognitive decline in senior adults (National Institutes of Health, Office of Dietary Supplements, 2019b).
Folate	Cancer	Evidence suggests adequate *dietary* folate may decrease the risk of some cancers but the effects of supplemental folic acid on cancer are not clear (NIH, ODS, 2019c).
	Alzheimer's disease, dementia	Most clinical trial research has not shown that folic acid supplementation affects cognitive function or the development of Alzheimer's disease or dementia (NIH, ODS, 2019c).
Choline	Cardiovascular disease, peripheral artery disease, Alzheimer's disease, nonalcoholic fatty liver disease	Some observational studies show a link between choline intake and these disorders, and others do not. More research is needed (NIH, ODS, 2019d).
Vitamin C	Cancer prevention	Evidence from most randomized clinical trials suggests that vitamin C supplementation, alone or in combination with other micronutrients, does not affect cancer risk (NIH, ODS, 2019e).
	Cardiovascular disease	Findings from most intervention trials do not provide convincing evidence that the supplements of vitamin C decrease the risk of cardiovascular disease or lower its morbidity or mortality (NIH, ODS, 2019e).
MVM	Cardiovascular disease	A systematic review and meta-analysis of existing systematic reviews and meta-analyses and single randomized controlled trials found no consistent benefit between MVM use and the prevention of cardiovascular disease, myocardial infarction, stroke, or all-cause mortality during the study period. Researchers speculate that a longer period of study may be needed to observe lower risk because chronic diseases develop over a long period of time (Jenkins et al., 2018).

- The Food and Drug Administration (FDA) requires a standardized "Supplement Facts" label on all supplements.
  - Like the "Nutrition Facts" label, the supplement label is intended to provide consumers with better information.
- According to the FDA, "high potency" may be used to describe individual vitamins or minerals that are present at ≥100% of the Reference Daily Intakes.
- When possible, people should choose an MVM appropriately tailored to their age, sex, or condition, such as pregnancy. For instance, MVM for older adults may provide more vitamin D and vitamin B_{12} than MVM for younger adults.

How Do You Respond?

Is it better to take vitamin supplements with meals or between meals? In general, it is better to take supplements with meals because food enhances the absorption of some vitamins.

What does "USP" on the vitamin label mean? USP (U.S. Pharmacopeia) means the product passes tests for disintegration, dissolution, strength, and purity. It does not ensure that the supplement is safe or beneficial to health.

Is price an indication of quality? Should I buy the most expensive vitamins? No, cost is not an indication of quality. Large retail chains are high-volume customers and can demand their own top-quality, private label supplements that are comparable to brand-name varieties in content and quality. Content and freshness are key considerations with vitamins.

REVIEW CASE STUDY

Michael is a 22-year-old college student who lives off campus. He has a kitchen in his apartment, but he has neither time nor interest in making or stocking his own food. All three of his daily meals come from fast-food restaurants. A typical day's intake is shown to the right.

- What vitamins is Michael probably lacking in his diet? What vitamins is he probably getting enough of?
- Are there better choices he could make at fast-food restaurants that would improve his vitamin intake?
- What suggestions would you make for keeping *quick* and *easy* food in his apartment that would improve his vitamin intake without being too much *bother*?
- Michael asks, "Can I just take a multivitamin so I don't have to make changes in my eating habits?" How would you respond?

Breakfast: Two egg and bacon sandwiches on English muffins, large coffee with creamer and sugar.
Lunch: Two cheeseburgers with ketchup, large french fries, soft drink, and cookies.
Dinner: A foot-long submarine with deli meats, cheese, mayonnaise, lettuce, tomato, onion, and pickles; bag of potato chips; and soft drink.
Snacks: Chocolate bar, chips and salsa, and popcorn.

STUDY QUESTIONS

1 When developing a teaching plan for a client who is on warfarin (Coumadin), which of the following foods would the nurse suggest that the client consume consistently because of their vitamin K content?
   a. Vegetable oils, fruit, and seafood
   b. Brussels sprouts, cauliflower, and spinach
   c. Fortified cereals, whole grains, and nuts
   d. Dried peas and beans, wheat germ, and seeds

2 A client asks if it is better to consume folic acid from fortified foods or from a vitamin pill. What is the nurse's best response?
   a. "It is better to consume folic acid through fortified foods because it will be better absorbed than through pill form."
   b. "It is better to consume folic acid through vitamin pills because it will be better absorbed than through fortified foods."
   c. "Fortified foods and vitamin pills have the same form of folic acid, so it does not matter which source you use because they are both well absorbed."
   d. "It is best to consume naturally rich sources of folate because that form is better absorbed than the folic acid in either fortified foods or vitamin pills."

3 Which population is at risk for combined deficiencies of thiamin, riboflavin, and niacin?
   a. Pregnant women
   b. Vegetarians
   c. Alcoholics
   d. Athletes

4 Which vitamin is given in large doses to facilitate wound and bone healing?
   a. Vitamin A
   b. Vitamin D
   c. Vitamin C
   d. Niacin

5 Which statement indicates that the client understands the instructions given about using a vitamin supplement?
   a. "USP on the label guarantees safety and effectiveness."
   b. "Natural vitamins are always better for you than synthetic vitamins."
   c. "Vitamins are best absorbed on an empty stomach."
   d. "Taking a multivitamin cannot fully make up for poor food choices."

6 The client asks if taking supplements of beta carotene will help reduce risk of cancer. What is the nurse's best response?
   a. "Supplements of beta carotene may help reduce the risk of heart disease but not of cancer."
   b. "Supplements of beta carotene have not been shown to lower the risk of cancer and may even promote cancer in certain people."
   c. "Although evidence is preliminary, taking beta-carotene supplements is safe and may prove to be effective against cancer in the future."
   d. "Natural supplements of beta carotene are generally harmless; synthetic supplements of beta carotene may increase cancer risk and should be avoided."

7 A client is diagnosed with pernicious anemia. What vitamin are they not absorbing?
   a. Folic acid
   b. Vitamin B_6
   c. Vitamin B_{12}
   d. Niacin

8 A client with hyperlipidemia is prescribed niacin. The client asks if they can simply include more niacin-rich foods in their diet in order to forgo niacin in pill form. What is the nurse's best response?
   a. "The dose of niacin needed to treat hyperlipidemia is far more than can be consumed through eating a niacin-rich diet."
   b. "You can't get the therapeutic form of niacin through food."
   c. "Niacin from food is not as well absorbed as niacin from pills."
   d. "If you are able to consistently choose niacin-fortified foods in your diet, then your doctor may allow you to forgo the pills and rely on dietary sources of niacin."

CHAPTER SUMMARY VITAMINS

Vitamins do not provide calories but are involved in the metabolism of energy.

- Only small amounts are needed: microgram or milligram quantities.
- They are essential in the diet because they cannot be made by the body or they are synthesized in inadequate amounts.
- Fortification and enrichment have virtually eliminated vitamin deficiencies in healthy Americans.
- If a variety of nutritious foods are consumed, then vitamin intake will likely be adequate for most people.
- Vitamins are organic compounds that are soluble in either water or fat. Their solubility determines how they are absorbed, transported through the blood, stored, and excreted.

(continued)

CHAPTER SUMMARY VITAMINS (continued)

Fat-Soluble Vitamins

Vitamins A, D, E, and K are the fat-soluble vitamins. They do not need to be consumed daily because they are stored in the liver and adipose tissue.

Vitamin A is preformed or from the precursor beta carotene, and involved in vision, growth, development, and immune system functioning. Preformed vitamin A is toxic in large amounts and can cause birth defects during pregnancy.

Vitamin D naturally occurs in few foods. A major source is endogenous synthesis from sunlight on the skin. Lack of adequate sunlight is the biggest cause of deficiency. It maintains serum calcium and phosphorus concentrations to maintain bone integrity. Excessive intakes can cause hypercalcemia, hypercalciuria, and vascular and soft-tissue calcification.

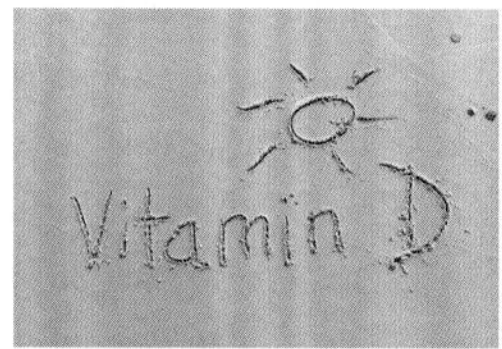

Vitamin E acts as an antioxidant to protect vitamin A and polyunsaturated fats. Richest sources are vegetable oils, green leafy vegetables, and fortified cereals. It is relatively nontoxic.

Vitamin K is a coenzyme for reactions involved in blood clotting and bone metabolism. It is synthesized by intestinal microbiota. Dietary sources include green leafy vegetables, other vegetables, and eggs. Certain anticoagulants and antibiotics interfere with vitamin K metabolism or synthesis.

Water-Soluble Vitamins

The B-complex vitamins and vitamin C are water-soluble. A daily intake is necessary because they are generally not stored in the body. They are considered nontoxic because they are excreted when consumed in excess.

Thiamin (B_1), riboflavin (B_2), and niacin (B_3) share similar sources (e.g., refined grains) and function as coenzymes in energy metabolism. Americans consume more than required. People who abuse alcohol are most at risk for deficiency.

Vitamin B_6 is involved in amino acid and fatty acid metabolism and helps produce several body compounds. It is stored extensively in muscle tissue. Large doses over long periods of time cause neurological symptoms.

Folate is the umbrella name for food form (folate) and synthetic form (folic acid) that occurs in fortified foods and supplements. It acts as a coenzyme in DNA synthesis. It helps prevent neural tube defects when taken in adequate amounts before conception and through the first trimester.

Vitamin B_{12} occurs only in animal products. It needs IF in the stomach for absorption. The liver stores may last 5–10 years. Deficiency symptoms include anemia and neurologic impairments that can be permanent.

Other B vitamins, such as pantothenic acid and biotin, are widespread in the diet and act as coenzymes in energy metabolism. It is assumed that the average American diet provides adequate amounts of both.

Choline is often categorized with B vitamins. It is necessary for structural integrity of cell membranes. The best sources are milk, liver, and eggs. The emulsifier lecithin provides choline.

Vitamin C is important for collagen formation, wound healing, and immune system functioning and acts as an antioxidant. Best sources are citrus fruits and juices. Scurvy can occur after a month of poor vitamin C intake and can be fatal but is quickly and easily cured with supplements.

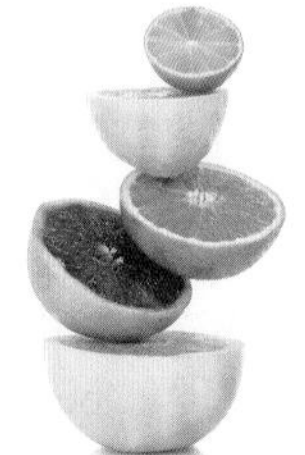

Vitamins in Health Promotion

Vitamin needs should be met primarily from food, not from supplements.

Shortfall Nutrients and Vitamin-Rich Eating Patterns: Vitamins that are under-consumed by American adults are vitamins A, D, E, C, and choline.

- Key food groups that supply these vitamins—vegetables, fruits, whole grains, and dairy—are under-consumed by the majority of Americans.
- To obtain adequate amounts of these shortfall vitamins, Americans are urged to eat more fruit, preferably whole fruits; more vegetables in greater variety; whole grains in place of refined grains; more seafood; vitamin A- and D-fortified dairy products; and oils in place of solid fats.

Phytonutrients. Phytonutrients are bioactive plant chemicals that promote health by various methods, such as acting as antioxidants, detoxifying enzymes, stimulating the immune system, and regulating hormones.

- Not enough is known about phytonutrients to elevate them to the status of essential nutrients.
- Different plants have different phytochemicals: Eating a variety of plants provides a variety of phytochemicals.

Vitamin Supplements: More than half of American adults take a supplement. Usage increases among older people. Most people who take them say they have excellent health but take supplements to improve their health.

CHAPTER SUMMARY VITAMINS (continued)

- MVM supplements can bridge the gap in meeting vitamin needs in people who do not have a vitamin-rich eating pattern. They do not provide all the healthful substances found in food.
- Vegans, older adults, people with certain chronic diseases, and people dependent on alcohol are among the groups who may benefit from MVM.
- Taking an MVM that provides no more than 100% of the DV is usually better than taking individual nutrients.
- People should use supplements tailored to their sex, age, and condition (e.g., pregnancy).
- More is not better. Studies using supplements to reduce the risk of chronic disease generally have not shown benefits, with the exception of reducing the risk of AMD in certain groups.

Figure sources: *shutterstock.com/Happy Zoe, shutterstock.com/Gts, and shutterstock.com/RudchenkoLiliia*

Student Resources on thePoint®
For additional learning materials, activate the code in the front of this book at https://thePoint.lww.com/activate

Websites

Dietary Reference Intakes from the Institute of Medicine at www.nap.edu
National Institutes of Health Office of Dietary Supplements at ods.od.nih.gov
Produce for Better Health Foundation at www.fruitsandveggiesmorematters.org
U.S. Department of Agriculture Nutrient Data Laboratory at fnic.nal.usda.gov/food-composition/usda-nutrient-data-laboratory

References

Age-Related Eye Disease Study Research Group. (2001). A randomized, placebo-controlled, clinical trial of high-dose supplementation with vitamins C and E, beta carotene, and zinc for age-related macular degeneration and vision loss: AREDS report no. 8. *Archives of Ophthalmology, 119*(10), 1417–1436. https://doi.org/10.1001/archopht.119.10.1417

The Alpha-Tocopherol, Beta-Carotene Cancer Prevention Study Group. (1994). The effect of vitamin D and beta carotene on the incidence of lung cancer and other cancers in male smokers. *The New England Journal of Medicine, 330*, 1029–1035. https://doi.org/ 10.1056/NEJM199404143301501

Bailey, R. L., Fulgoni, V. L. 3rd, Keast, D. R., & Dwyer, J. T. (2012). Examination of vitamin intakes among US adults by dietary supplement use. *Journal of the Academy of Nutrition and Dietetics, 112*(5), 657–663.e4. https://doi.org/10.1016/j.jand.2012.01.026

Chan, C., Low, L., & Lee, K. (2016). Oral vitamin B_{12} replacement for the treatment of pernicious anemia. *Frontiers in Medicine, 3*, 38. https://doi.org/10.3389/fmed.2016.00038

Food and Nutrition Board, Institute of Medicine. (1998). *Dietary reference intakes for thiamin, riboflavin, niacin, vitamin B_6, folate, vitamin B_{12}, pantothenic acid, biotin, and choline.* The National Academies Press.

Food and Nutrition Board, Institute of Medicine. (2000). *Dietary reference intakes for vitamin C, vitamin E, selenium, and carotenoids.* The National Academies Press.

Food and Nutrition Board, Institute of Medicine. (2011). *Dietary reference intakes for calcium and vitamin D.* The National Academies Press.

Hemilä, H., & Chalker, E. (2013). Vitamin C for preventing and treating the common cold. *Cochrane Database of Systematic Reviews, 1*, CD000980. https://doi.org/10.1002/14651858.CD000980.pub4

Holick, M. (2007). Vitamin D deficiency. *The New England Journal of Medicine, 357*, 266–281. https://doi.org/10.1056/NEJMra070553

Huang, H.-Y., Caballero, B., Chang, S., Alberg, A. J., Semba, R. D., Schneyer, C., Wilson, R. F., Cheng, T.-Y., Prokopowicz, G., Barnes, G. J., Vassy, J., & Bass, E. B. (2007). Multivitamin/mineral supplements and prevention of chronic disease: Executive summary. *American Journal of Clinical Nutrition, 85*(1), 265S–268S. https://doi.org/10.1093/ajcn/85.1.265S

Jenkins, D., Spence, J., Giovannucci, E., Kim, Y.-I., Josse, R., Vieth, R., Mejia, S. B., Viguiliouk, E., Nishi, S., Sahye-Pudaruth, S., Paquette, M., Patel, D., Mitchell, S., Kavanagh, M., Tsirakis, T., Bachiri, L., Maran, A., Umatheva, N., McKay, T., … Sievenpiper, J. L. (2018). Supplemental vitamins and minerals for CVD prevention and treatment. *Journal of the American College of Cardiologists, 71*(22), 2570–2584. https://doi.org/10.1016/j.jacc.2018.04.020

Kantor, E., Rehm, C., Du, M., White, E., &Giovannucci, E. L. (2016). Trends in dietary supplement use among U.S. adults from 1999–2012. *JAMA, 316*(14), 1464–1474. https://doi.org/10.1001/jama.2016.14403

Klein, E., Thompson, I., Tangen, C., Crowley, J. J., Lucia, M. S., Goodman, P. J., Minasian, L. M., Ford, L. G., Parnes, H. L., Gaziano, M., Karp, D. D., Lieber, M. M., Walther, P.J., Klotz, L., Parsons, J. K., Chin, J. L., Darke, A. K., Lippman, S. M., Goodman, G. E., & Baker, L. H. (2011). Vitamin E and the risk of prostate cancer: The Selenium and Vitamin E Cancer Prevention Trial (SELECT). *JAMA, 306*, 1549–1556. https://doi:10.1001/jama.2011.1437

Kulkantrakorn, K. (2014). Pyridoxine-induced sensory ataxic neuronopathy and neuropathy: Revisited. *Neurological Sciences, 35*, 1827–1830. https://doi.org/10.1007/s10072-014-1902-6

Lewerin, C., Jacobsson, S., Lindstedt, G., & Nilsson-Ehle, H. (2008). Serum biomarkers for atrophic gastritis and antibodies against Helicobacter pylori in the elderly: Implication for vitamin B_{12}, folic acid and iron status and response to oral vitamin therapy. *Scandinavian Journal of Gastroenterology, 43*, 1050–1056. https://doi.org/10.1080/00365520802078341

Manson, J., Cook, N., Lee, I.-M., Christen, W., Bassuk, S. S., Mora, S., Gibson, H., Gordon, D., Copeland, T., D'Agostino, D., Friedenberg, G., Ridge, C., Bubes, V., Giovannucci, E. L., Willett, W. C., & Buring, J. E. for the VITAL Research Group. (2019). Vitamin D supplements and prevention of cancer and cardiovascular disease. *New England Journal of Medicine, 380*, 33–44. https://doi.org/10.1056/NEJMoa1809944

Marra, M., & Bailey, R. (2018). Position of the academy of nutrition and dietetics: Micronutrient supplementation. *Journal of the Academy of Nutrition and Dietetics, 118*(11), 2162–2173. https://doi.org/10.1016/j.jand.2018.07.022

Medical Research Council Vitamin Study Research Group. (1991). Prevention of neural tube defects: Results of the Medical Research Council Vitamin Study. *Lancet, 338*(8760), 131–137. https://doi.org/10.1016/0140-6736(91)90133-A

Moyer, V. on behalf of the U.S. Preventive Services Task Force. (2014). Vitamin, mineral, and multivitamin supplements for the primary prevention of cardiovascular disease and cancer: U.S. Preventive Services Task Force Recommendation Statement. *Annals of Internal Medicine, 160*(8), 558–564.

Nair, R., & Maseeh, A. (2012). Vitamin D: The "sunshine" vitamin. *Journal of Pharmacology and Pharmacotherapeutics, 3*(2), 118–126. https://doi.org/10.4103/0976-500X.95506

National Institutes of Health, Office of Dietary Supplements. (2019a). *Vitamin D: Fact sheet for health professionals.* https://ods.od.nih.gov/factsheets/VitaminD-HealthProfessional/

National Institutes of Health, Office of Dietary Supplements. (2019b). *Vitamin B6: Fact sheet for health professionals.* https://ods.od.nih.gov/factsheets/VitaminB6-HealthProfessional/

National Institutes of Health, Office of Dietary Supplements. (2019c). *Folate: Fact sheet for health professionals.* https://ods.od.nih.gov/factsheets/Folate-HealthProfessional/

National Institutes of Health, Office of Dietary Supplements. (2019d). *Choline: Fact sheet for health professionals.* https://ods.od.nih.gov/factsheets/Choline-HealthProfessional/

National Institutes of Health, Office of Dietary Supplements. (2019e). *Vitamin C: Fact sheet for health professionals.* https://ods.od.nih.gov/factsheets/VitaminC-HealthProfessional/

Niebyl, J. (2010). Clinical practice: Nausea and vomiting in pregnancy. *New England Journal of Medicine, 363*, 1544–1550. https://doi.org/10.1056/NEJMcp1003896

Nuangchamnong, N., & Niebyl, J. (2014). Doxylamine succinate-pyridoxine hydrochloride (Diclegis) for the management of nausea and vomiting in pregnancy: An overview. *International Journal of Women's Health, 6*, 401–409. https://doi.org/10.2147/IJWH.S46653

Omenn, G. S., Goodman, G. E., Thornquist, M. D., Balmes, J., Cullen, M. R., Glass, A., Keogh, J. P., Meyskens, F. L., Valanis, B., Williams, J. H., Barnhart, S., & Hammar, S. (1996). Effects of a combination of beta carotene and vitamin A on lung cancer and cardiovascular disease. *The New England Journal of Medicine, 334*, 1150–1155. https://doi.org/10.1056/NEJM199605023341802

Pawlak, R., Lester, S., &Babatunde, T. (2014). The prevalence of cobalamin deficiency among vegetarians assessed by serum vitamin B12: A review of literature. *European Journal of Clinical Nutrition, 68*, 541–548. https://doi.org/10.1038/ejcn.2014.46

Pfotenhauer, K. M., & Shubrook, J. H. (2017). Vitamin D deficiency, its role in health and disease, and current supplementation recommendations. *The Journal of the American Osteopathic Association, 117*(5), 301–305. https://doi.org/10.7556/jaoa.2017.055

Saini, R., Nile, S., & Kerum, Y.-S. (2016). Folates: Chemistry, analysis, occurrence, biofortification and bioavailability. *Food Research International, 89*(part 1), 1–13. https://doi.org/10.1016/j.foodres.2016.07.013

Stevens, G., Bennett, J., Hennocq, Q., Lu, Y., De-Regil, L.M., Rogers, L., Danaei, G., Li, G., White, R. A., Flaxman, S. R., Oehrle, S.-P., Finucane, M.M., Guerrero, R., Bhutta, Z. A., Then-Paulino, A., Fawzi, W., Black, R. E., & Ezzati, M. (2015). Trends and mortality effects of vitamin A deficiency in children in 138 low-income and middle-income countries between 1991 and 2013: A pooled analysis of population-based surveys. *The Lancet Global Health, 3*(9), e528–e536. https://doi.org/10.1016/S2214-109X(15)00039-X

Theodoratou, E., Tzoulaki, I., Zgaga, L., & Ioannidis, J. P. (2014). Vitamin D and multiple health outcomes: Umbrella review of systematic reviews and meta-analyses of observational studies and randomised trials. *British Medical Journal (Clinical research ed.), 348*, g2035. https://doi.org/10.1136/bmj.g2035

U.S. Department of Agriculture, Agricultural Research Service. (2018). Nutrient intakes from food and beverages: Mean amounts consumed per individual, by gender and age. *What We Eat in American, NHANE 201*. www.ars.usda.gov.nea/blnrc/fsrg

U.S. Department of Agriculture, U.S. Department of Health and Human Services. (2020, December). *Dietary guidelines for Americans, 2020–2025.* https://www.dietaryguidelines.gov

U.S. Preventive Services Task Force. (2014, February, 15). *Vitamin supplementation to prevent cancer and CVD: Preventive medication.* https://www.uspreventiveservicestaskforce.org/uspstf/recommendation/vitamin-supplementation-to-prevent-cancer-and-cvd-counseling#fullrecommendationstart

U.S. Preventive Services Task Force. (2017). Folic acid supplementation for the prevention of neural tube defects. *Journal of the American Medical Association, 317*(2), 183–189. https://doi.org/10.1001/jama.2016.19438

Wang, L., Sesso, H. D., Glynn, R. J., Christen, W. G., Bubes, V., Manson, J. E., Buring, J. E., & Gaziano, J. M. (2014). Vitamin E and C supplementation and risk of cancer in men: Posttrial follow-up in the Physician's Health Study II randomized trial. *The American Journal of Clinical Nutrition, 100*(3), 915–923. https://doi.org/10.3945/ajcn.114.085480

Chapter 7 Water and Minerals

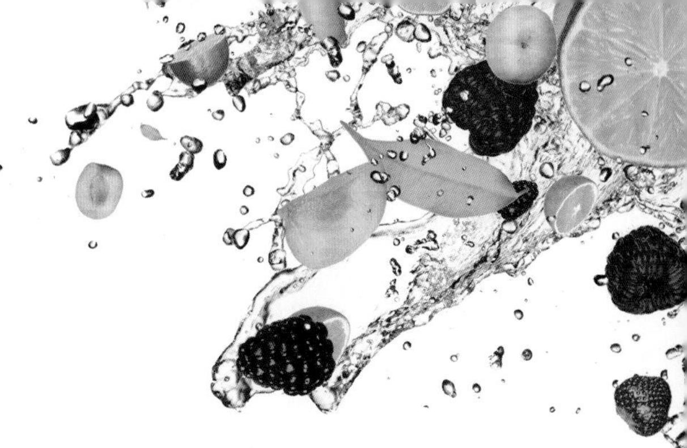

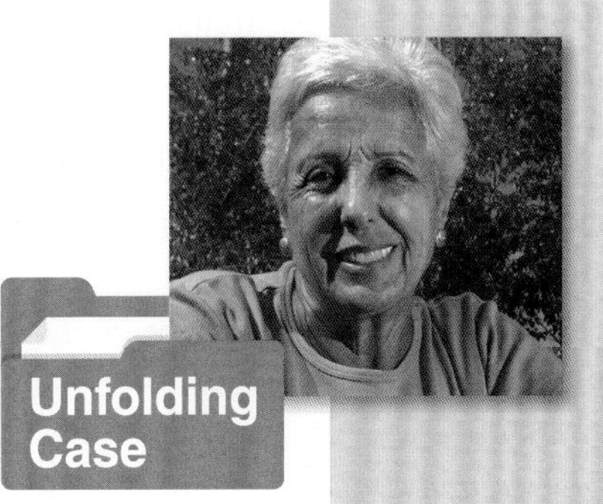

Unfolding Case

Myra Johnson

Myra is a healthy, active 83-year-old woman who is conscientious about healthy eating and exercise. She read about the many health benefits from using aloe to detox and decided to give them a try. Over a period of diligent use, she developed diarrhea but passed it off as part of the detox process. Her family took her to the emergency department when she exhibited what they thought were signs of a stroke: weakness, exhaustion, and delirium. What may be causing her symptoms?

Learning Objectives

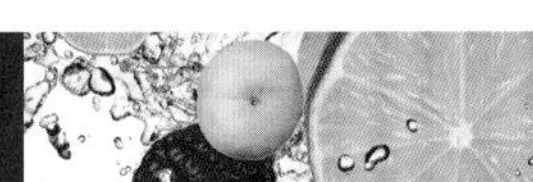

Upon completion of this chapter, you will be able to:

1 Discuss a healthy person's fluid requirement.
2 Give examples of mechanisms by which the body maintains mineral homeostasis.
3 Identify sources of minerals.
4 Discuss functions of minerals.
5 Explain why Americans should eat less sodium.
6 Discuss the potential benefits from increasing calcium and potassium intake.
7 Describe the Dietary Approaches to Stop Hypertension (DASH) diet.

Inorganic
not containing carbon or concerning living things.

Body fluids consist of water and chemicals. Among those chemicals are **inorganic** elements that arise from the earth's crust, known as minerals. Although minerals account for only about 4% of the body's total weight, they are found in all body fluids and tissues. Some minerals are electrolytes that dissociate (dissolve) into ions in water and are able to conduct electricity. Although minerals—including electrolytes—are micronutrients, they are vital for life and essential in the diet.

This chapter discusses water, electrolytes, major minerals, and trace minerals. Minerals in health promotion are presented.

WATER

Water is fundamental to life. It is the single largest constituent of the human body, averaging approximately 60% of the total body weight. It is the medium in which all biochemical reactions take place. Although most people can survive 6 weeks or longer without food, death occurs in a matter of days without water.

Water occupies essentially every space within and between body cells and is involved in virtually every body function. Water performs the following functions:

- *Provides shape and structure to cells:* Approximately two thirds of the body's water is located within cells (intracellular fluid). Muscle cells have a higher concentration of water (70% to 75%) than fat, which is only about 25% water. Men generally have more muscle mass than women and, therefore, have a higher percentage of body water.
- *Regulates body temperature:* Because water absorbs heat slowly, the large amount of water contained in the body helps to maintain body temperature homeostasis despite fluctuations in environmental temperatures. Evaporation of water (sweat) from the skin cools the body.
- *Aids in the digestion and absorption of nutrients:* Approximately 7 to 9 L of water is secreted in the gastrointestinal (GI) tract daily to aid in digestion and absorption. Except for the approximately 100 mL of water excreted through the feces, all of the water contained in the GI secretions (saliva, gastric secretions, bile, pancreatic secretions, and intestinal mucosal secretions) is reabsorbed in the ileum and colon.
- *Transports nutrients and oxygen to cells:* By moistening the air sacs in the lungs, water allows oxygen to dissolve and move into blood for distribution throughout the body. Approximately 92% of blood plasma is water.
- *Serves as a solvent for vitamins, minerals, glucose, and amino acids:* The solvating property of water is vital for health and survival.
- *Participates in metabolic reactions:* For instance, water is used in the synthesis of hormones and enzymes.
- *Eliminates waste products:* Water helps to excrete body wastes through urine, feces, and expirations.
- *Is a major component of mucus and other lubricating fluids:* Water reduces friction in joints where bones, ligaments, and tendons come in contact with each other, and it cushions contacts between internal organs that slide over one another.

Water Balance

Water balance is the dynamic state between water output and water intake. Under normal conditions, output and intake are approximately equal (Fig. 7.1).

Water Output

Insensible Water Loss immeasurable losses.

Sensible Water Loss measurable losses.

On average, adults lose approximately 1750 to 3000 mL of water daily. Extreme environmental temperatures (very hot or very cold), high altitude, low humidity, and strenuous exercise increase **insensible water losses** from respirations and the skin. Water evaporation from the skin is also increased by prolonged exposure to heated or recirculated air, for example, during long airplane flights. **Sensible water losses** from urine and feces make up the remaining water loss. Because the body needs to excrete a minimum of 500 mL of urine daily to rid itself of metabolic wastes, the minimum daily total fluid output is approximately 1500 mL. To maintain water balance, intake should approximate output.

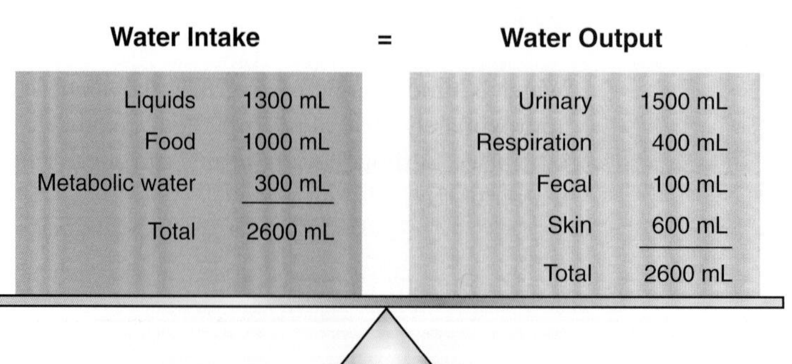

Water Intake
=
Water Output
Liquids 1300 mL
Food 1000 mL
Metabolic water 300 mL
Total 2600 mL
Urinary 1500 mL
Respiration 400 mL
Fecal 100 mL
Skin 600 mL
Total 2600 mL

Figure 7.1 ► **Water balance approximations.**

Water Intake

Metabolic Water
water produced as a by-product from the breakdown of carbohydrates, protein, and fat for energy.

Liquids, solid foods, and metabolism are all sources of water. Water intake averages about 2.5 L/day, of which approximately 80% is from fluids and 20% from solid food (Institute of Medicine [IOM], 2005). Except for oils, almost all foods contain water, with fruits and vegetables providing the most (Fig. 7.2). Depending on total calorie intake, the body produces approximately 250 to 350 mL of **metabolic water** daily from the catabolism of carbohydrates, protein, and fat.

Water Recommendations

Water is an essential nutrient because the body cannot produce as much water as it needs. There is no Recommended Dietary Allowance (RDA) for water because of insufficient evidence linking a specific amount of water intake to health; actual requirements vary depending on diet, physical activity, environmental temperatures, and humidity. The Adequate Intake (AI) for total water, which includes drinking water, water in beverages, and water in food, is based on the median total water intake from U.S. food consumption survey data (IOM, 2005).

- For men age 19 and older, the AI is 3.7 L/day, which includes 3 L as fluids.
- For women of the same age, the AI is 2.7 L, which includes approximately 2.2 L from fluids.
- Similar to AIs set for other nutrients, daily intakes below the AI may not be harmful to healthy people because normal hydration is maintained over a wide range of intakes. Amounts higher than the AI are recommended for rigorous activity in hot climates.
- Because the body cannot store water, it should be consumed throughout the day.

For healthy people, the universal, age-old advice has been to drink at least eight 8-oz glasses of water daily.

- Although that may be excellent advice, there is little scientific evidence to support this recommendation (Valtin, 2002).
- For healthy people, hydration is unconsciously maintained with ad lib access to water. In healthy adults, thirst is usually a reliable indicator of water need, and fluid intake is assumed to be adequate when the color of urine produced is pale yellow.

Figure 7.2 ▶
Percentage of water content of various foods.

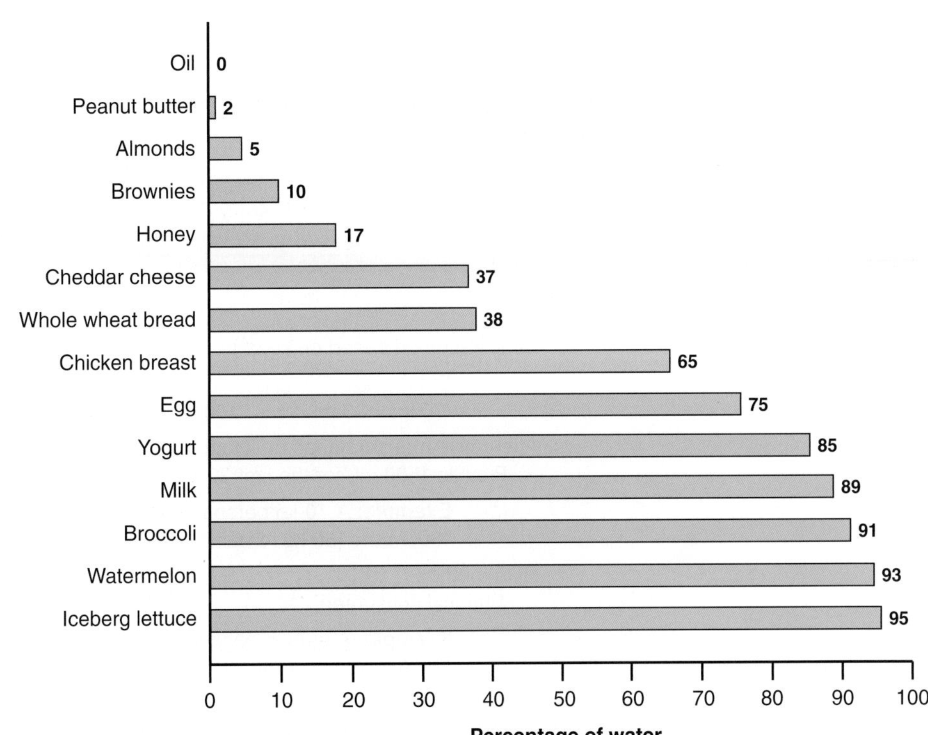

- In some conditions and for some segments of the population, the sensation of thirst is blunted and may not be a reliable indicator of need. For the senior adults and children, and during hot weather or strenuous exercise, drinking fluids should not be delayed until the sensation of thirst occurs because by then fluid loss is significant.

Estimating Fluid Requirements

Box 7.1 outlines several methods for estimating fluid requirements. However, according to the Academy of Nutrition and Dietetics Evidence Analysis Library, there is no evidence to validate any of these equations despite their widespread use in clinical practice (Academy of Nutrition and Dietetics, Evidence Analysis Library, 2007).

Excessive Fluid Intake

A chronic high intake of water has not been shown to cause adverse effects in healthy people who consume a varied diet as long as intake approximates output (IOM, 2005). An excessive water intake may cause hyponatremia, but it is rare in healthy people who consume a typical diet. Athletes in endurance events who drink too much water, fail to replace lost sodium, or both are at risk of hyponatremia. See Table 7.1 for excess fluid related to clinical conditions.

Inadequate Fluid Intake

An inadequate intake of water can lead to dehydration, characterized by impaired mental function, impaired motor control, increased body temperature during exercise, increased resting heart rate when standing or lying down, and an increased risk of life-threatening heat stroke. A net water loss of 1% to 2% of body weight causes thirst, fatigue, weakness, vague discomfort, and loss of appetite. A loss of 7% to 10% leads to dizziness, muscle spasticity, loss of balance, delirium, exhaustion, and collapse. If left untreated, dehydration ends in death.

Clinical situations in which water losses are increased—and thus water needs are elevated—include vomiting, diarrhea, fever, thermal injuries, uncontrolled diabetes, hemorrhage, certain renal disorders, and the use of drainage tubes (Table 7.1).

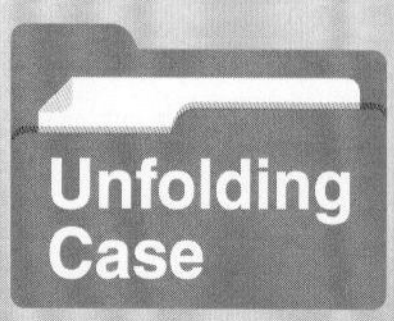

Recall Myra. She lost excessive amounts of fluid from diarrhea and is diagnosed with dehydration. Why didn't she feel thirsty as she became dehydrated?

BOX 7.1 Methods to Estimate Fluid Needs

Method

- Simple method based on kg of body weight 30 mL/kg body weight for average adults

  Example: A 70-kg person needs 2100 mL/day
  (70 kg × 30 mL/kg = 2100 mL/day)
- Alternative method based on kilogram of body weight
  - Provide 1500 mL for the first 20 kg of weight and 20 mL/kg for each remaining kilogram.

    Example: A 70-kg person needs 2500 mL/day
    1500 mL + (50 kg remaining × 20 mL/kg) = 1500 mL + 1000 mL = 2500 mL
- RDA method
  - 1 mL/cal consumed

    Example: A person consuming 2000 cal/day needs 2000 mL/day
    (2000 cal/day × 1 mL/cal = 2000 mL/day)
- Fluid balance method
  - Urine output/d + 500 mL

Table 7.1 Causes, Signs and Symptoms, and Treatment of Fluid, Sodium, and Potassium Imbalances

Nutrient	Imbalance	Causes	Signs and Symptoms	Treatment
Fluid	Hypervolemia: fluid overload	Sodium retention, excessive fluid supplementation that the body cannot handle; liver, kidney, and heart failure	Hypertension, dyspnea, shortness of breath, breath sounds such as rales and crackles, abdominal ascites, distended jugular veins, peripheral edema, tachycardia, and bounding/strong pulse	Correct underlying cause Fluid and sodium restrictions Diuretics
	Hypovolemia: deficit of body fluids	Severe dehydration; vomiting and diarrhea; secondary to bleeding and hemorrhage	Can lead to decreased cardiac output, hypovolemic shock, metabolic acidosis, multisystem failure, coma, and death	Correct underlying cause Intravenous (IV) rehydration, such as lactated Ringers, administration of plasma expanders, and blood and blood products if necessary
Sodium (Na) Normal range: 135–145 mEq/L Major extracellular cation	Hypernatremia Na > 145 mEq/L Reflects deficit of total body water relative to body sodium	Dehydration, which may be caused by fever, profuse diarrhea, inadequate water intake, severe burns, long exposure to environmental heat; Cushing's syndrome; diabetes insipidus	Agitation, thirst, restlessness, dry mucous membranes, decreased urine output, lethargy, and confusion Can progress to seizures and coma	Correct underlying cause Oral or IV water (hypotonic solution) replacement Possible sodium restriction
	Hyponatremia Na < 135 mEq/L Reflects excess of total body water relative to sodium	Diarrhea, excessive water intake or administration of nonelectrolyte IV fluids, diuretics, syndrome of inappropriate antidiuretic hormone; water intoxication resulting from various diseases and disorders, including cirrhosis, kidney failure, heart failure	Confusion, nausea, vomiting, muscle weakness, fatigue, headache, fatigue, restlessness	Correct underlying cause Diuretics, fluid restriction, oral or IV sodium depending on severity
Potassium (K) Normal range: 3.7–5.2 mEq/L Potassium is primarily found within cells	Hyperkalemia K > 5.2 mEq/L	Most often related to acute kidney disease; may occur secondary to some medications or potassium supplements	Muscular weakness, paralysis, nausea, possible life-threatening cardiac dysrhythmia	Correct underlying cause Life-threatening hyperkalemia is treated with dialysis and potassium-lowering medications Less severe cases may respond to dietary potassium restriction
	Hypokalemia K < 3.7 mEq/L Deficit of total body potassium or abnormal movement of potassium into cells	Potassium-wasting diuretics, severe vomiting or diarrhea, diabetic ketoacidosis, diaphoresis	Mild causes may be asymptomatic Moderate-to-severe cases: muscular weakness, muscle spasms, tingling, numbness, fatigue, dysrhythmias. Cardiac arrest can occur in severe cases	Correct underlying cause Administration of supplemental potassium

Source: Burke, A. (2020, May 24). *Fluid and electrolyte imbalances: NCLEX-RN*. https://www.registerednursing.org/nclex/fluid-electrolyte-imbalances

FLUID AND ELECTROLYTE BALANCE

Fluids in each body compartment are regulated by membranes (e.g., cell membranes and capillary membranes), the concentration of electrolytes, and hydrostatic pressure. In all electrolyte solutions, the number of negative and positive charges is equal. If an anion enters a cell, a cation must also enter or another anion must leave in order to maintain electrical neutrality. This balance of negative and positive ions occurs both within cells and outside cells, although the amounts and proportions of ions differ in each compartment.

Cations are positively charged ions such as sodium and potassium. Anions, such as chloride, are negatively charged. These electrolytes help regulate nerve and muscle function, acid–base balance, and water balance.

Electrolytes Attract Water

Sodium and chloride are found primarily in extracellular fluid and potassium and phosphates are located mostly in the intracellular fluid. The fluid levels within each compartment are maintained by the concentration of electrolytes in each. If the concentration of electrolytes is high, fluid moves into that compartment through the process of osmosis. Electrolytes can actively move in and out of cells to adjust fluid levels because electrolytes attract water.

Electrolyte Balance

Electrolyte concentrations in the body are held at a nearly constant level by feedback mechanisms involving the kidneys. The kidneys maintain electrolyte balance by filtering electrolytes and water from the blood and excreting excesses into the urine. Electrolyte imbalances, and accompanying fluid imbalance, occur when the body is unable to compensate for deficits or excesses, such as in the case of dehydration or over hydration; the use of certain medications; heart, kidney, or liver disorders; or inappropriate IV or enteral feedings. Table 7.1 summarizes imbalances of sodium and potassium.

UNDERSTANDING MINERALS

Unlike the macronutrients and vitamins, minerals are inorganic elements from the earth, not organic substances from plants or animals. Minerals do not undergo digestion nor are they broken down or rearranged during metabolism. Although they combine with other elements to form salts (e.g., sodium chloride) or with organic compounds (e.g., iron in hemoglobin), they always retain their chemical identities. Unlike vitamins, minerals are not destroyed by light, air, heat, or acids during food preparation. Minerals are lost only when they leach from foods soaked in water. When food is completely burned, minerals are the ash that remains.

Mineral Classifications

The classification as major minerals or trace minerals (elements) is based on the quantity in the body and amount needed, not by their importance. Both groups are essential for life.

- Calcium, phosphorus, magnesium, sulfur, sodium, potassium, and chloride are considered major minerals because they are present in the body in amounts greater than 5 g (the equivalent of 1 tsp).
- Iron, iodine, zinc, selenium, copper, manganese, fluoride, chromium, and molybdenum are classified as trace minerals, or trace elements, because they are present in the body in amounts less than 5 g.
- As many as 30 other potentially harmful minerals are present in the body, including lead, gold, and mercury. Their presence appears to be related to environmental contamination.

General Functions

Minerals function to provide structure to body tissues and to regulate body processes such as fluid balance, acid–base balance, nerve cell transmission, muscle contraction, and vitamin, enzyme, and hormonal activities (Table 7.2).

Table 7.2 General Functions of Minerals

Functions	Examples
Provide structure	Calcium, phosphorus, and magnesium provide structure to bones and teeth. Phosphorus, potassium, iron, and sulfur provide structure to soft tissues. Sulfur is a constituent of skin, hair, and nails.
Fluid balance	Sodium, potassium, and chloride maintain fluid balance.
Acid–base balance	Sodium hydroxide and sodium bicarbonate are part of the carbonic acid–bicarbonate system that regulates blood pH. Phosphorus is involved in buffer systems that regulate kidney tubular fluids.
Nerve cell transmission and muscle contraction	Sodium and potassium are involved in transmission of nerve impulses. Calcium stimulates muscle contractions. Sodium, potassium, and magnesium stimulate muscle relaxation.
Vitamin, enzyme, and hormone activity	Cobalt is a component of vitamin B_{12}. Magnesium is a cofactor for hundreds of enzymes. Iodine is essential for the production of thyroxine. Chromium enhances the action of insulin.

Mineral Balance

The body has several mechanisms by which it maintains mineral balance, depending on the mineral involved, such as the following:

- *Releasing minerals from storage for redistribution:* Calcium is released from the bone to maintain serum levels when intake is inadequate.
- *GI absorption:* For example, iron absorption increases when the body is deficient.
- *Urinary excretion:* For instance, virtually all of the sodium consumed in the diet is absorbed. The only way the body can rid itself of excess sodium is to increase urinary sodium excretion. For most people, the higher the intake of sodium, the greater is the amount of sodium excreted in the urine.

Mineral Toxicities

Minerals that are easily excreted, such as sodium and potassium, do not accumulate to toxic levels in the body under normal circumstances. Stored minerals can produce toxicity symptoms when intake is excessive, but excessive intake is not likely to occur from eating a balanced diet. Instead, mineral toxicity is related to excessive use of mineral supplements, environmental or industrial exposure, human errors in commercial food processing, or alterations in metabolism. For instance, in 2008, the most serious selenium toxicity outbreak that has ever occurred in the United States was caused by an improperly manufactured dietary supplement that contained 200 times the labeled concentration of selenium (Morris & Crane, 2013).

Mineral Interactions

Mineral balance is influenced by hundreds of interactions that occur among minerals and between minerals and other dietary components or medications. Mineral status must be viewed as a function of the total diet, not just from the standpoint of the quantity consumed. Examples follow:

- Vitamin D and lactose promote calcium absorption.
- Vitamin C enhances the absorption of nonheme iron.

Table 7.3 Major Sources[a] of Selected Minerals by Food Group[b]

Food Group	Potassium	Calcium	Phosphorus	Magnesium	Iron	Zinc	Selenium
Vegetables	✓						
Fruit	✓						
Grains				✓ (whole grains)	✓		✓ (whole grains)
Dairy	✓	✓	✓	✓		✓	✓
Protein Foods				✓	✓	✓	

[a] Major sources according to MyPlate.gov
[b] Oils do not provide minerals.

- High-dose iron supplements can impair zinc absorption.
- High-dose zinc supplements can inhibit copper absorption.
- Corticosteroids can deplete calcium.
- Thiazide diuretics, proton pump inhibitors, and some antibiotics can deplete magnesium.

Sources of Minerals

Key minerals are found in all food groups; items within each group vary in the amount and kind of minerals they provide (Table 7.3).

- Generally, unrefined or unprocessed foods have more minerals than refined foods.
- Trace mineral content varies with the content of soil from which the food originates.
- Within most food groups, processed foods are high in sodium and chloride.
- Drinking water contains varying amounts of calcium, magnesium, and other minerals; sodium is added to soften water. Fluoride may be a natural or added component of drinking water.

Mineral Supplements

Mineral supplements, alone or combined with vitamins, contribute to mineral intake.

- To the greatest extent possible, nutrient needs should be met through food, not through supplements.
- The degree to which a supplement can improve nutrient adequacy depends on the nutrients contained in the supplement. For instance, multivitamin and mineral supplements often contain low amounts of potassium, calcium, and magnesium (Marra & Bailey, 2018).
- The effectiveness of mineral supplements is affected by their form and the amount of the elemental mineral in the mineral salt (Marra & Bailey, 2018). For instance, calcium carbonate has the highest concentration of calcium but needs an acidic medium for optimal absorption and maximum absorption occur at doses ≤500 mg.

MAJOR ELECTROLYTES

Sodium, chloride, and potassium are major minerals that are also major electrolytes in the body. Table 7.4 highlights recommended intakes, sources, functions, deficiency symptoms, and toxicity symptoms of these minerals. Additional features follow.

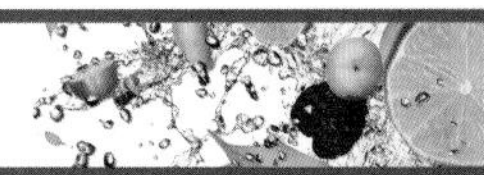

Table 7.4 Summary of Major Electrolytes

Electrolyte and Sources	Functions	Deficiency/Toxicity Signs and Symptoms
Sodium (Na) Adult AI: 19 y and older: 1.5 g UL: not determined CDRR: 14 y and older: Reduce intake if above 2300 mg/day • Processed foods; canned meat, vegetables, and soups; convenience foods; and restaurant and fast foods	Fluid and electrolyte balance, acid–base balance, maintains muscle irritability, regulates cell membrane permeability and nerve impulse transmission	**Deficiency** Rare, except with chronic diarrhea or vomiting and certain renal disorders; nausea, dizziness, muscle cramps, and apathy **Toxicity** Hypertension and edema
Potassium (K) Adult AI: Men 19 y and older: 3400 mg Women 19 y and older: 2600 mg No UL No CDRR • Baked potato with skin, canned tomato products, sweet potatoes, prunes, clams, molasses, milk, yogurt, tomato juice, prune juice, legumes, bananas, artichokes, fish, avocados, raisins, spinach, kiwifruit	Major cation of intracellular fluid Maintains fluid balance, maintains acid–base balance, transmits nerve impulses, catalyzes metabolic reactions, aids in carbohydrate metabolism and protein synthesis, controls skeletal muscle contractility	Deficiency Muscular weakness, paralysis, anorexia, and confusion (occurs with dehydration) Toxicity (from supplements/drugs) Muscular weakness, vomiting
Chloride (Cl) Adult AI: 19–50 y: 2.3 g 50–70 y: 2.0 g >70 y: 1.8 g Adult UL: 3.6 g • 1 tsp salt = 3600 mg Cl • Same sources as sodium	Fluid and electrolyte balance, acid–base balance, component of hydrochloric acid in stomach	Deficiency Rare, may occur secondary to chronic diarrhea or vomiting and certain renal disorders: muscle cramps, anorexia, apathy Toxicity Normally harmless; can cause vomiting

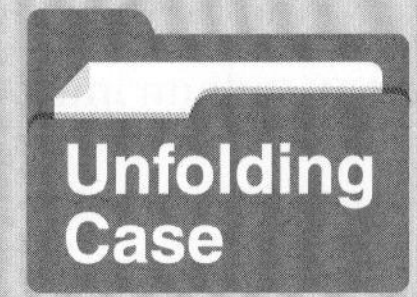

Think of Myra. The speed with which her food moved through the GI tract interfered with the absorption of fluid, electrolytes, and nutrients. She was given IV replacement fluid, an antidiarrheal medication, and oral fluids. What should Myra understand about the need for "detox" and its potential risks?

Sodium

By weight, salt (sodium chloride) is approximately 40% sodium; 1 tsp of salt provides 2325 mg of sodium. Of the total average intake of sodium among U.S. adults (Harnack et al., 2017)

- approximately 71% is sodium added to food outside the home, such as from processing or at eating establishments. Box 7.2 gives examples of sodium additives added to foods.
- only 14% is sodium that occurs naturally in foods such as milk, meat, poultry, and vegetables.
- 5.6% is salt added to food during cooking.
- 5% is from salt added at the table.
- less than 0.5% comes from home tap water consumed as a beverage and dietary supplements.

BOX 7.2 Examples of Sodium Additives

To enhance flavor

- Sodium chloride
- Monosodium glutamate
- Soy sauce
- Teriyaki sauce

To preserve freshness

- Brine
- Sodium sulfite (for dried fruits)

To prevent the growth of yeast and/or bacteria

- Sodium benzoate
- Sodium nitrate or sodium nitrite
- Sodium lactate
- Sodium diacetate

To prevent the growth of mold

- Sodium propionate

As an antioxidant

- Sodium erythorbate

As a sweetener

- Sodium saccharin

As a binder/thickener

- Sodium caprate
- Sodium caseinate

As a leavening agent

- Sodium bicarbonate (baking soda)
- Baking powder

As a stabilizer

- Sodium citrate
- Disodium phosphate

Almost 98% of all sodium consumed is absorbed; yet, humans are able to maintain homeostasis over a wide range of intakes, largely through urinary excretion.

- A salty meal causes a transitory increase in serum sodium, which triggers thirst.
- Drinking fluids dilutes the sodium in the blood to normal concentration, even though the volume of both sodium and fluid is increased.
- The increased volume stimulates the kidneys to excrete more sodium and fluid together to restore normal blood volume.
- Conversely, low blood volume or low extracellular sodium stimulates the hormone aldosterone to increase sodium reabsorption by the kidneys.
- In people who have minimal sweat losses, sodium intake and sodium excretion are approximately equal.

The Dietary Reference Intake (DRI) recommendations for sodium were recently revised since being established in 2005 (Food and Nutrition Board, National Academies of Sciences, Engineering, and Medicine, 2019).

- The AI for sodium is 1500 mg for everyone aged 14 and older, which is less than half of the average sodium intake (see following section).
- The Dietary Guidelines recommend sodium intake to be less than 2300 mg/day for everyone aged 14 and older (U.S. Department of Agriculture [USDA] & U.S. Department of Health and Human Services [USDHHS], 2020). This is the same level of intake cited in the new DRI category, Chronic Disease Risk Reduction (CDRR), which was set based on evidence of the benefits of lowering sodium intake on cardiovascular disease (CVD) risk, hypertension risk, systolic blood pressure, and diastolic blood pressure (Food and Nutrition Board, National Academies of Sciences, Engineering, and Medicine, 2019).

Wide variations in sodium intake exist between cultures and between individuals within a culture, based on the amount of processed foods consumed. On average, Americans consume far more sodium than needed or recommended.

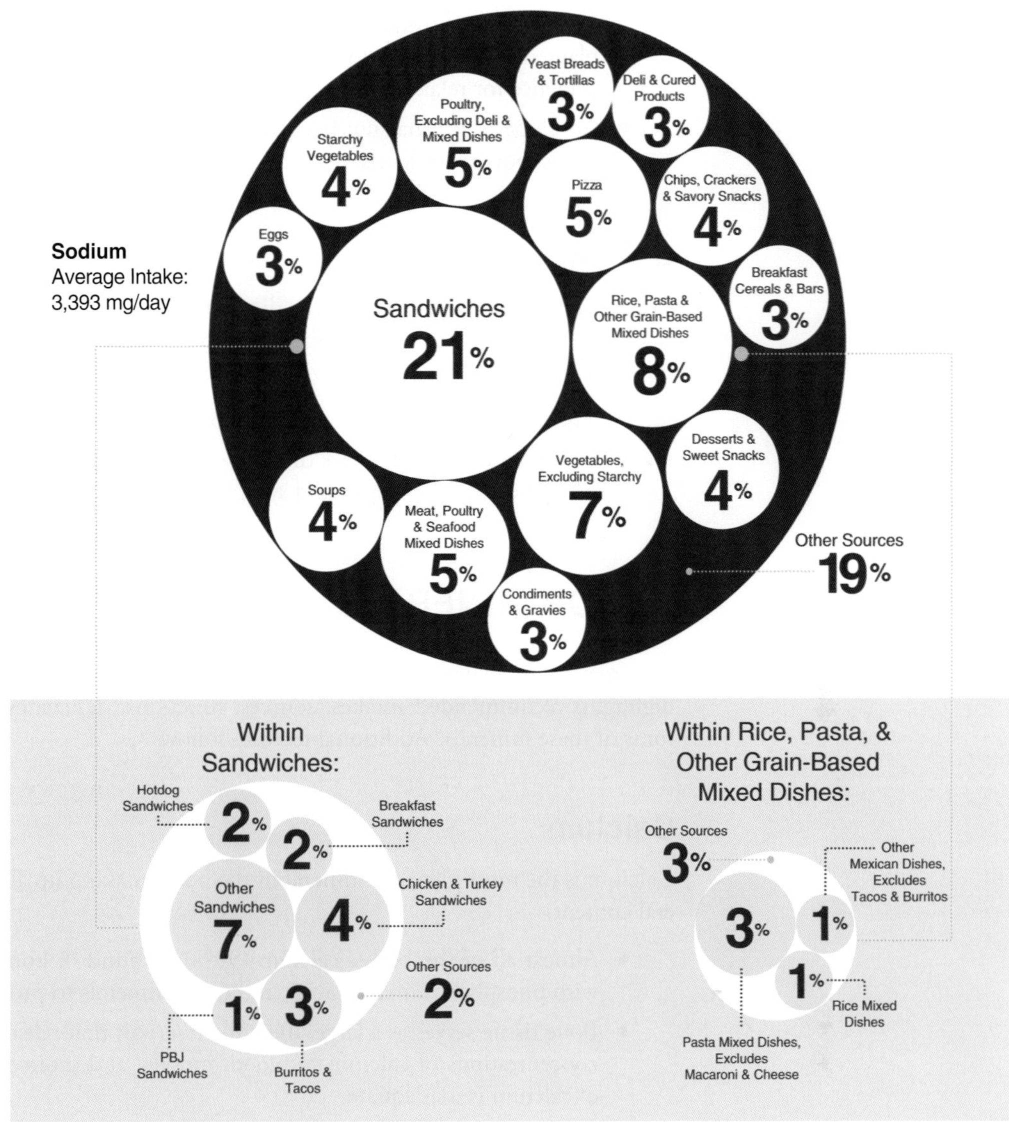

Figure 7.3 ▶

Top sources and average intakes of sodium: U.S. population ages 1 and older. (*Source:* U.S. Department of Agriculture & U.S. Department of Health and Human Services [2020]. *Dietary guidelines for Americans, 2020–2025.* https://www.dietaryguidelines.gov; Data Source: Analysis of What We Eat in America, NHANES, 2013–2016, ages 1 and older, 2 days, dietary intake data, weighted.)

- Average intakes of sodium for people ages 1 and older is 3393 mg/day, with a range of approximately 2000 to 5000 mg/day (USDA & USDHHS, 2020).
- Top sources of sodium in the U.S. population ages 1 and older are depicted in Figure 7.3.

Potassium

Like sodium, the DRIs for potassium were updated in 2019 (Food and Nutrition Board, National Academies of Sciences, Engineering, and Medicine, 2019). As with all AIs, they are estimates for an intake level in apparently healthy people rather than an estimate of potassium requirement.

- Due to a lack of a specific indicator of potassium adequacy, the AIs are based on the highest median potassium intake of adults with normal blood pressure and no reported history of CVD across two nationally representative surveys (Food and Nutrition Board, National Academies of Sciences, Engineering, and Medicine, 2019).
- The newest AI reflects an overall decrease for people age 1 and older.
- Despite moderately strong evidence that potassium supplements lower blood pressure, especially in hypertensive adults, a CDRR, which would have identified the intake level

below which chronic disease risk increases, was not established. This is because of unexplained inconsistency in the evidence, a lack of intake–response relationship, and limited evidence for relationships between potassium intake and chronic disease endpoints.

- An Upper Limit has not been set because in healthy people high intake increases urinary losses, not serum levels.

Chloride

Because almost all the chloride in the diet comes from salt (sodium chloride), the AI for chloride is set at a level equivalent (on a molar basis) to that of sodium. Unlike sodium, the DRIs for chloride have not changed since they were established in 2005.

- The AI for adults ages 19 to 50 is 2.3 g/day, the equivalent to 1500 mg sodium.
- Sodium and chloride share dietary sources, conditions that cause them to become depleted in the body, and signs and symptoms of deficiency.

MAJOR MINERALS

The remaining major minerals are calcium, phosphorus, magnesium, and sulfur. Table 7.5 highlights recommended intakes, sources, functions, deficiency symptoms, and toxicity symptoms of these minerals. Additional features follow.

Calcium

Calcium is the most plentiful mineral in the body, making up about half of the body's total mineral content.

- Almost all of the body's calcium (99%) is found in bones and teeth, where it combines with phosphorus, magnesium, and other minerals to provide rigidity and structure.
- Bone tissue serves as a large, dynamic reservoir that releases calcium to maintain constant concentrations of calcium in blood, muscle, and intercellular fluids when dietary intake of calcium is inadequate.
- Continuous remodeling of bone occurs naturally throughout life as calcium is deposited and resorbed.
- The balance between bone formation and bone breakdown changes with aging. From birth through adolescence, bone formation exceeds bone breakdown. In young adults, the processes occur at approximately the same rate. After the age of about 30, net bone loss occurs in all people.
- A high calcium intake may help maximize bone density.

Calcium balance—or, more accurately, calcium balance in the blood—is achieved through the action of vitamin D and hormones.

- When blood calcium levels fall, the parathyroid gland secretes parathormone (PTH), which promotes calcium reabsorption in the kidneys and stimulates the release of calcium from bones.
- Vitamin D has the same effects on the kidneys and bones and additionally increases the absorption of calcium from the GI tract.
- Together, the actions of PTH and vitamin D restore low blood calcium levels to normal, even though bone calcium content may fall.
- A chronically low calcium intake compromises bone integrity without affecting blood calcium levels. When blood calcium levels are too high, the thyroid gland secretes calcitonin, which promotes calcium deposition in the bone using excess calcium from the blood.

Table 7.5 Summary of Major Minerals

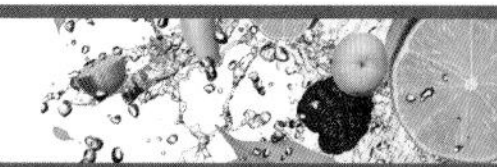

Mineral and Sources	Functions	Deficiency/Toxicity Signs and Symptoms
Calcium (Ca) Adult RDA Men: 19–70 y: 1000 mg >70: 1200 mg Women: 19–50 y: 1000 mg 51 and older: 1200 mg Adult UL: 19–50 y: 2500 mg >50 y: 2000 mg • Milk, yogurt, hard natural cheese, pasteurized processed American cheese, bok choy, broccoli, Chinese/Napa cabbage, collards, kale, okra, turnip greens, fortified breakfast cereal, fortified orange juice, legumes, fortified soy milk, almonds • Less well-absorbed sources: spinach, beet greens, Swiss chard	Bone and teeth formation and maintenance, blood clotting, nerve transmission, muscle contraction and relaxation, cell membrane permeability, blood pressure	Deficiency Children: impaired growth Adults: osteoporosis Toxicity Constipation, increased risk of renal stone formation, impaired absorption of iron and other minerals
Phosphorus (P) Adult RDA Men and women: 700 mg Adult UL: 70 y: 4 g/day >70 y: 3 g/day • All animal products (meat, poultry, eggs, milk), ready-to-eat cereal, dried peas and beans; bran and whole grains; raisins, prunes, dates	Bone and teeth formation and maintenance, acid–base balance, energy metabolism, cell membrane structure, regulation of hormone and coenzyme activity	Deficiency Unknown Toxicity Low blood calcium
Magnesium (Mg) Adult RDA Men: 19–30 y: 400 mg >30 y: 420 mg Women: 19–30 y: 310 mg >30 y: 320 mg Adult UL: 350 mg/day from supplements only (does not include intake from food and water) • Spinach, beet greens, okra, Brazil nuts, almonds, cashews, bran cereal, dried peas and beans, halibut, tuna, chocolate, cocoa	Bone formation: cofactor for >300 enzymes; involved in muscle and nerve function, protein synthesis, blood glucose control, blood pressure regulation, RNA and DNA synthesis	Deficiency Weakness, confusion; growth failure in children Severe deficiency: convulsions, hallucinations, tetany Toxicity No toxicity demonstrated from food Supplemental Mg can cause diarrhea, nausea, and cramping. Excessive Mg from magnesium in Epsom salts causes diarrhea
Sulfur(S) No recommended intake or UL • All protein foods (meat, poultry, fish, eggs, milk, dried peas and beans, nuts)	Component of disulfide bridges in proteins; component of biotin, thiamin, and insulin	Deficiency Unknown Toxicity In animals, excessive intake of sulfur-containing amino acids impairs growth.

Phosphorus

After calcium, the most abundant mineral in the body is phosphorus. Approximately 85% of the body's phosphorus is combined with calcium in bones and teeth. The rest is distributed in every body cell. As with calcium, phosphorus metabolism is regulated by vitamin D and PTH. Normally, about 40% to 60% of natural phosphorus from food sources is absorbed. Animal proteins, dairy products, and legumes are rich natural sources of phosphorus.

Phosphate food additives—which are used to extend shelf life, improve taste, improve texture, or retain moisture—are present in many processed foods.

- Phosphate additives are estimated to contribute approximately 10% to 50% of phosphorus intakes in Western countries (Itkonen et al., 2018). Their absorption rate is approximately 70% (Scanni et al., 2014).
- Most Americans consume more phosphorus than recommended. While some studies have found an association between high phosphorus intakes and adverse effects on cardiovascular, kidney, and bone health as well as increased risk of death (Chang et al., 2014), others have found no link between high intakes and increased disease risk (National Institutes of Health [NIH], Office of Dietary Supplements [ODS], 2019a).
- Phosphate content is not listed on the "Nutrition Facts" label, so consumers are not able to compare brands to find lower phosphate choices.

Magnesium

Magnesium is the fourth most abundant mineral in the body; approximately 50% to 60% of the body's magnesium content is deposited in bone with calcium and phosphorus and most of the rest is stored in various soft tissues and muscles. Less than 1% of total magnesium is in the blood, which is tightly regulated and not indicative of total body magnesium. The kidneys maintain magnesium balance by altering the amount excreted in the urine.

The National Health and Nutrition Examination Survey (NHANES) data for 2015 to 2016 show the mean intake of magnesium for adults age 20 and older is less than the RDAs (USDA & Agricultural Research Service [ARS], 2018). However, intake data do not include the magnesium content of water, which is significant in water classified as "hard." However, as much as 80% to 90% of the magnesium in food is lost in processing (de Baaij et al., 2015). For instance, an average slice of white (refined) bread provides 7 mg of magnesium compared to 24 mg found in whole wheat bread.

Symptomatic magnesium deficiency from a low intake in otherwise healthy people is uncommon because the kidneys limit urinary excretion.

- Magnesium deficiency is more commonly the result of certain disorders that increase urinary excretion of magnesium, such as type 2 diabetes, or impair its absorption, such as celiac disease and small intestine bypass or resection.
- People who abuse alcohol are at risk of magnesium deficiency secondary to poor intake, altered absorption, and/or excess urinary excretion.
- Aging is associated with lower magnesium intake, decreased absorption, and increased excretion.
- Certain medications, such as thiazide diuretics, proton pump inhibitors, and some antibiotics, can lead to magnesium depletion (de Baaij et al., 2015).

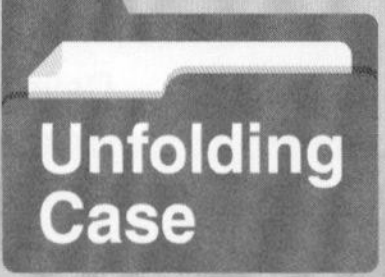

Recall Myra. Her fluid and electrolyte status was the immediate priority. However, general malabsorption of nutrients also occurred due to the diarrheal effect of the aloe. What would you tell Myra about what she should eat and how much fluid she should consume? What strategies may help her drink enough fluid given that she doesn't experience thirst?

Sulfur

Sulfur does not function independently as a nutrient, but it is a component of biotin, thiamin, and the amino acids methionine and cysteine.

- The proteins in skin, hair, and nails are made more rigid by the presence of sulfur.
- Although food and various sources of drinking water provide significant amounts of sulfur, the major source of inorganic sulfate for humans is body protein turnover of the amino acids methionine and cysteine.
- The need for sulfur is met when the intake of sulfur amino acids is adequate. A sulfur deficiency is likely only when protein deficiency is severe.

TRACE MINERALS

Although the presence of trace minerals in the body is small, their impact on health is significant. Each trace mineral has its own range over which the body can maintain homeostasis (Fig. 7.4). People who consume an adequate diet derive no further benefit from supplementing their intake with minerals and may induce a deficiency by upsetting the delicate balance that exists between minerals. Even though too little of a trace mineral can be just as deadly as too much, routine supplementation is not recommended. Factors that complicate the study of trace minerals are as follows:

- The high variability of trace mineral content of foods. The mineral content of the soil from which a food originates largely influences trace mineral content. Other factors that influence a food's trace mineral content are the quality of the water supply and degree of food processing. Because of these factors, the trace mineral content listed in food composition databases may not represent the actual amount in a given sample.
- Food composition data are not available for all trace minerals. Food composition databases generally include data on the content of iron, zinc, manganese, and selenium, but data on other trace minerals, such as iodine, chromium, and molybdenum, are not readily available.
- Bioavailability varies within the context of the total diet. Even when trace element intake can be estimated, the amount available to the body may be significantly less because the absorption and metabolism of individual trace elements is strongly influenced by mineral interactions and other dietary factors.
- Reliable and valid indicators of trace element status (e.g., measured serum levels, results of balance studies, and enzyme activity determinations) are not available for all trace minerals, so assessment of trace element status is not always possible.

Table 7.6 highlights recommended intakes, sources, functions, deficiency symptoms, and toxicity symptoms of trace minerals. Additional features follow.

Iron

Approximately two thirds of the body's 3 to 5 g of iron is contained in the heme portion of hemoglobin. Iron is also found in transferrin, the transport carrier of iron, and in enzyme

Figure 7.4 ▶ Health effects seen over a range of trace mineral intakes.

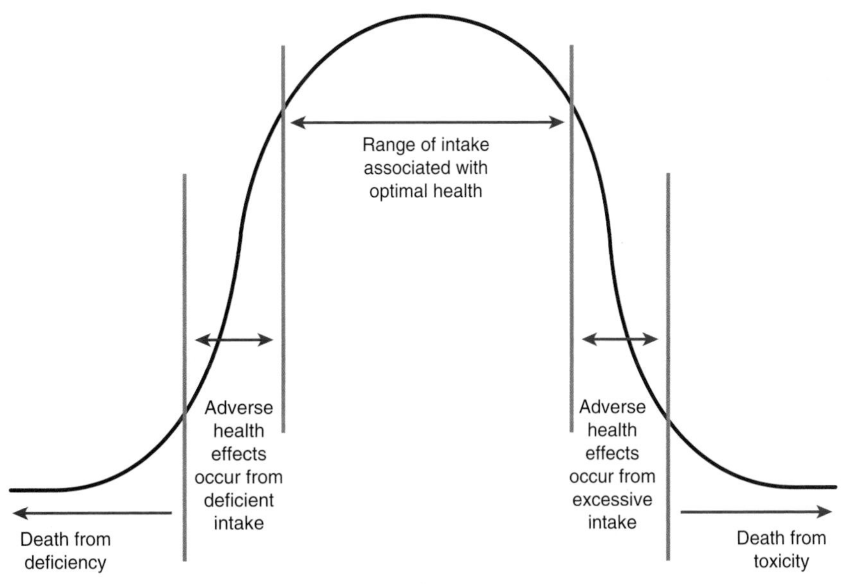

Table 7.6 Summary of Trace Minerals

Mineral and Sources	Functions	Deficiency/Toxicity Signs and Symptoms
Iron (Fe) Adult RDA Men: 8 mg Women: 19–50 y: 18 mg >50 y: 8 mg Adult UL: 45 mg • Beef liver, red meats, fish, poultry, clams, tofu, oysters, lentils, dried peas and beans, fortified cereals, bread, dried fruit	Oxygen transport via hemoglobin and myoglobin; constituent of enzyme systems	Deficiency Impaired immune function, decreased work capacity, apathy, lethargy, fatigue, itchy skin, pale nail beds and eye membranes, impaired wound healing, intolerance to cold temperatures Toxicity Increased risk of infections, apathy, fatigue, lethargy, joint disease, hair loss, organ damage, enlarged liver, amenorrhea, impotence Accidental poisoning in children causes death
Zinc (Zn) Adult RDA Men: 11 mg Women: 8 mg Adult UL: 40 mg • Oysters, red meat, poultry, dried peas and beans, fortified breakfast cereals, yogurt, cashews, pecans, milk	Required for the catalytic activity of approximately 100 enzymes; involved in immune function, protein synthesis, wound healing, DNA synthesis, cell division, normal growth and development, sense of taste and smell	Deficiency Growth retardation, hair loss, diarrhea, delayed sexual maturation and impotence, eye and skin lesions, anorexia, delayed wound healing, taste abnormality, mental lethargy Toxicity Anemia, elevated low-density lipoprotein, lowered high-density lipoprotein, diarrhea, vomiting, impaired calcium absorption, fever, renal failure, muscle pain, dizziness, reproductive failure
Iodine Adult RDA 150 mcg Adult UL: 1100 mcg • Iodized salt, seafood, bread, dairy products	Component of thyroid hormones that regulate growth, development, and metabolic rate	Deficiency Goiter, weight gain, lethargy During pregnancy may cause severe and irreversible mental and physical retardation (cretinism) Toxicity Enlarged thyroid gland, decreased thyroid activity
Selenium (Se) Adult RDA Men and women: 55 mcg Adult UL: 400 mcg/day • Brazil nuts, seafood, organ and muscle meats, poultry, cereals and other grains, dairy products, eggs	Component of >2 dozen selenoproteins that are involved in reproduction, thyroid hormone metabolism, DNA synthesis, and are antioxidants	Deficiency Enlarged heart, poor heart function, impaired thyroid activity Toxicity Rare; nausea, vomiting, abdominal pain, diarrhea, hair and nail changes, nerve damage, fatigue
Copper (Cu) Adult RDA 900 mcg Adult UL: 10,000 mcg • Organ meats, seafood, nuts, seeds, whole grains, cocoa products, drinking water	Cofactor of enzymes is involved in energy production, iron metabolism, neuropeptide activation, connective tissue synthesis, and neurotransmitter synthesis	Deficiency Rare; anemia, bone abnormalities Toxicity Vomiting, diarrhea, liver damage
Manganese (Mn) Adult AI Men: 2.3 mg Women: 1.8 mg Adult UL: 11 mg • Widely distributed in foods; top sources in U.S. diets are grain products, tea, and vegetables	Cofactor of many enzymes is involved in amino acid, cholesterol, glucose, and carbohydrate metabolism; bone formation, reproduction, immune functioning, blood clotting	Deficiency Rare Toxicity Rare; nervous system disorders
Fluoride (Fl) Adult AI Men: 4 mg Women: 3 mg Adult UL: 10 mg • Fluoridated water, water that naturally contains fluoride, tea, seafood	Formation and maintenance of tooth enamel, promotes resistance to dental decay, role in bone formation and integrity	Deficiency Susceptibility to dental decay; may increase risk of osteoporosis Toxicity Fluorosis (mottling of teeth), nausea, vomiting, diarrhea, chest pain, itching

Table 7.6 **Summary of Trace Minerals (continued)**

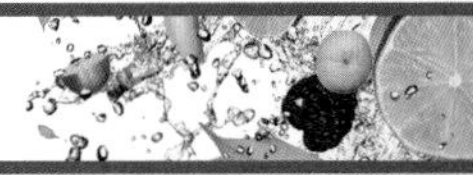

Mineral and Sources	Functions	Deficiency/Toxicity Signs and Symptoms
Chromium (Cr) Adult AI Men: 19–50 y: 35 mcg >50 y: 30 mcg Women: 19–50 y: 25 mcg >50 y: 20 mcg Adult UL: Undetermined • Widely distributed but most foods provide only in 1–2 mcg/serving; meat, whole grains, some fruits, and vegetables are good sources	Enhances the action of insulin; appears to be involved in the metabolism of carbohydrates, protein, and fat	Deficiency Rare; insulin resistance, impaired glucose tolerance Toxicity Dietary toxicity unknown
Molybdenum (Mo) Adult RDA 45 mcg Adult UL: 2000 mcg • Milk, legumes, bread, grains	Component of many enzymes; works with riboflavin to incorporate iron into hemoglobin	Deficiency Unknown Toxicity Occupational exposure to molybdenum dust causes gout-like symptoms.

systems that are active in energy metabolism. Ferritin, the storage form of iron, is located in the liver, bone marrow, and spleen.

Iron in foods exists in two forms: heme iron and nonheme iron.

- The majority of iron in the diet is nonheme iron. Plants and iron-fortified foods contain only nonheme iron.
- Nonheme iron absorption is inhibited by phytates found in legumes and grains and oxalates found in spinach and chard. Its absorption is promoted by the presence of heme iron and vitamin C (e.g., orange juice, tomatoes). However, within the context of a varied, mixed eating pattern, nonheme iron enhancers and inhibitors have little impact on most people's iron status (NIH, ODS, 2019b).
- Heme iron is found in meats, seafood, and poultry. Heme iron has higher bioavailability than nonheme iron and is less affected by other dietary components.

Based on average absorption rates and to compensate for daily (and monthly) iron losses, the RDA for iron is set at 8 mg for men and postmenopausal women and 18 mg for premenopausal women.

- Most adult men and postmenopausal women consume adequate amounts of iron.
- Iron requirements increase during growth and in response to heavy or chronic blood loss.
- Because the typical American diet provides only 6 to 7 mg of iron per 1000 cal, many menstruating women simply do not consume enough calories to satisfy their iron requirements.

Iron deficiency is the most common cause of anemia and infants and young children are at the highest risk (NIH, ODS, 2019b).

- Women of reproductive age and pregnant women are also at risk of iron deficiency.
- Nonnutritional risk factors for iron deficiency, particularly among older populations, include blood loss, malabsorption disorders, kidney disease, and cancer.

Iron deficiency anemia, a microcytic, hypochromic anemia, occurs when total iron stores become depleted. Symptoms include extreme fatigue, weakness, pale skin, and dizziness or light-headedness. A complete blood count usually shows low hemoglobin and hematocrit, low mean cellular volume, low ferritin, low serum iron, high transferrin or total iron-binding capacity, and low iron saturation.

- Iron deficiency during pregnancy is associated with poor pregnancy outcome, such as premature delivery, low birth weight, and increased perinatal infant mortality and maternal death.
- In young children, iron deficiency increases the risk of developmental delays and behavioral disturbances. Because very little iron is excreted from the body, the potential for toxicity is moderate to high when iron absorption is excessive.
- The most common cause of iron overload is hemochromatosis, one of the most common genetic disorders in the United States.
  - The absorption of excessive amounts of iron leads to iron accumulation in body tissues, especially the liver, heart, brain, joints, and pancreas. If left untreated, excess iron can cause heart disease, liver cancer, cirrhosis, diabetes, and arthritis.
  - Phlebotomies or chelation are used to reduce body iron. A low-iron diet is not recommended as part of treatment, nor could it be realistically achieved given the prevalence of iron enrichment and iron fortification in the U.S. food supply.
- Excessive dietary iron intake poses very little risk in adults with normal GI function because the body adjusts the rate of iron absorption accordingly.

Zinc

The small amount of zinc contained in the body (about 2 g) is found in almost all the cells and is especially concentrated in the eyes, bones, muscles, and prostate gland. Zinc in tissues is not available to maintain serum levels when intake is inadequate, so an adequate daily intake is necessary.

There is no single laboratory test that adequately measures zinc status, so zinc deficiency is not readily diagnosed.

- Risk factors for zinc deficiency include poor calorie intake, alcoholism, sickle cell disease, and malabsorption syndromes such as celiac disease, Crohn's disease, and short bowel syndrome.
- Vegetarians are also at increased risk because zinc is only half as well absorbed from plants as it is from animal sources.

Iodine

Iodine is found in the muscles, the thyroid gland, the skin, the skeleton, endocrine tissues, and the bloodstream. It is an essential component of thyroxine (T_4) and triiodothyronine (T_3), the thyroid hormones responsible for regulating metabolic rate, body temperature, reproduction, growth, the synthesis of blood cells, and nerve and muscle function. It may also play a role in immune response (IOM, 2001).

Most foods are naturally low in iodine.

- The iodine content of vegetables and grains varies with the soil content. Iodine-deficient soil around the Great Lakes was known as a "goiter belt" region in the United States.
- Processed foods almost always contain salt that is not iodized (NIH, ODS, 2019c).
- Milk is naturally low in iodine but has become an important source of iodine partly because of the use of iodine feed supplements and iodine-containing disinfectants used to sanitize udders, milking machines, and milk tanks.
- Some breads provide iodine due to the use of iodate dough conditioners.
- Seaweed (e.g., kelp, nori, and kombu) is one of the best food sources of iodine but its content is highly variable.
- The United States has generally been considered iodine sufficient since table salt began to be voluntarily iodized in 1924 (Perrine et al., 2010).
- Iodine deficiency has multiple adverse effects on growth and development (NIH, ODS, 2019c).

Goitrogens
thyroid antagonists found in cruciferous vegetables (e.g., cabbage, cauliflower, broccoli), soybeans, and sweet potatoes.

- Hypothyroidism occurs when iodine intake falls below 10 to 20 mcg/day. It may be accompanied by goiter, which is often the earliest sign of iodine deficiency. The effect of **goitrogens** on iodine balance is clinically insignificant except when iodine deficiency exists.
- Iodine deficiency in pregnant women can cause major neurodevelopmental deficits and growth retardation in the fetus, as well as miscarriage and stillbirth. Cretinism, characterized by a lack of physical and mental development, can be caused by severe iodine deficiency in utero.
- Less severe iodine deficiency in infants and children can also cause neurodevelopmental deficits.
- Adults with mild-to-moderate iodine deficiency may have goiter, impaired mental function, and reduced work productivity secondary to hypothyroidism (NIH, ODS, 2019c).

Concept Mastery Alert

Few foods naturally provide iodine. Nurses should be aware that iodized salt has iodine added to it. The iodine is not naturally occurring. Seafood has naturally occurring iodine due to the iodine in sea water.

Selenium

Selenium is a component of a group of enzymes, called glutathione peroxidases, that function as antioxidants to disarm free radicals produced during normal oxygen metabolism.

- The selenium content in plant foods varies widely depending on where they were grown.
- Most Americans consume more than the RDA for selenium according to NHANES data (USDA & ARS, 2018).
- Selenium deficiency is very rare in the United States. It is most likely to occur in people undergoing hemodialysis due to removal of selenium from the blood and poor selenium intake. People with human immunodeficiency virus may be at risk due to diarrhea and malabsorption.

Copper

Copper is distributed in muscles, liver, brain, bones, kidneys, and blood. Americans typically consume adequate amounts of copper.

- Excess zinc intake has the potential to induce copper deficiency by impairing its absorption, but copper deficiency is rare.
- Supplements, not food, may cause copper toxicity, as do some rare genetic disorders, such as Wilson disease.

Manganese

Mean manganese intake among American adults is well above the AI, and dietary deficiencies have not been noted.

- Manganese toxicity is a well-known occupational hazard for miners who inhale manganese dust over a prolonged period of time, leading to central nervous system abnormalities with symptoms similar to those of Parkinson disease.
- There is some evidence to suggest that high manganese intake from drinking water, which may be more bioavailable than manganese from food, also produces neuromotor deficits similar to Parkinson disease.

Fluoride

Fluoride promotes the mineralization of developing tooth enamel prior to tooth eruption and the remineralization of surface enamel in erupted teeth.

Cariogenic
cavity promoting.

- It concentrates in plaque and saliva to inhibit the process by which **cariogenic** bacteria metabolize carbohydrates to produce acids that cause tooth decay.
- Fluoridation of municipal water is credited with a major decline in the prevalence and severity of dental caries in the U.S. population and is deemed one of the 10 great public health achievements of the 20th century (Centers for Disease Control and Prevention [CDC], 1999). Water fluoridation has been credited with reducing tooth decay by 25% in children and adults (CDC, 2019a).

- Numerous organizations endorse fluoridation of municipal water, including the American Academy of Pediatrics, the American Association of Public Health Dentistry, the American Dental Association, and the U.S. Task Force on Community Preventive Services.
- Young children are susceptible to mottled tooth enamel if they ingest several times more fluoride than the recommended amount during the time of tooth enamel formation. The swallowing of fluoridated toothpaste is to blame.

Chromium

Although chromium is an essential trace mineral, its functions and requirements are not well defined (NIH, ODS, 2019d).

- Chromium enhances the action of insulin; however, there is no clear scientific evidence that supplements are effective in improving glucose control in patients with existing type 2 diabetes (Costello et al., 2016).
- Because existing databases lack information on chromium, few food intake studies utilizing few laboratories are available to estimate usual intake. However, it appears that average intake is adequate.

Molybdenum

Molybdenum is a cofactor for certain enzymes. Usual intake is well above the RDA. Dietary deficiencies and toxicities are unknown.

Other Trace Elements

Limited human studies suggest arsenic, boron, nickel, silicon, and vanadium may have a role in human health. However, there is insufficient data to set RDAs or AIs for any of these trace minerals. Based on animal studies, UL were set for boron, nickel, and vanadium.

WATER AND MINERALS IN HEALTH PROMOTION

Health is "promoted" when water (beverage) choices are healthy and when the intake of minerals is not excessive (e.g., sodium) or inadequate (e.g., calcium and potassium).

Choose Healthy Beverages

Beverages are often overlooked when people consider their food intake, but they are an important part of eating patterns. Some beverages provide nutrients such as protein, vitamins, minerals, and phytonutrients; others are considered empty calories because they provide calories with few or no nutrients.

- The primary beverages consumed should be calorie free, such as water, or contribute beneficial nutrients, such as non fat and low-fat milk and 100% juice.
- Coffee, tea, and flavored waters that are free of added sugar and cream are also options. Healthy adults can consume up to 400 mg/day of caffeine without dangerous effects (USDA & USDHHS, 2020), which is approximately equivalent to four 8-oz cups of coffee.
- If consumed at all, sugar-sweetened beverage intake should be limited. Sugar-sweetened beverage intake has been linked to obesity in adults and children (Luger et al., 2017) and increased risk of type 2 diabetes and atherosclerotic CVD (Arnett et al., 2019).
- Substituting artificially sweetened beverages may help adults who habitually consume large amounts of sugar-sweetened beverages transition to water easier (Arnett et al., 2019).
- If consumed at all, alcohol intake should be limited to a moderate intake or less. Moderate is defined as up to one drink per day for women and up to two drinks per day for men and only by adults of legal drinking age.

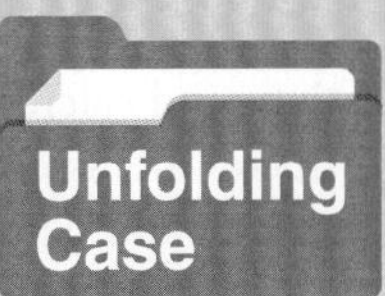

Consider Myra. Which fluids should she be encouraged to use to satisfy her fluid recommendation? Would more than 8 glasses of fluid a day be excessive?

Reduce Sodium Intake

According to the Agency for Healthcare Research and Quality (2018), a review of studies on the effects of decreasing sodium intake and increasing potassium showed the following:

- Reducing sodium intake lowers blood pressure in normotensive adults and more so in adults with hypertension.
- Higher sodium intake may be related to higher risk of developing hypertension.
- Using potassium-containing salt substitutes to lower sodium intake likely reduces blood pressure in adults.
- Sodium intake may be associated with all-cause mortality.
- Lowering sodium intake may lower the risk of combined CVD morbidity and mortality.

Since its inception in 1980, every edition of the *Dietary Guidelines for Americans* has urged Americans to lower their sodium intake to prevent and treat hypertension, CVD, and stroke. Despite the long-standing advice to eat less sodium, the average sodium intake (3393 mg/day) remains well above recommended amounts (<2300 mg/day) (USDA & USDHHS, 2020). Figure 7.3 shows the top sources of sodium among Americans ages 1 and older. Tips for reducing sodium intake are shown in Box 7.3.

BOX 7.3 Tips for Lowering Sodium Intake

Know what labeling terms mean:

- *Sodium-free* has less than 5 mg sodium per serving.
- *Very low sodium* has less than 35 mg per serving.
- *Low sodium* has less than 140 mg per serving.
- *Reduced or less sodium* has at least 25% less sodium per serving than the traditional food.
- *Light in sodium* has 50% less sodium than the traditional food.
- *Salt-free* has less than 5 mg of salt.
- *Unsalted or no added salt* means no salt was added during processing, although the food itself may contain natural sodium.

Make better choices

- Avoid or limit convenience foods, such as boxed mixes, frozen dinners, and canned foods.
- Eat home-cooked meals more often.
- Eat more fresh or frozen vegetables.
- Compare labels to choose brands or varieties with the lowest amount of sodium.
- Replace processed meats with fresh meats
- Use cheese sparingly.
- Choose nut butters with no sodium added.
- Cook rice and pasta without salt.
- Use lower-salt condiments, such as vinegar or reduced sodium ketchup or Worcestershire sauce.
- Substitute homemade vinegar and oil dressing for bottled varieties.
- If you use canned vegetables, drain away liquid and rinse thoroughly.
- Limit salty snacks.
- Instead of salt, season food with spices, herbs, lemon, vinegar, or salt-free seasonings.

Shortfall Minerals

The Dietary Guidelines have identified potassium and calcium as shortfall minerals that are considered public health concerns because low intakes are associated with health issues (USDA & USDHHS, 2020). Low intakes of vegetables, fruits, and dairy contribute to the underconsumption of these two minerals. Menstruating and pregnant women may also not consume enough iron. Figure 7.5 depicts the mean intake of these minerals as a percent of the DRI for adults 20 and older. Health concerns related to low intakes of potassium and calcium as well as suggestions for improving the intake of each are presented in the following.

Potassium

Lower intakes of potassium and higher intakes of sodium are associated with higher blood pressure (Jackson et al., 2018).

- This finding supports the dietary advice to lower sodium intake and increase potassium intake because hypertension is a key modifiable risk factor for CVD.
- Increasing potassium intake also most likely lowers blood pressure in adults with existing hypertension (AHRQ, 2018).

Potassium is widespread across food groups, but not all foods within a group have high potassium levels. Variety helps ensure adequacy. High potassium choices include the following:

- Fruits: prune juice, kiwifruit, dried fruit (e.g., dates, prunes, raisins), banana, avocado, purple passion fruit
- Vegetables: baked potato with the skin, other types of cooked potatoes, sweet potato baked in the skin, fresh spinach, beets, artichoke, tomato paste and sauce, winter squash

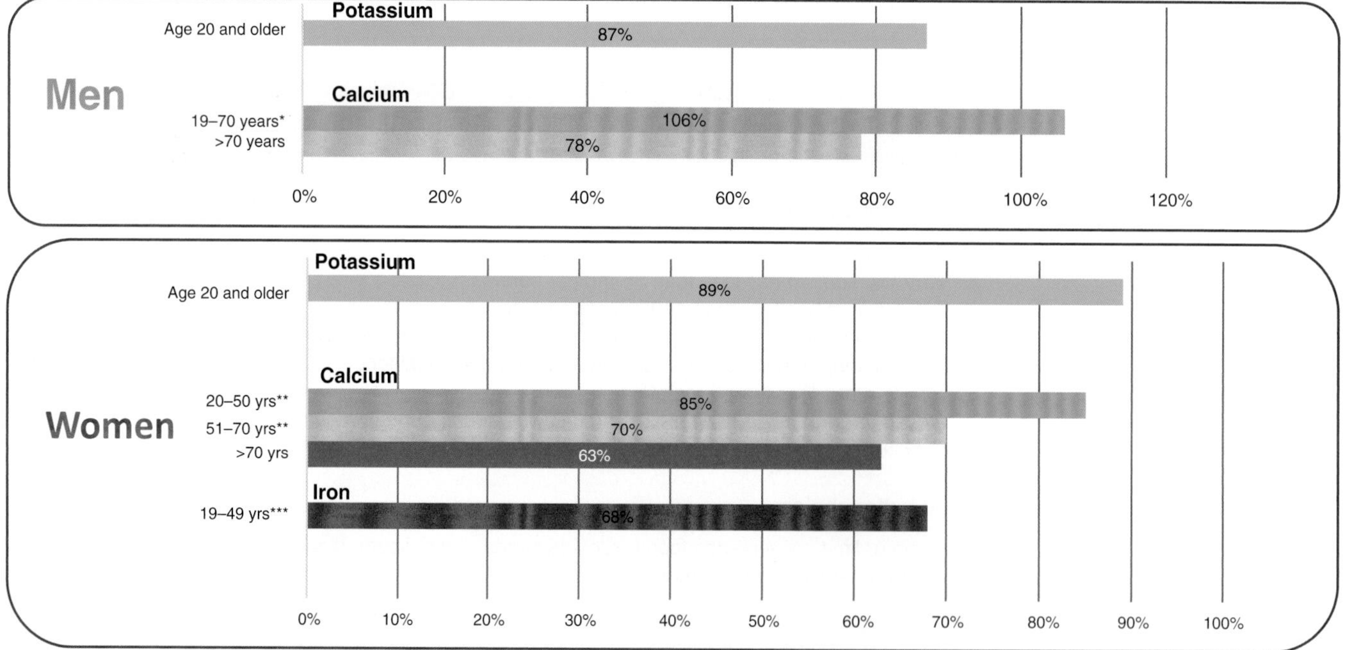

Figure 7.5 ▲ Mean intake of shortfall minerals as a percentage of the dietary reference intakes in adult men and women aged 20 and older.

(*Source:* U.S. Department of Agriculture & Agricultural Research Service. [2018]. Nutrition intakes from food: Mean amounts consumed per individual, by gender and age. *What We Eat in America, NHANES 2015–2016.* www.ars.usda.gov/bc/bhnrcfsrg; https://www.ars.usda.gov/ARSUserFiles/80400530/pdf/1516/tables_1-56_2015-2016.pdf)

- Grains: bran and certain bran cereals
- Dairy: milk (nonfat, low fat, whole, buttermilk), yogurt
- Protein foods: beans (e.g., baked, navy, pinto, refried), lentils, salmon, pollock

Calcium

There are no short-term adverse effects of low calcium intake because serum calcium levels are tightly regulated by vitamin D and parathyroid hormone.

- Hypocalcemia occurs primarily from alterations in calcium metabolism (e.g., parathyroid disorders, kidney disease) or the use of certain medications.
- The long-term risk of low calcium intake is osteopenia, a condition characterized by a significant decrease in bone mineral density. If left untreated, osteopenia can progress to osteoporosis.
- Low calcium intake is associated with low bone mass, rapid bone loss, and high fracture rates (NIH Osteoporosis and Related Bone Diseases National Resource Center, 2018).

Milk is a nearly perfect source of calcium because it contains vitamin D and lactose, which promote calcium absorption.

- People who are lactose intolerant can obtain calcium from lactose-reduced milk, acidophilus milk, and lactose-free yogurt.
- Low-oxalate green vegetables, such as broccoli, bok choy, collard greens, and kale, are good sources of calcium.
- Significant amounts of calcium can also be found in calcium-fortified foods, such as fruit juices, tomato juice, and ready-to-eat breakfast cereals.

Healthy Eating Patterns

The healthy eating patterns repeated throughout this book, such as the Healthy U.S.-Style Eating Pattern, the Mediterranean diet, and the generic "plant-based diet," can be used to help ensure AIs of minerals, specifically the shortfall minerals potassium and calcium. These patterns are also lower in sodium. According to the *Dietary Guidelines for Americans*, another eating pattern, the Dietary Approaches to Stop Hypertension (DASH) diet, is healthy eating pattern that has many of the same characteristics as the Healthy U.S.-Style Eating Pattern (USDA & USDHHS, 2020). The most notable difference is that the DASH diet recommends ⅓ to ½ less oils.

- The DASH diet was designed to see if a healthy eating pattern, not specifically individual nutrients, could lower high blood pressure (Appel et al., 1997).
- The results clearly showed that, even without lowering sodium intake, an eating pattern rich in fruit, vegetables, low-fat dairy products, and whole grains; moderate in poultry, fish, and nuts; and low in fat, red meat, and added sugar lowered blood pressure and also low-density lipoprotein cholesterol (LDL-C). Adding a sodium restriction improves its blood pressure–lowering effect.
- Its blood pressure–lowering effect likely comes from a combination of factors, including its high content of potassium, calcium, and magnesium.
- Table 7.7 features a 2000-cal DASH eating pattern

Table 7.7 Daily and Weekly Eating Plan for a 2000-Cal Dietary Approaches to Stop Hypertension Diet

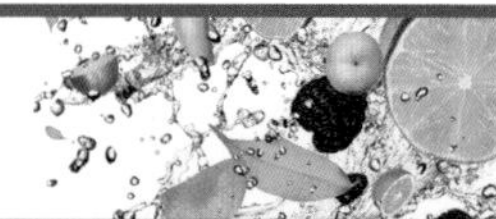

Food Group and Serving Size	Daily Servings
Fruit, ½ c	4–5
Vegetables, 1 c leafy greens or ½ c other vegetables cooked or raw	4–5
Grains, preferably whole grains, 1 ounce equivalents	6–8
Protein	6 oz or less
Dairy (nonfat or low fat), 1 cup	2–3
Oils	8–12 g
Sodium	2300 mg
	Weekly servings
Nuts (1/3 c), seeds (2 tbsp), legumes (1/2 c cooked)	4–5
Sweets	5 or less

Source: National Institutes of Health National Heart, Lung, and Blood Institute. DASH Eating Plan. https://www.nhlbi.nih.gov/health-topics/dash-eating-plan

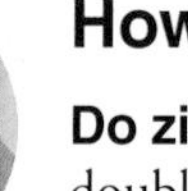

How Do You Respond?

Do zinc lozenges cure the common cold? Meta-analyses of randomized, double-blind, placebo-controlled trials show that zinc lozenges may reduce the duration of colds by approximately 33% (e.g., Hemila, 2017). More research is needed to determine the optimal dosage, formulation, and duration of treatment. However, the safety of intranasal zinc has been questioned based on numerous reports linking their use to a loss of the sense of smell, which in some cases has been long-lasting or permanent (NIH, ODS, 2019e).

Does chlorine in drinking water cause cancer? Chlorine is added to drinking water as a disinfectant to control microbial contaminants. It is allowed at levels up to 4 ppm, a level at which no harmful health effects are likely to occur. Concern arises from trihalomethanes (THM), a group of organic chemicals that often occur in drinking water from the reaction between naturally occurring organic and inorganic matter and chlorine. The Environmental Protection Agency (EPA) has established a Maximum Contaminant Level (MCL) for total THMs in public drinking water to ensure that any potential adverse effects are outweighed by the benefit of reducing the risk of acute GI diseases related to contamination. The MCL for total THMs is 80 ppb. The small quantities of THMs allowed in water are not enough to cause cancer risk because they fall far below where risk is determined to begin. The benefits of chlorine in preventing outbreaks of cholera, hepatitis, and other diseases far outweigh the negligible effects of THM.

What are chelated minerals? A chelated mineral is a mineral that has been chemically combined with an amino acid to protect it from other food components such as oxalates and phytates that can bind to the mineral and prevent it from being absorbed. There is no evidence to support claims that chelated minerals are better than non-chelated minerals.

REVIEW CASE STUDY

Bill is a 45-year-old bachelor who eats a grab-and-go breakfast, eats all of his lunches out, and has takeout or "something easy" for dinner. Bill's doctor is concerned that his blood pressure is progressively rising with every office visit and has advised him to "cut out the salt" to lower his sodium intake. Bill rarely uses salt from a salt shaker and is unsure what else he can do to lower his sodium intake. A typical day's intake is shown on the right:

- What foods did Bill eat yesterday that were high in sodium? What foods were relatively low in sodium? What would be better choices for him when eating out? How could he lower his sodium intake while still relying on "something easy" when he prepares food at home?
- Knowing that potassium may help blunt the effect of a high sodium intake on blood pressure, what foods would you recommend he add to his diet that would increase his potassium intake?
- In overweight people, weight loss helps lower high blood pressure. Bill is "a little heavy." What changes/substitutions would help him lose weight?

Breakfast: Black coffee and two jelly doughnuts
Midmorning snack: Black coffee and cookies
Lunch: Two fast-food tacos with tortilla chips and salsa or a 6-in cold cut submarine with potato chips, cola
Midafternoon snack: Candy bar
Dinner: If takeout, then Chinese food or pizza. If "something easy," then boxed macaroni and cheese with a couple of hot dogs, canned soup with a cold cut sandwich, or frozen TV dinners.
Dessert: Instant pudding, ice cream, or candy bars
Evening snacks: Cereal and milk or potato chips and dip

STUDY QUESTIONS

1 A healthy, young adult client asks how much water he should drink daily. Which of the following would be the nurse's best response?
   a. "The old adage is true: Drink eight 8-oz glasses of water daily."
   b. "Drink to satisfy thirst and you will consume adequate fluid."
   c. "You can't overconsume water, so drink as much as you can spread out over the course of the day."
   d. "It is actually not necessary to drink water at all. It is equally healthy to meet your fluid requirement with sugar-free soft drinks."

2 When developing a teaching plan for a client who is lactose intolerant, which of the following foods would the nurse suggest as sources of calcium the client could tolerate?
   a. cheddar cheese, bok choy, broccoli
   b. spinach, beet greens, nonfat milk
   c. poultry, meat, eggs
   d. whole grains, nuts, cocoa

3 The client asks what makes the DASH diet different from a Healthy U.S.-Style Eating Pattern. What is the best response?
   a. "They are basically the same except that the DASH diet is lower in calories."
   b. "The DASH diet is low in dairy products and grains."
   c. "The DASH diet recommends significantly less oils."
   d. "The DASH diet is lower in protein foods."

4 Which of the following recommendations would be most effective at increasing potassium intake?
   a. Choose enriched grains in place of whole grains.
   b. Consume more fruits, vegetables, and dairy.
   c. Eat more red meat in place of poultry.
   d. Because there are few good dietary sources of potassium, it is best obtained by taking potassium supplements.

5 A client asks why eating less sodium is important for healthy people. Which of the following is the nurse's best response?
   a. "Low-sodium diets tend to be low in fat and therefore may reduce the risk of heart disease."
   b. "Low-sodium diets are only effective at preventing high blood pressure, not lowering existing high blood pressure, so the time to implement a low-sodium diet is when you are healthy."
   c. "Lowering sodium intake lowers blood pressure in healthy people and may also decrease the risk of atherosclerotic heart disease."
   d. "Low-sodium diets are inherently low in calories and help people lose weight, which can help prevent a variety of chronic diseases."

6 Which of the following foods provides iron in a form that would be absorbed best?
   a. red meat
   b. iron-fortified cereal
   c. legumes
   d. enriched bread

7 A client says he never adds salt to any foods that his wife serves, so he believes he is consuming a low-sodium diet. Which of the following is the nurse's best response?
a. "If you don't add salt to any of your foods, you are probably eating a low-sodium diet. Continue with that strategy."
b. "Even though you aren't adding salt to food at the table, your wife is probably salting food as she cooks. She should stop doing that."
c. "Lots of foods are naturally high in sodium, such as milk and meat; in addition to not using a salt shaker, you must also limit foods that are naturally high in sodium."
d. "The major sources of sodium are processed and convenience foods. Limiting their intake makes the biggest impact on overall sodium intake."

8 What should you tell the client about taking mineral supplements?
a. "Most Americans are deficient in minerals, so it is wise to take a multimineral supplement."
b. "Like water-soluble vitamins, if you consume more minerals than your body needs, you will excrete them in the urine, so do not worry about taking in too much."
c. "If you do not have a mineral deficiency, supplements are not necessary and can lead to a potentially excessive intake that can cause adverse health effects."
d. "Mineral deficiencies do not exist in the United States, so you do not need to waste your money on them."

CHAPTER SUMMARY WATER AND MINERALS

Body fluids consist of water and chemicals, such as minerals. Because water is involved in almost every body function, is not stored, and is excreted daily, it is more vital to life than food.

Water

Under normal conditions, water intake equals water output to maintain water balance.

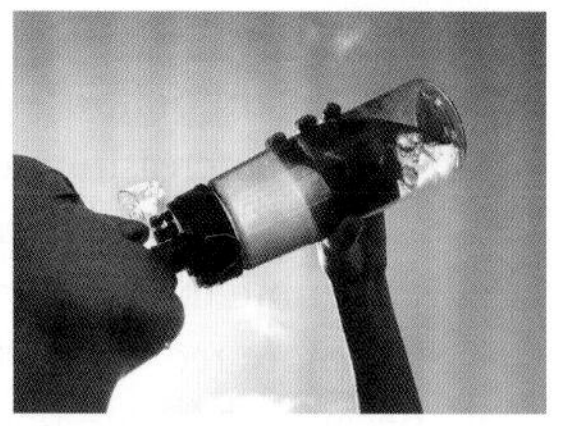

- In most healthy people, thirst is a reliable indicator of need.
- activity, climate, and health affect the body's need for water.

Fluid and Electrolyte Balance

Some minerals are electrolytes that dissociate (dissolve) into ions in water and are able to conduct electricity. Membranes (e.g., cell membranes, capillary membranes), the concentration of electrolytes, and hydrostatic pressure work to regulate the fluids in each body compartment.

Understanding Minerals

Minerals are found in all body fluids and tissues. Minerals are inorganic elements from the earth's crust.

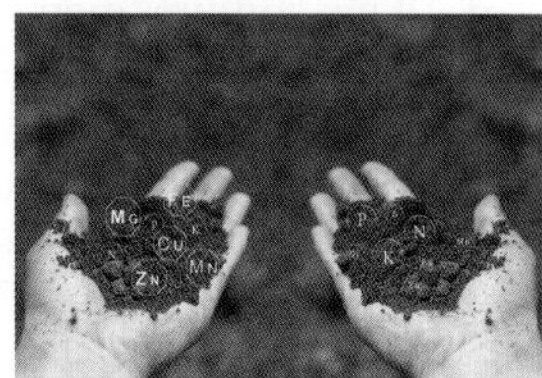

- provide structure to body tissues and regulate body processes
- vary in how they are regulated by the body, such as by the rate of absorption, urinary excretion, or storage.
- can be toxic but generally only from excess supplemental intake or environmental exposure.
- are found in all food groups to varying degrees.
- should only be taken in supplemental form if needed.

Major Electrolytes

Sodium, potassium, and chloride are major minerals in addition to being electrolytes.

- **Sodium:** Approximately 71% of sodium is added to food outside the home. Americans eat too much sodium.
- **Potassium:** Most Americans do not consume enough potassium. Wholesome foods provide more potassium than processed foods.
- **Chloride:** Almost all dietary chloride comes from salt (sodium chloride).

Major Minerals

Major minerals are present in the body in amounts >5 g.

- **Calcium:** The most plentiful mineral in the body. Bone tissue serves as a dynamic reservoir to release calcium as needed to maintain serum levels.
- **Phosphorus:** The phosphorus content of foods goes up with processing. Americans may be eating more than required.
- **Magnesium:** A cofactor for more than 300 enzymes in the body.
- **Sulfur:** Does not function independently as a nutrient but is a component of some amino acids and vitamins.

Trace Minerals

A delicate balance exists between trace minerals: too much of one can create a deficiency of another.

- **Iron:** Bioavailability varies with the type of iron consumed. Iron deficiency is not uncommon.
- **Zinc:** Because there is no single lab test that measures zinc status, zinc deficiency is not readily diagnosed.
- **Iodine:** Most foods are low in iodine. Iodized salt enables Americans to consume adequate iodine.

CHAPTER SUMMARY WATER AND MINERALS (continued)

- Selenium, Copper, Manganese, and Molybdenum: Americans consume adequate amounts of these minerals. Dietary deficiencies are rare.
- **Fluoride:** Fluoridated water has dramatically reduced the prevalence and severity of cavities in the United States population.
- **Chromium:** Enhances the action of insulin.

Water and Minerals in Health Promotion

- Water, low-fat or non fat milk, and 100% juice should be the primary beverages of choice.
- Americans are urged to eat less sodium to lower blood pressure and possibly CVD morbidity and mortality.

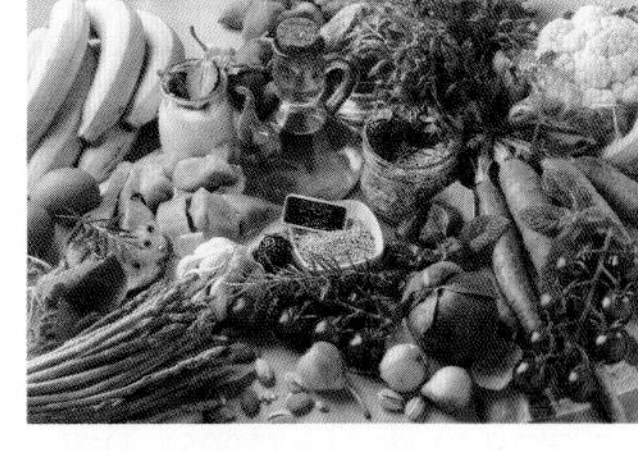

- Potassium and calcium are shortfall nutrients of concern because not eating enough of these minerals is associated with health problems. Iron intake may be inadequate in young children, menstruating women, and pregnant women.
- The DASH diet is an eating pattern rich in potassium, calcium, and magnesium and limited in sodium. It has been shown to lower high blood pressure and LDL-C.

Figure Sources: *shutterstock.com/KieferPix, shutterstock.com/SNP_SS, shutterstock.com/Antonina Vlasova*

Student Resources on thePoint®
For additional learning materials, activate the code in the front of this book at https://thePoint.lww.com/activate

Websites

Dietary supplement fact sheets from the National Institutes of Health, Office of Dietary Supplements at https://ods.od.nih.gov/HealthInformation/healthprofessional.aspx

National Academy of Sciences, Institute of Medicine for Reference Dietary Intakes at www.nap.edu

National Dairy Council at www.nationaldairycouncil.org

Nutrient content of foods at the UDA's Food Data central website at https://fdc.nal.usda.gov/

References

Academy of Nutrition and Dietetics, Evidence Analysis Library. (2007). *Hydration: Estimating fluid needs.* https://www.andeal.org/topic.cfm?cat=3217&evidence_summary_id=250714&highlight=fluid%20requirement&home=1

Agency for Healthcare Research and Quality. (2018). Sodium and potassium intake: Effects on chronic disease outcomes and risks. Evidence Summary. *Comparative Effectiveness Review*, Number 206. https://effectivehealthcare.ahrq.gov/sites/default/files/cer-206-evidence-summary-sodium-potassium_0.pdf

Appel, L. J., Moore, T. J., Obarzanek, E., Vollmer, W. M., Svetkey, L. P., Sacks, F. M., Bray, G. A., Vogt, T. M., Cutler, J. A., Windhauser, M. M., Lin, P.-H., Karanja, N., Simons-Morton, D., McCullough, M., Swain, J., Steele, P., Evans, M. A., Miller, E. R., & Harsha, D. W. for the DASH Collaborative Research Group. (1997). A clinical trial of the effects of dietary patterns on blood pressure. *The New England Journal of Medicine*, *336,* 1117–1124. https://doi.org/10.1056/NEJM199704173361601

Arnett, D. K., Blumenthal, R. S., Albert, M. A., Buroker, A. B., Goldberger, Z. D., Hahn, E. J., Himmelfarb, C. D., Khera, A., Lloyd-Jones, D., McEvoy, J. W., Michos, E. D., Miedema, M. D., Munoz, D., Smith, S. C. Jr., Virani, S. S., Williams, K. A. Sr., Yeboah, J., & Ziaeian, B. (2019). 2019 ACC/AHA guideline on the primary prevention of cardiovascular disease: A report of the American College of Cardiology/American Heart Association Task Force on Clinical Practice Guidelines. *Circulation*, *140*(11), e596–e646. https://doi.org/10.1161/CIR.0000000000000678

Centers for Disease Control and Prevention. (1999). Ten great public health achievements—United States, 1990–1999. *Morbidity and Mortality Weekly Report*, *48*(50), 1141. https://www.cdc.gov/mmwr/preview/mmwrhtml/mm4850bx.htm

Centers for Disease Control and Prevention. (2019a). *Water fluoridation basics.* https://www.cdc.gov/fluoridation/basics/

Centers for Disease Control and Prevention. (2019b). *Water fluoridation data and statistics.* https://www.cdc.gov/fluoridation/statistics/index.htm

Chang, A., Lazo, M., Appel, L., Gutiérrez, O. M., & Grams, M. E. (2014). High dietary phosphorus intake is associated with all-cause mortality: Results from NHANES III. *The American Journal of Clinical Nutrition*, *99*(2), 320–327. https://doi.org/10.3945/ajcn.113.073148

Costello, R. B., Dwyer, J. T., & Bailey, R. L. (2016). Chromium supplements for glycemic control in type 2 diabetes: Limited evidence of effectiveness. *Nutrition Reviews*, *74*(7), 455–468. https://doi.org/10.1093/nutrit/nuw011

de Baaij, J. H. F., Hoenderop, J. G. J., & Bindels, R. J. M. (2015). Magnesium in man: Implications for health and disease. *Physiological Reviews*, *95*(1), 1–46. https://doi.org/10.1152/physrev.00012.2014

Food and Nutrition Board, National Academies of Sciences, Engineering, and Medicine. (2019). Consensus study report highlights. *Dietary reference intakes for sodium and potassium.* https://www.nap.edu/resource/25353/030519DRISodiumPotassium.pdf

Harnack, L. J., Cogswell, M. E., Shikany, J. M., Gardner, C. D., Gillespie, C., Loria, C., Zhou, X., Yuan, K., & Steffan, L. M. (2017). Sources of sodium in US adults from 3 geographic regions. *Circulation, 135*(19), 1775–1783. https://doi.org/10.1161/CIRCULATIONAHA.116.024446

Hemila, H. (2017). Zinc lozenges and the common cold: A meta-analysis comparing zinc acetate and zinc gluconate, and the role of zinc dosage. *Journal of the Royal Society of Medicine Open*, *8*(5), 1–7. https://doi.org/10.1177%2F2054270417694291

Institute of Medicine. (2001). *Dietary reference intakes for vitamin A, vitamin K, arsenic, boron, chromium, copper, iodine, iron, manganese, molybdenum, nickel, silicon, vanadium, and zinc.* National Academy Press.

Institute of Medicine. (2005). *Dietary reference intakes for water, potassium, sodium, chloride, and sulfate.* http://www.nap.edu/catalog.php?record_id=10925#

Itkonen, S. T., Karp, H. J., & Lamberg-Allardt, C. J. (2018). Bioavailability of phosphorus. In: J. Uribarri & M.S. Calvo (Eds.), *Dietary phosphorus: Health, nutrition, and regulatory aspects* (pp. 221–233). CRC Press.

Jackson, S. L., Cogswell, M. D., Zhao, L., Terry, A. L., Wang, C.-Y., Wright, J., Coleman King, S. M., Bowman, B., Chen, T.-C., Merritt, R., & Loria, C. M. (2018). Association between urinary sodium and potassium excretion and blood pressure among adults in the United States: National health and Nutrition Examination Survey, 2014. *Circulation, 137*(3), 237–246. https://doi.org/10.1161/CIRCULATIONAHA.117.029193

Luger, M., Lafontan, M., Bes-Rastrollo, M., Winzer, E., Yumuk, V., & Farpour-Lambert, N. (2017). Sugar-sweetened beverages and weight gain in children and adults: A systematic review from 2013–2015 and a comparison with previous studies. *Obesity Facts, 10*(6), 674–693. https://doi.org/10.1159/000484566

Marra, M. V., & Bailey, R. L. (2018). Position of the academy of nutrition and dietetics: Micronutrient supplementation. *Journal of the Academy of Nutrition and Dietetics, 118*(11), 2162–2173. https://doi.org/10.1016/j.jand.2018.07.022

Morris, J. S., & Crane, S. B. (2013). Selenium toxicity from a misformulated dietary supplement, adverse health effects, and the temporal response in the nail biologic monitor. *Nutrients, 5*(4), 1024–1057. https://doi.org/10.3390/nu5041024

National Institutes of Health, Office of Dietary Supplements. (2019a). *Phosphorus: Fact sheet for health professionals.* https://ods.od.nih.gov/factsheets/Phosphorus-HealthProfessional/#en65

National Institutes of Health, Office of Dietary Supplements. (2019b). *Iron: Fact sheet for health professionals.* https://ods.od.nih.gov/factsheets/Iron-HealthProfessional/#en2

National Institutes of Health, Office of Dietary Supplements. (2019c). *Iodine: Fact sheet for health professionals.* https://ods.od.nih.gov/factsheets/Iodine-HealthProfessional/

National Institutes of Health, Office of Dietary Supplements. (2019d). *Chromium: Dietary supplement fact sheet.* https://ods.od.nih.gov/factsheets/Chromium-HealthProfessional/

National Institutes of Health, Office of Dietary Supplements. (2019e). *Zinc: Fat sheet for health professionals.* https://ods.od.nih.gov/factsheets/Zinc-HealthProfessional/

National Institutes of Health Osteoporosis and Related Bone Diseases National Resource Center. (2018). *Osteoporosis overview.* https://www.bones.nih.gov/health-info/bone/osteoporosis/overview#-Prevention

Perrine, C. G., Herrick, K., Serdula, M. K, & Sullivan, K. M. (2010). Some subgroups of reproductive age women in the United States may be at risk for iodine deficiency. *The Journal of Nutrition, 140*(8), 1489–1494. https://doi.org/10.3945/jn.109.120147

Scanni, R., vonRotz, M., Jehle, S., Hulter, H. N., & Krapf, R. (2014). The human response to acute enteral and parenteral phosphate loads. *Journal of the American Society of Nephrology, 25*(12), 2730–2739. https://doi.org/10.1681/ASN.2013101076

U.S. Department of Agriculture & Agricultural Research Service. (2018). *Nutrient intakes from food and beverages: Mean amounts consumed per individual, by gender and age. What we eat in America, NHANES 2015–2016.* www.ars.usda.gov/nea/bhnrc/fsrg

U.S. Department of Agriculture & U.S. Department of Health and Human Services. (2020, December). *Dietary guidelines for Americans, 2020–2025.* https://www.dietaryguidelines.gov

Valtin, H. (2002). "Drink at least eight glasses of water a day." Really? Is there scientific evidence for "8 × 8"? *American Journal of Physiology: Regulatory, Integrative and Comparative Physiology, 283*(5), R993–R1004. https://doi.org/10.1152/ajpregu.00365.2002

Chapter 8 Energy Balance

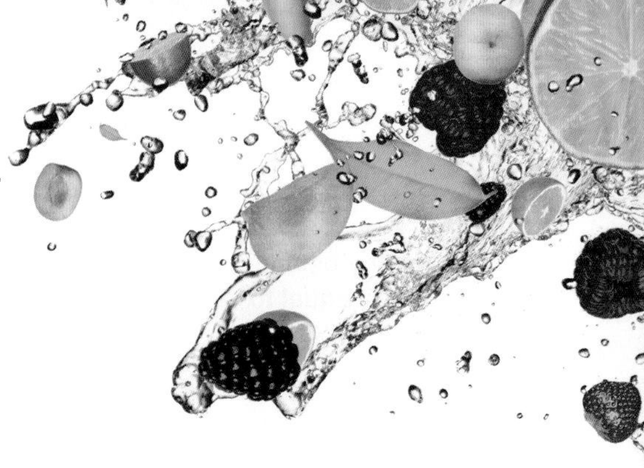

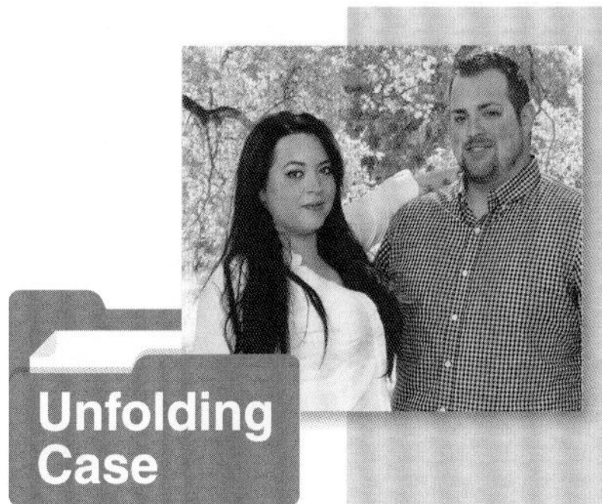

Unfolding Case

Kyla and Garrett Wilkinson

Kyla and Garrett are both 25 years old and have been married 6 months. Since then, Kyla has gained 10 to 15 pounds and Garrett has gained 40 pounds, which they attribute to eating dinner out three to four times a week and getting takeout the other days of the week. They are shocked at how quickly "things got out of control" and want to adopt a healthier lifestyle before embarking on parenthood.

Learning Objectives

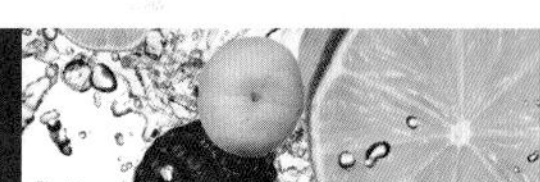

Upon completion of this chapter, you will be able to:

1 Discuss the three factors that contribute to total calorie expenditure.
2 Calculate an individual's basal metabolic rate.
3 Calculate a person's total calorie requirement.
4 Determine an individual's body mass index (BMI).
5 Evaluate weight status based on BMI.
6 Explain the value of measuring a person's waist circumference.
7 Discuss strategies that promote portion control.
8 Give examples of healthier substitutes for calorically dense foods.
9 Calculate the calorie value of a food or eating pattern based on the macronutrient composition.
10 Summarize key physical activity guidelines for adults.

The state of energy balance is determined by comparing the number of calories consumed to the number of calories expended. Body weight changes over time when the ratio of calorie intake to calorie output changes. This chapter discusses states of energy balance, energy intake, energy output, and how total calorie requirements are estimated. Methods of evaluating body weight are presented. Energy in health promotion focuses on consuming the appropriate number of calories, being physically active, and reducing sitting time.

STATE OF ENERGY BALANCE

Energy balance occurs when the number of calories consumed is approximately equal to the number of calories expended over time. Body weight remains stable (Fig. 8.1).

- A positive energy balance occurs when calorie intake exceeds calorie expenditure, whether the imbalance is caused by overeating, low activity, or both (Fig. 8.2). Over time, the

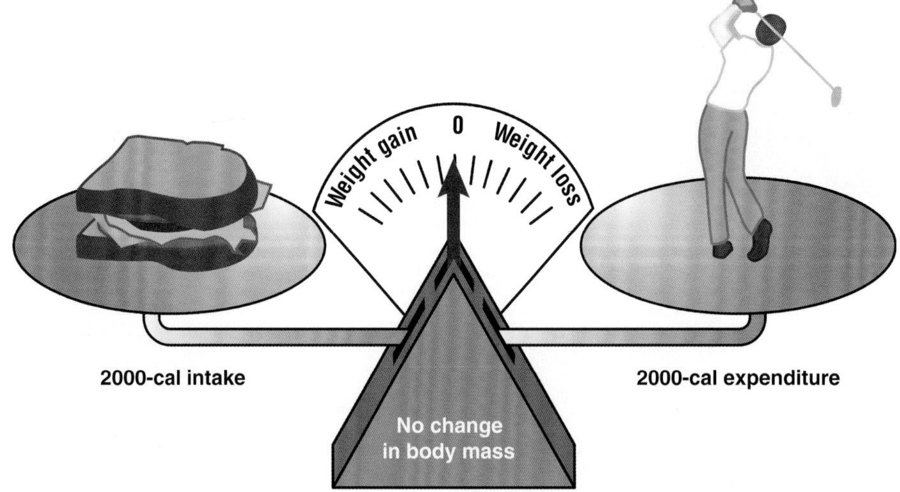

Figure 8.1 ▶ **A state of energy balance: Calorie intake is equal to calorie expenditure.**

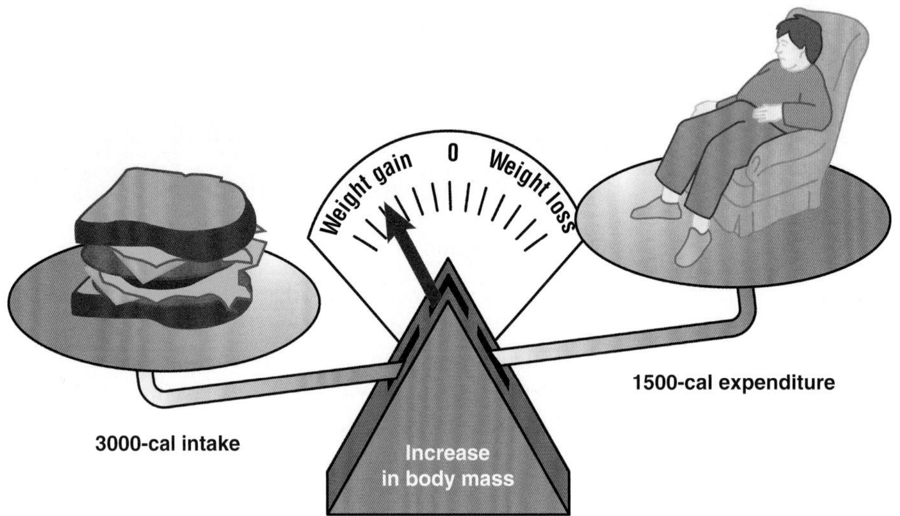

Figure 8.2 ▶ **A positive energy balance: Calorie intake is greater than calorie expenditure.**

calories consumed in excess of expenditure contribute to weight gain. Because a pound of body fat is equivalent to 3500 calories, a surplus of 500 cal/day over a 7-day period theoretically results in a 1-pound weight gain.

- Conversely, a negative calorie balance occurs when calorie expenditure exceeds intake, whether the imbalance is from decreasing calorie intake, increasing physical activity (PA), or (preferably) both (Fig. 8.3).

Energy Intake

The energy value of food is measured in kilocalories, which is commonly shortened to **calories**. Nutrients that provide calories are carbohydrates, protein, and fat (Fig. 8.4). Alcohol also provides calories. The total number of calories in a food or eating pattern can be estimated by multiplying the total grams of these nutrients by the appropriate calories per gram—namely, 4 cal/g for carbohydrates and protein, 9 cal/g for fat, and 7 cal/g for alcohol. Box 8.1 features an example.

> **Calorie**
> unit by which energy is measured; the amount of heat needed to raise the temperature of 1 kg of water by 1°C. Technically, calorie is actually kilocalorie or kcal.

Counting Calories

"Counting calories" can be practiced in a number of ways—manually, online, or with a mobile phone app.

- It is a tedious and imprecise process dependent on knowing or accurately measuring the amount of all foods consumed.

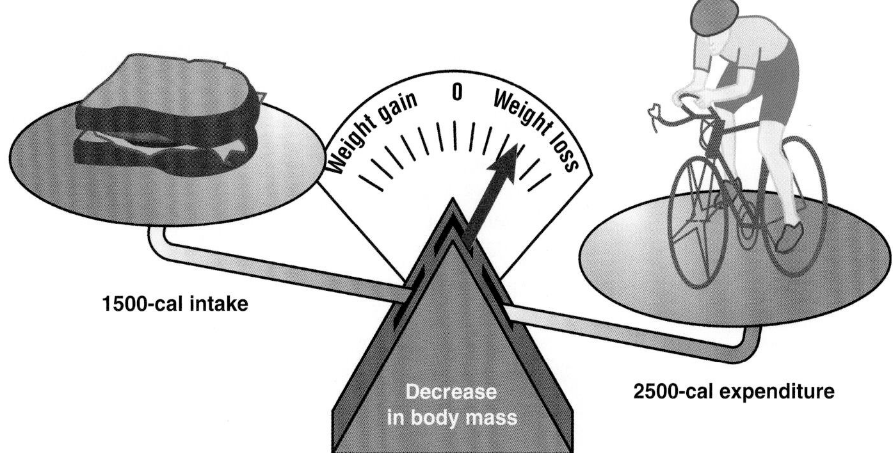

Figure 8.3 ▶
A negative energy balance: Calorie intake is less than calorie expenditure.

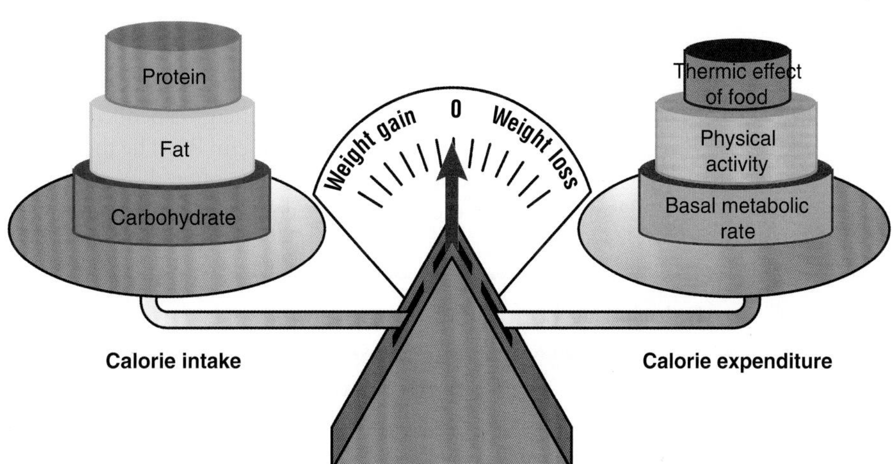

Figure 8.4 ▶
Sources of calorie intake and calorie expenditure.

- Another drawback is that food composition databases used to assign nutrient and calorie values to food represent *average* analysis of a number of food samples, not the actual specific food consumed.

Estimating Calories

An imprecise but easy way to estimate calorie intake is to use a food group approach, such as the Food Lists for Weight Management (American Diabetes Association & Academy of Nutrition and Dietetics, 2019).

- Each food group is assigned average calorie content for a specified serving size (Table 8.1).
- After counting servings consumed from each food group, the approximate total calories can be calculated.
- Separate lists exist for combination foods such as casseroles, sandwiches, and fast foods that do not fit into a single food group.
- Counting actual portion sizes (e.g., the amount eaten), not just serving sizes (generally the amount recommended), is vital for accuracy. For instance, 6 almonds are considered a serving, not ¼ c that may be listed on the Nutrition Facts label.

The drawback of counting calories by any method is that appropriate calories are only one aspect of a healthy eating pattern and nutritional adequacy is not guaranteed. For instance, an individual can consume the appropriate number of calories, but if the calories come from burgers and fries rather than from fruit, vegetables, and whole grains, the eating pattern is not healthy, even though it is calorie appropriate.

BOX 8.1 Calculating the Calories in Food

A double fast-food burger provides 49 g carbohydrate, 67 g protein, and 75 g fat.

49 g CHO × 4 cal/g = 196 cal
67 g pro × 4 cal/g = 268 cal
75 g fat × 9 cal/g = 675 cal
Total calories = 1139 cal

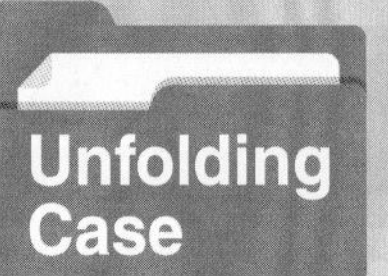

Recall Kyla and Garrett. A food record would help identify the types, amounts, and pattern of food they eat so that a strategy to improve intake can be formulated. What other factors need to be assessed before recommending changes to their intake?

Energy Expenditure

Calories are also the unit by which energy expended by the body is measured. The body uses energy for involuntary activities and purposeful PA. The thermic effect of food is another category of energy expenditure, although in practice it is often disregarded. The total of these expenditures represents an estimate of the number of calories a person expends in a day (Fig. 8.4).

Table 8.1 Calories by Food Lists

Food Group	Representative Serving Size	Average Calories per Serving
Starch (breads, grains, cereals, starchy vegetables, dried peas, and beans)	1 oz bread	80
Fruits	1 small fresh fruit, ½ cup canned or frozen fruit	60
Milk	1 cup	
Fat-free, low-fat, 1%		100
Reduced fat, 2%		120
Whole		160
Non-starchy vegetables	½ cup cooked or 1 cup raw	25
Protein foods	1 oz	
Plant-based protein		Varies
Lean		45
Medium fat		75
High fat		100
Fat/oils	1 tsp butter or margarine	45
Sweets, desserts	Varies	Varies
For example:		
Number of Servings Consumed	**Calories per Serving**	**Calories Consumed per Food Group**
6 grains	80	480
4 fruit	60	240
5 vegetables	25	125
2½ cup nonfat milk	80	200
6 oz medium-fat protein	75	450
3 tsp oils	45	135
	Total calories per day	1630

Basal Metabolism

Basal Energy Expenditure (BEE) or Basal Metabolic Rate (BMR) the number of calories expended in a 24-hour period to fuel the involuntary activities of the body at rest and after a 12-hour fast.

Resting Metabolic Rate (RMR) or Resting Energy Expenditure (REE) the number of calories expended in a 24-hour period to fuel the involuntary activities of the body at rest. RMR does not adhere to the criterion of a 12-hour fast, so it is slightly higher than BEE because it includes energy spent on digesting, absorbing, and metabolizing food.

Basal energy expenditure (BEE) or basal metabolic rate (BMR) is the number of calories required to fuel the involuntary activities of the body at rest after a 12-hour fast.

- Involuntary body activities include maintaining body temperature and muscle tone, producing and releasing secretions, propelling the gastrointestinal tract, inflating the lungs, and beating the heart.
- For most American adults, BEE accounts for 60% to 70% or more of total calories expended. The less active a person is, the greater is the proportion of calories used for BEE.
- The term *BEE* is often used interchangeably with **resting metabolic rate (RMR) or resting energy expenditure (REE)**, even though they are slightly different measures.
- Online tools are available to calculate BEE (e.g., https://www.omnicalculator.com/health/BEE).
- BEE can also be manually calculated using any number of formulas, such as the Mifflin-St Jeor equation (Box 8.2).
- A drawback of using predictive formulas based on weight is that they do not account for other variables that affect BEE, such as body composition (Table 8.2).

Physical Activity

Physical activity (PA), or voluntary muscular activity, generally accounts for approximately 30% of total calories used, although it may be as low as 20% in sedentary people and as high as 50% in people who are very active.

- The actual amount of energy expended on PA depends on the intensity and duration of the activity and the weight of the person performing the activity. The more intense and longer the activity, the greater the number of calories burned.

BOX 8.2 Estimating Total Calorie Requirements: Basal Energy Expenditure + Calories for Physical Activity

1. Estimate BEE with the Mifflin-St Jeor formula (simplified equation)

   Men: BEE = 10 × weight (kg) + 6.25 × height (cm) – 5 × age (years) + 5
   Women: BEE = 10 × weight (kg) + 6.25 × height (cm) – 5 × age (years) – 161

2. Multiply BEE by the appropriate factor for usual intensity of activity to determine total calories needed.

   Sedentary (little or no exercise): BEE × 1.2
   Lightly active (light exercise/sports 1–3 days/week): BEE × 1.375
   Moderately active (moderate exercise/sports 3–5 days/week): BEE × 1.55
   Very active (hard exercise/sports 6–7 days/week): BEE × 1.725
   Extra active (very hard exercise/sports and physical job): BEE × 1.9

Example: A 25-year-old sedentary woman is 5 ft 5 in. tall (165 cm) and weighs 142 pounds (65 kg).

1. Use Mifflin-St Jeor formula for women to calculate BEE.
   Women: BEE = 10 × weight (kg) + 6.25 × height (cm) – 5 × age (years) – 161

   (10 × 65) + (6.25 × 165) – (5 × 25) – 161
   650 + 1031 – 125 – 161
   BEE = 1395 cal

2. Multiply by BEE activity factor to determine total calorie requirements

   Total calorie requirements for sedentary activity: BEE × 1.2
   1395 × 1.2
   Total calorie requirements = 1674 cal

Table 8.2 Factors That Affect Basal Energy Expenditure

Variables	Effect on Metabolism
Age	Loss of lean body mass with age lowers BEE.
Growth	The formation of new tissue, as seen in children and during pregnancy, increases BEE.
Stresses	Stresses, such as infection and many diseases, raise BEE.
Thyroid hormones: tetraiodothyronine (thyroxine, or T_4) and triiodothyronine (T_3)	An oversecretion of thyroid hormones (hyperthyroidism) speeds up BEE; undersecretion of thyroid hormones (hypothyroidism) lowers BEE. The change may be as great as 50%.
Fever	BEE increases 7% for each degree Fahrenheit above 98.6.
Height	When considering two people of the same gender who weigh the same, the taller one has a higher BEE than the shorter one because of a larger surface area.
Extreme environmental temperatures	Very hot and very cold environmental temperatures increase the BEE because the body expends more energy to regulate its own temperature.
Starvation, fasting, and malnutrition	Part of the decline in BEE that occurs with these conditions is attributed to the loss of lean body tissue. Hormonal changes may contribute to the decrease in metabolic rate.
Weight loss from calorie deficits	With smaller body mass, less energy is required to fuel metabolism.
Smoking	Nicotine increases BEE.
Caffeine	Caffeine increases BEE.
Certain drugs, such as barbiturates, narcotics, and muscle relaxants	Decrease BEE.
Sleep, paralysis	Decrease BEE.

- Heavier people who have more weight to move use more energy than lighter people to perform the same activity.
- A rule-of-thumb method for estimating daily calories expended on PA is to calculate the percentage increase above BEE on the basis of estimated intensity of usual daily activities (Box 8.2).
- Wearable fitness tracking devices and smart watches can record fitness-related metrics using algorithms and sensors, such as temperature sensors and optical sensors. Trackers measure motion, which is then converted into steps and activity; from there, calories and sleep quality are estimated. Apps present the data after more fine-tuning with algorithms. Due to differences in sensors and algorithms, reported statistics vary among individual devices even when the same data are used. Tracking devices provide an estimate, not an actual reading.

Thermic Effect of Food

The **thermic effect of food** represents the calories spent on processing food.

Thermic Effect of Food an estimation of the amount of energy required to digest, absorb, transport, metabolize, and store nutrients.

- In a normal mixed diet, the thermal effect of food is estimated to be about 10% of the total calorie intake. For instance, people who consume 1800 cal/day use about 180 calories to process their food.
- The actual number of calories spent varies with the composition of food eaten, the frequency of eating, and the size of meals consumed.
- Although it represents an actual and legitimate use of calories, the thermic effect of food in practice is often disregarded when calorie requirements are estimated because it constitutes such a small amount of energy and is imprecisely estimated.

ESTIMATING TOTAL CALORIE REQUIREMENTS

Total calorie needs can be imprecisely estimated by using predictive equations, of which more than 200 have been published. The following are different approaches for estimating calorie needs; all yield estimates, not precise measurements.

- Use BEE and activity factor to estimate total calories (Box 8.2).
- Use a simple formula based on kilogram of body weight. For nonobese adults, a standard of 25 to 30 cal/kg is often used.
- Use a standard reference that lists estimated daily calorie needs based on gender, age, and activity (Table 8.3).

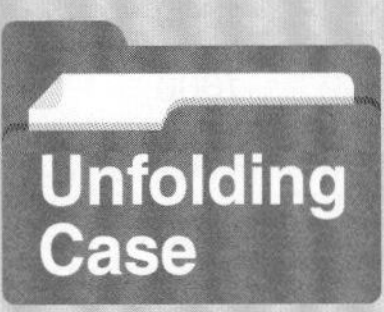

Think of Kyla and Garrett. They want to lose weight, and they also want to eat healthy. Often, people forget about health and just concentrate on calories and weight. Although their estimated calories as sedentary 25-year-olds are 2000 calories for Kyla and 2400 calories for Garrett, they do not want to count calories or measure serving sizes. What strategies can they use to eat a healthy, calorie-appropriate eating pattern that will promote weight loss without actually counting calories?

Table 8.3 **Estimated Calorie Needs per Day by Age, Sex, and Physical Activity Level, Ages 2 and Older**

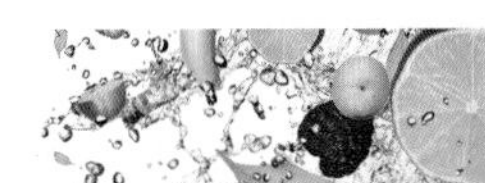

	Male			Female[a]		
	Activity Level[b]					
	Sedentary	Moderately Active	Active	Sedentary	Moderately Active	Active
Age (years)						
2	1000	1000	1000	1000	1000	1000
3	1200	1400	1400	1000	1200	1400
4	1200	1400	1600	1200	1400	1400
5	1200	1400	1600	1200	1400	1600
6	1400	1600	1800	1200	1400	1600
7	1400	1600	1800	1200	1600	1800
8	1400	1600	2000	1400	1600	1800
9	1600	1800	2000	1400	1600	1800
10	1600	1800	2200	1400	1800	2000
11	1800	2000	2200	1600	1800	2000
12	1800	2200	2400	1600	2000	2200
13	2000	2200	2600	1600	2000	2200
14	2000	2400	2800	1800	2000	2400
15	2200	2600	3000	1800	2000	2400
16	2400	2800	3200	1800	2000	2400
17	2400	2800	3200	1800	2000	2400
18	2400	2800	3200	1800	2000	2400
19–20	2600	2800	3000	2000	2200	2400
21–25	2400	2800	3000	2000	2200	2400

(continued)

Table 8.3 **Estimated Calorie Needs per Day by Age, Sex, and Physical Activity Level, Ages 2 and Older (continued)**

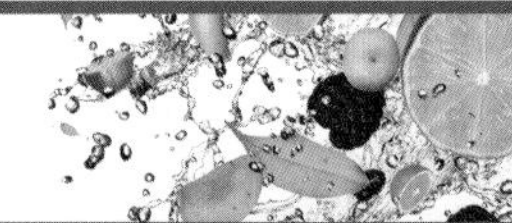

	Male			Female[a]		
	Activity Level[b]					
	Sedentary	Moderately Active	Active	Sedentary	Moderately Active	Active
26–30	2400	2600	3000	1800	2000	2400
31–35	2400	2600	3000	1800	2000	2200
36–40	2400	2600	2800	1800	2000	2200
41–45	2200	2600	2800	1800	2000	2200
46–50	2200	2400	2800	1800	2000	2200
51–55	2200	2400	2800	1600	1800	2200
56–60	2200	2400	2600	1600	1800	2200
61–65	2000	2400	2600	1600	1800	2000
66–70	2000	2200	2600	1600	1800	2000
71–75	2000	2200	2600	1600	1800	2000
76+	2000	2200	2400	1600	1800	2000

[a]Estimates for females do not include women who are pregnant or breastfeeding.
[b]*Sedentary* means a lifestyle that includes only the physical activity of independent living. *Moderately active* means a lifestyle that includes physical activity equivalent to walking about 1.5 to 3 miles per day at 3 to 4 miles per hour, in addition to the activities of independent living. *Active* means a lifestyle that includes physical activity equivalent to walking more than 3 miles per day at 3 to 4 miles per hour, in addition to the activities of independent living.
Source: Institute of Medicine. (2002). *Dietary reference intakes for energy, carbohydrate, fiber, fat, fatty acids, cholesterol, protein, and amino acids*. The National Academies Press; U.S. Department of Agriculture & U.S. Department of Health and Human Services. (2020). *Dietary guidelines for Americans, 2020–2025*. https://www.dietaryguidelines.gov

EVALUATING WEIGHT STATUS

From a health perspective, healthy or desirable weight is that which is statistically correlated to good health. But the relationship between body weight and good health is more complicated than simply the number on the scale. For instance, although increased body weight is a risk factor for type 2 diabetes, the actual risk is more accurately related to the quantity and distribution of body fat (Després, 2012). However, methods to accurately assess quantity of body fat and its distribution are not readily available or cost effective (Hsu et al., 2015). Body mass index (BMI), waist circumference, and waist-to-height ratio (WHR) may be used to identify risk for obesity and obesity-related comorbidities.

Body Mass Index

Ideal Body Weight
the formula given here is a universally used standard in clinical practice to quickly estimate a person's reasonable weight based on height and sex, even though this and all other methods are not absolute.

Historically, a quick and easy method of calculating **ideal body weight** and evaluating weight for height is the Hamwi method (Table 8.4). However, since the early 1980s, weight status has been assessed by BMI.

- BMI is calculated by dividing weight in kilograms by height in meters squared (kg/m^2).
- Nomograms and tables that plot height and weight to determine BMI eliminate complicated mathematical calculations (Table 8.5).
- Established cutoffs identify overweight as a BMI ≥25 and obese as a BMI ≥30, which are based on the rationale that adults with a BMI ≥25 have increased risks for both morbidity and mortality (National Heart, Lung, and Blood Institute Obesity Task Force, 1998). Those risks include coronary heart disease, hypertension, hypercholesterolemia, type 2 diabetes, and other diseases.

Table 8.4 Evaluating Weight

Standard	Calculation	Interpretation
Percentage of "ideal" body weight as determined by the Hamwi method.	Hamwi method calculation for ideal body weight Women: Allow 100 pounds for the first 5 ft of height; add 5 pounds for each additional inch. Men: Allow 106 pounds for the first 5 ft of height; add 6 pounds for each additional inch.	• ≤69% severe malnutrition • 70%–79% moderate malnutrition • 80%–89% mild malnutrition • 90%–110% within normal range • 110%–119% overweight • ≥120% obese • ≥200% morbidly obese
Body mass index	For men and women: weight in kg ÷ height in meters squared	• ≤18.5, may ↑ health risk • 18.5–24.9, healthy weight • 25–29.9, overweight • 30–34.9, obesity class 1 • 35–39.9, obesity class 2 • ≥40, obesity class 3

Controversy Surrounding Body Mass Index

Despite its widespread use as a screening tool, BMI is not without controversy.

- The BMI levels that define overweight and obesity are somewhat arbitrary because the relationship between increasing weight and risk of disease is continuous.
- BMI does not take sex into account, nor body composition; a lean athlete may have well-developed muscle mass and little fat tissue, yet if their BMI is high, they would fall under the designation of overweight or obese. Conversely, a senior adult may have a normal BMI and be deemed "healthy" despite a low percentage of muscle mass masked by a high amount of body fat.
- BMI does not take body fat distribution into account.
- Health risks related to BMI occur at different cutoff points for certain populations. For instance, the American Diabetes Association recommends that testing for diabetes be considered for all Asian and Asian American adults who have a BMI ≥23 (Hsu et al., 2015).

Body Fat Distribution

Central Obesity
proportionally greater amount of fat in the upper body compared to the hips and lower extremities.

As far back as the 1940s, researchers noted that **central obesity** fat distribution, commonly referred to as an apple shape, posed greater health risks than when fat was deposited peripherally, or a pear shape (Fig. 8.5). Even after controlling for BMI, people who have a primarily upper-body fat distribution are at increased risk of type 2 diabetes, cardiovascular disease, cancer, and death (Sun et al., 2019; Zhang et al., 2008). Within the last few decades, it has been shown that health risks, predominately hypertension, cardiovascular disease, and type 2 diabetes, are more accurately determined by assessing the relative distribution of excess fat rather than by total fat amount (Després, 2012). Waist circumference and WHR are screening tools for identifying central obesity.

Waist Circumference

- The current waist circumference cutoff points in common use are >40 in. for men and >35 in. for women (National Institutes of Health, National Heart Lung and Blood Institute, 2000).
- The World Health Organization/International Diabetes Foundation uses the cutoff points of >37 in. in men and >31.5 in. in women (WHO, 2008).

Table 8.5 **Body Mass Index**

Body Mass Index	Normal						Overweight					Obese					
	19	20	21	22	23	24	25	26	27	28	29	30	31	32	33	34	35
Height (inches)	Body Weight (pounds)																
58	91	96	100	105	110	115	119	124	129	134	138	143	148	153	158	162	167
59	94	99	104	109	114	119	124	128	133	138	143	148	153	158	163	168	173
60	97	102	107	112	118	123	128	133	138	143	148	153	158	163	168	174	179
61	100	106	111	116	122	127	132	137	143	148	153	158	164	169	174	180	185
62	104	109	115	120	126	131	136	142	147	153	158	164	169	175	180	186	191
63	107	113	118	124	130	135	141	146	152	158	163	169	175	180	186	191	197
64	110	116	122	128	134	140	145	151	157	163	169	174	180	186	192	197	204
65	114	120	126	132	138	144	150	156	162	168	174	180	186	192	198	204	210
66	118	124	130	136	142	148	155	161	167	173	179	186	192	198	204	210	216
67	121	127	134	140	146	153	159	166	172	178	185	191	198	204	211	217	223
68	125	131	138	144	151	158	164	171	177	184	190	197	203	210	216	223	230
69	128	135	142	149	155	162	169	176	182	189	196	203	209	216	223	230	236
70	132	139	146	153	160	167	174	181	188	195	202	209	216	222	229	236	243
71	136	143	150	157	165	172	179	186	193	200	208	215	222	229	236	243	250
72	140	147	154	162	169	177	184	191	199	206	213	221	228	235	242	250	258
73	144	151	159	166	174	182	189	197	204	212	219	227	235	242	250	257	265
74	148	155	163	171	179	186	194	202	210	218	225	233	241	249	256	264	272
75	152	160	168	176	184	192	200	208	216	224	232	240	248	256	264	272	279
76	156	164	172	180	189	197	205	213	221	230	238	246	254	263	271	279	287

Source: Adapted from U.S. Department of Health and Human Services. (1998). *Clinical guidelines on the identification, evaluation, and treatment of overweight and obesity in adults: The evidence report.*

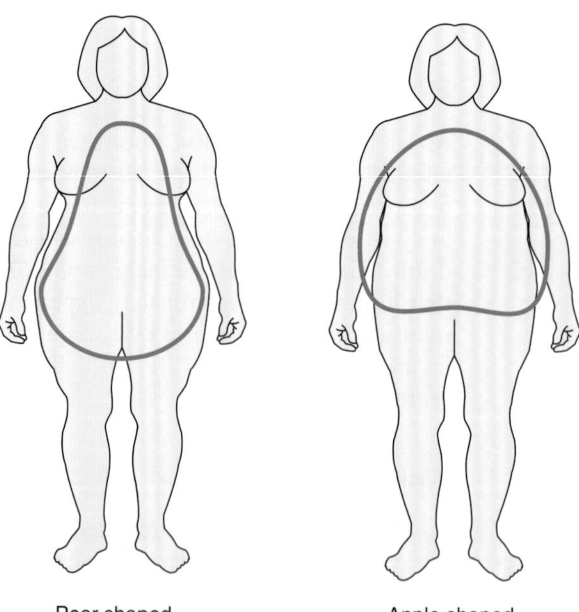

Figure 8.5 ▶
Pear shape versus apple shape.

Extreme Obesity																		
36	37	38	39	40	41	42	43	44	45	46	47	48	49	50	51	52	53	54
Body Weight (pounds)																		
172	177	181	186	191	196	201	205	210	215	220	224	229	234	239	244	248	253	258
178	183	188	193	198	203	208	212	217	222	227	232	237	242	247	252	257	262	267
184	189	194	199	204	209	215	220	225	230	235	240	245	250	255	261	266	271	276
190	195	201	206	211	217	222	227	232	238	243	248	254	259	264	269	275	280	285
196	202	207	213	218	224	229	235	240	246	251	256	262	267	273	278	284	289	295
203	208	214	220	225	231	237	242	248	254	259	265	270	278	282	287	293	299	304
209	215	221	227	232	238	244	250	256	262	267	273	279	285	291	296	302	308	314
216	222	228	234	240	246	252	258	264	270	276	282	288	294	300	306	312	318	324
223	229	235	241	247	253	260	266	272	278	284	291	297	303	309	315	322	328	334
230	236	242	249	255	261	268	274	280	287	293	299	306	312	319	325	331	338	344
236	243	249	256	262	269	276	282	289	295	302	308	315	322	328	335	341	348	354
243	250	257	263	270	277	284	291	297	304	311	318	324	331	338	345	351	358	365
250	257	264	271	278	285	292	299	306	313	320	327	334	341	348	355	362	369	376
257	265	272	279	286	293	301	308	315	322	329	338	343	351	358	365	372	379	386
265	272	279	287	294	302	309	316	324	331	338	346	353	361	368	375	383	390	397
272	280	288	295	302	310	318	325	333	340	348	355	363	371	378	386	393	401	408
280	287	295	303	311	319	326	334	342	350	358	365	373	381	389	396	404	412	420
287	295	303	311	319	327	335	343	351	359	367	375	383	391	399	407	415	423	431
295	304	312	320	328	336	344	353	361	369	377	385	394	402	410	418	426	435	443

- As with BMI, ethnic groups differ in regard to where risk begins in relation to waist circumference. For instance, thresholds for central obesity among people of South Asian, Japanese, and Chinese origin are 35.5 in. for men and 31.5 in. for women (Purnell, 2018).
- These cutoff points are somewhat arbitrary because the relationship between cardiovascular risk and waist circumference is continuous: the greater the waist circumference, the greater the risks.

Waist-to-Height Ratio

- Waist-to-height ratio (WHR) may be a better screening tool than both waist circumference and BMI for cardiometabolic risk factors such as hypertension, diabetes, dyslipidemia, metabolic syndrome, and cardiovascular disease (Ashwell et al., 2012).
- WHR is a simple, easy, and practical tool that can identify "early health risk" (Ashwell & Gibson, 2014).
- WHR is calculated by dividing waist measurement by height measurement. The suggested cutoff value of 0.5 translates to the practical advice of "keep your waist to less than half your height," which the authors suggest can be cheaply and easily determined by a single piece of string (Ashwell et al., 2012).
- This boundary value of 0.5 has been used around the world, and findings in many populations support the premise that WHR is an effective index to identify health risks. It also has a clearer relationship with mortality than BMI (Ashwell & Gibson, 2016).

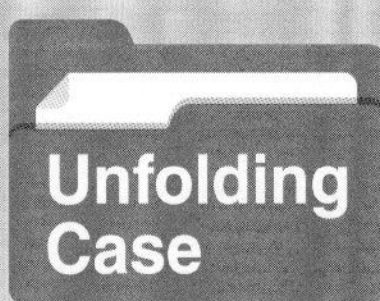

Recall Kyla and Garrett. Kyla is 5 ft 5 in. tall, currently weighs 150 pounds, and has a waist size of 31 in. Garrett is 6 ft tall, currently weighs 210 pounds, and has a waist size of 36 in. Evaluate their BMI, waist circumference, and WHR.

ENERGY BALANCE IN HEALTH PROMOTION

Guidelines put forth by public health agencies consistently urge Americans to attain and maintain a healthy body weight. Factors involved in achieving that goal are to consume the appropriate number of calories, be physically active, and reduce sitting time.

Consume Appropriate Calories

An "appropriate" calorie level is one in which the individual is able to attain and maintain a healthy weight. Table 8.3 can be used as a reference to choose a reasonable calorie level based on age, sex, and activity; the appropriateness of the calorie level is determined by monitoring body weight over time.

- After the appropriate calorie level is determined, it can be translated into daily servings per food group using a healthy eating pattern, such as the Healthy U.S.-Style Eating Pattern, Healthy Mediterranean-Style Eating Pattern, or Healthy Vegetarian Eating Pattern, described in Chapter 2. Another option is the DASH diet (Chapter 7).
- Choosing appropriate serving sizes is vital to ensuring the appropriate calorie intake. Table 8.6 illustrates how portion sizes have grown over the last 20 years. Even over-consumption of healthy food can lead to a positive calorie balance and weight gain over time.
- Changing the environment that promotes large portion sizes may help people "right size" portions (Box 8.3).

Beyond Calories: Diet Quality

Although the appropriate calorie intake is important for weight, a healthy eating pattern must also provide adequate amounts of all essential nutrients while limiting foods or nutrients linked to an increased risk of chronic disease.

- A simple strategy to achieve a balanced mix of foods is to use the MyPlate depiction of filling ½ the plate with fruits and vegetables, approximately ¼ with grains, and ¼ with protein with a choice of dairy on the side.

BOX 8.3 Strategies to Promote Portion Control

Focus on efforts to make food less accessible and less visible.

- Switch to smaller plates, bowls, and glasses.
- Buy smaller packages of food at the grocery store; forgo the jumbo size.
- Buy prepackaged, portion-controlled items, such as 100 calorie packs.
- Store food out of sight.
- Order smaller portions at restaurants.
- Fill a doggie bag before beginning to eat.

Table 8.6 Portion Distortion: A Comparison between Portion Sizes 20 Years Ago and Today

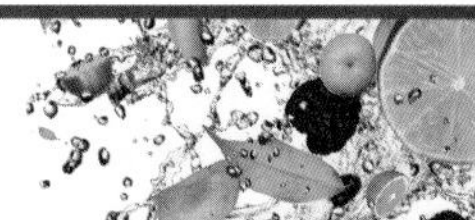

	20 Years Ago	Today
Bagel	3 in. diameter 140 calories	6 in. diameter 350 calories
Pepperoni pizza	1–2 slices 500 calories	2 slices 850 calories
Chocolate chip cookies	1.5 in. diameter 55 calories	3.5 in. diameter 275 calories
Coffee	8 oz with whole milk and sugar 45 calories	16 oz with whole milk and mocha syrup 350 calories
French fries	2.4 oz 210 calories	6.9 oz 610 calories
Soda	6.5 oz 85 calories	20 oz 250 calories
Spaghetti with meatballs	1 cup pasta with sauce and 3 meatballs 500 calories	2 cups pasta with sauce and 3 large meatballs 1025 calories
Popcorn	5 cups 270 calories	11 cups 630 calories

Source: U.S. Department of Health and Human Services, National Heart Lung and Blood Institute, National Institutes of Health. (2015). *Portion distortion*. http://www.nhlbi.nih.gov/health/educational/wecan/eat-right/portion-distortion.htm

- Growing evidence suggests that overall nutrient composition is important in determining overeating and weight gain (Stinson et al., 2018). Eating a relatively larger percentage of foods high in fat (≥45% calories from fat) and high in simple sugars (≥30% of calories) appears to promote overeating and weight gain.
- Higher intake of ultra-processed food has also been associated with excess weight, and the association is more pronounced in women (Juul et al., 2018).
    - Foods that qualify as ultra-processed include "junk food" (sugar-sweetened beverages, potato chips, candy), commercial baked goods, commercial breads, canned soups, flavored yogurt, and low-calorie frozen dinners.
    - Although these foods may contribute essential nutrients, they tend to be high in saturated fat, added sugar, and sodium and are considered poor in nutrition quality.
    - "Fat-free" or "sugar-free" versions of ultra-processed foods do not make them "healthier," nor do they necessarily lower their calorie content.
- Conversely, substituting healthier alternatives for calorie-dense foods within all food groups can help ensure nutrient needs are met without exceeding calorie limits (Box 8.4).
- Plant-based diets may help reduce the risk of chronic diseases, such as cardiovascular disease, certain types of cancer, and diabetes.

Be Physically Active

Physical activity is one of the most important actions people of all ages can do to improve their health, yet 80% of American adults are not meeting the key guidelines for both aerobic and muscle-strengthening activity (Box 8.5) (U.S. Department of Health and Human Services [USDHHS], 2018). An estimated 10% of premature mortality is linked to lack of physical activity.

BOX 8.4 Healthier Alternatives

Here are some foods that contain extra calories from solid fats and/or added sugars and some healthier alternatives. Choices on the right side are more nutrient dense—lower in solid fats and added sugars. Try these new ideas instead of your usual choices. This guide gives sample ideas; it is not a complete list. Use the "Nutrition Facts" label to help identify more alternatives.

More Calorically Dense Foods	Healthier Alternatives
Milk Group	
Sweetened fruit yogurt	Plain fat-free yogurt with fresh fruit or vanilla flavoring
Whole milk	Low-fat or fat-free milk
Natural or processed cheese	Low-fat or reduced-fat cheese
Protein Foods	
Beef (corned beef, prime cuts of beef, short ribs, 85% lean or lower ground beef)	Beef round steaks and roasts (eye of round, top round), top sirloin, top loin, 90% lean or higher ground beef
Chicken legs with skin	Chicken breast without skin
Lunch meats (such as bologna)	Low-fat lunch meats (95%–97% fat free)
Hot dogs (regular)	Hot dogs (lower fat)
Bacon or sausage	Canadian bacon or lean ham
Refried beans	Cooked or canned kidney or pinto beans
Grain Group	
Granola	Reduced-fat granola
Sweetened cereals	Unsweetened cereals with cut-up fruit
Pasta with cheese sauce	Pasta with vegetables (primavera)
Pasta with white sauce (alfredo)	Pasta with red sauce (marinara)
Croissants or pastries	Toast or bread (try whole-grain types)
Fruit Group	
Apple or berry pie	Fresh apple or berries
Sweetened applesauce	Unsweetened applesauce
Canned fruit packed in syrup	Canned fruit packed in juice or "lite" syrup
Vegetable Group	
Deep-fried french fries	Oven-baked french fries
Baked potato with cheese sauce	Baked potato with salsa
Fried vegetables	Steamed or roasted vegetables
Solid Fats	
Cream cheese	Light or fat-free cream cheese
Sour cream	Plain low-fat or fat-free yogurt
Regular margarine or butter	Light-spread margarines, diet margarine
Added Sugars	
Sugar-sweetened soft drinks	Seltzer mixed with 100% fruit juice
Sweetened tea or drinks	Unsweetened tea or water
Syrup on pancakes or french toast	Unsweetened applesauce or berries as a topping
Candy, cookies, cake, or pastry	Fresh or dried fruit
Sugar in recipes	Experiment with reducing amount and adding spices (cinnamon, nutmeg, etc.)

BOX 8.5 Key Physical Activity Guidelines for Adults

Adults should move more and sit less throughout the day. Some physical activity is better than none. Adults who sit less and do any amount of moderate to vigorous physical activity gain some health benefits.

For substantial health benefits, adults should do at least 150 minutes (2 hours and 30 minutes) to 300 minutes (5 hours) a week of moderate-intensity aerobic physical activity or 75 minutes (1 hour and 15 minutes) to 150 minutes (2 hours and 30 minutes) a week of vigorous-intensity aerobic physical activity or an equivalent combination of moderate- and vigorous-intensity aerobic activity. Preferably, aerobic activity should be spread throughout the week.

Additional health benefits are gained by engaging in physical activity beyond the equivalent of 300 minutes (5 hours) of moderate-intensity physical activity a week.

Adults should also do muscle-strengthening activities of moderate or greater intensity and those that involve all major muscle groups on 2 or more days a week, as these activities provide additional health benefits.

Source: U.S. Department of Health and Human Services. (2018). *Physical activity guidelines for Americans*. https://health.gov/paguidelines/default.aspx

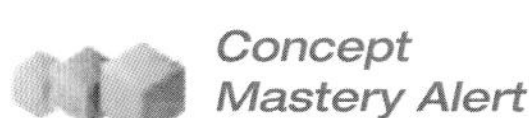

Although exercise should be spread across the week if possible, muscle-strengthening activities for recently ill clients who need to increase their physical activity to prevent further deterioration should be undertaken at least twice a week.

The chronic disease prevention and health promotion benefits of regular physical activity are many (Box 8.6). Research shows the following benefits of physical activity:

- Regular moderate to vigorous physical activity reduces the risk of many adverse health outcomes.
- Some physical activity is better than none.
- For most health outcomes, additional benefits occur as the amount of physical activity increases through higher intensity, greater frequency, and/or longer duration. Tips for increasing activity appear in Box 8.7.
- Substantial health benefits for adults occur with 150 to 300 minutes a week of moderate-intensity physical activity, such as brisk walking. Additional benefits occur with more physical activity.
- Both aerobic and muscle-strengthening physical activity is beneficial.

BOX 8.6 Health Benefits Associated with Regular Physical Activity

Strong or moderate evidence shows that adults and older adults receive the following health benefits from regular physical activity:

- lower risk of all-cause mortality
- lower risk of cardiovascular disease mortality
- lower risk of cardiovascular disease (including heart disease and stroke)
- lower risk of hypertension
- lower risk of type 2 diabetes
- lower risk of adverse blood lipid profile
- lower risk of cancers of the bladder, breast, colon, endometrium, esophagus, kidney, lung, and stomach
- improved cognition
- reduced risk of dementia (including Alzheimer's disease)
- improved quality of life
- reduced anxiety
- reduced risk of depression
- improved sleep
- slowed or reduced weight gain
- weight loss, particularly when combined with reduced calorie intake
- prevention of weight regain following initial weight loss
- improved bone health
- improved physical function
- lower risk of falls (older adults)
- lower risk of fall-related injuries (older adults)

Source: U.S. Department of Health and Human Services. (2018). *Physical activity guidelines for Americans*. https://health.gov/paguidelines/default.aspx

BOX 8.7 Tips for Increasing Physical Activity

- **Find something enjoyable:** The best chance of success comes from choosing a physical activity that is enjoyable to the individual. The best activity or exercise is one that is performed, not just contemplated.
- **Use the buddy system:** Committing to an exercise program or increased physical activity with a friend makes the activity less of a chore and helps to sustain motivation.
- **Spread activity over the entire day if desired:** This recommendation is particularly important for people who "don't have time to exercise." Many people find it easier to fit three 10-minute activity periods into a busy lifestyle than to find 30 uninterrupted minutes to dedicate to activity.
- **Start slowly and gradually increase activity:** For people who have been inactive, it is prudent to start with only a few minutes of daily activity, such as walking, and gradually increase the frequency, duration, and then intensity. People with existing health problems such as diabetes, heart disease, and hypertension should consult a physician before beginning a program, as should all men older than 40 years and all women older than 50 years.
- **Move more:** Just moving more can make a cumulative difference in activity. Take the stairs instead of the elevator, park at the far end of the parking lot, mow the lawn with a push mower, do gardening, yardwork, walk around while talking on the phone, walk instead of driving short distances, play golf without a golf cart or caddy, or fidget.
- **Track it:** Just as people tend to underestimate the amount of food they eat, people usually overestimate the amount of physical activity they perform. Monitoring physical activity provides objective data for evaluating progress.

- Health benefits occur for children and adolescents, young and middle-aged adults, older adults, and those in every studied racial and ethnic group.
- The health benefits of physical activity occur for people with chronic conditions or disabilities.
- The benefits of physical activity generally outweigh the risk of adverse outcomes or injury.

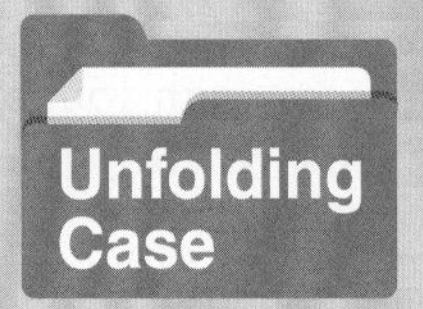

Think of Kyla and Garrett. They admit that they get hungry after doing cardio at the gym and may be sabotaging themselves by eating too much afterward. What would you suggest they consume after working out if they cannot wait until the next meal to eat?

Reduce Sitting Time

A relatively new area of research is the health effects of sedentary behavior. Although the 2018 Advisory Committee found a strong relationship between sedentary behavior time and the risk of all-cause mortality and cardiovascular disease mortality in adults, evidence has been insufficient to recommend a specific sedentary time target for adults or youth. This is because the risk from sedentary behavior is dependent upon the amount of moderate to vigorous physical activity performed.

Figure 8.6 illustrates the relationship between sedentary behavior, moderate to vigorous physical activity, and the risk of all-cause mortality.

- The risk of all-cause mortality improves from red (highest risk) → orange → yellow → green (lowest risk).
- The all-cause mortality risk is greater with the highest daily sitting time (red, upper left corner) but begins to improve (becomes orange) with only small amounts of moderate to vigorous physical activity. This suggests that sedentary adults can reduce their risk of all-cause mortality by replacing some sitting time with even light physical activity.
- At the greatest volume of moderate to vigorous physical activity, the risk is low even for people who sit the most (green, upper right corner).
- Even adults who sit the least (orange, lower left corner) are at increased risk if they do not perform any moderate to vigorous activity.
- Because Americans do not meet physical activity guidelines and have high levels of sitting time, most Americans would benefit from moving more and sitting less.

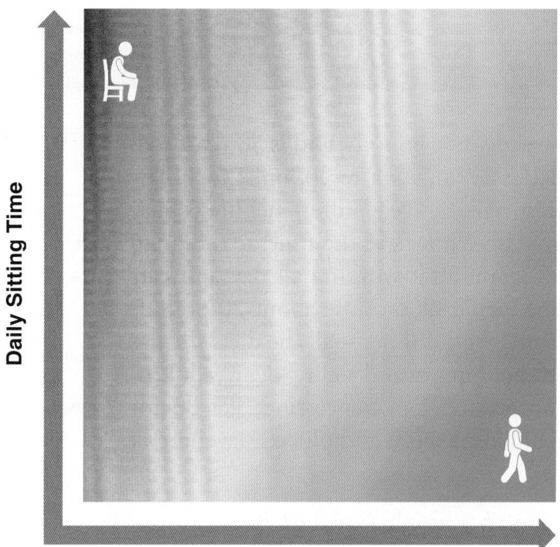

Figure 8.6 ▲ Relationship among moderate to vigorous physical activity, sitting time, and risk of all-cause mortality in adults. (*Source:* U.S. Department of Health and Human Services *Physical Activity Guidelines for Americans* from Ekelund, U., Steene-Johannessen, J., & Brown, W. J. [2016, September]. Does physical activity attenuate or even eliminate, the detrimental association of sitting time with mortality? A harmonized metaanalysis of data from more than 1 million men and women. *Lancet, 388*[10051], 1302–1310. https://doi.org/10.1016/S0140-6736(16)30370-1)

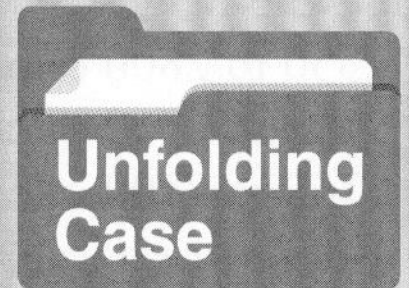

Consider Kyla and Garrett. In addition to the cardio exercise they are already doing, what other PA recommendations may be helpful? They have sedentary jobs. What suggestions would you make to help them become more active during the work day?

How Do You Respond?

Is eating breakfast helpful for losing weight? Although often extolled as "the most important meal of the day," there is increasing evidence that eating breakfast does not improve weight loss (St-Onge et al., 2017). In fact, recommending breakfast to adults to promote weight loss may have the opposite effect due to an increase in total daily calorie intake (Sievert et al., 2019). Although eating breakfast may not promote weight loss in adults, it should still be encouraged as part of an overall healthy lifestyle.

Is intermittent fasting a good way to lose weight? Intermittent fasting has been labeled "the next big weight loss fad" (Collier, 2013). *Intermittent fasting* is a broad term that includes many variations of taking a break from eating, such as fasting for up to 24 hours once or twice a week with ad lib food for the remaining days; eating only for 8 hours and then fasting for the other 16 hours of the day; and alternate-day fasting. There is evidence that both alternate-day fasting and periodic fasting may be effective for weight loss, although there are no data to indicate whether the weight loss can be sustained over the long term (St-Onge et al., 2017). A review of animal studies and recent clinical trials also suggests that intermittent fasting may have beneficial effects on cardiovascular biomarkers and may decrease inflammation and oxidative stress (Stockman et al., 2018). Intermittent fasting appears to be a viable weight loss method, though a continuous calorie-restricted diet may be as effective (Stockman et al., 2018). Further long-term human studies are needed using a consistent definition of intermittent fasting.

REVIEW CASE STUDY

Tonya is 5 ft 3 in. tall, weighs 151 pounds, and is 38 years old. Her waist circumference is 37 in. As a receptionist for a law firm and mother of two socially active children, her life is busy but sedentary. She simply does not have the time or energy to stay with an exercise program after working all day and caring for her children. She would like to lose about 20 pounds but knows "dieting" doesn't work for her—all the diets she has tried in the past have left her hungry and feeling deprived. Losing weight has taken on greater importance since her doctor told her that both her blood pressure and glucose level are at "borderline" high levels.

- What is her BMI? Assess her weight based on BMI.
- Estimate her total calorie requirements using the Mifflin-St Jeor method of calculating BEE and adding calories for a sedentary lifestyle. How does it compare to the level of calories recommended in Table 8.3 for a woman of her age and sedentary lifestyle?
- Which calorie level do you think is most accurate? Why?
- How many calories would she need to eat to lose 1 pound of weight per week if her activity level stays the same? Two pounds per week? Is a 2-pound weight loss per week a reasonable goal?
- To help her avoid feeling hungry while eating fewer calories, what foods would you recommend she consume more of? She knows she should drink fewer soft drinks. What advice would you give her to help her do that?

STUDY QUESTIONS

1 For most Americans, the largest percentage of their total calories expended daily is from
  a. Physical activity.
  b. thermal effect of food.
  c. basal energy expenditure.
  d. sitting.

2 A nurse knows that their instructions about portion control have been effective when the client verbalizes that they will
  a. prepare a doggie bag after they feel they are full enough while eating out.
  b. use a smaller dinner plate.
  c. be careful not to overfill their cereal bowl when they serve themselves from the large, family-sized box.
  d. remind themselves not to overeat.

3 A client asks how they can speed up their metabolism. Which of the following is the best response?
  a. "You can't. Metabolic rate is genetically determined."
  b. "Ask your doctor to check your thyroid hormone levels. Taking thyroid hormone will stimulate metabolism."
  c. "Include strength training in your exercise program because adding muscle tissue will increase metabolic rate."
  d. "Eat fewer calories because that will stimulate metabolic rate."

4 How much weight will a person lose in a week if they eat 500 fewer cal/day than they need and increase their exercise expenditure by 500 cal/day?
  a. 1 pound per week.
  b. 2 pounds per week.
  c. 3 pounds per week.
  d. There isn't enough information provided to estimate weekly weight loss.

5 Using a simple formula based on calories per kilogram of body weight, how many calories per day would a healthy-weight adult who weighs 70 kg need?
  a. 2350 to 2800 calories
  b. 2100 to 2350 calories
  c. 1750 to 2100 calories
  d. 1400 to 1750 calories

6 Waist circumference is an indicator of
  a. percentage of body fat.
  b. central obesity.
  c. the ratio of body fat to muscle mass.
  d. BMI.

7 Which of the following substitutions results in a less calorically dense choice?
  a. Canadian bacon in place of bacon
  b. refried beans instead of cooked or canned pinto beans
  c. natural cheese instead of low-fat cheese
  d. baked potato with cheese sauce instead of baked potato with salsa

8 A BMI of 26 is classified as
  a. normal
  b. overweight
  c. class 1 obesity
  d. class 2 obesity

CHAPTER SUMMARY ENERGY BALANCE

Calories are derived from the metabolism of carbohydrates, protein, fat, and alcohol. Calories are expended to fuel basal metabolic functions, physical activity, and digesting, absorbing, and metabolizing food.

State of Energy Balance

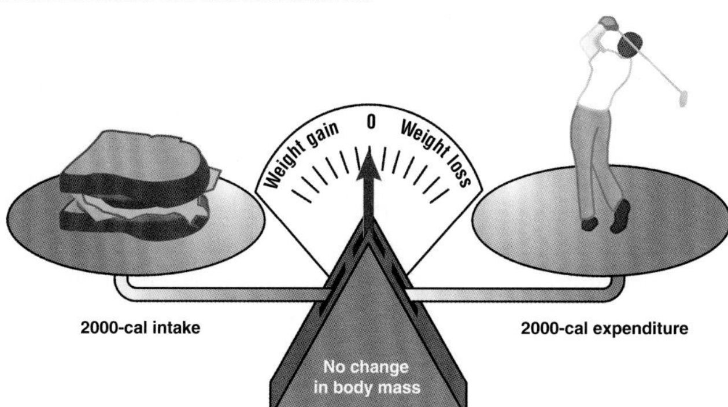

The relationship between calorie intake and calorie expenditure determines energy balance.

- A neutral balance occurs when calorie intake and expenditure are approximately equal. Body weight stays stable.
- A positive balance occurs when calorie intake exceeds expenditure. Over time, body weight increases.
- A negative balance occurs when calorie intake is less than expenditure. Over time, weight loss occurs.

Estimating Total Calorie Requirements

Ways to estimate total calorie requirement include

- using a predictive equation based on gender, height, weight, age, and activity level, such as the Mifflin-St Jeor formula,
- using a standard of 25 to 30 cal/kg for healthy adults,
- referring to a list of estimated calorie needs based on age, gender, and activity level.

Evaluating Weight Status

Methods to evaluate body weight include the following:

- BMI, which uses height and weight, does not distinguish between genders, nor does it compensate for body composition (e.g., muscle mass) or body weight distribution.
- Waist circumference assesses fat distribution to identify central obesity, which increases the risk of cardiovascular disease, type 2 diabetes, and all-cause mortality.
- WHR divides waist circumference by height. Results >0.5 indicate central obesity risk. Simple advice is to "keep your waist to less than half your height."

Energy Balance in Health Promotion

Health is promoted when individuals consume the appropriate number of calories, are physically active, and limit sitting time.

Consume an appropriate number of calories.

- After the appropriate number of calories has been determined by any of the previously discussed methods, a heatlhy eating pattern can be used to determine the number of servings per food group recommended to meet nutrient needs without exceeding calorie limits.
- Some foods, such as foods high in added fat, high in added sugar, and ultra-processed foods, may promote weight gain more than wholesome foods that characterize a healthy plant-based eating pattern.
- Portion control is inherent in achieving the appropriate number of calories.
- Making food less visible and accessible may help control overeating.

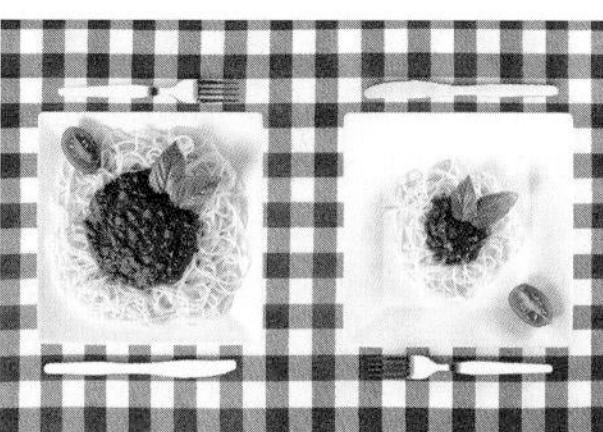

Be physically active.

- Any exercise is better than none.
- Generally, the more activity the better.
- Moderate to vigorous activity should occur on most days of the week.
- Health benefits from physical activity are physical, emotional, and even cognitive.
- Strength training twice a week is recommended.

Sit less.

- There is a strong relationship between sedentary behavior time and the risk of all-cause mortality and cardiovascular disease mortality in adults.
- The risk from sedentary behavior is dependent upon the amount of moderate to vigorous physical activity performed.
- The all-cause mortality risk is greatest with the highest daily sitting time in combination with the least moderate-to-vigorous physical activity.
- Sedentary adults can reduce their risk of all-cause mortality by replacing some sitting time with even light physical activity.

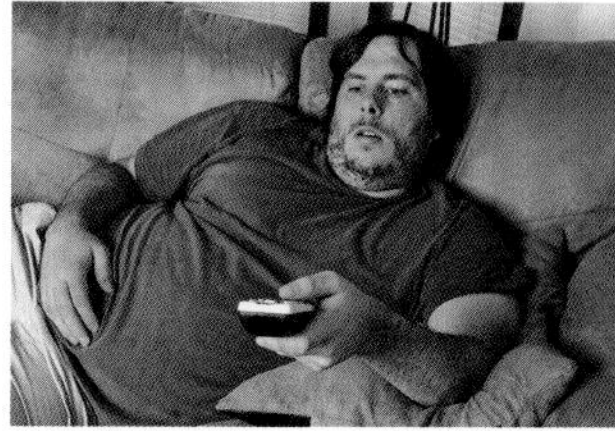

Figure sources: *shutterstock.com/Jose Luis Stephens and shutterstock.com/txking*

Student Resources on thePoint®
For additional learning materials, activate the code in the front of this book at https://thePoint.lww.com/activate

Websites

American College of Sports Medicine at www.acsm.org

Calculate your own calories at https://www.mayoclinic.org/healthy-lifestyle/weight-loss/in-depth/calorie-calculator/itt-20402304

National Institute of Diabetes and Digestive and Kidney Diseases, Weight-Control Information Network at https://www.niddk.nih.gov/health-information/health-communication-programs/win/Pages/community-groups-organizations.aspx

Physical Activity Guidelines for Americans at https://health.gov/paguidelines/default.aspx

President's Council on Physical Fitness and Sports at www.fitness.gov

References

American Diabetes Association & Academy of Nutrition and Dietetics. (2019). *Choose your foods: Food lists for weight management*. American Diabetes Association.

Ashwell, M., & Gibson, S. (2014). A proposal for a primary screening tool: "Keep your waist circumference to less than half your height." *BMC Medicine, 12*(207). https://doi.org/10.1186/s12916-014-0207-1

Ashwell, M., & Gibson, S. (2016). Waist-to-height ratio as an indicator of "early health risk": Simpler and more predictive than using a "matrix" based on BMI and waist circumference. *BMJ Open, 6*, e010159. https://doi.org/10.1136/bmjopen-2015-010159

Ashwell, M., Gunn, P., & Gibson, S. (2012). Waist-to-height ratio is a better screening tool than waist circumference and BMI for adult cardiometabolic risk factors: Systematic review and meta-analysis. *Obesity Reviews, 13*(3), 275–286. https://doi.org/10.1111/j.1467-789X.2011.00952.x

Collier, R. (2013). Intermittent fasting: The science of going without. *Canadian Medical Association Journal, 185*(9), E363–E364. https://doi.org/10.1503/cmaj.109-4451

Després, J. (2012). Body fat distribution and risk of cardiovascular disease: An update. *Circulation, 126*(10), 1301–1313. https://doi.org/10.1161/CIRCULATIONAHA.111.067264

Hsu, W., Araneta, M., Kanaya, A., Chiang, J., & Fujimoto, W. (2015). BMI cut points to identify at-risk Asian Americans for type 2 diabetes screening. *Diabetes Care, 38*(1), 150–158. https://doi.org/10.2337/dc14-2391

Juul, F., Martinez-Steele, E., Parekh, N., Monteiro, C. A., & Chang, V. W. (2018). Ultra-processed food consumption and excess weight among US adults. *British Journal of Nutrition, 120*(1), 90–100. https://doi.org/10.1017/S0007114518001046

National Heart, Lung, and Blood Institute Obesity Task Force. (1998). Clinical guidelines on the identification, evaluation, and treatment of overweight and obesity in adults—The evidence report. *Obesity Research, 6*(Suppl. 2), 51S–209S.

National Institutes of Health, National Heart Lung and Blood Institute. (2000). The practical guide identification, evaluation, and treatment of overweight and obesity in adults. NIH Publication Number 00-4084. https://www.nhlbi.nih.gov/files/docs/guidelines/prctgd_c.pdf#page=19

Purnell, J. (2018). Definitions, classification, and epidemiology of obesity. [Updated April 12, 2018]. In K. R. Feingold, B. Anawalt, A. Boyce, et al. (Eds.), *Endotext* [Internet]. MDText.com, Inc.; 2000-. https://www.ncbi.nlm.nih.gov/books/NBK279167/

Sievert, K., Hussain, S. M., Page, M. J., Wang, Y., Hughes, H. J., Malek, M., & Cicuttini, F. M. (2019). Effect of breakfast on weight and energy intake: Systematic review and meta-analysis of randomised controlled trials. *British Medical Journal, 364*, 142. https://doi.org/10.1136/bmj.l42

Stinson, E. J., Piaggi, P., Ibrahim, M., Venti, C., Krakoff, J., & Votruba, S. B. (2018). High fat and sugar consumption during ad libitum intake predicts weight gain. *Obesity, 26*(4), 689–695. https://doi.org/10.1002/oby.22124

Stockman, M.-C., Thomas, D., Burke, J., & Apovian, C. (2018). Intermittent fasting: Is the wait worth the weight? *Current Obesity Reports, 7*, 172–185. https://doi.org/10.1007/s13679-018-0308-9

St-Onge, M.-P., Ard, J., Baskin, M., Chiuve, S., Johnson, H., Kris-Etherton, P., & Varady, K., & on behalf of the American Heart Association Obesity Committee of the Council on Lifestyle and Cardiometabolic Health; Council on Cardiovascular Disease in the Young; Council on Clinical Cardiology; and Stroke Council. (2017). Meal timing and frequency: Implications for cardiovascular disease prevention—A scientific statement from the American Heart Association. *Circulation, 135*(9), e96–e121. https://doi.org/10.1161/CIR.0000000000000476

Sun, Y., Liu, B., Snetselaar, L. G., Wallace, R. B., Caan, B. J., Rohan, T. E., Neuhouser, M. L., Shadyab, A. H., Chlebowski, R. T., Manson, J. E., & Bao, W. (2019). Association of normal-weight central obesity with all-cause and cause-specific mortality among postmenopausal women. *The Journal of the American Medical Association Network Open, 2*(7), e197337. https://doi.org/10.1001/jamanetworkopen.2019.7337

U.S. Department of Health and Human Services. (2018). *Physical activity guidelines for Americans*. https://health.gov/sites/default/files/2019-09/Physical_Activity_Guidelines_2nd_edition.pdf

World Health Organization. (2008). *Waist circumference and waist-hip ratio: Report of a WHO expert consultation*. https://apps.who.int/iris/bitstream/handle/10665/44583/9789241501491_eng.pdf?sequence=1

Zhang, C., Rxrode, K. M., van Dam, R. M., Li, T. Y., & Hu, F. B. (2008). Abdominal obesity and the risk of all-cause cardiovascular, and cancer mortality. Sixteen years of follow-up in US Women. *Circulation, 117*(13), 1658–1667. https://doi.org/10.1161/CIRCULATIONAHA.107.739714

UNIT TWO

Nutrition in Health Promotion

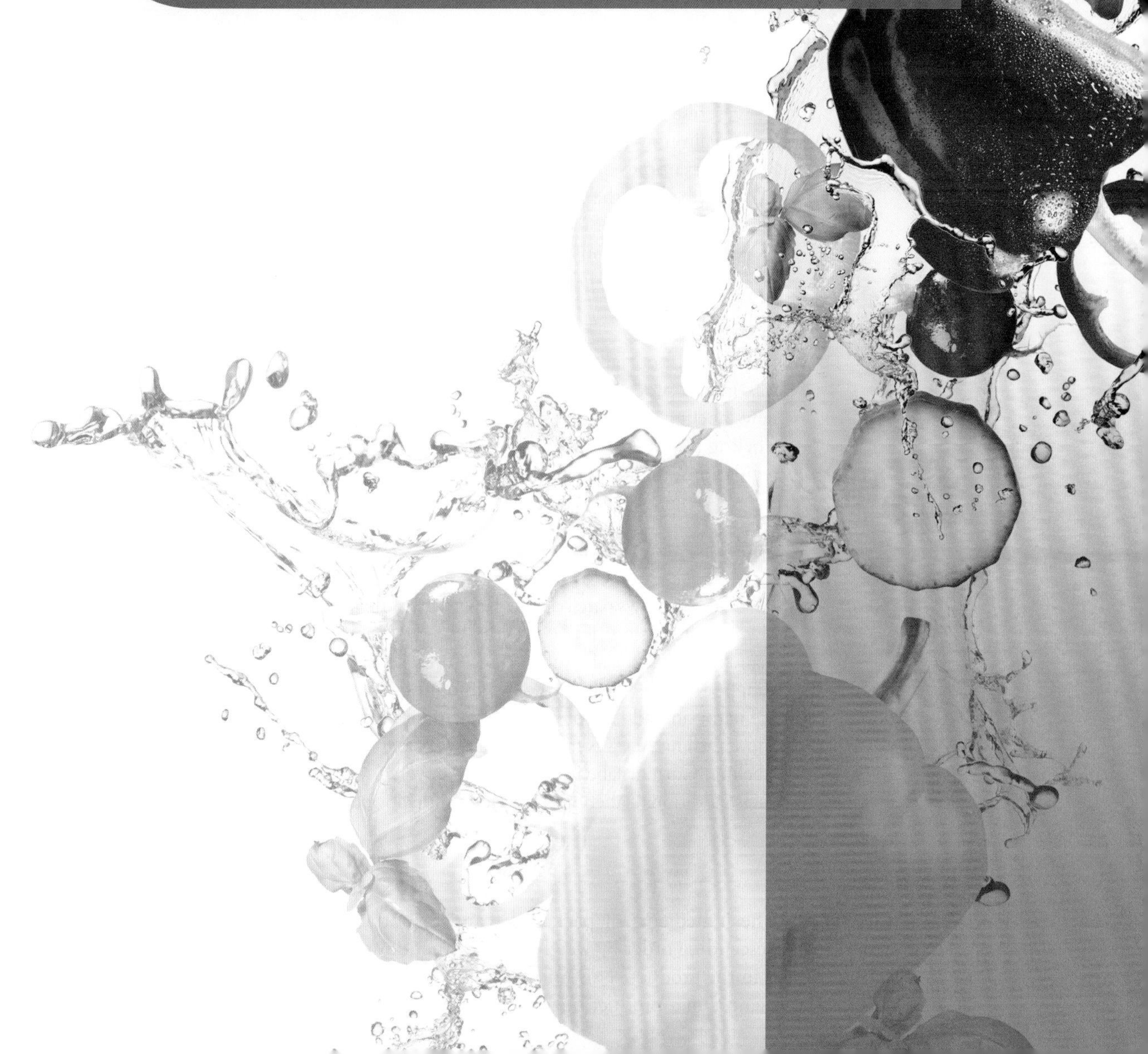

Chapter 9

Food and Supplement Labeling

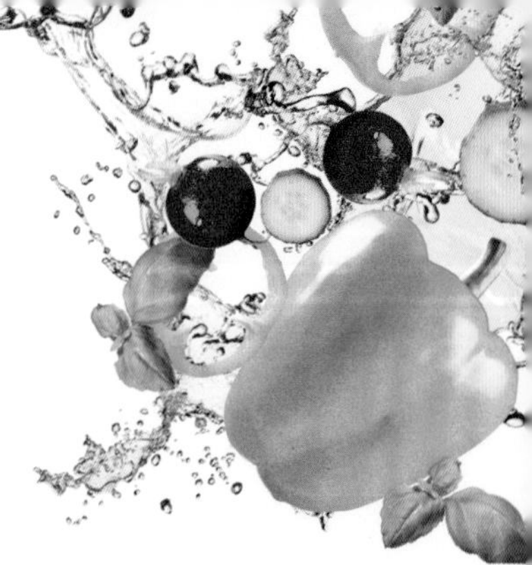

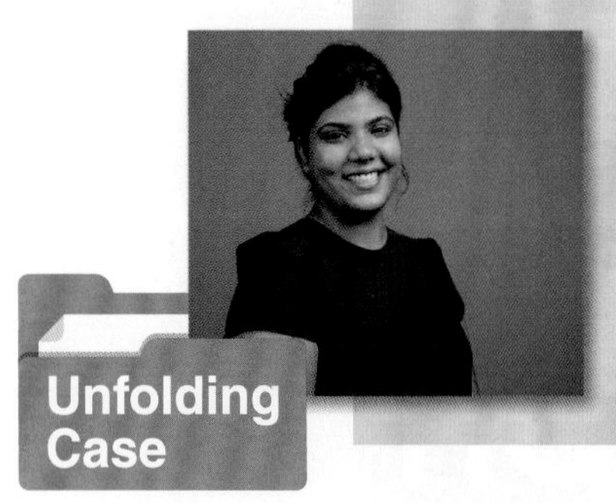

Unfolding Case

Rebecca McNally

Rebecca McNally is recently graduated from college. As an undergraduate, she gained 25 pounds, which she attributes to fast food, irregular eating patterns, convenience foods, snacking, and alcohol. Now that she is living in her own apartment, Rebecca wants to get her weight under control and eat healthier so she has more energy.

Learning Objectives

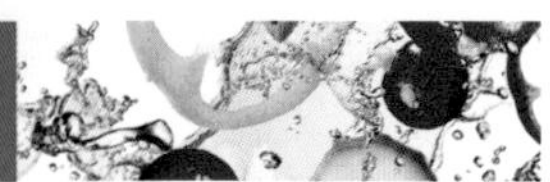

Upon completion of this chapter, you will be able to:

1 Describe requirements for listing ingredients on the label.
2 Explain how the Nutrition Facts label can help consumers make better food choices.
3 Give examples of an unqualified health claim and a qualified health claim.
4 Describe how the regulation and marketing of dietary supplements differ from regulation and marketing of drugs.
5 Suggest precautions supplement users should take to limit the potential for adverse effects.
6 Discuss the use of cannabidiol.

Interest in food labeling began in the 1960s, when consumers became concerned about what was in the processed foods they were eating (Brown, 2019). The government responded with new labeling regulations, which have evolved over time to the labels we have today. Nutrition labeling is a tool consumers can use to choose a healthy diet. This chapter presents food labeling regulations, dietary supplement regulations, and the growing popularity of cannabidiol (CBD).

FOOD LABELING

Food labeling laws date back to 1967, when the Fair Packaging and Labeling Act directed the Federal Trade Commission (FTC) and the U.S. Food and Drug Administration (FDA) to issue regulations mandating that specific information be included on the food label: the name and form (e.g., sliced or chopped) of the product; the net amount of the food or beverage by weight, measure, or count; and the name and address of the manufacturer, packer, or distributor. The purpose of the Fair Packaging and Labelling Act was to enable value comparisons and to prevent unfair or deceptive packaging and labeling. Current labeling regulations covered in the next section include ingredient lists, Nutrition Facts, additional labeling regulations and allowed claims, and industry-originated labeling.

Ingredient List

The ingredients of packaged (canned, bottled, boxed, and wrapped) foods must be listed in descending order by weight. The further down the list an item appears, the less of that ingredient is in the product. This information gives the consumer a relative idea of how much of each ingredient is in a product but not the proportion. Ingredients present in amounts of ≤2% by weight can be listed after a quantifying statement such as "contains 2% or less of . . ."; however, this 2% rule does not remove the requirement that ingredients be declared regardless of their level.

Nutrition Facts

In the spring of 2016, the FDA published final rules on an updated Nutrition Facts panel that reflects new scientific information, including the link between diet and chronic disease such as obesity and heart disease (U.S. Food and Drug Administration [FDA], 2020a). Most foods were required to bear the new label by January 1, 2020. Smaller food manufacturers have until January 1, 2021, to comply. Manufacturers of single ingredient sugars (e.g., honey, maple syrup) have until July 1, 2021, to make the changes. Figure 9.1 features the updated Nutrition Facts label. Changes are summarized in the following section.

Percent Daily Value (%DV) amount of nutrients to consume, or not exceed, which is used on both food and dietary supplement labels. The %DV refers to the percentage of the nutrient in one serving of food based on the daily goal in a 2000-calorie diet.

Daily Values (DVs) reference values established by the FDA for use on food labels. For some nutrients (e.g., sodium), they are amounts that should not be exceeded; for others (e.g., fiber), they are amounts to strive toward. For nutrient intakes that are based on the percentage of calories consumed, 2000 calories is the standard used.

Greater Understanding of Nutrition Science

The Nutrition Facts label reflects what is currently known about nutrition and health. Added sugars are included in both grams and as the **percent daily value (%DV)**, based on the guideline that the daily intake of calories from added sugars not exceed 10% of total calories consumed. Added sugars were previously not included.

- The **Daily Values (DVs)** for sodium, dietary fiber, and vitamin D are based on newer scientific evidence.
- The micronutrients required in both gram amount and %DV are vitamin D, calcium, iron, and potassium. Potassium and vitamin D are new to the label because they are nutrients of public health significance. Vitamin A and C content are no longer required because deficiencies of these nutrients in the general population are not common.
- "Calories from fat" is eliminated based on evidence that the type of fat consumed is more important than total fat intake.

Updated Serving Sizes

Changes to the label reflect how people currently eat and drink.

- Serving sizes must be based on amounts of foods and beverages that people are actually eating, not what they should be eating or the previous serving size requirements published

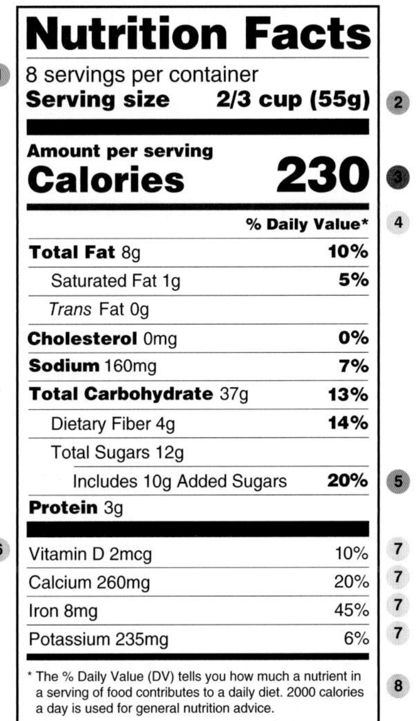
Nutrition Facts
1 8 servings per container
Serving size 2/3 cup (55g) 2

Amount per serving
Calories 230 3

	% Daily Value* 4
Total Fat 8g	**10%**
Saturated Fat 1g	**5%**
Trans Fat 0g	
Cholesterol 0mg	**0%**
Sodium 160mg	**7%**
Total Carbohydrate 37g	**13%**
Dietary Fiber 4g	**14%**
Total Sugars 12g	
Includes 10g Added Sugars	**20%** 5
Protein 3g	
6 Vitamin D 2mcg	10% 7
Calcium 260mg	20% 7
Iron 8mg	45% 7
Potassium 235mg	6% 7

* The % Daily Value (DV) tells you how much a nutrient in a serving of food contributes to a daily diet. 2000 calories a day is used for general nutrition advice. 8

Changes to the Nutrition Facts label:

1. Servings per container and the serving size in larger bold type
2. Serving sizes updated to reflect how much people typically eat at one time
3. Calories in larger bold type
4. % Daily Values updated
5. Added sugars included in grams and as a % Daily Value
6. Change in required vitamins and minerals reflects nutrients that, when deficient, are associated with risk of chronic disease:
   Vit D and potassium added
   Vit C and Vit A deleted
7. Actual amounts of nutrients declared, not just the % Daily Value
8. The footnote better explains the % Daily Value

Figure 9.1 ▶
The new nutrition facts label and key changes to nutrition facts. (*Source:* U.S. Food and Drug Administration. [2020a, July 10]. *Changes to the nutrition facts label.* https://www.fda.gov/food/food-labeling-nutrition/changes-nutrition-facts-label)

in 1993. For instance, the reference amount for a serving of soda is now 12 oz, not 8 oz, and the reference amount for a serving of ice cream has increased to 2/3 cup from ½ cup.

- Packaged foods and beverages that are typically consumed in one sitting are labeled as a single serving; therefore, calories and nutrient information listed are for the entire package. For instance, a 20-oz soft drink, typically consumed in one sitting, is labeled as one serving, not 2½ servings.
- A dual-column label is required on certain larger packages that could be consumed in either one or multiple sittings, such as a 24-oz bottle of soft drink or a pint of ice cream. One column is per serving and one per package.

Refreshed Design

The iconic look of the label was slightly changed to ensure consumers have access to information they need to make informed decisions. The font size is larger for calories, servings per container, and serving size.

- The number of calories and the serving size declaration are in bold type to emphasize their importance in public health concerns such as obesity, diabetes, and cardiovascular disease.
- The footnote more clearly explains the meaning of the %DV. It reads, "The % Daily Value tells you how much a nutrient in a serving of food contributes to a daily diet. Two thousand calories a day is used for general advice."

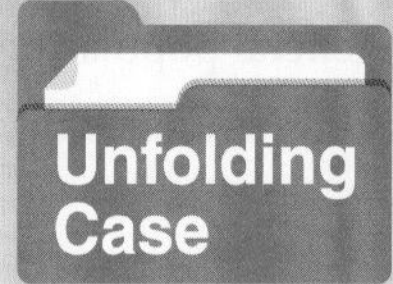

Recall Rebecca. She has begun to read labels now that she is doing her own grocery shopping and meal prep. What are the most important Nutrition Facts for her to focus on to make healthy choices?

Food Labeling Exemptions

Almost 90% of all packaged foods provide nutrition information. Some foods are exempt from labeling.

- raw foods: fresh fruits, vegetables, and fish
- foods containing insignificant amounts of nutrients, such as coffee, tea, and spices
- bulk food
- foods in packages with a surface area for labeling of <12 square inches, such as breath mints

Additional Label Declarations

Regulations regarding allergens, gluten-free products, and the country of origin have been enacted through various other labeling acts.

Allergens

Manufacturers are required to clearly state if a food product contains any ingredients that contain protein from the eight major food allergens listed in Box 9.1. These eight allergens are responsible for 90% of all food allergies.

Gluten-Free

Regulations require that a product must contain <20 ppm of gluten to be labeled as gluten-free. Products that are naturally gluten-free, such as tomatoes, may be labeled gluten-free. Although some consumers think the 20 ppm threshold is too high, the Celiac Disease Foundation supports 20 ppm as a suitable safety threshold (Celiac Disease Foundation, 2014).

BOX 9.1 Major Allergens That Must Be Declared on the Food Label

Milk
Eggs
Fish
Crustacean shellfish
Tree nuts
Peanuts
Wheat
Soybeans

Country of Origin

The USDA requires Country of Origin labeling on beef, lamb, pork, chicken, fish, shellfish, peanuts, fresh and frozen fruits and vegetables, pecans, macadamia nuts, and ginseng. Certain exemptions apply. Although Country of Origin does not provide information regarding food safety, it does enable consumers to make informed decisions about purchasing items from countries that may not regulate pesticides or antibiotic use as closely as the United States. Three categories are defined:

- U.S.-only origin
- foreign-only origin
- mixed origin (This category must be labeled with the country of birth, raising, and slaughter.)

Nutrient Content Claims label descriptions of the amount of a nutrient or substance provided in a food or beverage.

Health Claim a statement that describes a relationship between a food, food substance, or dietary supplement ingredient and a reduced risk of disease or a disease-related condition.

Structure/Function Claims statements identifying relationships between nutrients or dietary ingredients and a body function.

FDA-Allowed Claims

The FDA allows three types of claims on food and dietary supplement labels: **nutrient content claims**, **health claims**, and **structure/function claims**.

Nutrient Content Claims

Terms such as *low*, *free*, and *high* describe the level of a nutrient or substance in a food. The terms are legally defined, so they are reliable and valid. Nutrient claims may also compare the level of a nutrient to that of comparable food with terms such as *more*, *reduced*, or *light*. Box 9.2 defines the terms used in nutrient claims.

BOX 9.2 Definitions of Terms Used in Nutrient Claims

Free: the product contains virtually none of that nutrient. *Free* can refer to calories, sugar, sodium, salt, fat, saturated fat, and cholesterol.
Low: there is a small enough amount of a nutrient that the product can be used frequently without concern about exceeding dietary recommendations. Low sodium, low calorie, low fat, low saturated fat, and low cholesterol are all defined as to the amount allowed per serving. For instance, to be labeled low cholesterol, a product must have no more than 20 mg cholesterol per serving.
Very low: refers to sodium only. The product cannot have >35 mg sodium per serving.
Reduced or less: the product has at least a 25% reduction in a nutrient compared to the regular product.
Light or lite: the product has fewer calories than a comparable product or 50% of the fat found in a comparable product.
Good source: the product provides 10% to 19% of the DV for a nutrient.
High, rich in, or excellent source: the product has at least 20% of the DV for a nutrient.
More: the product has at least 10% more of a desirable nutrient than does a comparable product.
Lean: meat or poultry products with <10 g fat, <4 g saturated fat, and <95 mg cholesterol per standardized serving and per 100 g.
Extra lean: meat or poultry products with <5 g fat, <2 g saturated fat, and <95 mg cholesterol per standardized serving and per 100 g.

Health Claims

A health claim proposes a relationship between a food or substance in a food and a disease or health-related condition. There are two types of health claims, and they differ in the degree of scientific evidence that supports the claim.

Unqualified Health Claims

Unqualified Health Claim a type of health claim supported by significant scientific agreement.

Unqualified health claims, also known as *authorized health claims*, are supported by significant scientific agreement (SSA) among experts who have examined the evidence (Box 9.3).

- These claims are referred to as unqualified health claims because they do not require a disclaimer about the strength of evidence supporting the claim.
- Foods must contain enough of the nutrient to contribute at least 10% of the DV and must not contain any nutrient of substance that increases the risk of a disease or health condition (Brown, 2019). For instance, whole milk cannot make the claim regarding calcium and osteoporosis because its saturated fat content is high.

Qualified Health Claims

Qualified Health Claim a type of health claim that must be qualified by a statement that specifies the degree of scientific evidence that supports it. These claims are based on the weight of evidence but are not considered to be backed by significant scientific agreement.

The FDA allows certain **qualified health claims** when the relationship between food, a food component, or a supplement is not strong enough to meet SSA or published authoritative standards.

- The term *qualified* as it relates to health claims means that the claim is limited in some way.
- FDA-approved language allowed for these claims is very specific, and companies must petition the FDA for prior written permission to make a qualified health claim.
- The weakest claim is as follows: "Very limited and preliminary scientific research suggests [health claim]. The FDA concludes that there is little scientific evidence supporting this claim."
- Examples of qualified health claims are listed in Box 9.4.

BOX 9.3 Examples of Approved Unqualified Health Claims That Are Supported by Significant Scientific Agreement

Cancer Risk

- Dietary fat
- Fruits and vegetables
- Fiber-containing grain products

Coronary Heart Disease Risk

- Saturated fat and cholesterol
- Fruits, vegetables, and grain products that contain fiber, particularly soluble fiber
- Plant sterol/stanol esters
- Soluble fiber, such as that found in whole oats and psyllium seed husk
- Soy protein

Useful in Not Promoting Dental Caries

- Dietary noncariogenic carbohydrate sweeteners (e.g., sugar alcohols such as xylitol and sorbitol and the nonnutritive sweetener sucralose)

Hypertension Risk

- Sodium

Neural Tube Defect Risk

- Folate

Osteoporosis Risk

- Calcium
- Calcium and vitamin D

BOX 9.4 Examples of Qualified Health Claims

Cancer Risk

- Green tea
- Selenium
- Antioxidant vitamins
- Tomatoes and/or tomato sauce (prostate, ovarian, gastric, and pancreatic cancers)

Cardiovascular Disease Risk

- Nuts
- Walnuts
- Monounsaturated fatty acids from olive oil
- Omega-3 fatty acids
- B vitamins
- Unsaturated fatty acids from canola oil
- Corn oil

Hypertension Risk and Pregnancy-Induced Hypertension and Preeclampsia

- Calcium

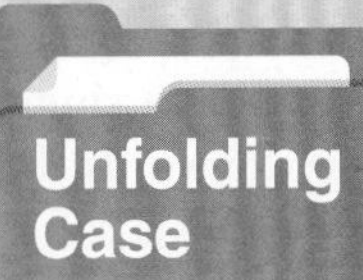

Remember Rebecca. She is unsure of the value of health claims she has seen on nuts. She's been avoiding them because they are high in calories, but Rebecca heard the claim that they may reduce the risk of heart disease. She's wondering if she should add them to her diet. What would you tell Rebecca?

Structure/Function Claims

Structure/function claims suggest the possibility that a food may improve or support body function, which is a fine distinction from the approved health claims that relate a food or nutrient to a disease.

- An example of a disease claim needing approval is "suppresses appetite to treat obesity," whereas a function claim that does not need approval is "suppresses appetite to aid weight loss."
- These structure claims had previously been used primarily by supplement manufacturers with the following disclaimer: "These statements have not been evaluated by the FDA. This product is not intended to diagnose, treat, cure, or prevent any disease."
- Structure/function claims are now appearing on food labels and do not require a disclaimer.
- Unlike health claims that can appear only on foods that meet other nutritional criteria (e.g., they cannot be high in fat, cholesterol, sodium), structure/function claims can appear on junk foods.
- Structure/function claims do not require FDA approval, so there may be no evidence to support the claim.
- See Box 9.5 for structure/function claims that do not need prior approval.

BOX 9.5 Structure/Function Claims That Do Not Need Approval

Improves memory
Improves strength
Improves digestion
Boosts stamina
For common symptoms of premenstrual syndrome
For hot flashes
Helps you relax
Helps enhance muscle tone or size
Relieves stress
Helps promote urinary tract health
Maintains intestinal flora
For hair loss associated with aging
Prevents wrinkles
For relief of muscle pain after exercise
To treat or prevent nocturnal leg muscle cramps
Helps maintain normal cholesterol levels
Provides relief of occasional constipation
Supports the immune system

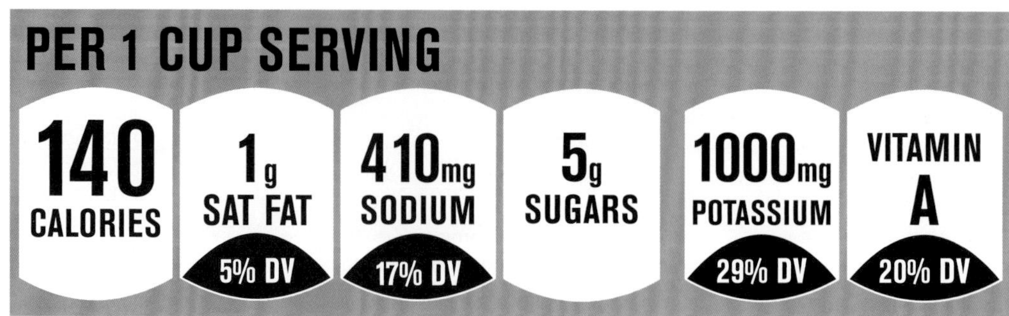

Figure 9.2 ▶ Facts Up Front.

Industry-Originated Labeling

Over the last decade, many food manufacturers and some health organizations have added a variety of nutrition symbols and rating systems to the front of food packages to show how nutritious they are. For instance, to guide consumers toward heart healthy choices, the American Heart Association Heart-Check utilizes a single symbol that features a red heart with a check mark in it and accompanied by the words *American Heart Association Certified.* The Whole Grain Council's Whole Grain Stamp is a front-of-package symbol used to indicate the presence of a food group or ingredient. Although intended to simplify choices for consumers, having too many types of front-of-package labels may actually increase confusion.

Facts Up Front

The Grocery Manufacturers Association and Food Marketing Institute created a voluntary front-of-package labeling initiative known as Facts Up Front.

- In a standardized format, four basic icons provide information from the Nutrition Facts panel on calories, saturated fat, sodium, and sugar. All four basic icons must appear.
- Up to two additional nutrients that have positive health benefits—namely, potassium, fiber, protein, vitamin A, vitamin C, vitamin D, calcium, and iron—may be added (Fig. 9.2). These additional nutrients can be placed on a package only when one serving provides 10% or more of the DV.
- Smaller packages may limit the icon to just calories.

DIETARY SUPPLEMENTS

As defined by law, a dietary supplement is a product other than tobacco that

- is intended to supplement the diet,
- contains one or more dietary ingredients, including vitamins, minerals, herbs or other botanicals, amino acids, and other substances or their constituents,
- is taken by mouth as a pill, capsule, tablet, or liquid, and
- must be labeled as a dietary supplement on the front panel (Fig. 9.3).

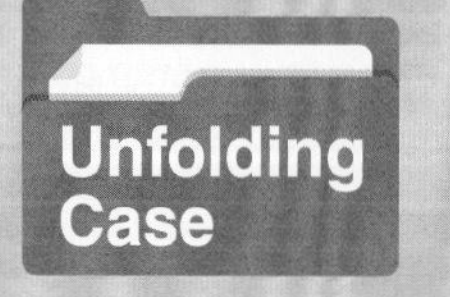

Think of Rebecca. She bought melatonin supplements because she read online that melatonin promotes sleep. What would you tell Rebecca about supplements in general?

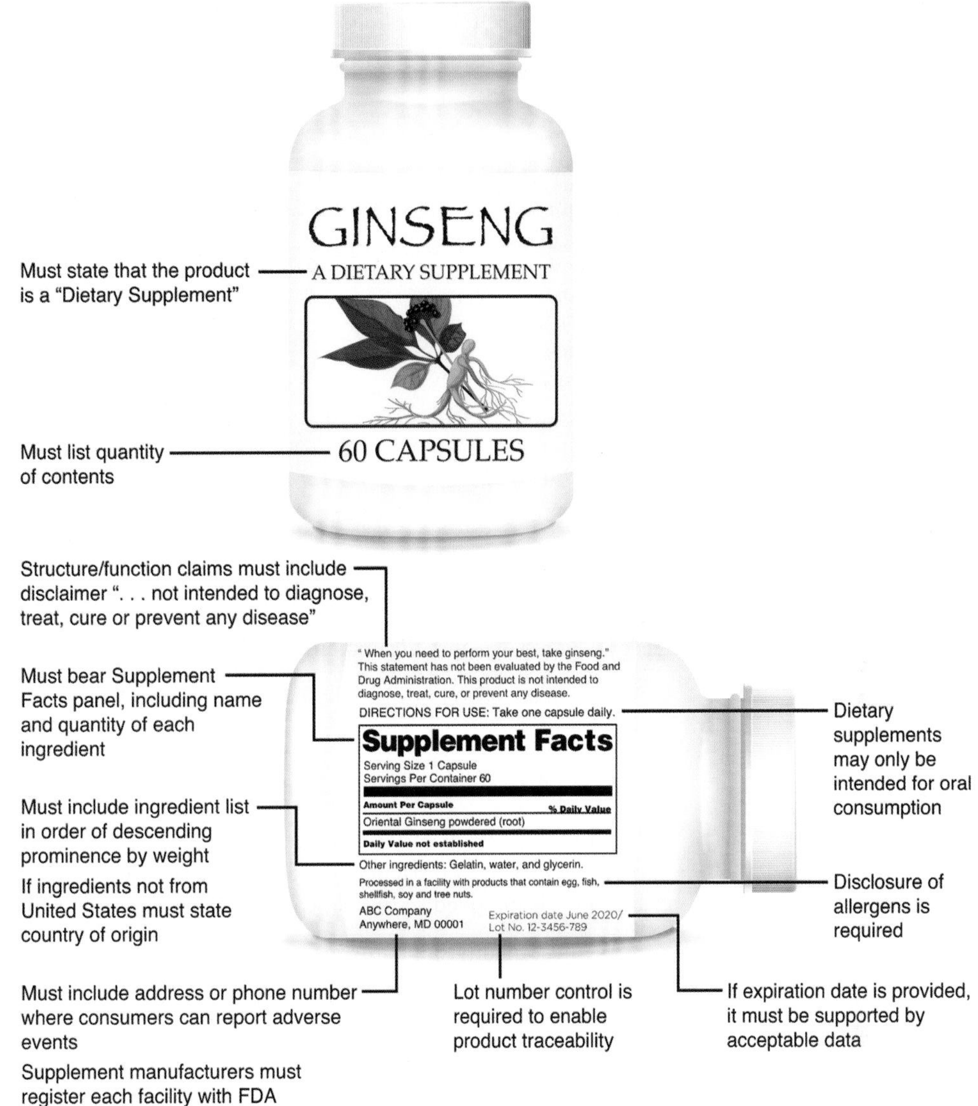
GINSENG
A DIETARY SUPPLEMENT
Must state that the product is a "Dietary Supplement"
60 CAPSULES
Must list quantity of contents
Structure/function claims must include disclaimer ". . . not intended to diagnose, treat, cure or prevent any disease"
" When you need to perform your best, take ginseng." This statement has not been evaluated by the Food and Drug Administration. This product is not intended to diagnose, treat, cure, or prevent any disease.
DIRECTIONS FOR USE: Take one capsule daily.
Supplement Facts
Serving Size 1 Capsule
Servings Per Container 60
Amount Per Capsule
% Daily Value
Oriental Ginseng powdered (root)
Daily Value not established
Other ingredients: Gelatin, water, and glycerin.
Processed in a facility with products that contain egg, fish, shellfish, soy and tree nuts.
ABC Company
Anywhere, MD 00001
Expiration date June 2020/
Lot No. 12-3456-789
Must bear Supplement Facts panel, including name and quantity of each ingredient
Must include ingredient list in order of descending prominence by weight
If ingredients not from United States must state country of origin
Dietary supplements may only be intended for oral consumption
Disclosure of allergens is required
Must include address or phone number where consumers can report adverse events
Supplement manufacturers must register each facility with FDA
Lot number control is required to enable product traceability
If expiration date is provided, it must be supported by acceptable data

Figure 9.3 ▶ Supplement label.
(*Source:* Council for Responsible Nutrition. [2017]. *Dietary supplement labeling.* https://www.crnusa.org/sites/default/files/pdfs/DS-RegsLabel-2017.pdf)

Supplement Popularity

In 2018, Americans spent $42.6 billion on dietary supplements (Reports and Data, 2019). Potential health benefits (Box 9.6), an aging population, increasing healthcare costs, and medical discoveries are among the factors fueling consumer interest in dietary supplements. Supplement use is widespread because they are readily accessible, are low in cost, appeal to people as natural cures, are presumed to be safe and effective, and allow consumers to take charge of their own health (Starr, 2015).

BOX 9.6 Top Reasons[a] Adults Cite for Taking Supplements

For overall health/wellness benefits: 30%
For energy: 24%
For immune health: 20%
To fill nutrient gaps: 19%
For heart health: 18%
For healthy aging: 18%

[a]*Reasons are not limited to one response per survey participant.*
Source: Council for Responsible Nutrition (CRN). (2019). *Who takes dietary supplements? And why?* 2019 CRN Consumer Survey on Dietary Supplements. https://www.crnusa.org/2019survey

BOX 9.7 The Top 10 Selling Herbal Dietary Supplements in U.S. Natural Channels

1. CBD
2. Turmeric
3. Elderberry
4. Wheatgrass/barley grass
5. Flax seed/flax oil
6. Aloe vera
7. Ashwagandha
8. Milk thistle
9. Echinacea
10. Oregano

Source: Smith, T., Gillespie, M., Eckl, V., & Reynolds, C. M. (2019). Herbal supplement sales in U.S. increase by 9.4% in 2018. *HerbalGram, Fall 2019*(123), 62–73. http://cms.herbalgram.org/herbalgram/issue.html?Issue=123

While vitamins account for the largest share of the supplement market, sales of herbs and botanicals continue to grow at the fastest pace among supplement categories and represent the second largest category of supplement sales (Nutrition Business Journal, 2019). The top 10 selling herbal dietary supplements in U.S. Natural Channels (e.g., natural and health food specialty retail outlets) are listed in Box 9.7.

Good Manufacturing Practices

The FDA requires dietary supplements to be produced using current good manufacturing practices. Identity, purity, strength, and composition are required to be accurately reflected on the label. This is intended to protect consumers by requiring supplements to

- meet quality standards for manufacturing processes,
- be free of contaminants or impurities such as natural toxins, bacteria, pesticides, glass, lead, or other substances,
- be manufactured to ensure identity, purity, and composition, and
- have an accurate listing of ingredients.

Supplement Regulations: Similarities with Food Labeling

By law, supplement labels share certain characteristics with food labels.

- The Supplement Facts panel is similar to the Nutrition Facts panel (Fig. 9.1).
- Nondietary ingredients such as fillers, artificial colors, sweeteners, flavors, or binders must be listed in descending order by weight.
- Health claims, nutrient content claims, or structure/function claims (as discussed under the FDA-allowed claims for food labeling in the previous section) are allowed.
- Supplements that make a structure/function claim must also include the disclaimer that reads, *This statement has not been evaluated by the FDA. This product is not intended to diagnose, treat, cure, or prevent any disease.*

User Beware: Herbs Are Like Unapproved Drugs

In their medicinal sense, herbs are technically unapproved drugs. Approximately 30% of drugs used today originated from plants (e.g., paclitaxel, aspirin, digoxin). In the United States, dietary supplements do not have to meet the same standards as drugs and over-the-counter medications. However, dietary supplements cannot claim to be used for the diagnosis, treatment, cure, or prevention of disease. Supplements differ greatly from conventional drugs in how they are marketed and regulated.

Herbal Supplements
supplements from plants or parts of plants used to alleviate health problems or promote wellness.

Concept Mastery Alert

Some **herbal supplements** (such as cranberry) have few or no drug–supplement interactions whereas others, such as ginseng, St. John's work, and ginkgo biloba, have significant interaction potential. Because herbal supplements may have significant interactions with each other or with prescribed medications, users should consult their healthcare provider before using.

New Dietary Ingredient
supplement ingredient not marketed in the United States before October 15, 1994.

Safety and Effectiveness Are Not Proven

Although the functions and requirements of vitamins and minerals are fairly well understood, scientific research is lacking for many herbal products. Many people mistakenly believe *natural* is synonymous with *safe*. They assume that herbs must be harmless because they come from flowers, leaves, and seeds. In truth, herbs are not guaranteed to be safe or effective.

- Before a drug can be marketed, the FDA must authorize its use based on the results of clinical studies performed to determine safety, effectiveness, possible interactions with other substances, and appropriate doses.
- In contrast, the regulations regarding dietary supplements are lax.
  - Ingredients sold in the United States before October 15, 1994, are assumed to be safe and so do not require FDA review for safety before they are marketed. The FDA is limited in regulating these supplements.
  - Dietary supplement manufacturers that want to market a **new dietary ingredient** must submit information to the FDA that supports their conclusion that *reasonable* evidence exists that the product is safe for human consumption.
  - Manufacturers do not have to *prove* to the FDA that dietary supplements are safe or effective; however, they are not supposed to market unsafe or ineffective products and are required to report all serious dietary supplement adverse events to the FDA.
  - Once a product is marketed, the responsibility lies with the FDA to take action against supplement manufacturers if one of their products is a significant or unreasonable risk of illness or injury when used as recommended; poses an imminent hazard to public health or safety; is a new ingredient for which there is inadequate safety information; or has been adulterated (Resnik, 2017). The burden of proof falls on the FDA to demonstrate that a product meets one of these conditions before taking action against a manufacturer.
  - When the FDA determines that a supplement is unsafe, it issues a consumer advisory discouraging its use.
  - One study estimated that at least 1 in 12 American adults take an herbal supplement known to cause kidney damage. Other supplements are known carcinogens, hepatotoxins, and hormone modulators (Starr, 2015).

Standardized
a manufacturing process that ensures product consistency from batch to batch.

Strength and Dosages Are Not Standardized

Dietary supplements are not required to be **standardized** in the United States. This means there is no safeguard to ensure batch-to-batch consistency in products.

- The concentration of active compounds in different batches of supposedly identical plant material can vary greatly.
- Factors that influence concentration include the variety of plant used, the part of the plant used (e.g., the stems or leaves), and the maturity of the plant at harvest.
- Supplements may theoretically be marketed in any concentration as long as the daily recommended value, if applicable, is specified on the label.
- Recommended dosages vary among manufacturers because there is no premarket testing to determine optimum dosage or maximum safe dosage.
- Other than manufacturer responsibility to ensure safety, there are no regulations that limit a serving size of any supplement.
- Many people believe that if a little is good, then more is better. They proceed to megadoses, which raises additional safety concerns (Starr, 2015).

Warnings Are Not Required

Unlike drugs, supplements are not required to carry warning labels about potential side effects, adverse effects, or supplement–drug interactions. Due to lack of extensive research, problems with supplements are not even known. There are also no advisories about who should not use the product.

Supplements Are Self-Prescribed

A major concern with self-medication is that consumers may misdiagnose their condition or forsake effective conventional medical care to treat themselves in a way that they regard as *natural.*

- Patients may not inform their physicians about their use of herbs, so side effects and herb–drug interactions go undiagnosed and unreported.
- The responsibility for determining whether a product has been recalled by the FDA rests with the user.
- Suggested precautions for supplement users are summarized in Box 9.8.

Cannabidiol

One relatively new product to the marketplace is CBD. Beginning in 2018, sales of CBD skyrocketed, making it the top selling product in the natural channel as well as the fastest growing ingredient (Smith et al., 2019). Currently, CBD may be found in hundreds of supplements, foods, and other products such as drinks, pet products, lotions, and chewable gummies. The marketplace for CBD products is growing faster than the science behind it and federal laws to regulate it (MacCleery, 2019).

CBD is the second most prevalent active ingredient in cannabis (marijuana), second only to tetrahydrocannabinol or THC. Although CBD is a component of medical marijuana, it is derived from the hemp plant. According to the World Health Organization, "In humans, CBD exhibits no effects indicative of any abuse or dependence potential. ... There is no evidence of public health related problems associated with the use of pure CBD" (World Health Organization [WHO], 2017; p.5). Unlike THC, CBD does not cause euphoria—or a *high*. However, it does change consciousness, promoting a mellow feeling, diminishing the sensation of pain, and increasing comfort (Harvard Health Publishing, 2019).

The strongest evidence for using CBD is its effectiveness in treating certain epilepsy syndromes that usually do not respond to antiseizure medications. The FDA has approved only one CBD product, the prescription drug Epidiolex, for treatment of two severe seizure disorders in children. There is moderate evidence that CBD can improve sleep disorders, fibromyalgia pain, muscle spasticity related to multiple sclerosis, and anxiety (Harvard Health Publishing, 2019).

The legal status of CBD is murky. The FDA has concluded that THC and CBD products do not meet the definition of dietary supplement because CBD is an active ingredient in an approved drug (Epidiolex). The FDA further states that it is "illegal to market CBD by adding it to a food or labeling it as a dietary supplement" (FDA, 2020b).

In the meantime, the FDA claims it is cracking down on companies that are using "egregious and unfounded claims" to market their products to "vulnerable populations" (Harvard Health Publishing, 2019). Because it is illegal to advertise that CBD-infused products can prevent, treat, or cure human disease without competent and reliable scientific evidence to support such claims,

BOX 9.8 Suggested Precautions for Supplement Users

Clients who choose to use supplements should

- evaluate the potential benefits compared to the potential risks using scientific evidence,
- recognize that *natural* does not necessarily mean *safe* and the terms *standardized*, *verified*, and *certified* do not guarantee quality or consistency,
- understand that if it sounds too good to be true, then it probably is,
- check with the FDA website for consumer advisories on supplements to avoid,
- discuss supplement use with the physician,
- be aware that some supplements have been found to be contaminated with prescription drugs or other compounds, especially supplements marketed for weight loss, sexual health, and athletic performance,
- take only single supplement products and keep the dose small to prevent and manage adverse side effects and supplement–drug interactions,
- take supplements at different times from prescribed medications to help reduce the potential for supplement–drug interactions,
- discontinue supplements immediately if adverse side effects or supplement–drug interactions occur, and
- avoid herbs and other botanical supplements if they are pregnant or lactating women or children under the age of 6 years.

the FTC has issued warning letters to companies that have advertised their CBD-infused products can treat or cure a variety of serious diseases and health conditions, including cancer, Alzheimer's disease, multiple sclerosis, fibromyalgia, colitis, autism, bipolar disorder, and traumatic brain injuries (Federal Trade Commission [FTC], 2019).

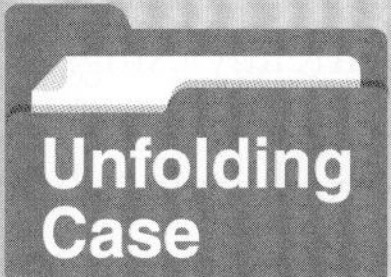

Think of Rebecca. She is not satisfied with the results of using melatonin. She is curious about whether CBD can improve her sleep issues. What would you tell her about using CBD?

The consumer watchdog organization Center for Science in the Public Interest (CSPI) has filed comments with the FDA asking the agency to play a more active role in ensuring these products are safe, accurately labeled, free of adulterants and contaminants, and that consumers are aware of relevant risks (MacCleery, 2019). CSPI urges the FDA to especially take action on products that pose the greatest public health risks such as products that appeal to children and youth and products found to be mislabeled or contaminated.

Caution is advised (Harvard Health Publishing, 2019):

- Buy only from a dispensary (if marijuana is legal in your state) because the amount of CBD in the product must be labeled as well as whether it contains any THC.
- Like other supplements, CBD products are not standardized, so the dosing may vary.
- The safest way to take CBD is orally via a tablet, chewable, or tincture.
- Although CBD appears to be safe, it can produce nausea, fatigue, and irritability and may interact with certain medications.
- Regular use is not appropriate for anyone under the age of 21.

How Do You Respond?

I need only 1600 calories a day. How can I make the Nutrition Facts label work for me when it is based on a 2000-calorie diet? Recognize that the %DV listed for total fat, saturated fat, total carbohydrate, dietary fiber, and added sugars—nutrients whose DV is based on calories—will *underreport* the percent contribution when daily intake is <2000 calories. For instance, Americans are urged to limit their intake of added sugars to 10% of total calories, which is 50 g/day in a 2000-calorie eating pattern, but only 40 g in a 1600-calorie pattern (1600 × 10% = 160 cal ÷ 4 cal/g = 40 g). A serving of fruited yogurt lists added sugars at 9 g with a DV of 18% (because labels are based on a 2000-calorie eating pattern) but in a 1600-calorie eating pattern, 9 g translates to 22.5% DV of added sugar (9 g ÷ 40 g × 100 = 22.5%). Use calorie-based %DV to get a relative idea of what a serving will contribute to your intake and compare %DV among brands if possible. Nutrients with a DV that are not based on calorie intake, such as cholesterol and sodium, will accurately reflect their percent contribution to all eating patterns regardless of the total calorie content.

Can a dietary supplement help me lose weight? The FDA does not regulate supplements for weight loss with the same standards applied do prescription or over-the-counter medications for weight loss. Manufacturers are responsible for ensuring their supplements are safe and that the labels are not misleading but supplements do not need to prove efficacy. Even if there was evidence of efficacy, if the composition and quality of ingredients cannot be reliably ensured, effectiveness may be altered (Starr, 2015). The FDA faces multiple challenges in enforcing existing regulations, so consumers are not well protected against supplements that are ineffective or potentially harmful.

REVIEW CASE STUDY

Maria is 52 years old, has a healthy body mass index, and does not have any health problems. She prides herself on her knowledge of holistic treatments and goes to the doctor only when her attempts to treat herself fail. She occasionally takes one aspirin a day because she has heard that it can prevent heart attacks. She tries to eat a healthy diet and uses supplements to give her added protection against chronic diseases, especially heart disease, which runs in her family. Currently, she takes turmeric, garlic, and fish oil supplements to keep her blood thin. She routinely drinks omega-3–fortified orange juice. She attributes the bruises on her legs to being clumsy. She is thinking about adding vitamin E to her regimen because she heard it may also lower the risk of heart disease by thinning the blood. She is thinking about discontinuing her use of garlic pills and fish oil supplements and eating more garlic and fish in her diet instead.

- What are the dangers of her present regimen? What may be responsible for the bruising she is experiencing?
- What would you tell Maria about the use of supplements in general? About the types and combination of supplements she is currently using? What specific changes would you suggest she make?
- What would you tell her about using juice fortified with omega-3?
- Is it safer for her to eat more garlic and fish instead of taking them as supplements? Is it as effective as taking them as supplements? Could she overdose on garlic and fish oil from food?
- What questions would you ask about her diet to see if there are any improvements in her eating habits she could make to reduce the risk of heart disease?

STUDY QUESTIONS

1 Which statement indicates that the client needs further instruction about reading nutrition labels?
   a. "The %DV is based on a 2000-calorie eating pattern."
   b. "The %DV represents the percentage of calories from carbohydrate, protein, and fat in that food."
   c. "The dual-column labels show information per serving and per package."
   d. "The serving size listed on the label is based on how much people actually consume, not on what they should be eating."

2 The nurse knows her instructions about label reading have been effective when the client verbalizes that fat-free on the label means
   a. the product is free of any ingredients that contain any fat.
   b. the product does not contain any fat or saturated fat.
   c. there is <0.5 g of fat in a serving.
   d. there is <1 g of fat in a serving.

3 The nurse knows her instructions about nutrient claims on the label have been effective when the client says,
   a. "'Excellent source' is not defined, so it cannot be trusted."
   b. "'Excellent source' means a serving of the food must provide at least 20% of the DV for that nutrient."
   c. "'Excellent source' means a serving of the food must provide a day's worth of that nutrient."
   d. "'Excellent source' means a serving of the food provides 10% more of a desirable nutrient than does a comparable product."

4 What is the component in allergens that is responsible for triggering an allergic attack in susceptible people?
   a. sugar
   b. starch
   c. protein
   d. fat

5 The nurse knows her instructions about gluten-free labeling are understood when the client verbalizes one of the following statements:
   a. "Only foods that have been specially made gluten-free, not foods that are naturally gluten-free, can be labeled gluten-free."
   b. "Gluten-free means there are no detectable amounts of gluten in the product."
   c. "Products labeled gluten-free are limited to foods that are naturally gluten-free."
   d. "Gluten-free products provide <20 ppm of gluten per serving."

6 The client asks if a tea that claims to improve memory really works. Which of the following would be the nurse's best response?
   a. "If the tea claims to improve memory, then it has been tested and proven effective at improving memory."
   b. "The tea probably works but you need to try it to know."
   c. "Function claims like 'improve memory' can be used on labels without supporting proof that they are accurate."
   d. "That type of claim is illegal and should not appear on any food label."

7 Which statement about supplements is accurate?
   a. All supplements must be tested for safety and effectiveness before they can be marketed.
   b. Supplement dosages are standardized.
   c. Proper handling of supplement ingredients is required by law.
   d. Warnings about potential side effects or interactions must be stated on the packaging.

8 Which of the following statements about CBD is accurate?
   a. The FDA defines CBD as a dietary supplement.
   b. CBD is the most active ingredient in marijuana.
   c. CBD may be addictive over time.
   d. CBD is the active ingredient in a drug approved by the FDA.

CHAPTER SUMMARY FOOD AND SUPPLEMENT LABELING

Food Labeling

Food labels are a learning tool to help consumers make healthier food choices.

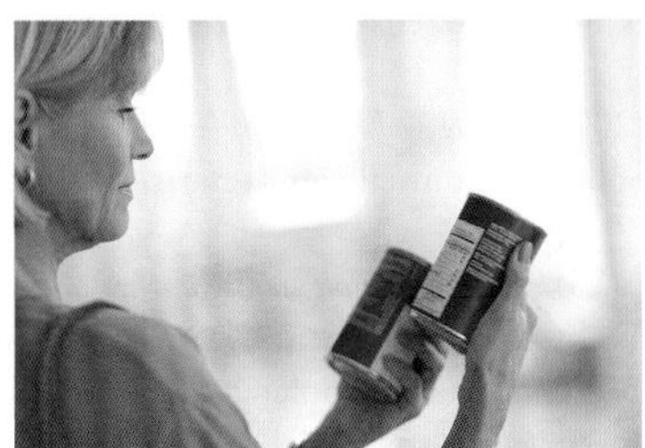

- **Ingredient list:** all ingredients are listed in descending order by weight. Relative amounts are identified but not the proportion of ingredients.
- **Nutrition Facts label:** intended to provide consumers with reliable and useful information to help avoid nutritional excesses.
  - Serving sizes: updated to reflect the amounts people typically eat, not what they "should" eat.
  - A dual column of Nutrition Facts appears on some packages that may be consumed in one or more sittings.
  - Vitamin D and potassium are now required to be listed in gram and %DV quantities because these are nutrients of public health concern.
  - Vitamins A and C content is no longer required because deficiencies of these vitamins are uncommon.
  - Added sugars are a newly added feature.
- Additional labeling regulations are to inform consumers about what they are eating.
  - Foods containing any of the eight major allergens that are responsible for 90% of all allergies must declare them on the label.
  - Gluten-free labeling is allowed for products that provide <20 ppm of gluten.
  - Country of Origin applies to certain foods defined by three categories.
- FDA-allowed claims
  - Nutrition content claims defines the level of a nutrient or substance in a food, such as *free*, *good source*, or *lean*.
  - Health claims describe a relationship between a food or substance in a food and a disease or health-related condition.
  - Unqualified health claims do not require a disclaimer because they are backed by SSA.
  - Qualified health claims are supported by weaker evidence and must be accompanied by a disclaimer.
- **Structure/function claims:** offer possibility that a food may improve or support body function. They must be accompanied by the disclaimer, *these statements have not been evaluated by the FDA*.
- Facts Up Front is an industry-driven labeling system that gives basic Nutrition Facts information for calories, saturated fat, sodium, and sugar. Up to two more specified optional nutrients may be added.

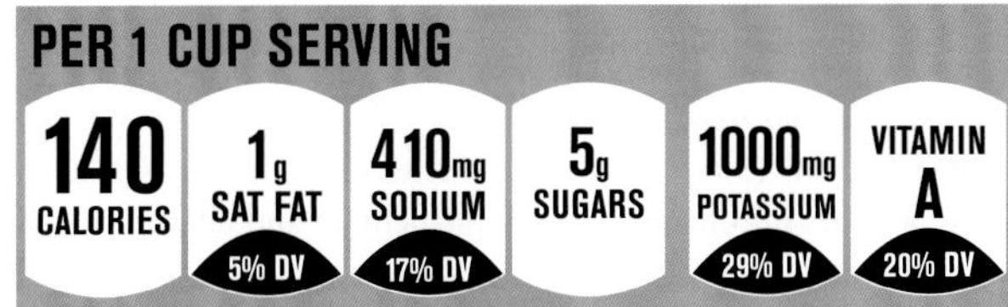

PER 1 CUP SERVING
140 CALORIES
1g SAT FAT 5% DV
410mg SODIUM 17% DV
5g SUGARS
1000mg POTASSIUM 29% DV
VITAMIN A 20% DV

Dietary Supplements

Dietary supplements are intended to add to (not replace) a healthy eating pattern, if necessary.

- Supplements are widely used. Consumers often confuse *natural* with *safe* or *effective*.
- Supplements must be labeled as supplements, include a Supplement Facts panel, and list ingredients, if applicable.
- Supplement regulation differs greatly from how drugs are regulated.
  - Safety and efficacy are not proven.
  - Strength and dosing are not standardized.
  - Warnings about side effects or supplement–drug interactions are not required.
  - Supplements are self-prescribed and megadosing may be a problem.
  - The burden of proof to remove a product from the market rests with the FDA, not with the manufacturer.
  - The statement *buyer beware* is good advice for people thinking of using a supplement.

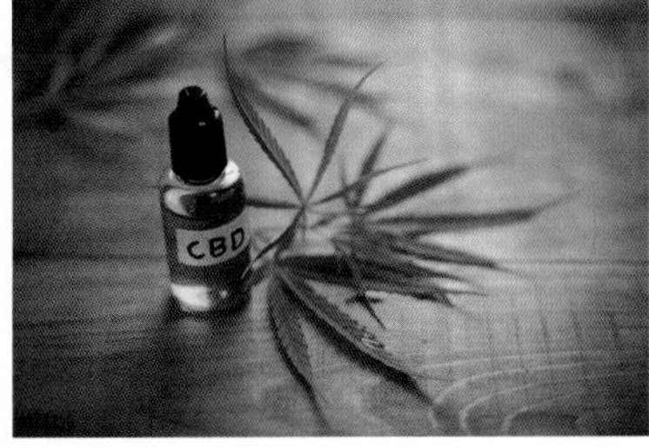

- CBD is a relatively new product that is being marketed as a supplement, although the FDA has ruled that it is not a supplement. Science and regulations have not kept pace with its fast growing popularity.

Figure sources: *shutterstock.com/tmcphotos and shutterstock.com/Infinity Time*

Student Resources on thePoint®
For additional learning materials, activate the code in the front of this book at https://thePoint.lww.com/activate

Websites

Nutrition Facts Information

Changes to the Nutrition Facts Label at https://www.fda.gov/food/food-labeling-nutrition/changes-nutrition-facts-label

Supplement Information

National Center for Complementary and Alternative Medicine Clearinghouse provides information on complementary and alternative medication at www.nccam.nih.gov

Office of Dietary Supplements (ODS) of the National Institutes of Health at http://ods.od.nih.gov/

Tips for dietary supplement users at https://www.fda.gov/food/information-consumers-using-dietary-supplements/tips-dietary-supplement-users

References

Brown, A. C. (2019). *Understanding food principles and preparation* (6th ed.). Cengage Learning.

Celiac Disease Foundation. (2014, August 5). *10 fast facts about the FDA gluten-free labeling rule.* https://celiac.org/about-the-foundation/featured-news/2014/08/fda-gluten-free-food-labeling-information-page

Federal Trade Commission. (2019, September 10). *FTC sends warning letters to companies advertising their CBD-infused products as treatments for serious diseases, including cancer, Alzheimer's, and multiple sclerosis.* https://www.ftc.gov/news-events/press-releases/2019/09/ftc-sends-warning-letters-companies-advertising-their-cbd-infused

Harvard Health Publishing. (2019, August). *CBD products are everywhere. But do they work?* https://www.health.harvard.edu/staying-healthy/cbd-products-are-everywhere-but-do-they-work

MacCleery, L. (2019, July 19). *CSPI urges FDA to take steps to reduce risks of cannabis use.* Center for Science in the Public Interest. https://cspinet.org/news/cspi-urges-fda-take-steps-reduce-risks-cannabis-use-20190716

Nutrition Business Journal. (2019). *2018 NBJ supplement business report.* https://www.nutritionbusinessjournal.com/reports/2018-nbj-supplement-business-report

Reports and Data. (2019, March 25). *Dietary supplements market to reach USD 210.3 billion by 2026.* http://www.globenewswire.com/news-release/2019/03/25/1760423/0/en/Dietary-Supplements-Market-To-Reach-USD-210-3-Billion-By-2026-Reports-And-Data.html

Resnik, D. B. (2017). Proportionality in public health regulation: The case of dietary supplements. *Food Ethics, 2,* 1–6. https://doi.org/10.1007/s41055-017-0023-3

Smith, T., Gillespie, M., Eckl, V., Knepper, J., & Reynolds, C. M. (2019). *Herbal supplement sales in U.S. increase by 9.4% in 2018.* http://cms.herbalgram.org/herbalgram/issue123/files/HG123-HMR.pdf

Starr, R. R. (2015). Too little, too late: Ineffective regulation of dietary supplements in the United States. *American Journal of Public Health, 105*(3), 478–485. https://doi.org/10.2105/AJPH.2014.302348

U.S. Food and Drug Administration. (2020a, July 10). *Changes to the nutrition facts label.* https://www.fda.gov/food/food-labeling-nutrition/changes-nutrition-facts-label

U.S. Food and Drug Administration. (2020b, March 5). *What you need to know (and what we're working to find out) about products containing cannabis or cannabis-derived compounds, including CBD.* https://www.fda.gov/consumers/consumer-updates/what-you-need-know-and-what-were-working-find-out-about-products-containing-cannabis-or-cannabis

World Health Organization. (2017). *Cannabidiol (CBD).* https://www.who.int/medicines/access/controlled-substances/5.2_CBD.pdf

Chapter 10

Consumer Interests and Concerns

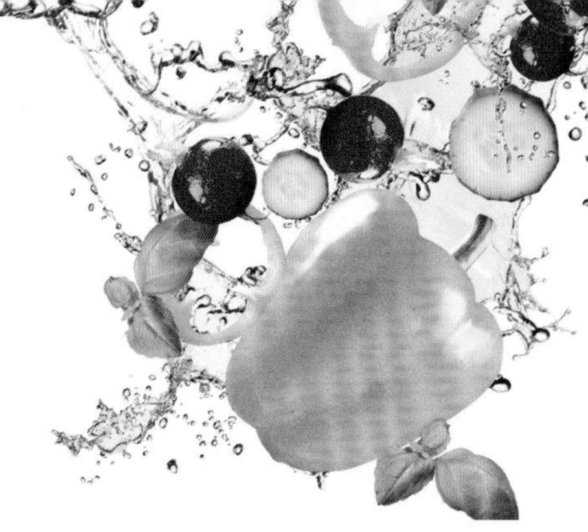

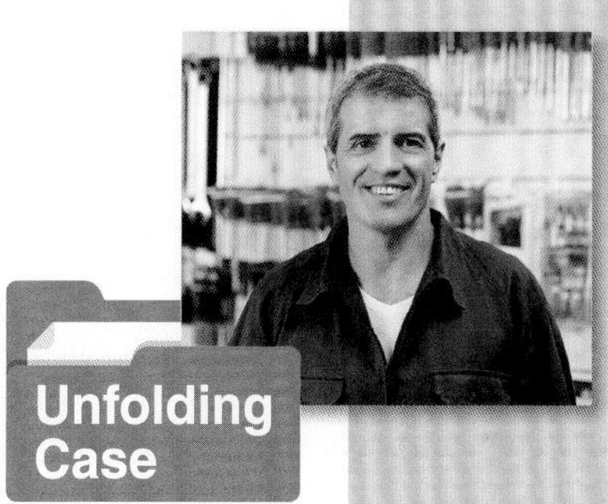

Unfolding Case

Paul Youngblood

Paul is a 63-year-old single man with mild developmental and cognitive impairments who has lived with his mother for his entire life. He has held the same part-time entry-level position at a local hardware store for 40 years. His mother's recent death means he will be living independently for the first time in his life. He has no life skills pertaining to shopping or cooking because his mother always took care of that.

Learning Objectives

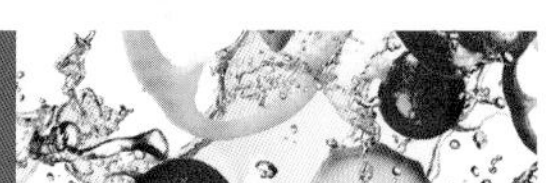

Upon completion of this chapter, you will be able to:

1 Discuss points to consider when evaluating the credibility of nutrition information.
2 Give examples of conventional and modified functional foods.
3 Interpret labeling on organic products.
4 Discuss the benefits and disadvantages of consuming organic foods.
5 Teach clients about the four simple steps to keep food safe.
6 Debate the safety of genetically modified food.
7 Explain the reason why some foods are irradiated.
8 Define issues of food access: food insecurity and food deserts.

Functional Foods
commonly (not legally) defined as foods that provide health benefits beyond basic nutrition.

Food Irradiation
treatment of food with approved levels of ionizing radiation for a prescribed period of time and a controlled dose to destroy bacteria and parasites that would otherwise cause foodborne illness.

The proliferation of cyberspace information—and misinformation—gives millions of Americans ready access to nutritional concepts. Advances in food technology have brought us **functional foods**, bioengineering, and **food irradiation** as well as new questions about food safety and optimal nutrition. The ever-evolving science of nutrition has progressed from three square meals a day and a well-rounded diet to MyPlate. This is an era that presents old and new challenges for health professionals.

This chapter begins with consumer information and misinformation. Consumer interests discussed include functional food, organic foods, foodborne illnesses, biotechnology, antibiotics in the food supply, and irradiation. Issues of food access, namely, food insecurity and food deserts, are presented.

CONSUMER INFORMATION AND MISINFORMATION

The role of food has shifted from simply a means to prevent deficiency diseases to a tool for optimizing health, preventing chronic disease, and delaying aging. Several factors are driving this "food as medicine" paradigm, including

- consumer interest in managing their own health,
- increasing age of the population,
- escalating health care costs,

- technologic advances, such as biotechnology,
- the obesity epidemic, and
- evidence-based science that links healthy eating patterns to a reduced risk of chronic disease.

BOX 10.1 Points to Consider When Evaluating the Credibility of Information

- Was the research conducted at a reputable institution or an impressive-sounding but unknown facility?
- The distinction between correlation and causation may be blurred, and inappropriate conclusions may be made from study results.
- Generally, if it sounds too good to be true, it usually is.
- Features or articles that fail to identify how much or little of a food should be eaten, how often it should be eaten, or to whom the advice applies do not give consumers enough information to appropriately judge what the study means to them personally.
- Other types of media inaccuracy include generalizing a study to a broader population than was actually studied and overstating the size of the effect.
- URLs ending in .edu (educational institutions), .org (organizations), or .gov (government agencies) are more credible than those ending in .com (commercial). A commercial website's main objective may be to sell a product.
- Anyone who stands to benefit economically by promoting a food, supplement, or diet is not likely to be an objective resource.

Combating Misinformation

Nutrition misinformation abounds. Breaking news stories may be little more than *spin* (a favorable slant in news articles) or incomplete coverage of preliminary results from scientific studies, which are often discounted later as more research is completed. Although information available on the Internet is vast, there are no regulatory safeguards in place to ensure the information is accurate. Junk science coexists with legitimate data. It is the responsibility of each individual consumer to evaluate the reliability of information (Box 10.1).

Many people treat nutrition as a belief system rather than as a science and formulate opinions in response to emotional appeals rather than scientific evidence. Others assume that anything that appears in print form (e.g., in a book, magazine, or newspaper) is accurate and not everyone recognizes the shortcomings of the Internet. If client beliefs are unsupported but harmless, then you may risk alienating them for no reason by trying to convince them that they're misinformed. Determine how much of an emotional investment the client has in believing harmless misinformation. Be aware that casual or judgmental dismissal of misinformation can cause clients to become defensive and distrustful; clients may conclude that you are not as up to date as they are about nutrition, and they may reject you as a credible reference.

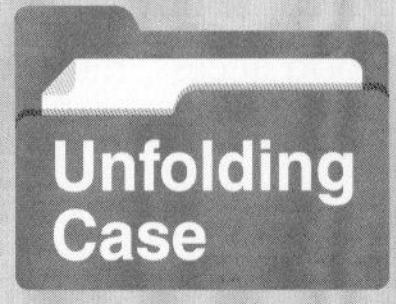

Recall Paul. He is used to treating himself to fast-food meals and eating the food that mom buys—without thought about nutrition and health. He is not capable of applying critical thinking to news about nutrition, and he is easily directed by his eagerness to please. What points should a learning plan include that enable Paul to purchase and prepare food for himself?

CONSUMER-RELATED INTERESTS

As knowledge of nutrition in health and disease continues to grow, consumers interested in self-directed care look to food- and nutrition-related strategies to ensure health and wellness. Some of those strategies are discussed in the following sections.

Functional Foods

Functional foods are one of the fastest growing segments of the food industry. The term has no legal meaning in the United States; it is currently a marketing, not a regulatory, term. In reality, all food is in essence "functional" in that it provides calories and nutrients necessary to sustain life; however, functional food is generally considered a food or food component that provides health benefits beyond basic nutrition.

The Academy of Nutrition and Dietetics defines functional foods as "whole foods along with fortified, enriched, or enhanced foods that have a potentially beneficial effect on health when consumed as part of a varied diet on a regular basis at effective levels" (Crowe & Francis, 2013; p. 1097). Whole or natural functional foods are foods that are not modified in any way. Examples include whole fruits, vegetables, whole grains, nuts, legumes, and fish. Table 10.1 gives examples of natural functional foods and their potential health benefits. Modified functional foods have one or more functional ingredients added, which can occur through enrichment, fortification, or other means (e.g., enzymatic, chemical, technological). Examples include calcium-fortified orange juice, fermented dairy products, and omega-3 fatty acid–enriched eggs.

Functional food definitions may also include **nutraceuticals**, dietary supplements, and **medical foods** (Litwin et al., 2018).

Nutraceuticals
isolated, modified, and/or synthetic bioactive components that are typically given as a dietary supplement.

Medical Foods
foods formulated to meet nutrient needs of a patient, such as an enteral tube feeding formula; used in the dietary management of a disease and/or medical condition under the supervision of the physician.

Table 10.1 Natural Functional Foods

Food	Active Ingredient	Potential Health Benefits
Berries: strawberries, cranberries, blueberries, raspberries, black berries	Anthocyanins	May reduce the risk of Alzheimer's disease through anti-inflammatory and antioxidant properties
Soy foods	Soy protein	Lower total and low-density lipoprotein (LDL) cholesterol; may inhibit tumor growth
Oats, oatmeal, barley, rye	Soluble fiber (beta-glucan)	Lower total and LDL cholesterol
Fatty fish	Omega-3 fatty acids	Lower triglycerides, lower heart disease, lower cardiac deaths, and lower fatal and nonfatal heart attacks
Purple grape juice or red wine	Resveratrol	Decreases platelet aggregation
Cranberry juice, strawberries, cinnamon	Proanthocyanidins and procyanidins	Reduce bacteriuria
Green tea	Catechins	Reduces the risk of certain cancers, such as breast and prostate cancer
Tomatoes and tomato products	Lycopene	Reduce the risk of prostate, ovarian, gastric, and pancreatic cancer
Yogurt and fermented dairy products	Probiotics	Promote gastrointestinal, immune, cardiovascular, and metabolic health
Nuts, olive oil	Monounsaturated fatty acids and vitamin E	Reduce the risk of cardiovascular disease
Citrus fruits	Flavanones	Neutralize free radicals; promote cellular antioxidant defenses
Cruciferous vegetables (e.g., broccoli, cauliflower, cabbage)	Sulforaphane	Reduce the risk of certain types of cancer
Garlic, onions, leeks, scallions	Sulfur compounds	Lower total and LDL cholesterol; may promote healthy immune function
Orange, red, and dark green fruits and vegetables	Beta carotene	Neutralize free radicals, which may damage cells; may inhibit cancer growth; may improve immune response
Spinach, kale, collard greens, corn	Lutein, zeaxanthin	Lower risk of age-related macular degeneration

Source: Litwin, N., Clifford, J., & Johnson, S. (2018). *Functional foods for health*. https://extension.colostate.edu/topic-areas/nutrition-food-safety-health/functional-foods-for-health-9-391; American Institute for Cancer Research. *Phytochemicals: The cancer fighters in your foods*. https://www.aicr.org/reduce-your-cancer-risk/diet/elements_phytochemicals.html

It is likely that more foods will be considered functional and the supply of manufactured functional foods will expand exponentially as scientific evidence mounts in the role of specific nutrients or food substances in preventing chronic diseases such as heart disease, cancer, diabetes, hypertension, and osteoporosis. Natural functional foods—namely, fruits, vegetables, nuts, whole grains, and fatty fish—are the foundation of a healthy eating pattern. Modified functional foods should be viewed as an option to optimize a healthy eating plan but not as a miracle food to compensate for poor food choices.

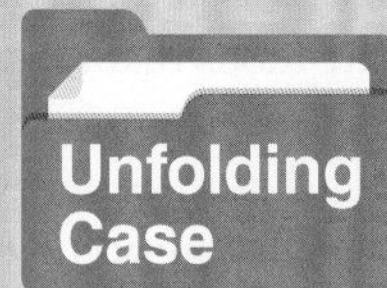

Recall Paul. He heard about functional foods but has been unable to find them on food labels in the grocery store. What would you tell Paul about natural and modified functional foods?

Organically Grown Foods

Sale of organic food in the United States has grown from $1 billion in 1990 to over $47.9 billion in 2018 and represents approximately 5.7% of total food sales (Organic Trade Association, 2019). Fresh fruits and vegetables have been the top-selling category of organically grown food since retail sale of organic food began more than 30 years ago. Consumers have the impression that organic vegetables and fruits are *safer*, *more nutritious*, and *healthier*, but findings are complicated and dependent upon how those terms are defined.

Safety

Although consumers often have the perception that organic foods are safer than conventionally produced foods, organic standards do not specifically address safety issues such as microbial or chemical hazards (Harvey et al., 2016).

- Foodborne illness outbreaks reported from organic food have increased in recent years. This parallels the increase in organic food intake.
- Unfortunately, the risk of outbreaks due to organic foods compared to that of conventional foods cannot be assessed because foodborne outbreak surveillance does not systematically collect information about food production methods.
- Reviews that assessed whether organic produce is more or less susceptible to microbial contamination compared to conventional produce did not find any significant difference (Gomiero, 2018).
- Food safety precautions are necessary with all food—organic *and* conventional foods.
- Raw milk and fresh produce, whether conventionally or organically produced, are common vehicles for pathogens.

Organic: In a chemical sense, *organic* means containing carbon. Generally, *organic* refers to living organisms; as such, all plants and animals are technically organic. Organic foods are grown and processed according to federal guidelines that cover soil quality, animalraising practices, pest and weed control, and the use of additives. Organic produce is grown on soil that had no prohibited synthetic fertilizers and pesticides. Organic meat requires that animals have the ability to graze on pasture, are fed 100% organic feed, and do not receive antibiotics or hormones. Organic processed foods must be free of artificial preservatives, colors, and flavors and be made from organic ingredients, with few exceptions.

Nutritional Value

Evidence that organic food is more nutritious than conventional food is relatively scarce. It is difficult to reliably measure nutritional differences due to many variables, including an exact definition of *conventional*, the maturity of the samples used, the varieties of individual plants chosen, the study designs (e.g., farm surveys, retail surveys), and the question whether produce has been grown in the same region and climatic conditions (Gomiero, 2018). A review by Hurtado-Barroso et al. (2019) cites numerous studies, which show the following:

- Organic produce provides higher levels of phytonutrients (e.g., polyphenols, anthocyanin, flavonoids, quercetin), vitamin C, and carotenoids than conventional produce. The clinical significance is unknown.
- Organic animal products, such as meat and milk, have higher levels of omega-3 fatty acid than conventionally grown animals, but the differences and amounts are too low to have any effect on human health (Hurtado-Barroso et al., 2019).

Impact on Health

The impact of organic foods on health is potentially multifaceted.

- Even though antioxidant levels are higher in organic produce than conventional produce, nutrition intervention studies performed so far have not shown a clear association between antioxidant levels in people and whether they consume organic or conventionally grown foods (Hurtado-Barroso et al., 2019).
- Organic diets unequivocally expose consumers to fewer pesticides and with residues of much lower toxicity compared to conventional foods (Gomiero, 2018). Large prospective cohort studies are needed to assess the relationship between pesticide exposure in conventional foods and human disease.
- Organic animals have the potential to reduce antibiotic-resistant infections in humans.
- All milk contains growth hormone. Whether present naturally or given to increase milk production, growth hormone is a peptide hormone that is digested in the human gastrointestinal (GI) tract.

Organic Labeling

The U.S. Department of Agriculture (USDA) ensures that the production, processing, and certification of organically grown foods adhere to strict national standards and that organic labeling meets criteria that define the four official organic categories (Table 10.2).

Final Considerations

Organic food is usually more expensive because of higher production costs, greater losses, and smaller yields. For instance, a gallon of organic milk typically costs twice as much as a gallon of store-brand or name-brand milk. However, not all organic foods are appreciably more expensive than their conventional counterparts, such as oranges, grapes, and bread.

Despite the controversy regarding the risks of pesticide residues in food, both sides agree that the benefits of eating a diet rich in plants outweigh any potential risks of pesticide exposure. Each year, the Environmental Working Group (EWG) compiles a list of the *Dirty Dozen*™ and the *Clean 15*™, which identify fruits and vegetables with the most and least levels of pesticides, respectively (EWG, 2019) (Table 10.3). This list may help consumers save money while lowering pesticide exposure by helping them choose conventionally grown "clean" items and selecting organic versions of the "dirtiest" produce.

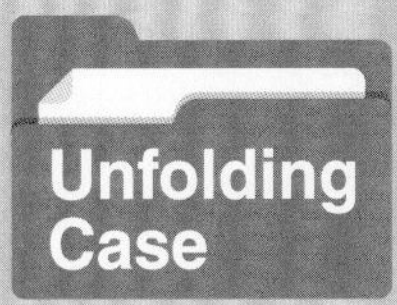

Think of Paul. He watched a documentary on pesticides in the food supply and is convinced he will get cancer if he eats conventionally grown produce. However, he can't afford organic fruits and vegetables, so he has decided he is better off not eating *any* fruits and vegetables rather than eating conventional ones. What would you say to Paul?

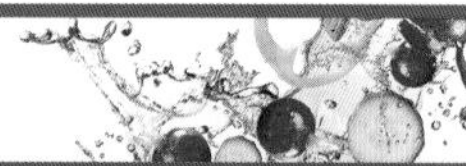

Table 10.2 U.S. Department of Agriculture Criteria for Labeling Organic Products

Organic Term and Definition	Labeling Allowed
• **100% Organic:** all of the ingredients must be certified organic (except salt and water). Crops must be grown without synthetic fertilizers and pesticides. Natural products like manure, compost, and naturally occurring chemicals in the environment (e.g., nicotine, sulfur) may be used when growing the food. • Food irradiation, sewage sludge, and GMOs are not allowed. • Organic livestock must be raised on 100% organic feed, allowed to graze at pasture at least 4 months of the year, and obtain 30% of their feed through grazing. • Hormones and antibiotics are prohibited. • Organic milk must come from cows not treated with antibiotics or hormones.	May include USDA organic seal and/or "100% organic" claim. 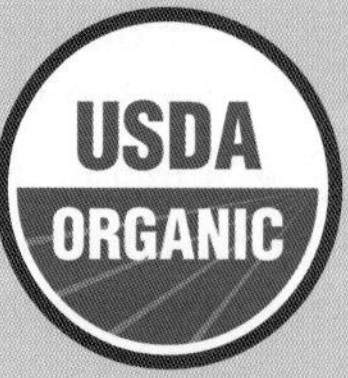
Organic: at least 95% of ingredients must be certified organic.	May include USDA organic seal and/or "organic" claim. 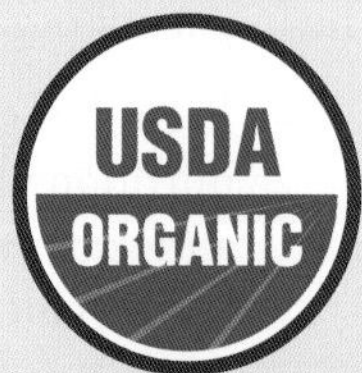
Made with organic ingredients: at least 70% of the ingredients must be certified organic.	May state "made with organic …" *(insert up to 3 ingredients or ingredient categories)* Cannot use organic seal, represent finished product as organic, or state "made with organic ingredients."
Contains organic: less than 70% of ingredients are certified organic.	May only list organic ingredients on the ingredient list—for example, "Ingredients: water, barley, organic beans …" Cannot use organic seal or the word *organic* on the display panel

Source: U.S. Department of Agriculture. (n.d.). *Organic labeling standards*. https://www.ams.usda.gov/grades-standards/organic-labeling-standards

Table 10.3 *The Dirty Dozen*™ and *The Clean 15*™

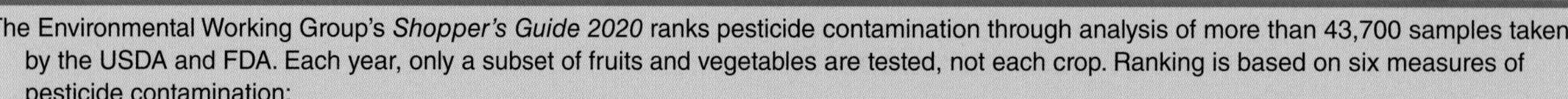

The Environmental Working Group's *Shopper's Guide 2020* ranks pesticide contamination through analysis of more than 43,700 samples taken by the USDA and FDA. Each year, only a subset of fruits and vegetables are tested, not each crop. Ranking is based on six measures of pesticide contamination:

- Percentage of samples with detectable pesticides
- Percentage of samples with two or more detectable pesticides
- Average number of pesticides found on a single sample
- Average amount of pesticides found; measured in parts per million
- Maximum number of pesticides found on a single sample
- Total number of pesticides found on the crop

The Dirty Dozen™ (with 1 being "dirtiest")	The Clean 15™ (with 1 being "cleanest")
1. Strawberries	1. Avocados
2. Spinach	2. Sweet corn
3. Kale	3. Pineapples
4. Nectarines	4. Onions
5. Apples	5. Papayas
6. Grapes	6. Sweet peas (frozen)
7. Peaches	7. Eggplant
8. Cherries	8. Asparagus
9. Pears	9. Cauliflower
10. Tomatoes	10. Cantaloupe
11. Celery	11. Broccoli
12. Potatoes	12. Mushrooms
	13. Cabbage
	14. Honeydew melon
	15. Kiwi

Source: Environmental Working Group Science Team. (2020). *EWG's 2020 shopper's guide to pesticides in produce*. https://www.ewg.org/foodnews/summary.php.

Figure 10.1 ▶
Pathogens identified as the cause of illness in confirmed, single-etiology foodborne illness outbreaks, 2017. (*Source:* Centers for Disease Control and Prevention [CDC]. [2019]. *Surveillance for foodborne disease outbreaks, United States, 2017, annual report.* https://www.cdc.gov/fdoss/pdf/2017_FoodBorneOutbreaks_508.pdf?deliveryName=DM9453)

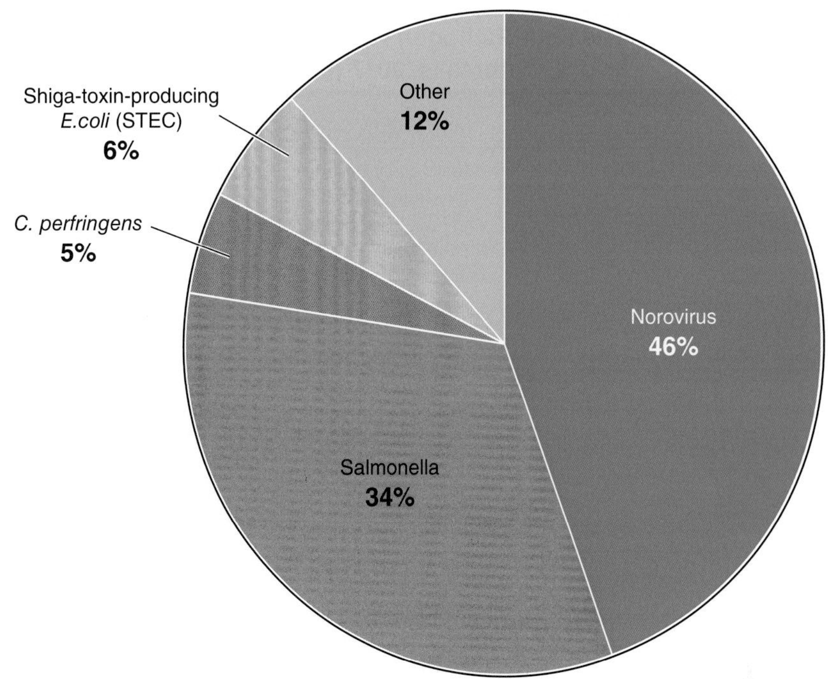

Foodborne Illness

In a 2019 survey, foodborne illness from bacteria was selected as the top food safety concern among polled Americans (International Food Information Council Foundation, 2019). The Centers for Disease Control and Prevention (CDC) estimates that every year, approximately 48 million Americans experience a foodborne illness, resulting in 128,000 hospitalizations and 3000 deaths (Centers for Disease Control and Prevention [CDC], 2018). Relatively few of these illnesses occur in a recognized outbreak, yet outbreaks provide insight into the pathogens and foods that cause illness (CDC, 2019). In 2017, 841 foodborne disease outbreaks were reported, resulting in 14,481 illnesses, 827 hospitalizations, 20 deaths, and 14 food product recalls. More than 90% of confirmed, single-etiology **outbreak** illnesses were caused by only four pathogens (Fig. 10.1). Table 10.4 summarizes details of these four pathogens. It also includes *Listeria* because it is one of the leading causes of death from **foodborne illness**.

Outbreak
the occurrence of two or more cases of a similar illness resulting from ingestion of a common food.

Foodborne Illness
an illness transmitted to humans via food.

Food Vehicles of Transmission

The microorganisms that cause foodborne illness are found widely in nature and are transmitted to people from within food (e.g., meat, fish), from on food (e.g., eggshell, vegetables), from unsafe

Table 10.4 **The Four Pathogens Linked to Nearly 90% of Foodborne Illness in U.S. Outbreaks, 2017**

Pathogen/Type	Onset	Common Food Vehicles	Symptoms	Risk Reduction Strategies
Norovirus/virus	24–48 hours	Fruit, vegetables, shellfish, any food prepared or handled by infected person.	Explosive vomiting, watery diarrhea, cramps, headache, mild fever, muscle aches. Usually lasts 1–2 days.	Wash fruits and vegetables. Avoid raw oysters and other shellfish. Wash hands with soap and water (hand sanitizer does not protect against norovirus).
Salmonella/bacteria	6–72 hours	Almost any food: beef, pork, poultry, eggs, fruits, vegetables, spices, nuts, sprouts.	GI: nausea, vomiting, diarrhea, cramps, fever that usually last a couple of days. Long-term arthritis may develop.	Cook meat, poultry, and eggs thoroughly. Keep raw foods separated from cooked foods. Refrigerate foods at 40° or below. Wash fruits and vegetables except for prewashed greens (which could become contaminated by washing in at home sink).

(continued)

Table 10.4 The Four Pathogens Linked to Nearly 90% of Foodborne Illness in U.S. Outbreaks, 2017 (continued)

Pathogen/Type	Onset	Common Food Vehicles	Symptoms	Risk Reduction Strategies
Shiga-toxin-producing *Escherichia coli* (STEC)/bacteria Most common form in North America is *E. coli* O157:H7, often shorted to just *E. coli* 0157.	3–4 days	Beef (especially ground), unpasteurized milk and juice, raw fruits and vegetables, sprouts.	Watery diarrhea, mild abdominal cramps. Some types of STEC frequently cause severe disease, including bloody diarrhea, severe abdominal pain, and vomiting. Around 5%–10% of people diagnosed with STEC infection develop hemolytic uremic syndrome (kidney failure). May cause permanent damage or death.	Wash hands thoroughly. Use a thermometer to cook ground beef to 160°. Avoid unpasteurized milk and juices. Avoid raw sprouts. Prevent cross contamination.
Clostridium perfringens/ bacteria	8–16 hours	Known as the *cafeteria germ* associated with steam table foods that are not kept hot enough (such as meat and poultry roasts or stews).	Commonly causes mild cramps and watery diarrhea that usually resolve in 24 hours. More serious illness, called *pig-bel* (*enteritis necroticans*), is much more severe and often fatal but is rare in the United States. Symptoms of *pig-bel* are abdominal pain and distention, diarrhea that is sometimes bloody, and vomiting.	Serve meat and poultry hot. Refrigerate leftovers within 2 hours. Divide leftovers into smaller containers for more rapid cooling.
Also important: *Listeria* is not among the top four but is one of the leading causes of death from foodborne illness				
Listeria monocytogenes/ bacteria	A few hours to 2–3 days. Invasive form of the illness can have a long incubation period, which may vary from 3 days to 3 months.	Raw milk, soft cheese, raw sprouts, smoked fish and other seafood, meats and deli meats, raw vegetables, melon. *Listeria* is hardy and tolerates salty and cold environments.	Mild-to-intense symptoms of nausea, vomiting, aches, fever, and sometimes diarrhea. *Listeria* usually resolves on its own. More deadly form occurs when the infection invades the nervous system and results in meningitis and other potentially fatal problems. Pregnant women are more susceptible to *Listeria* infection, which usually results in spontaneous abortion or stillbirth.	Avoid raw milk. Choose soft cheeses made only from pasteurized milk. Cook food thoroughly. Wash fruits and vegetables. Wash hands. Keep raw food away from cooked foods. Use refrigerated melon within a week of cutting.

Source: Centers for Disease Control and Prevention (CDC). (2019). *Surveillance for foodborne disease outbreaks, United States, 2017, annual report*. https://www.cdc.gov/fdoss/pdf/2017_FoodBorneOutbreaks_508.pdf?deliveryName=DM9453; U.S. Food and Drug Administration. (2017, October 24). *Big bad bug book (second edition)*. https://www.fda.gov/food/foodborne-pathogens/bad-bug-book-second-edition; Moyer, L. (2018). *The most common causes of foodborne illness outbreaks*. https://cspinet.org/tip/most-common-causes-foodborne-illness-outbreaks

BOX 10.2 Foods Causing the Highest Percentage of Illnesses Based on 2017 Outbreaks

Food Implicated	Percentage of Total Illnesses
Turkey	16
Chicken	13
Fruits	13
Pork	10
Leafy vegetables	9
Beef	9
Mollusks	7
Fish	4
Dairy	2
Eggs	2
Sprouts	2

Source: Centers for Disease Control and Prevention (CDC). (2019). *Surveillance for foodborne disease outbreaks, United States, 2017, annual report*. https://www.cdc.gov/fdoss/pdf/2017_FoodBorneOutbreaks_508.pdf?deliveryName=DM9453

water, or from human or animal feces. Any uncooked food that is handled by someone who is ill poses a risk. All food categories were involved in outbreaks, but the frequency varies for each category. Foods causing the most outbreak-associated illnesses in 2017 are listed in Box 10.2.

Symptoms

The most common symptoms of foodborne illness may be mistaken for the "stomach flu:" diarrhea, nausea, vomiting, fever, abdominal pain, and headaches.

- Most cases are self-limiting and run their course within a few days.
- Symptoms that warrant medical attention include bloody diarrhea (possible *Escherichia coli* 0157:H7 infection), a stiff neck with severe headache and fever (possible meningitis related to *Listeria*), excessive diarrhea or vomiting (possible life-threatening dehydration), and any symptoms that persist for more than 3 days.
- Infants, pregnant women, senior adults, and people with compromised immune systems (e.g., people with AIDS, cancer, organ transplant recipients, people taking corticosteroids) are particularly vulnerable to the effects of foodborne illness.

Prevention

The major cause of foodborne illnesses is unsanitary food handling. Box 10.3 features actions to reduce the risk of contamination.

BOX 10.3 Actions to Reduce the Risk of Foodborne Illness

- Wash hands thoroughly with soap and water for at least 20 seconds after using the restroom, before cooking, and after each touch of raw meat, poultry, seafood, or eggs.
- Avoid cross contamination. Wash cutting boards, counter, utensils, serving platters, etc. after they have been in contact with raw meats, poultry, seafood, or eggs. Do not reuse marinades that have been in contact with raw meats. Do not rinse raw poultry or meat.
- Cook food thoroughly. Check internal temperature with a thermometer.
- Chill leftovers and takeout foods within 2 hours.
- Refrigerate cold foods at 40° or less.
- Clean produce, except for prewashed greens. Gently rub under cold running water. Scrub firm produce with a clean vegetable brush, even when the rind will be cut away. Remove outer leaves, if appropriate.

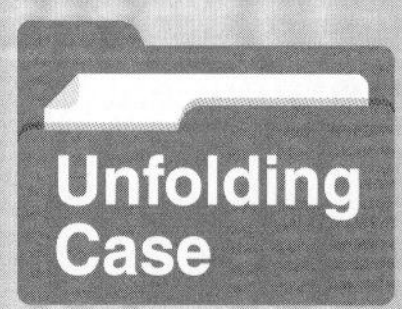

Consider Paul. He is very proud of his cooking accomplishment—a big pot of homemade chili. You learn that he keeps it on the stove all the time and heats it up when it is time for lunch and dinner so he doesn't have to wash the pan. What points would you include in teaching Paul about food safety?

Food Biotechnology

Food Biotechnology
a process that involves taking a gene with a desirable trait from one plant and inserting it into another with the goal of changing one or more of its characteristics; also called genetically engineered food.

Food biotechnology combines biotechnology and genetic engineering to improve food. Food biotechnology is usually described as genetically engineered (GE) or genetically modified organisms (GMO). In **food biotechnology**, recombinant deoxyribonucleic acid in genes associated with desirable characteristics are transferred from one plant to another. This is a quicker, more controlled, and more predicable version of old-fashioned crossbreeding.

In 1994, the Flavr Savr tomato became the first GE plant approved by the U.S. Food and Drug Administration (FDA) for human consumption in the United States. It was modified to delay ripening and improve resistance to rot. Today, 26 countries grow biotech crops on 191.7 million hectares (International Service for the Acquisition of Agri-Biotech Applications [ISAAA], 2018). The United States is the leading producer of biotech crops with more than 74 million hectares, according to the ISAAA (2018).

- The primary crops grown in the United States are corn, cotton, soybeans, alfalfa, sugar beets, canola, squash, papaya, potatoes, and apples.
- Ninety-three percent of all the corn, soybeans, and cotton in the United States are grown using biotechnology.
- Ingredients made from these top crops, such as soybean oil, corn oil, and corn syrup, are pervasive in processed foods available in U.S. grocery stores, such as cereals, frozen pizza, hot dogs, and soft drinks.
- In addition to permeating the food supply, biotechnology has provided breakthrough health care products and technologies, beginning with FDA approval of recombinant human insulin in 1982.
- Currently, there are more than 250 biotechnology health care products and vaccines available, many for previously untreatable diseases (Biotechnology Innovation Organization, 2016).

Benefits of Biotechnology

Perhaps the greatest potential benefit of GE foods is in increasing global crop yields to meet the world's increasing demand for food. The Food and Agricultural Organization projects the global population to expand to approximately 9.7 billion by 2050, an almost 50% increase from 2013 (Raman, 2018). Current agricultural practices alone cannot sustain the world's population and eradicate malnutrition and hunger on a global scale in the future (Raman, 2018). Producing more food on less acreage has the potential to better meet the world's need for food. Other potential benefits are listed in Box 10.4.

BOX 10.4 Potential Benefits of Biotechnology

- **Healthier crops:** Some plants are genetically modified to increase their resistance to plant viruses and other diseases. This means they can be raised using fewer pesticides to help reduce production costs and environmental residues.
- **Greater resistance to severe weather:** Crop loss will be reduced and year-round availability of fresh crops increases. One example is a biotech drought-tolerant corn.
- **Longer shelf life and increased freshness:** Plants can be made to ripen more slowly, staying fresher longer—a big plus for transportation.

BOX 10.4 Potential Benefits of Biotechnology (continued)

- **Higher nutritional value:** Plants can be genetically modified to contain more micronutrients or protein, or less fat. For instance, Golden Rice has been GE as a humanitarian project to provide beta carotene, the precursor of vitamin A. In developing countries where rice is the staple crop and where vitamin A deficiency is endemic, Golden Rice has the potential to prevent the 4500 daily child deaths caused by vitamin A deficiency (Dubock, 2017). Vitamin A deficiency mostly affects children under the age of 5; it is known as the major cause of childhood blindness globally and causes death related to impaired immune system functioning.
- **Healthier composition:** For instance, Innate potato has been approved for use in the United States. It has lower levels of acrylamide, a potential carcinogen in humans produced when potatoes are cooked at high temperatures.
- **Better flavor:** Genetic modification has produced sweeter melons and sweeter strawberries.
- **Improved characteristics:** An example is celery without strings.
- **New food varieties through crossbreeding:** Broccoflowers (a blend of broccoli and cauliflower) and tangelos (a tangerine–grapefruit hybrid) are examples.
- Products such as consistent, reliable, and highly purified enzymes used in cheese production can replace the more expensive and variable enzyme rennin that is obtained from calf's stomach.

How the U.S. Food and Drug Administration Regulates Genetically Engineered Foods

Foods from GE plants must meet the same requirements, including safety requirements, as foods from traditionally bred plants (U.S. Food and Drug Administration [FDA], 2020).

- A voluntary consultation process with developers of GE plants culminates in the GE plant developer completing a safety assessment and submitting the summary to the FDA.
- Any safety and other regulatory concerns expressed by the FDA must be resolved before the food product can be brought to market.
- As of 2018, more than 150 GE plant varieties have been evaluated.

Acceptance

Major health organizations that endorse the responsible use of genetic engineering as a safe and effective means to improve food security and reduce negative effects of agriculture include the American Medical Association, the National Academy of Sciences, the American Association for the Advancement of Science (AAAS), the American Council on Science and Health, and the World Health Organization (American Council on Science and Health [ACSH], 2016).

- These endorsements are based on the research of independent groups worldwide that concludes that GE foods are safe for consumers.
- According to a Pew Research Center survey, 88% of scientists in the AAAS think that GE foods are safe to eat, yet only 37% of the general public shares this thought (Pew Research Center, 2015).

Public Concerns Regarding Health

Commonly expressed concerns are how GMOs may affect consumer health, such as unwanted changes in nutritional content, the creation of allergens, and toxic effects on bodily organs.

- GMO fears are still theoretical, like the possibility that an inserted gene could have a negative impact on other desirable genes naturally present in the crop.
- According to Edward Parson, a codirector of the Emmett Institute on Climate Change and the Environment at University of California, Los Angeles, after more than a quarter

century of growing GMO crops in North America, no detrimental impacts have been detected in North America compared to Europe, where people have little exposure to GMOs (Brown, 2016).

- Parson also adds that it is not possible to prove a food is safe. It is only possible to say that no hazard has been shown to exist (Brown, 2016).

Research on Safety

GMOs appear as a class to be no more likely to cause harm than traditionally bred and grown food sources, though each new product will require careful analysis and safety assessment (Norris, 2015). Findings from worldwide independent researchers on various aspects of GMO safety, especially as it pertains to consumer health and toxicity, are as follows (Norris, 2015):

- No relationship between GMOs and mutations exists.
- Fertility, pregnancy, and offspring are unaffected by GMOs.
- Organ health and function are unaffected by GMOs.
- There is no evidence for gene transfer between GMOs and consumers.

Environmental Concern

Glyphosate (also known by its brand name Roundup) is a broad-spectrum herbicide that kills weeds by preventing them from making an essential protein. The problem is that it works on crops as well as weeds, which led researchers to develop GE "Roundup Ready crops" (soybeans, cotton, corn) that contain a gene from bacteria that makes them immune to the herbicide.

- The widespread use of Roundup eventually led to the development of glyphosate-resistant weeds, causing farmers to resort to spraying herbicides that were much more toxic than Roundup in an attempt to keep superweeds from spreading.
- Greater use of herbicides increases the likelihood of higher concentrations of chemicals running off into nearby ecosystems and damaging the environment.
- In order for GMOs to live up to their potential, conscientious research on negative environmental risks must occur.
- The goal should be to support only safe products that represent an improvement over the original product and focus opposition to products that carry risks (Brody, 2018).

Labeling Regulations

In July 2016, Congress passed a law directing the USDA to establish a national mandatory standard for disclosing foods that are or may be bioengineered (U.S. Department of Agriculture [USDA], 2019).

- Bioengineered foods are defined as foods that contain detectable genetic material that has been modified through certain lab techniques and cannot be created through conventional breeding or found in nature. They may be identified by a symbol, words, scannable links, or by other means.
- The mandatory compliance date is January 1, 2022, on all food products that require disclosure.
- In the meantime, many national food manufacturers are voluntarily disclosing on the label that their products contain GE ingredients.
- Foods that carry a symbol that states *derived from bioengineering* or that disclose the product contains ingredients *derived from bioengineering* are not bioengineered foods because these foods do not contain detectable modified genetic material. Specific voluntary disclosures for these type of products apply.

Antibiotics in the Food Supply

Antibiotics are valuable for treating infections in both humans and animals. Antibiotics are approved for use in food animals under specific situations: to treat disease in animals that are sick, to control disease in a group of animals when some of the animals are sick, and to prevent disease in animals that are at risk for becoming sick (CDC, 2018). Previously, antibiotics were often routinely given in low doses to healthy animals for the purpose of promoting growth, increasing feed efficiency, or preventing disease in crowded, unhygienic living conditions. This ultimately contributed to the emergence of antibiotic-resistant bacteria.

Antibiotic-resistant bacteria can be transmitted to humans through the food supply and can cause antibiotic-resistant infections (Fig. 10.2).

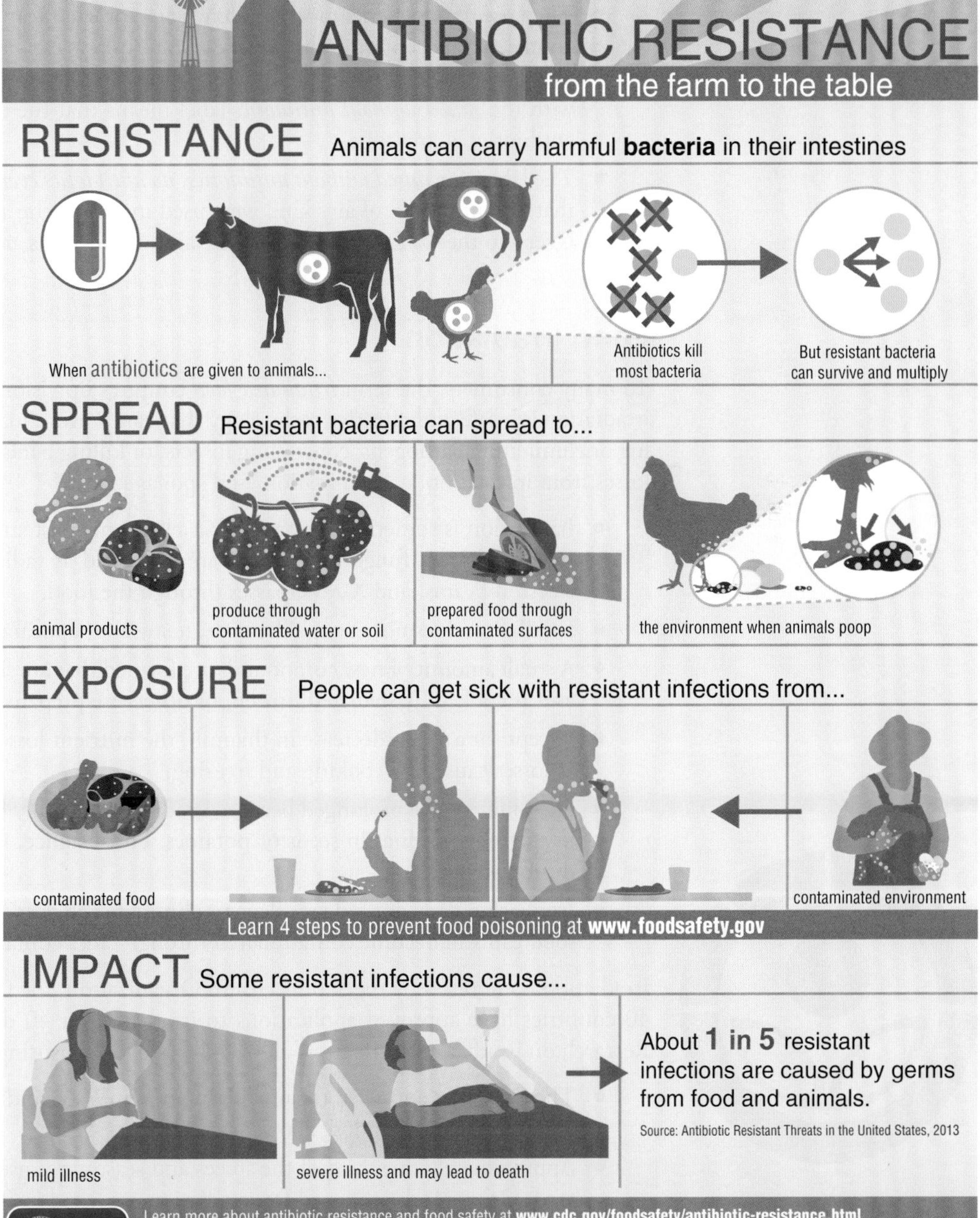

Figure 10.2 ▶ Antibiotic resistance from the farm to the table. (*Source:* Centers for Disease Control and Prevention. [2019, December 11]. *Antibiotic resistance and food safety.* http://www.cdc.gov/foodsafety/challenges/from-farm-to-table.html)

- When food animals are slaughtered, antibiotic-resistant bacteria from the gut can contaminate meat and other animal products.
- Antibiotic-resistant bacteria in manure can contaminate irrigation water, which in turn can contaminate fruits and vegetables.

Since January 2017, federal regulations have prohibited the use of antibiotics in healthy animals for the purpose of promoting weight gain and require a veterinarian's approval before using antibiotics that are important for human health.

Antibiotic-Free Labeling

All animal farming must adhere to strict rules to ensure there are no antibiotic residues in the animal prior to slaughter. *Antibiotic-free* on food labels is not officially defined.

- *Antibiotic-free* does not guarantee the animal does not carry antibiotic-resistant bacteria. All animals have bacteria in their gut, some of which may be resistant.
- The *Organic* label on a meat, poultry, dairy, or egg means no antibiotics were given to the animal. The exception is that chickens and turkeys can be given antibiotics in the hatchery while the chick is still in the egg and on its first day of life. The *Organic* label combined with the *raised without antibiotics* label means that the chicken or turkey were not given antibiotics at any time.
- The labels for *raised without antibiotics, no antibiotics ever,* and *never given antibiotics* mean that no antibiotics of any kind were used in raising the animal. Although documentation is sent to the USDA to support the claim, inspections are not conducted.

Food Irradiation

To many consumers, the term *irradiated food* conjures up visions of radioactive fallout. In truth, irradiation is a safe and effective technology that can prevent many foodborne illnesses by reducing or eliminating pathogens, controlling insects, or killing parasites. Irradiation also reduces food losses from infestation, contamination, and spoilage.

- Irradiation is sometimes referred to as electronic pasteurization, but it does not use heat. Bacteria, mold, fungi, and insects are destroyed as radiant energy, such as gamma rays, electron beams, and X-rays, passes through the food.
- Irradiation does not change the taste, texture, or appearance of food.
- A small amount of new compounds are formed that are similar to the changes seen in food as it is cooked, pasteurized, frozen, or otherwise prepared.
- Except for a slight decrease in thiamin, the nutrient losses are less than or about the same as losses caused by cooking and freezing.
- Shelf life may be prolonged because irradiation kills any living cells that may be contained in the food, such as in seeds or potatoes. For instance, irradiated potatoes do not sprout during storage.
- Irradiation does not hide spoilage or eliminate the need for safe food handling; irradiated food can still become contaminated through cross contamination.

Irradiation is endorsed by the World Health Organization, the CDC, and the USDA. More than 40 countries have approved applications to irradiate over 40 different foods (McHugh, 2019). Research on irradiation as a part of an overall system of ensuring food safety is ongoing.

- The FDA first approved the use of radiation in 1963 and is responsible for establishing the maximum radiation dose allowed on foods.
- Approximately one third of the spices and seasonings used in the United States are irradiated. Other foods approved for irradiation are listed in Box 10.5.
- Federal law requires irradiated food to be labeled with the international symbol of the Radura (Fig. 10.3) and state "treated with irradiation" or "treated by irradiation."

Figure 10.3 ▲
Radura: the international symbol for irradiation.

BOX 10.5 Foods Approved for Irradiation in the United States

- Wheat flour
- Beef and pork
- Crustaceans
- Fresh fruits and vegetables
- Poultry
- Seeds for sprouting
- Shell eggs
- Shellfish
- Spices and seasonings

Source: McHugh, T. (2019). *Realizing the benefits of food irradiation*. https://www.ift.org/news-and-publications/food-technology-magazine/issues/2019/september/columns/processing-food-irradiation

FOOD ACCESS

Food access is influenced by the affordability and proximity of food retailers—concepts that are relative to a consumer's socioeconomic status and access to transportation. The ability to choose a healthy diet is impaired when there is limited access to a variety of culturally appropriate, healthy, affordable foods. Food insecurity and food deserts describe problems of food access.

Food Insecurity

Household food insecurity describes households whose access to adequate food is limited by a lack of money and other resources (Coleman-Jensen et al., 2019). The extent and severity of food insecurity are monitored by the USDA via a nationally representative annual survey. Referring to the year 2018, Coleman-Jensen et al. have reported the following findings:

- An estimated 11.1% of U.S. households were food insecure at least some time during 2018. This figure represents a decline in food insecurity from 11.8% in the previous year.
- In households with very low food security among children, children were hungry, skipped a meal, or did not eat for a whole day because there was not enough money for food.
- Rates of food insecurity were higher than the national average for certain groups: households with incomes near or below the federal poverty line, households with children and particularly households with children headed by single women or men, women and men living alone, Black- and Hispanic-headed households, and households in principal cities.
- About 56% of food-insecure households in the survey reported that within the previous month they had participated in one or more of the three largest federal nutrition assistance programs, including Supplemental Nutrition Assistance Program (SNAP, formerly the Food Stamp Program); Special Supplemental Nutrition Program for Women, Infants, and Children (WIC); and National School Lunch Program.

Food Deserts

Food deserts occur predominately in low-income areas, where a substantial proportion of the residents experience a lack of access to a supermarket. A food desert is defined as living at least half a mile from the nearest supermarket, supercenter, or large grocery store in an urban area or more than 10 miles from a supermarket in a rural area (USDA, ERS, 2019). Without ready access to supermarkets, access to fresh fruits, vegetables, whole grains, low-fat milk, and other healthy whole foods is low. Poor access to healthy foods could lead to poor diet quality and increased risk of chronic diseases such as obesity or diabetes.

Data from USDA's National Household Food Acquisition and Purchase Survey revealed that both low-income and higher-income households consider store characteristics other than proximity when deciding where to shop (Ver Ploeg & Rahkovsky, 2016). Households often do not shop at the nearest supermarket to obtain groceries regardless of whether the mode of transportation is driving, walking, biking, or public transit (Ver Ploeg & Rahkovsky, 2016).

SNAP households are more sensitive to price than proximity, which may explain why households bypass the closest store for stores farther away that offer lower prices (Ver Ploeg & Rahkovsky, 2016).

- The prices of different food groups have a larger effect on what is purchased than does access. In fact, the effects of food access were negligible when price and demographic factors were accounted for.
- Low income is more strongly associated with buying unhealthy food than living in an area with limited access to supermarkets (Rahkovsky & Snyder, 2015).
- Results suggest that improving access to healthy foods itself will not likely have a major impact on diet quality (Ver Ploeg & Rahkovsky, 2016).
- The cost of food, income available to spend on food, consumer knowledge about nutrition, and food preferences may be more important factors in food purchase decisions than access.

Remember Paul. He drives to a big-box store to buy groceries in order to make his food dollars stretch. He is a novice cook at best, so he relies on sandwiches made from deli meats, boxed macaroni and cheese, and frozen dinners, which he knows are expensive. What advice would you give Paul about food purchasing? What federal nutrition assistance programs may he be eligible for?

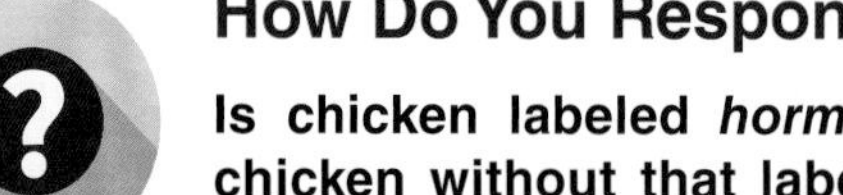

How Do You Respond?

Is chicken labeled *hormone-free* safer and more healthy than chicken without that label? All animals naturally produce hormones, so there is no such thing as *hormone-free* chicken or any other animals. However, the USDA prohibits the use of hormones in raising chicken, so no chickens are given hormones—whether or not that is stated on the label. To increase transparency, any chicken label that states *no hormones added* must also include the phrase *federal regulations prohibit the use of hormones.*

Can you prevent foodborne illness by washing produce? Although washing produce—even varieties that you peel—is recommended, it cannot guarantee food safety. For instance, it is difficult to remove sticky bacteria from leafy greens like spinach. Even triple-washed or thoroughly washed ready-to-eat bags of spinach, lettuce, and mixed greens may be contaminated with bacteria because cleaning processes that use chlorinated water kill only 90% to 95% of microbes when performed correctly. And with other produce, such as melon, mango, or apple, bacteria might have migrated to the inside of the fruit, such as traveling through the apple core to the interior, so washing will not remove it. Safe food handling at home is important but cannot guarantee safety.

REVIEW CASE STUDY

You have been asked to present a class on consumer-related interests regarding food for young mothers. They want to hear about organic foods, GMOs, antibiotics, and foodborne illness.

- List the major points you would cover for each topic.
- What points would you emphasize?
- Do you have a bias on any of these topics?
- How do you deal with personal bias when imparting information?
- What additional information do you think you need to make a complete and balanced presentation on the topics?
- Are there any additional topics of interest you think should be included? Why?

STUDY QUESTIONS

1 What percentage of ingredients must be organic for a product to bear the USDA organic seal and state that it is *organic*?
   a. 70%
   b. 80%
   c. 95%
   d. 100%

2 A client wants to eat more conventional functional foods. Which of the following would the nurse recommend?
   a. omega-3 fatty acid–enriched milk and orange juice
   b. yogurt and cheese
   c. rice and enriched pasta
   d. berries and green leafy vegetables

3 The client asks the nurse whether GMOs are safe. Which of the following is the nurse's best response?
   a. "Not enough is known about GMOs to know if they have a negative impact on health."
   b. "GMOs probably cause reproductive health issues and may cause gene mutations. It is best to avoid them."
   c. "As a group, GMOs do not pose health risks."
   d. "It is best to try to avoid them if you can."

4 Which pathogen is not killed by hand sanitizers?
   a. norovirus
   b. *Salmonella*
   c. *E. coli*
   d. *Listeria*

5 A client asks how they can minimize their risk of foodborne illness. Which of the following should the nurse include in their response as the best way to reduce the risk? Select all that apply.
   a. "Wash your hands before and after handling food."
   b. "Rely on organically grown foods as much as possible."
   c. "Cook foods thoroughly."
   d. "Avoid cross contamination by using separate surfaces for meats and foods that will be eaten raw."

6 What is the best response to a client's question about if organic food is worth the extra cost?
   a. "Is there anything more important to spend money on than your health?"
   b. "There is no difference in pesticide levels and nutritional value of organically grown foods compared to conventional foods."
   c. "Buying organic foods is an individual decision; some may have more nutritional value than their conventional counterparts, and they do have lower pesticide levels."
   d. "It is worth it to buy organic produce but not organic meats."

7 A client asks how they can avoid meat and poultry that are given antibiotics. What is the nurse's best response?
   a. "Meat and poultry labeled as *organic* cannot be given antibiotics."
   b. "There is no way to avoid meat and poultry that have been given antibiotics."
   c. "Buy meat and poultry labeled as *natural* or *all natural*."
   d. "Buy meat and poultry labeled as *American Humane Association*."

8 A client asks how they can avoid buying foods that are GE. What is the nurse's best response?
   a. "Foods labeled as *organic* cannot be genetically engineered."
   b. "There is no way to avoid genetically engineered foods."
   c. "Buy foods that have the Radura symbol on them. This symbol means they cannot be genetically engineered."
   d. "Buy foods labeled as *natural* because they cannot be genetically engineered."

CHAPTER SUMMARY CONSUMER INTERESTS AND CONCERNS

Consumer Information and Misinformation

The field of nutrition is rapidly changing and growing. Nutrition misinformation is everywhere and can be difficult to refute in a client who is convinced that what they know is accurate.

Consumer-Related Interests

- Functional foods contain substances that appear to enhance health beyond their basic nutritional value. Plants that are rich in phytochemicals are natural functional foods.
- Organically grown foods are regulated by USDA standards.
  - They are not bacteriologically safer than their conventional counterparts.
  - They have more phytochemicals and maybe other nutrients, but it is difficult to measure and the clinical significance is unknown.
  - They have lower levels of pesticides than conventionally grown foods and cannot be GMOs.
  - Organic animals cannot be given antibiotics or hormones and must be raised on 100% organic feed.

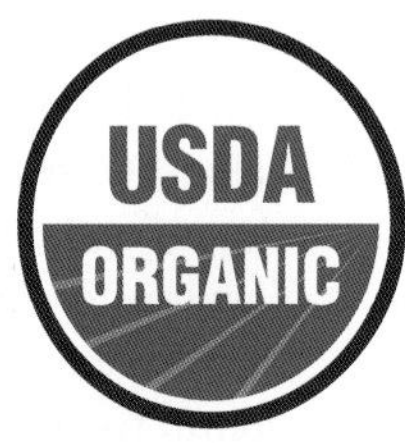

- Foodborne illnesses sicken thousands of Americans annually.
  - Norovirus is often the most implicated pathogen in foodborne illness outbreaks.
  - Common food vehicles for foodborne illnesses are turkey, chicken, fruits, and green leafy vegetables.
  - Handwashing, temperature control, and avoiding cross contamination help prevent foodborne illness.

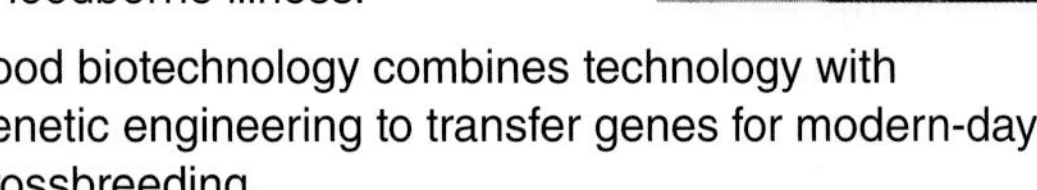

- Food biotechnology combines technology with genetic engineering to transfer genes for modern-day crossbreeding.
  - GE can produce more nutritious plants that are better at resisting disease, drought, and salty conditions.
  - The FDA controls GMO foods through a voluntary process of approval.
  - Numerous scientific organizations endorse GE; consumers are much less accepting.
  - Studies do not show that there are adverse health effects from GMOs.
  - Superweeds have developed from the overuse of pesticides delivered on GMO crops that have been made resistant to it.

Antibiotics. Routine use of antibiotics in healthy animals to promote growth or prevent infection has been linked to antibiotic resistance that can be passed to humans through the food supply. Antibiotic use in healthy animals for the purpose of promoting weight gain is now prohibited by federal law.

Irradiation is used to reduce or eliminate pathogens that can cause foodborne illness. The food remains uncooked and completely free of any radiation residues.

Food Access

Food access refers to the affordability and access to healthy food.

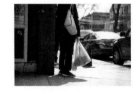

- Food-insecure households have limited access to food due to lack of money or other resources.
- Food deserts occur in low-income areas with limited access to supermarkets.
  - Increasing access to healthy food itself is not likely to improve diet quality.
  - The price of food, available income, nutrition knowledge, and food preferences may have a greater effect on food choices than access.

Figure sources: *shutterstock.com/wavebreakmedia and shutterstock.com/Erin Deleon*

Student Resources on thePoint®

For additional learning materials, activate the code in the front of this book at https://thePoint.lww.com/activate

Websites

Reliable Nutrition Information

Academy of Nutrition and Dietetics at www.eatright.org
American Cancer Society at www.cancer.org
American Council on Science and Health at www.acsh.org
American Diabetes Association at www.diabetes.org
Center for Science in the Public Interest at www.cspinet.org
Health on the Net Foundation at www.hon.ch
International Food Information Council at www.foodinsight.org
National Cancer Institute, National Institutes of Health at www.nci.nih.gov
National Heart, Lung, and Blood Institute, National Institutes of Health at www.nhlbi.nih.gov
New Wellness Consumer Health Information at www.netwellness.org
Nutrition.gov at www.nutrition.gov
U.S. Department of Agriculture Food and Nutrition Information Center at fnic.nal.usda.gov
U.S. Department of Health and Human Services Healthfinder at www.healthfinder.gov
U.S. Food and Drug Administration Center for Food Safety and Applied Nutrition at https://www.fda.gov/about-fda/office-foods-and-veterinary-medicine/center-food-safety-and-applied-nutrition-cfsan

Food Safety

Partnership for Food Safety Education at www.fightbac.org
U.S. Food and Drug Administration at www.fda.gov

References

American Council on Science and Health. (2016). *Why ACSH supports GMOs and biotechnology.* https://www.acsh.org/news/2016/11/18/why-acsh-supports-gmos-and-biotechnology-10459

Biotechnology Innovation Organization. (2016). *Biotechnology Industry Organization changes name to Biotechnology Innovation Organization.* https://www.businesswire.com/news/home/20160104006245/en/Biotechnology-Industry-Organization-Biotechnology-Innovation-Organization

Brody, J. (2018). Are GMOS foods safe? *New York Times.* https://www.nytimes.com/2018/04/23/well/eat/are-gmo-foods-safe.html

Brown, E. (2016). Go ahead: Eat your genetically modified vegetables. *Zocalo Public Square.* https://www.zocalopublicsquare.org/2016/12/15/go-ahead-eat-genetically-modified-vegetables/events/the-takeaway/

Centers for Disease Control and Prevention (CDC). (2018). *Food and food animals.* https://www.cdc.gov/drugresistance/food.html

Centers for Disease Control and Prevention (CDC). (2019). *Surveillance for foodborne disease outbreaks, United States, 2017, Annual report.* https://www.cdc.gov/fdoss/pdf/2017_FoodBorneOutbreaks_508.pdf

Coleman-Jensen, A., Rabbit, M., Gregory, C., & Singh, A. (2019). *Household food security in the United States in 2015 (ERR-275).* U.S. Department of Agriculture, Economic Research Service. https://www.ers.usda.gov/webdocs/publications/94849/err-270.pdf?v=963.1

Crowe, K., & Francis, C. (2013). Position of the academy of nutrition and dietetics: Functional foods. *Journal of the Academy of Nutrition and Dietetics, 113*(8), 1096–1103. https://doi.org/10.1016/j.jand.2013.06.002

Dubock, A. (2017). An overview of agriculture, nutrition and fortification, supplementation and biofortification: Golden Rice as an example for enhancing micronutrient intake. *Agriculture & Food Security, 6*(59). https://doi.org/10.1186/s40066-017-0135-3

Gomiero, T. (2018). Food quality assessment in organic vs. conventional agricultural produce: Findings and issues. *Applied Soil Ecology, 123,* 714–728. https://doi.org/10.1016/j.apsoil.2017.10.014

Harvey, R., Zakjour, C., & Gould, L. (2016). Foodborne disease outbreaks associated with organic foods in the United States. *Journal of Food Protection, 79*(11), 1953–1958. https://doi.org/10.4315/0362-028X.JFP-16-204

Hurtado-Barroso, S., Tresserra-Rimbau, A., Vallverdú-Queralt, A., & Lamuela-Raventós, R. M. (2019). Organic food and the impact on human health. *Critical Reviews in Food Science and Nutrition, 59*(4), 704–714. https://doi.org/10.1080/10408398.2017.1394815

International Food Information Council Foundation. (2019). *2019 food & health survey.* https://foodinsight.org/wp-content/uploads/2019/05/IFIC-Foundation-2019-Food-and-Health-Report-FINAL.pdf

International Service for the Acquisition of Agri-Biotech Applications. (2018). *ISAAA Brief54-2018: Executive summary.* http://www.isaaa.org/resources/publications/briefs/54/executivesummary/default.asp

Litwin, N., Clifford, J., & Johnson, S. (2018). *Functional foods for health.* https://extension.colostate.edu/topic-areas/nutrition-food-safety-health/functional-foods-for-health-9-391/

McHugh, T. (2019). *Realizing the benefits of food irradiation.* https://www.ift.org/news-and-publications/food-technology-magazine/issues/2019/september/columns/processing-food-irradiation

Norris, M. (2015). *Will GMOs hurt my body? The public's concerns and how scientists have addressed them.* http://sitn.hms.harvard.edu/flash/2015/will-gmos-hurt-my-body/

Organic Trade Association. (2019). *US organic sales break through $50 billion mark in 2018.* https://ota.com/news/press-releases/20699

Pew Research Center. (2015). *Public and scientists' view on science and society.* https://www.pewresearch.org/science/2015/01/29/public-and-scientists-views-on-science-and-society/

Rahkovsky, I., & Snyder, S. (2015). *Food choices and store proximity (EER-195).* http://www.ers.usda.gov/media/1909239/err195.pdf

Raman, R. (2018). The impact of Genetically Modified (GM) crops in modern agriculture: A review. *GM Crops & Food, 8*(4), 195–208. https://doi.org/10.1080/21645698.2017.1413522

U.S. Department of Agriculture. (2019). *BE disclosure.* https://www.ams.usda.gov/rules-regulations/be

U.S. Department of Agriculture, Economic Research Service. (2019). *Documentation.* https://www.ers.usda.gov/data-products/food-access-research-atlas/documentation/

U.S. Food and Drug Administration. (2020). *Understanding new plant varieties.* https://fda.gov/food/food-new-plant-varieties/understanding-new-plant-varieties

Ver Ploeg, M., & Rahkovsky, I. (2016). *Recent evidence on the effects of food store access on food choice and diet quality.* https://www.ers.usda.gov/amber-waves/2016/may/recent-evidence-on-the-effects-of-food-store-access-on-food-choice-and-diet-quality/

Chapter 11

Cultural and Religious Influences on Food and Nutrition

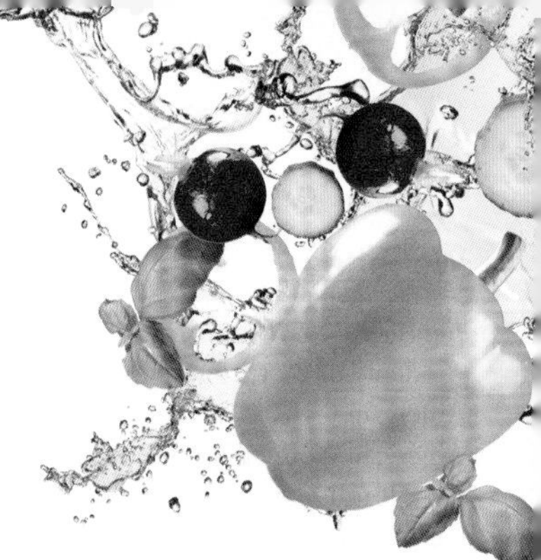

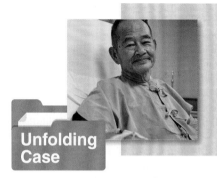

Unfolding Case

Phouvong Chanthavong

Phouvong is a 61-year-old man who immigrated with his wife and two daughters to the United States from Laos at the age of 35. He does not speak English, but his daughters are bilingual. He has just been admitted to the hospital for pneumonia, where it was discovered he also has type 2 diabetes.

Learning Objectives

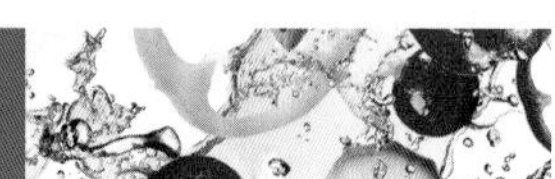

Upon completion of this chapter, you will be able to:

1 Suggest ways to eat healthy while eating out.
2 Describe the characteristics of traditional food practices for different cultural groups in the United States.
3 Discuss the nutrition-related health concerns of different cultural groups in the United States.
4 Explain the general ways in which people's food choices change as they become acculturated to a new area.
5 Summarize dietary laws followed by major world religions.

Food and nutrition rank on the same level as air as basic necessities of life in Maslow's hierarchy of needs. Obviously, death eventually occurs without food. But unlike air, food does so much more than simply sustain life. Food is loaded with personal, social, and cultural meanings that define our food values, beliefs, and customs. The concept that food nourishes the mind as well as the body broadens nutrition to an art as well as a science. Nutrition is not simply a matter of food or no food but rather a question of what kind, how much, how often, and why. It is important to balance wants with needs and pleasure with health in order to nourish the body, mind, and soul.

This chapter discusses what America eats and the impact of **culture** on food choices. Traditional food practices, changes in food practices related to acculturation, and nutrition-related health problems of major cultural subgroups in the United States are presented. Religious food practices are outlined.

Culture
encompasses the total way of life of a particular population or community at a given time.

AMERICAN CUISINE

American cuisine is a rich and complex melting pot of foods and cooking methods. They have been adapted and adopted from cuisines brought to the United States by immigrants beginning with early settlers from northern and southern Europe. Cuisines from around the globe melded as the influx of immigrants continued. Today, it is difficult to determine which foods are truly

Table 11.1 American Cuisine as Influenced by Advances in Technology, Societal Changes in Lifestyle, and Product Innovation

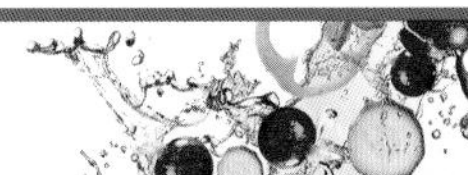

Time Period	Key Characteristics	Products Introduced	Popular Dishes
Late 1800s	Appliances (iceboxes, cook stoves), kitchen tools (apple parers), and tin (not heavy cast iron)	Fleischman's yeast, Coca-Cola, Heinz ketchup, Jell-O	Cornbread, meat stew, fried oysters, boiled mutton
1900–1940	New foods and flavors introduced by waves of immigrants Home economists instructed housewives about food nutrition, measuring ingredients, and meal planning	Crisco shortening, canned soups, canned tuna, Wonder Bread, Birdseye brand frozen foods, Spam	Pineapple upside-down cake, Jell-O molds, chop suey, baked ham, meat croquettes, meat loaf
1940s	Technology improved freezing, canning, and dehydration Food rationing from 1942 to 1947 required making do with less, such as meatless meals and eggless cakes	Pillsbury hot roll mix, cake mixes, M & Ms, frozen french fries, frozen orange juice concentrate	Goulash, chipped beef on toast, liver loaf, homemade soups, mashed potatoes, meat and potato patties
1950s	Postwar golden age. Keeping house and entertaining were in vogue, increased popularity of frozen foods	Rice-A-Roni, Minute rice, Swanson TV dinners, marshmallow peeps, Tang, Sweet 'n Low	Tuna noodle casserole, green bean casserole, Swedish meat balls, chicken or beef pot pie, Baked Alaska
1960s	Women began working outside the home, fast food is a dinner treat, Julia Child is popular	Instant mashed potatoes Cool Whip, Shake 'n Bake, SpaghettiOs, Gatorade, diet Pepsi	Coq au Vin, beef bourguignon, iceberg wedge salad, Buffalo wings, Beef Wellington
1970s	Natural food movement, vegetarianism, health food stores, TV cooking shows	Hamburger helper, stove top stuffing mix, Egg McMuffins, Quaker oats granola, Morton's salt substitute, Ben and Jerry's ice cream	Ziti casserole, pasta primavera, slow cooker beef stew, fondue meals, quiche, Watergate salad
1980s	Casual gourmet is popular, wine and cheese parties, upscale pizza, authentic ethnic, record number of women in the workforce	Boboli premade pizza crust, prewashed bagged salad greens, Jell-O pudding pops, Snapple	Blackened Cajun seafood, French onion soup, Tex-Mex tacos, Chinese chicken salad, pasta salad
1990s	The World Wide Web, Food Network channel, decadent desserts, fat-free grocery items	Snackwell cookies, Boca burgers (soy), Lay's baked potato crisps, Promise Ultra	Sushi, stuffed crust pizza, focaccia, sun-dried tomatoes, goat cheese on salads, molten chocolate cake
2000s	Comfort food comeback, Super-Size Me documentary, high obesity rates, organic and farm-to-table movements	Omega-3 eggs; turkey Spam, tuna and brown rice in pouches, G2 sports drink	Macaroni and cheese, anything bacon-wrapped, instant pot chicken, roasted beets, kale salad, sliders, avocado toast, poke

Source: Gagliardi, N. (n.d.). *Dinner through the decades*. https://www.familycircle.com/recipes/seasonal-recipes/dinner-through-the-decades/; Olver, L. (2015, February 27). *FAQs: Popular 20th century American foods*. Food Timeline. https://www.foodtimeline.org/fooddecades.html; Petreycik, C. (2018, August 14). *The 40 biggest food trends of the past 40 years*. Food & Wine. https://www.foodandwine.com/news/40-biggest-food-trends

American and which are an adaptation from other cultures. Swiss steak, Russian dressing, and chili con carne are American inventions. Cross-cultural food creations, such as Tex-Mex wontons and tofu lasagna, reaffirm the ongoing melting-pot nature of American cuisine. American cuisine is also shaped by advances in technology, societal changes in lifestyle, and product innovation (Table 11.1).

Food Away from Home

Convenience Food broadly defined as any product that saves time in food preparation, ranging from bagged fresh salad mixes to frozen packaged complete meals.

Convenience foods and meals from restaurants (either dine-in or takeout) are a driving force in current food trends. Food away from home (FAFH) accounts for more than 40% of food spending (Binkley & Liu, 2019). The National Health and Nutrition Examination Survey data show that among men and women age 20 and older, 33% of total calorie intake comes from food and beverages consumed away from home (U.S. Department of Agriculture, Agricultural Research Service, 2018).

Numerous studies have found that the nutritional quality of FAFH is lower than that of food consumed at home. For instance, Nguyen and Powel (2014) found that both fast-food and full-service restaurant food intake among adults is associated with significant increases in the intake of calories, sugar, saturated fat, and sodium. Conversely, eating home-cooked meals more

BOX 11.1 Food at Home and Food Away from Home: Nutrition Differences

- FAFH tends to consist of less healthy foods and more calorically dense types of food within all food groups, such as white potatoes instead of sweet potatoes and high-fat burgers instead of low-fat burgers.
- The higher caloric density of FAFH is partly due to higher-fat cooking methods such as frying instead of baking.
- Meat and soft drinks are more important in FAFH meals.
- Fruit and milk are seldom consumed as part of FAFH.
- FAFH is estimated to be responsible for the increasing consumption of potatoes, chicken, beef, lettuce, and cheese.
- Evidence shows that more frequent consumers of FAFH tend to have less healthy home diets than non-FAFH consumers, suggesting that FAFH diners select less healthy foods regardless of the source.

Source: Binkley, J., & Liu, Y. (2019). Food at home and away from home: Commodity composition, nutrition differences, and differences in consumers. *Agricultural and Resource Economics Review*, *48*(2), 221–252. https://www.cambridge.org/core/services/aop-cambridge-core/content/view/FD229E025ACD524B31C6D1DA48AFD2DF/S1068280519000017a.pdf/div-class-title-food-at-home-and-away-from-home-commodity-composition-nutrition-differences-and-differences-in-consumers-div.pdf

than five times per week is associated not only with better diet quality but also with a greater likelihood of having normal-range body mass index (BMI) and percentage of body fat (Mills et al., 2017). Box 11.1 features findings on FAFH.

Eating out has evolved from a special treat to a regular event, so planning and menu savvy are needed to ensure that eating out is consistent with eating healthy and not contrary to it. Tips for eating healthy while eating out appear in Box 11.2. *Best bet* choices from various ethnic restaurants are listed in Box 11.3.

BOX 11.2 Tips for Eating Healthy While Eating Out

Plan Ahead

- Choose the restaurant carefully so you know there are reasonable choices available.
- Check online or call ahead to inquire about menu selections. This is an especially important strategy when the location is not a matter of choice but, rather, a requirement such as for business luncheons or conferences. It may be possible to make a special request ahead of time.

Don't Arrive Starving

- People become much less discriminating in their food choices when they are hungry.
- Eating a small, high-fiber snack an hour or so before going out to dinner, such as whole wheat crackers with peanut butter or a piece of fresh fruit with milk, can take the edge off hunger without bankrupting healthy eating.

Balance the Rest of the Day

- When eating out *is* an occasion, such as for a birthday or anniversary celebration, make healthier choices the rest of the day to compensate for a planned indulgence.

Practice Portion Control

- Order the smallest size meat available.
- Create a doggie bag before eating; if you wait until the end of the meal, there may not be any left.
- Order regular size, not biggie size or supersize.
- Order a la carte. Is a value meal a "better value" if it undermines your attempt to eat healthily?
- Order a half portion when available.
- Order two (carefully chosen) appetizers in place of an entrée, or order an appetizer and split an entrée with a companion.

Know the Terminology

Calorie-laden words to watch out for include the following:

- Buttered
- Battered
- Breaded
- Deep fried
- Au gratin
- Creamy
- Crispy

(continued)

BOX 11.2 Tips for Eating Healthy While Eating Out (continued)

- Alfredo
- Bisque
- Hollandaise
- Parmigiana
- Béarnaise
- En croute
- Escalloped
- French fried
- Pan fried
- Rich
- Sautéed
- With gravy, with mayonnaise, with cheese

Less fatty terms are *baked*, *braised*, *broiled*, *cooked in its own juice*, *grilled*, *lightly sautéed*, *poached*, *roasted*, and *steamed*.

Beware of Hidden Fats, such as

- High-fat meats
- Nuts
- Cream and full-fat milk
- Full-fat salad dressings and mayonnaise
- Sauces and gravies

Make Special Requests

- Order sauces and gravies "on the side."
- Ask that lower-fat items be substituted for high-fat items (e.g., a baked potato instead of french fries).
- Substitute brown rice for white rice.
- Request an alternate cooking method (e.g., broiled instead of fried).

BOX 11.3 Best Bet Choices from Fast-Food and Ethnic Restaurants

Fast Foods

English muffins or bagels with spreads on the side
Oatmeal
Butter, margarine, or syrups on the side—not added to food
Baked potato—plain or with reduced-fat or fat-free dressings or salsa
Pretzels or baked chips
Regular, small, or junior sizes
Ketchup, mustard, relish, BBQ sauce, and fresh vegetables as toppings
Grilled chicken sandwiches without "special sauce"
Veggie burger
Small roast beef on roll
Corn tortilla burritos with chicken, beans, veggies, and guacamole
Grilled chicken nuggets
Fruit 'n yogurt parfait
Lean, 6-in. subs on whole-grain rolls with extra vegetables
Side salads with reduced-fat or fat-free dressings
Salads with grilled chicken
Low-fat or nonfat milk
Fresh fruit
Specialty coffees with skim milk

Pizza

Thin crust
Vegetables: onions, spinach, tomatoes, broccoli, mushrooms, peppers
Lean meats: Canadian bacon, ham, grilled chicken, shrimp, crab meat
Half-cheese pizza
Salad as a side dish

Mexican

Sauces: salsa, mole, picante, enchilada, pico de gallo
Guacamole in place of cheese and sour cream
Black bean soup, gazpacho
Soft, nonfried corn tortillas, as in bean burritos or enchiladas
Refried beans (without lard)
Arroz con pollo (chicken with rice)
Grilled meat, fish, or chicken
Steamed vegetables
Soft-shell chicken, shrimp, or veggie tacos
A la carte or half entrée
Fajitas: chicken, seafood, vegetable, beef
Flan (usually a small portion)

Chinese

Hot-and-sour soup, wonton soup
Chicken chow mein
Chicken or beef chop suey
Moo Shu vegetables
Moo Goo Gai Pan
Buddha's Delight
Chicken lettuce wraps
Shrimp with garlic sauce or black bean sauce
Stir-fried and teriyaki dishes
Steamed rice instead of fried
Steamed spring rolls
Tofu
Steamed dumplings and other dim sum instead of egg rolls
Sauce on the side

Italian

Minestrone
Garden salad; vinegar and oil dressing
Cioppino (seafood stew)
Breadsticks, bruschetta, Italian bread
Sauces: red clam, marinara, wine, cacciatore, fra diavolo, marsala
Fresh fish, shrimp, veal, chicken without breading
Pasta primavera

BOX 11.3 Best Bet Choices from Fast-Food and Ethnic Restaurants (continued)

Choose vegetables for a side dish instead of pasta or potatoes
Limit "unlimited" bread or breadsticks
Italian ice, sorbet, or fruit

Indian

Raw vegetable salads, Mulligatawny soup (lentil soup)
Tandoori meats
Condiments: fruits and vegetable chutneys, raita (cucumber and yogurt sauce)
Lentil and chickpea curries
Kebobs (with brown rice instead of pilaf)
Aloo Gobi
Chana Masala
Naan (bread baked in tandoori oven)
Dal

Japanese

Edamame
Miso soup (high in sodium)
Sashimi, sushi, norimaki, temaki
Sushi—cooked varieties include imitation crab, cooked shrimp, scrambled egg
Most combinations of grilled meats or seafood
Teriyaki chicken, tofu, or seafood
Soba noodles
Green tea

Greek

Gigantes Plaki (large white beans baked in tomato sauce)
Avgolemono (Greek chicken noodle soup)
Lentil soup
Greek salad, tabouli
Souvlaki salad or sandwich made with pork, chicken, lamb, or beef
Shish kebabs
Pita bread
Make a meal of appetizers: baba ghanoush (smoked eggplant), hummus (mashed chickpeas), dolma (stuffed grape leaves), and tabbouleh (cracked wheat salad). Olive oil is often poured on the baba ghanoush, hummus, and other foods, so ask for it on the side.

THE EFFECT OF CULTURE

Culture has a profound and unconscious effect on food choices. Yet, within, among, and across cultural groups, individuals or subgroups may behave differently from the socially standardized **foodway** because of age, sex, state of health, household structure, or socioeconomic status. Race, ethnicity, and geographic region are often inaccurately assumed to be synonymous with culture. This misconception leads to stereotypic grouping, such as assuming that all Jewish people adhere to orthodox food laws or that all Americans from the South eat sausage, biscuits, and gravy. **Subgroups** within a culture display a unique range of cultural characteristics that affect food intake and nutritional status. What is edible, the role of food, how food is prepared and seasoned, the symbolic use of food, and when and how food is eaten are among the many characteristics defined by culture.

Foodway
an all-encompassing term that refers to all aspects of food, including what is edible, the role of certain foods in the diet, how food is prepared, the use of foods, the number and timing of daily meals, how food is eaten, and health beliefs related to food.

Subgroups
unique cultural groups that exist within a dominant culture.

The characteristics of culture are that it

- has an inherent value system that defines what is considered "normal,"
- is learned, not instinctive,
- is passed from generation to generation,
- has an unconscious influence on its members, and
- resists change but is not static.

Culture Defines What Is Edible

Culture determines what is **edible** and what is **inedible.** To be labeled a food, an item must be readily available, safe, and nutritious enough to support reproduction. However, cultures do not define as *edible* all sources of nutrients that meet those criteria. For instance, in the United States, horse meat, insects, and dog meat are not considered food, even though they meet the food criteria. Culture overrides flavor in determining what is offensive or unacceptable. For example, you may like a food (e.g., rattlesnake) until you know what it is; this reflects disliking the *idea* of the food rather than the actual food itself. An unconscious food selection decision process appears in Figure 11.1.

Edible
foods that are part of an individual's diet.

Inedible
foods that are usually poisonous or taboo.

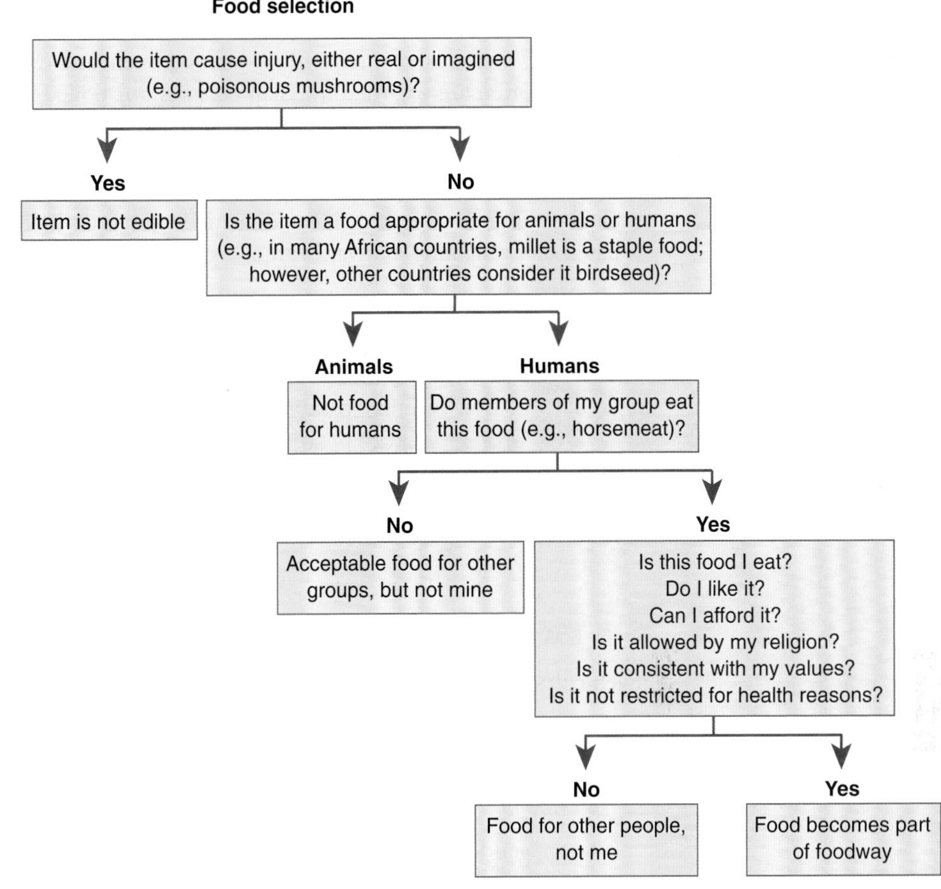

Figure 11.1 ▶ **Food selection and decision-making.**

The Role of Certain Foods in the Diet

Every culture ranks food based on cost and availability.

Core Foods
the important and consistently eaten foods that form the foundation of the diet. They are the dietary staples.

- Core or staple foods serve as the foundation of the diet. They are usually bland, inexpensive, easy to prepare, and provide a significant source of calories.
- **Core foods** are typically complex carbohydrates, such as cereal grains (rice, wheat, millet, corn), starchy tubers (potatoes, yams, taro, cassava), and starchy vegetables (plantain or green bananas).

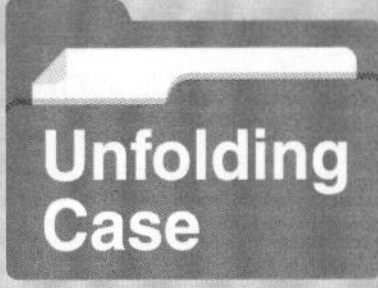

Consider Phouvong. A core food in his eating pattern is sticky rice, a type of rice referred to as glutinous because it holds together when picked up, not because it contains gluten. Through an interpreter, the nurse learns that Phouvong eats a traditional Laotian eating pattern and will not eat American food. The only food he eats that is not prepared by his wife is prepared by other Laotians in his tightly knit community. What information would be important to obtain in order to meet his nutritional needs in a culturally appropriate manner?

Secondary Foods
foods that are widespread in the diet but not eaten consistently.

Peripheral, or Occasional, Foods
foods that are infrequently consumed.

Secondary foods are foods that are widely consumed but not on a daily basis. Examples of secondary foods are vegetables, legumes, nuts, fish, eggs, and meats.

Peripheral, or occasional, foods are eaten sporadically and are typically based on an individual's preference, not on cultural norms. They may be foods that are reserved for special occasions, not readily available, or not generally well tolerated (as is the case with milk among Asian Americans).

How Food Is Prepared and Seasoned

Traditional methods of preparation vary between and within cultural groups. For instance, vegetables often are stir-fried in Asian cultures but boiled in Hispanic or Latinx cultures. What is deemed a healthy cooking method in the United States, such as baking and grilling, may be seen by other groups as causing an undesirable change in the nature of the food (Carr, 2012). Traditional seasonings may be the distinguishing feature between one culture's food and another's, such as garam masala in Indian cooking and lemon grass in Thai cuisine. The choice of seasonings is based on availability and varies among geographic regions and seasons.

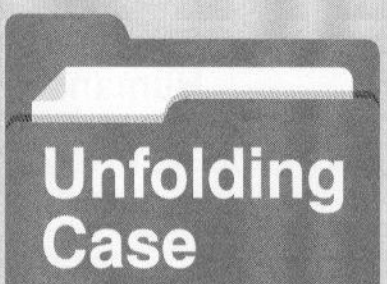

Recall Phouvong. A Laotian comfort food is pho, a beef broth–based soup that is made by boiling the broth and then adding sliced raw beef with the idea that the broth cooks the meat. His wife is smuggling pho, sticky rice, and a variety of other foods into the hospital because he will not eat American food. His wife has been hiding the food in his bedside table to avoid getting in trouble. What should the nurse do?

Symbolic Use of Foods

Each culture has food customs and bestows symbolism. Culture defines that foods

- are served as meals versus snacks,
- are used in celebration,
- provide comfort,
- are gendered as feminine (e.g., salad) or masculine (e.g., steak),
- express love, are used to reward or punish, display piety, or express moral sentiments, and
- demonstrate belongingness to a group or proclaim the separateness of a group.

When and How Food Is Eaten

All cultures eat at least once a day. Some may eat five or more meals each day. Food may be eaten with chopsticks, a knife and fork, or fingers. In the United States, eating with bad manners may be associated with animal behavior, as in eating like a pig, chewing like a cow, or wolfing down food.

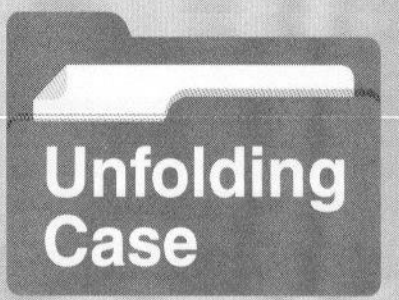

Think of Phouvong. He eats sticky rice with his hands and sometimes dips it in fish paste or pho. Are you able to remain non-judgmental in your reaction? What measures can you take to help minimize Phouvong's risk of foodborne illness?

Cultural Values

Cultural values define desirable and undesirable personal and public behavior and social interactions. Understanding the client's cultural values and their impact on health and food choices facilitates cross-cultural nutrition care. Table 11.2 highlights the contrast between selected American cultural values and values of more traditional cultures.

Role of Food in Health or Disease

Almost all cultures define certain foods that promote wellness, cure disease, or impart medicinal properties. For instance, many people who are Chinese believe that health is a balance between yin and yang forces in the body. Diseases caused by yin forces are treated with yang-force foods and *vice versa*.

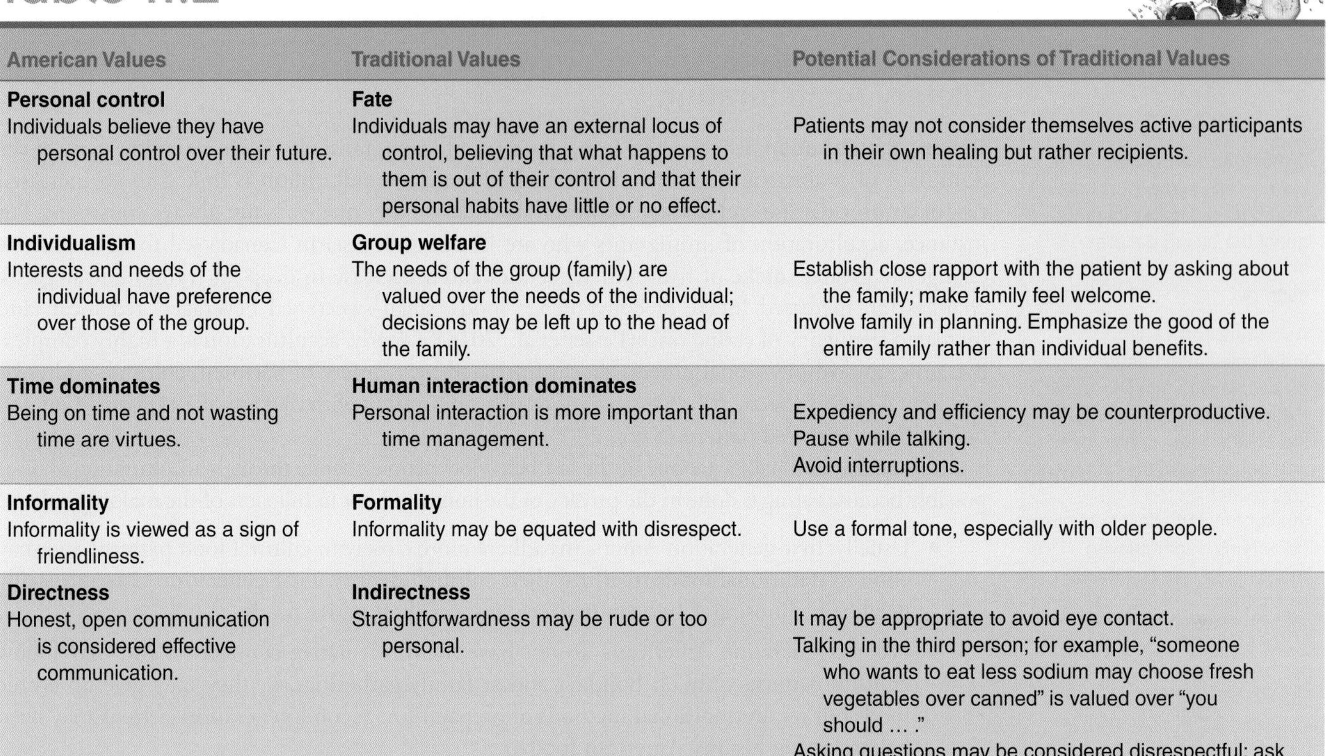

Table 11.2 A Contrast of Cultural Values

American Values	Traditional Values	Potential Considerations of Traditional Values
Personal control Individuals believe they have personal control over their future.	**Fate** Individuals may have an external locus of control, believing that what happens to them is out of their control and that their personal habits have little or no effect.	Patients may not consider themselves active participants in their own healing but rather recipients.
Individualism Interests and needs of the individual have preference over those of the group.	**Group welfare** The needs of the group (family) are valued over the needs of the individual; decisions may be left up to the head of the family.	Establish close rapport with the patient by asking about the family; make family feel welcome. Involve family in planning. Emphasize the good of the entire family rather than individual benefits.
Time dominates Being on time and not wasting time are virtues.	**Human interaction dominates** Personal interaction is more important than time management.	Expediency and efficiency may be counterproductive. Pause while talking. Avoid interruptions.
Informality Informality is viewed as a sign of friendliness.	**Formality** Informality may be equated with disrespect.	Use a formal tone, especially with older people.
Directness Honest, open communication is considered effective communication.	**Indirectness** Straightforwardness may be rude or too personal.	It may be appropriate to avoid eye contact. Talking in the third person; for example, "someone who wants to eat less sodium may choose fresh vegetables over canned" is valued over "you should … ." Asking questions may be considered disrespectful; ask questions judiciously.

Obtaining candid information about health beliefs requires health professionals to be culturally knowledgeable and sensitive and to ask questions that are open ended and nonjudgmental (Hagan et al., 2017) (Box 11.4).

Body Image

Culture also shapes body image. In the United States, you can never be too thin, and thinness, particularly in women, is often equated with beauty and status. Obesity and being overweight may be viewed as a character flaw. Conversely, thinness has historically been a risk factor for poor health or associated with poverty or insufficient food supplies. In many cultures today, including those

BOX 11.4 Questions That May Aid in Understanding Health Beliefs

- What does it mean to be healthy?
- What do you do to keep healthy?
- What do you teach your children about health?
- What health practices do you engage in that differ from what your ancestors did?
- What do you think makes a person sick?
- When a person is sick, do you think they are in control of making themselves better?
- What do you do when you are sick?
- Who helps you when you are sick?
- Have you been to a folk healer or used folk medicine when you are sick?
- Where do you get health information?

Source: Eggenberger, S., Grassley, J., & Restrepo, E. (2006). Culturally competent nursing care for families: Listening to the voices of Mexican-American women. *OJIN: The Online Journal of Issues in Nursing, 11*(3). https://doi.org/10.3912/OJIN.Vol11No03PPT01

of some African, Mexican, Native American, and Caribbean Islander cultures, being overweight is a sign of health, beauty, and prosperity (Kittler et al., 2012). To some people, healthy eating is synonymous with eating large quantities of food rather than making more nutritious food choices.

Dietary Acculturation

Dietary Acculturation the process that occurs as members of a minority group adopt the eating patterns and food choices of the host country.

Acculturation the process that occurs as people who move to a different cultural area adopt the beliefs, values, attitudes, and behaviors of the dominant culture; not limited to immigrants but affects anyone (to varying degrees) who moves from one community to another.

Dietary acculturation occurs when eating patterns of immigrants change to resemble those of the dominant or mainstream culture. In the United States, **acculturation** is linked to an increased risk of chronic disease and obesity; however, its effect on diet quality is not always consistent. For instance, acculturation of immigrants who are from South Asia in Canada led to both positive changes (a greater intake of fruit and vegetables and a decrease in deep fat frying) and negative changes (an increased intake of convenience foods, sugar-sweetened beverages, red meat, and increased frequency of eating out) (Lesser et al., 2014). Clearly, acculturation is a highly complex, dynamic, multidimensional process that is impacted by a variety of personal, cultural, and environmental factors (Satia, 2009). Associations of acculturation with diet are often inconsistent and do not fit an expected pattern (Satia, 2009).

Generally, food habits are one of the last behaviors people change through acculturation. This is possibly because eating is done in the privacy of the home and not in full view of the majority culture.

- Usually, first-generation Americans adhere more closely to cultural food patterns and may cling to traditional foods to affirm their cultural identity. First-generation citizens usually need help choosing American replacements for their native foods.
- Second-generation Americans do not have the direct native connection and may follow cultural patterns only on holidays and at family gatherings, or they may give up ethnic foods but retain traditional methods of preparation. Second-generation citizens may need help selecting healthy American foods.
- Children tend to adopt new ways quickly as they learn from other children at school.

Process of Acculturation

Ideally, people who acculturate will retain healthy traditional food practices, adopt healthy new food behaviors, and avoid less healthy American food habits. Actual food choices are influenced by income, education, urbanization, geographic region, and family customs. Points to keep in mind regarding dietary acculturation appear in Box 11.5.

- New foods are added to the diet.
  - Status, economics, information, taste, and exposure are some of the reasons why new foods are added to the diet.
  - Eating American food may symbolize status and make people feel more connected to their new culture.

BOX 11.5 Points to Consider Regarding Dietary Acculturation

- Generally with acculturation, the intake of sweets and fats increases, neither of which has a positive effect on health.
- Dietary acculturation is most likely to change food choices for breakfast and lunch rather than dinner, so focus on promoting healthy food choices available in America for those meals.
- Portion control is a better option than advising someone to eliminate an important native food from their diet. Lower-fat or lower-sodium options, when available, may also be an acceptable option for the client. Although giving up soy sauce may not be an option for an American of Chinese origin, using a reduced-sodium version may be doable.
- It is essential to determine how often a food is consumed in order to determine the potential impact of that food. For instance, lard is unimportant in the context of the total diet if it is used in cooking only on special occasions.
- Don't assume the client knows which American foods are considered healthy.
- Suggest fruits and vegetables that are similar in texture to those that are familiar but unavailable to the client.

  - Frequently, new foods are added because they are relatively inexpensive and widely available.
- Some traditional foods are replaced by new foods.
  - Traditional foods may be difficult to find, be too expensive, or have lengthy preparation times.
  - Breakfast and lunch are most likely to be composed of convenient American foods, whereas traditional foods are retained for the major dinner meal, which has greater emotional significance.
- Some traditional foods are rejected.
  - Children and adolescents are more likely than older adults to reject traditional foods to become more like their peers.
  - Traditional foods may be rejected because of an increased awareness of the role of nutrition in the development of chronic diseases. For instance, one reason why Indian immigrants who have resided in the United States for a relatively long period tend to eat significantly less ghee (clarified butter served with rice or spread on Indian breads) may be that they are trying to decrease their intake of saturated fat.

CULTURAL SUBGROUPS IN THE UNITED STATES

It is projected that by the year 2044, more than half of all Americans will belong to a cultural group (Colby & Ortman, 2015). The nutritional implication of this shift in cultural predominance is that cultural competence will become increasingly important to nursing care. Nutrition information that is technically correct but culturally inappropriate does not produce behavior change. Cultural competence facilitates nutrition care that is consistent with the individual's attitudes, beliefs, and values. Suggestions for conducting effective cross-cultural nutrition counseling are listed in Box 11.6.

The minimum categories of race and ethnicity were established by the U.S. Office of Management and Budget in 1997 and are still used today by the U.S. Census Bureau (2020).

- **Native North American or Alaska Native:** people having origins in any of the original peoples of North and South America, including Central America, who maintain tribal affiliation or community attachment.
- **Asian:** people having origins in any of the original peoples of the Far East, Southeast Asia, or the Indian subcontinent. Cambodia, China, India, Japan, Korea, Malaysia, Pakistan, the Philippine Islands, Thailand, and Vietnam are examples.
- **Black or African American:** people having origins in any of the Black racial groups of Africa.

BOX 11.6 Suggestions for Conducting Effective Cross-Cultural Nutrition Counseling

- Establish rapport and respect cultural differences.
- Be knowledgeable about cultural food habits and health beliefs.
- Relevant guidance must include advice on traditional foods and preparation methods to retain or reduce.
- Use culturally appropriate verbal and nonverbal communication.
- Determine the primary written and spoken language used in the client's home.
- Use trained interpreters when necessary.
- Determine whether the client prefers direct or indirect communication.
- Pare down information to only what the client needs to know.
- Emphasize the positive food practices of traditional health beliefs and food customs.
- Explain medical reasons for recommended changes.
- Provide written material only after determining reading ability.
- Communicate consistent messages.

- **Native Hawaiian or Other Pacific Islander:** people having origins in any of the original peoples of Hawaii, Guam, Samoa, or other Pacific islands.
- **White:** people having origins in any of the original peoples of Europe, the Middle East, or North Africa.
- **Hispanic, Latino, or Spanish:** people of Cuban, Mexican, Puerto Rican, South or Central American, or other Spanish culture or origin. The term *Spanish origin* can be used in addition to *Hispanic* or *Latino* regardless of race.

Each of these categories has multiple diverse subgroups. For instance, the category of Native Americans comprises more than 573 tribes legally recognized by the Bureau of Indian Affairs (Federal Register, 2019). In addition, multiracial individuals represent a growing population.

TRADITIONAL DIETS

Traditional diets are generally considered healthy because they contain large amounts of plant-based foods such as grains, vegetables, legumes, tubers, and fruit and low amounts of foods from animals, such as red meat (Valerino-Perea et al., 2019). However, it is difficult to define traditional diets because actual food choices vary greatly within subgroups on the basis of national, regional, and ethnic differences. For instance, foods eaten most often in traditional Mexican diet differ by geographical regions such as northern, central, and southern Mexico. Likewise, traditional diets change over time. While insects are no longer part of the traditional Mexican diet, eggs and milk appear to be recent additions (Valerino-Perea et al., 2019).

Generalizations about traditional eating practices and dietary changes related to acculturation for three major cultural subgroups in the United States are highlighted in the following sections. A summary of health statistics by cultural group appears in Table 11.3.

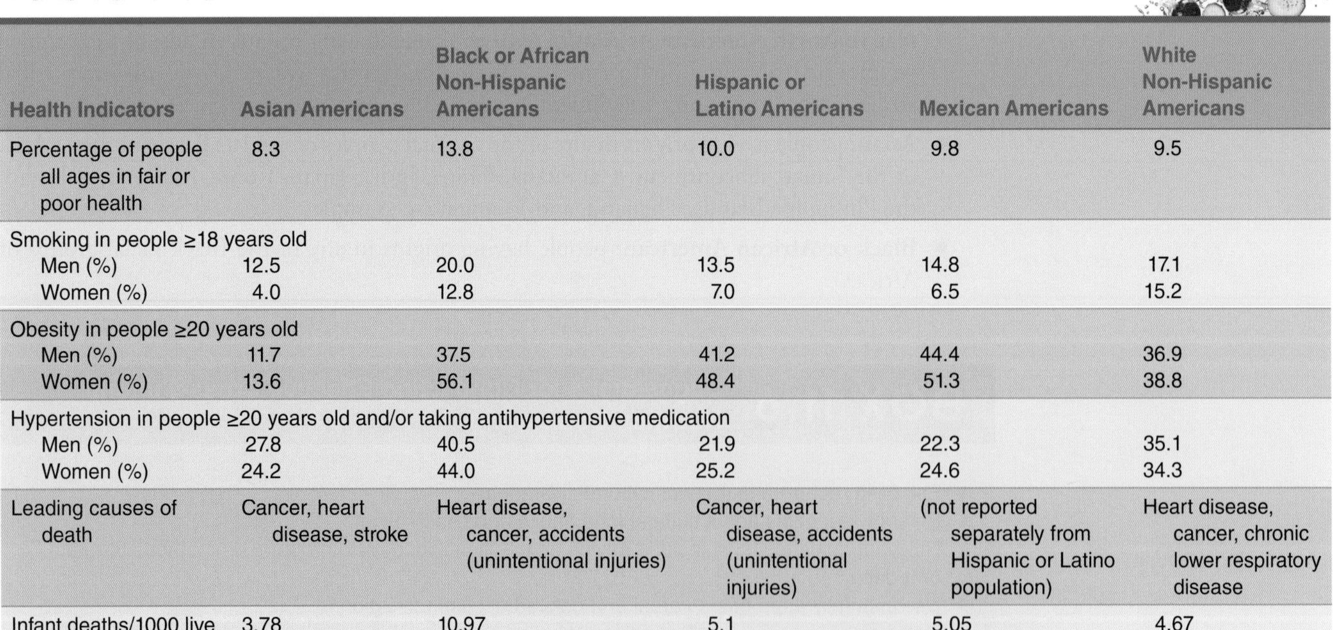

Table 11.3 Summary of Health Statistics by Cultural Group

Health Indicators	Asian Americans	Black or African Non-Hispanic Americans	Hispanic or Latino Americans	Mexican Americans	White Non-Hispanic Americans
Percentage of people all ages in fair or poor health	8.3	13.8	10.0	9.8	9.5
Smoking in people ≥18 years old					
Men (%)	12.5	20.0	13.5	14.8	17.1
Women (%)	4.0	12.8	7.0	6.5	15.2
Obesity in people ≥20 years old					
Men (%)	11.7	37.5	41.2	44.4	36.9
Women (%)	13.6	56.1	48.4	51.3	38.8
Hypertension in people ≥20 years old and/or taking antihypertensive medication					
Men (%)	27.8	40.5	21.9	22.3	35.1
Women (%)	24.2	44.0	25.2	24.6	34.3
Leading causes of death	Cancer, heart disease, stroke	Heart disease, cancer, accidents (unintentional injuries)	Cancer, heart disease, accidents (unintentional injuries)	(not reported separately from Hispanic or Latino population)	Heart disease, cancer, chronic lower respiratory disease
Infant deaths/1000 live births	3.78	10.97	5.1	5.05	4.67

Source: Centers for Disease Control and Prevention, National Center for Health Statistics. (2017, May 3). *Health of Asian or Pacific Islander population*. https://www.cdc.gov/nchs/fastats/asian-health.htm; Centers for Disease Control and Prevention, National Center for Health Statistics. (2017, May 3). *Health of Black or African American non-Hispanic population*. https://www.cdc.gov/nchs/fastats/black-health.htm; Centers for Disease Control and Prevention, National Center for Health Statistics. (2017, May 3). *Health of Hispanic or Latino population*. https://www.cdc.gov/nchs/fastats/hispanic-health.htm; Centers for Disease Control and Prevention, National Center for Health Statistics. (2017, May 3). *Health of Mexican American population*. https://www.cdc.gov/nchs/fastats/mexican-health.htm; Centers for Disease Control and Prevention, National Center for Health Statistics. (2017, May 3). *Health of White non-Hispanic population*. https://www.cdc.gov/nchs/fastats/white-health.htm

Black or African Americans

According to 2019 estimates, 13.4% of the population in 2018 was Black or African American alone (U.S. Census Bureau, 2019). The majority of people who are Black or African American can trace their ancestors to West Africa, although some have immigrated from the Caribbean, Central America, and East African countries. Since most are many generations away from their original homeland, much of their native heritage has been assimilated, lost, or modified. Box 11.7 highlights traditional food practices, changes in intake related to acculturation, and traditional health beliefs. Additional salient points are summarized in the following sections.

Soul Food

Soul food describes traditional Southern African American food eaten by people who are African American and cooking techniques that evolved from West African, slave, and post-abolition cuisine. The term *soul food* was first used in 1964 during the rise of the civil rights movement.

- Many soul food customs and practices are shared by in the Southern United States, particularly those of lower socioeconomic status or living in rural areas (Kulkarni, 2004).
- Soul food has become a symbol of identity for people who are African American and from African heritage; however, today, African American food habits usually reflect their current socioeconomic status, geographic location, and work schedule more than their African or Southern heritage (Kittler et al., 2012).
- Soul food may be reserved for special occasions and holidays.

Diet Quality

- In a study that examined dietary quality by race and ethnicity, the intake of total vegetables, whole grains, milk, fiber, potassium, and calcium is lower among people who are Black Americans than people who are White Americans and intakes of sugar-sweetened beverages and added sugars are higher (Hiza et al., 2013).

BOX 11.7 Food and Culture of People Who Are African American

Traditional Food and Eating Patterns

- The style of cooking that developed during the American slavery time period when slaves were given the leftover or less desirable cuts of meat. Farming, hunting, and fishing provided fish, wild game, and vegetables.
- Traditional soul foods tend to be high in fat, cholesterol, and sodium and low in protective nutrients, such as potassium (fruits and vegetables), fiber (whole grains and vegetables), and calcium (milk, cheese, and yogurt).
- Staples include corn and corn products (grits, cornmeal), rice, biscuits, black-eyed peas, butter beans, lima beans, catfish, chitterlings (cleaned and cooked intestines of hogs), breaded and fried beef, pork, poultry, variety meats (oxtail, pig's feet), pork rinds, *greens* (a variety of leafy vegetables), melons, peaches, pecans, sweet and white potatoes, butter, lard, bacon, fatback, fruit drinks, molasses, and sorghum.

Changes in Intake from Acculturation

- Greater intake of milk, at least among people who are Black Americans living in urban areas.
- Fruit intake remains low and is based on availability.
- Vegetable intake remains low but greens remain popular.
- Commercially made bread is substituted for homemade biscuits.
- Packaged and luncheon meats are popular, but intake of fatty meats, such as sausage and bacon, is high.

Traditional Health Beliefs

- Health beliefs of some are a blend of traditional African concepts and those encountered through early contact with Native North Americans and White Americans.
- Illnesses are classified as *natural* (stemming from the effects of cold, dirt, and improper diet or divine punishment) or *unnatural* (the result of witchcraft and conflict in the social network).
- Home remedies, natural therapies, and traditional healers may be used.
- Feelings of powerlessness may be evident among Black Americans living in poverty.

Source: African American Registry. (n.d.). *"Soul Food" in America: A brief history*. https://aaregistry.org/story/soul-food-a-brief-history; Snow, L. F. (1983). Traditional health beliefs and practices among lower class black Americans. *The Western Journal of Medicine, 139*(6), 820–828.

- Foreign-born people who are Black Americans are reported to have a higher Healthy Eating Index score and DASH diet scores compared with people who are Black Americans born in the United States. They were more likely to be in the top third for intake of vegetables, fruit, whole grains, and omega-3 fatty acids (Brown et al., 2018).

Nutrition-Related Health Issues

- People who are Black Americans have among the highest rates of morbidity and mortality from diet-related diseases (such as hypertension, heart disease, and stroke) compared to other racial/ethnic groups in the United States (Brown et al., 2018).
- Women who are Black Americans are less likely to perceive themselves as overweight than are women who are White Americans of the same BMI (Langellier et al., 2015a).
- Adults who are Black Americans have a significantly higher likelihood of developing diabetes than adults who are of White Americans—about 66 more cases of diabetes per 1000 people, with the greatest difference being between women who are Black Americans and White Americans (National Institutes of Health, 2018). Biological risk factors, including weight and fat around the abdomen, are primarily responsible for the higher rates.
- The percentage of people who are Black Americans whose health is fair or poor is greater than in any other ethnic group. This is also true for infant mortality.
- The death rate for people who are Black Americans is generally higher than that for people who are of White Americans for heart diseases, stroke, cancer, asthma, influenza and pneumonia, diabetes, HIV/AIDS, and homicide (Office of Minority Health, 2019a).

Hispanic or Latino Americans

People who are Hispanic or Latino Americans are a diverse group differing in native language, customs, history, and foodways. According to 2019 estimates, approximately 18.5% of the U.S. population are people of Hispanic or Latino ethnicity (U.S. Census Bureau, 2019). People of Mexican descent are the largest subgroup, at 63% of the American population of people who are of Hispanic or Latino descent. Box 11.8 highlights traditional food practices, changes in intake related to acculturation, and traditional health beliefs. Additional salient points are summarized in the following sections.

Diet Quality

- People of Hispanic origin who speak Spanish are more likely to report consuming foods in the Healthy Eating Index as compared to Hispanic people who are bilingual or prefer to speak English (Reininger et al., 2017).
- Acculturation is associated with lower diet quality scores from undesirable changes in the intake of vegetables, fruits, sodium, and empty calories (Yoshida et al., 2017).
- Mexican Americans who speak English (sign of greater acculturation) report eating more fast foods, pizza, non-homemade meals, and more meals at sit-down restaurants than other Mexican Americans who speak Spanish (Langellier et al., 2015b).

Nutrition-Related Health Issues

- People who are Hispanic or Latino Americans have a high prevalence of obesity and tend to be less physically active than people who are non-Hispanic White Americans (Centers for Disease Control and Prevention [CDC], 2019).
- People who are Hispanic or Latino Americans have a longer life expectancy than people who are White Americans, at 84.1 years for women and 79.6 years for men (Office of Minority Health, 2019b).
- People who are Hispanic or Latino Americans are more than twice as likely to develop type 2 diabetes as people who are non-Hispanic White Americans (CDC, 2019).
- Other health conditions that significantly affect people who are Hispanic or Latino Americans are asthma, chronic obstructive pulmonary disease, HIV/AIDS, suicide, and liver disease (Office of Minority Health, 2019b).

BOX 11.8 Mexican American Food and Culture

Traditional Food and Eating Patterns

- The traditional Mexican diet is influenced by Spanish and Native North American cultures. It is generally a low-fat and high-fiber diet rich in complex carbohydrates and vegetable proteins. There is an emphasis on corn (maize), corn products, beans, chili, and squash. Animal foods are limited.
- Individual foods cited most often include corn and corn products, amaranth, rice, potato, sweet potato, beans, tomatoes, squash, citrus fruits, guava, jicama, plums, prickly pear, turkey, chicken, duck, venison, rabbit, beef, chili, salt, and onion.
- Items less frequently mentioned are as follows: avocado, pumpkin and chia seeds, chocolate drinks, honey, sugar, and sugarcane.
- Tortillas are a staple and may be consumed at every meal.
- Chilies are a common main ingredient in meals.
- Rice is usually served first before the main meal.
- Four or five meals per day are consumed.
- Families gather at meals to build a sense of togetherness.
- Women prepare the food.

Changes in Intake from Acculturation

- Intake of fruits, vegetables, rice and beans, and fiber decreases.
- Use of lard and heavy cream decreases.
- Intake of traditional meat and vegetable preparations declines drastically.
- Flour tortillas replace corn. Sugar-sweetened beverages replace traditional fruit-based beverages.
- Intake of white bread, sweetened cereals, red meat, cheese, and saturated fat increases.
- Increase in FAFH.
- Intake of processed foods, refined carbohydrate, and added sugars increases.

Traditional Health Beliefs

- The majority of people who are Mexican are Roman Catholic. Religious and spiritual beliefs greatly influence health and illness practices, which result from a blend of European folk medicine introduced from rituals from Spain and Native North Americans.
- Illness is the result of punishment, worry, stress, fear, fatalism or luck, and/or the supernatural/evil eye.
- Herbal and folk remedies are often used for self-treatment. Drinks, tea, and ointments are common home remedies.
- Being overweight may be seem as a sign of wealth.
- The mother decides when an illness is beyond her ability to treat.
- Extended and nuclear families are highly valued and relied on for intergenerational help.
- Respect is based on status and hierarchy in the community.

Source: United Nations Educational, Scientific, and Cultural Organization. Intangible cultural heritage. (2010). *Traditional Mexican cuisine—ancestral, ongoing community culture, the Michoacan paradigm*. https://ich.unesco.org/en/RL/traditional-mexican-cuisine-ancestral-ongoing-community-culture-the-michoacan-paradigm-00400; Ohio State University Extension. (n.d.). *Mexican food and culture fact sheet*. https://dune.une.edu/cgi/viewcontent.cgi?article=1010&context=an_studedres; Sofianou, A., Fung, T., & Tucker, K. (2011). Differences in diet pattern adherence by nativity and duration of U.S. residence in the Mexican-American Population. *Journal of the American Dietetic Association*, *111*(10), 1563–1569. https://doi.org/10.1016/j.jada.2011.07.005; Valerino-Perea, S., Lara-Castor, L., Armstrong, M. E. G., & Papadaki, A. (2019). Definition of the traditional Mexican diet and its role in health: A systematic review. *Nutrients*, *11*(11), 2803. https://doi.org/10.3390/nu11112803

Asian Americans

Approximately 5.9% of the U.S. population are of people of Asian origin alone, according to 2019 census estimates (U.S. Census Bureau, 2019). People who are Chinese comprise the largest subgroup of people who are Asian American in the United States (Pew Research Center, 2019). The term *Asian Americans* encompasses a diverse population originating from at least 37 different ethnic groups; *Pacific Islander* includes about 25 nationalities (Kagawa-Singer et al., 2010). Two dietary commonalities exist between these diverse cultures: emphasis on rice and vegetables with relatively little meat and cooking techniques that include meticulous attention to preparing ingredients before cooking. Box 11.9 highlights traditional Chinese food practices, changes in intake related to acculturation, and traditional health beliefs. Additional salient points are summarized in the following sections.

Diet Quality

The traditional diet of people who are Chinese is low in fat and dairy products and high in complex carbohydrates and sodium (Kittler et al., 2012). With acculturation, the diet becomes higher in fat, protein, sugar, and cholesterol.

BOX 11.9 Chinese American Food and Culture

Traditional Food and Eating Patterns

- The traditional diet of people who are Chinese is low in fat and dairy products and high in complex carbohydrates and sodium.
- Rice is the staple for people living in the south of China. Products made of wheat flour (noodles, dumplings, pancakes, steamed bread) are staples in northern China.
- Vegetables are used extensively. Other foods commonly consumed include sea vegetables, nuts, seeds, beans, soy foods, vegetable and nut oils, herbs and spices, tea, wine, and beer.
- A variety of animal proteins are consumed. The use of fish and seafood depends on availability.
- Most Chinese food is cooked. The exception is fresh fruit, which is eaten infrequently.
- Few dairy products are consumed because lactose intolerance is common.
- Sodium intake is generally assumed to be high because of traditional food preservation methods (salting and drying) and condiments (e.g., soy sauce).
- Compared to other countries, people who are Chinese spend much more time on cooking. It generally takes 1 to 2 hours to make a dinner.
- Usually elders and the young are served first, followed by men, children, and women.
- Dinner is usually abundant and has 2 to 4 dishes and one soup.

Changes in Intake from Acculturation

- Rice remains a staple. Wheat bread and cereal intake increases.
- Intake of raw vegetables, salad, fruit, dairy, meat, sugar, and ethnic food increases.
- Fat intake increases as fast-food intake increases.
- Traditional vegetables are replaced by more commonly available ones.

Traditional Health Beliefs

- Illness and death may be viewed as a natural part of life.
- Health is maintained by balancing complementary energies such as cold and hot, dark and light. These forces are called *yin* and *yang*.
- Foods are thought to have medicinal purposes, and body parts may be healed by eating corresponding food parts, such as eating fish eyes to improve vision.
- Foods and herbs may be used to restore the *yin–yang* balance, as may other traditional remedies such as massage and acupuncture.
- Traditional approaches may be used before seeking Western medical care.
- There is less emphasis on individual feelings and more on loyalty to family and devotion to tradition. Decision-making may involve the whole family.

Source: Ma, G. (2015). Food, eating behavior, and culture in Chinese society. *Journal of Ethnic Foods*, 2(4), 195–199. https://doi.org/10.1016/j.jef.2015.11.004; University of Washington Medical Center. (2007, April). *Communicating with your Chinese patient*. https://depts.washington.edu/pfes/PDFs/ChineseCultureClue.pdf

Nutrition-Related Health Issues

- The cultural group of people who are Asian American has the lowest percentage of people in fair or poor health.
- Life expectancy among women who are of Asian origin is 82.0 years, and it is 77.5 years for men (Office of Minority Health, 2019c). This is longer than the average life expectancy of 81.1 years for women and 76.2 years for men among the total U.S. population (Murphy et al., 2018).
- People who are Asian Americans have the lowest prevalence of obesity among cultural groups in the United States.
- Epidemiologic studies show that diabetes risk in people who are of Asian Americans occurs at lower BMI values than in White Americans, partly because of the propensity for people of Asian origin to develop visceral, not peripheral, adiposity (King et al., 2012).
- At any given BMI level, men and women who are Asian Americans have a greater percentage of body fat than men and women who are White Americans.
- People who are Asian Americans have a high prevalence of chronic obstructive pulmonary disease, hepatitis B, HIV/AIDS, smoking, tuberculosis, and liver disease (Office of Minority Health, 2019c).
- Negative factors that may impact their health include infrequent medical visits for fear of deportation, language/cultural barriers, and lack of health insurance.

Recall Phouvong. His BMI is 24.5. Although that is considered healthy, risk of type 2 diabetes starts at a lower BMI in people of Asian descent than among other cultural groups. Attaining a BMI less than 23 will help control Phouvong's type 2 diabetes. Options to promote weight loss are to change the foods consumed, change the amounts, and/or increase activity. Which option (or options) would you recommend for Phouvong? How will you convey the information given the language barrier?

FOOD AND RELIGION

Kosher
a word commonly used to identify Jewish dietary laws that define *clean* and *unclean* foods, how food animals must be slaughtered, how foods must be prepared, and when foods may be consumed (e.g., the timing between eating milk products and meat products).

Religion tends to have a greater impact on food habits than nationality or culture. For example, Orthodox Jewish people follow **kosher** dietary laws regardless of their national origin. Religious food practices vary significantly even among denominations of the same faith. National variations also exist. A person's degree of orthodoxy affects how closely an individual follows dietary laws. An overview of religious food practices follows. Table 11.4 outlines major features of various religious dietary laws.

Christianity

The three primary branches of Christianity are Roman Catholicism, Eastern Orthodox Christianity, and Protestantism. Dietary practices vary from none to explicit.

- Roman Catholics do not eat meat on Ash Wednesday or on Fridays of Lent. Food and beverages are avoided for 1 hour before communion is taken. Devout Catholics observe several fast days during the year.
- Eastern Orthodox Christians observe numerous feast and fast days throughout the year.
- The only denominations in the Protestant faith with dietary laws are The Church of Jesus Christ of Latter-day Saints and Seventh-Day Adventists.
- Members of the Church of Jesus Christ of Latter-day Saints do not use coffee, tea, alcohol, or tobacco. Followers are encouraged to limit meats and consume mostly grains. Some Latter-day Saints fast 1 day a month.

Table 11.4 **Summary of Dietary Laws of Selected Religions**

	Orthodox Judaism	Islam	Hinduism	Buddhism
Meat	Cannot be eaten with dairy products	Kosher and halal animals are allowed	Beef is prohibited.	Avoided by the most devout
Pork and pork products	Prohibited	Prohibited	Avoided by the most devout	Avoided by the most devout
Lacto-ovo vegetarianism			Encouraged	Practiced by many
Seafood	Only fish with fins and scales are allowed		Restricted	Avoided by the most devout
Alcohol		Prohibited	Avoided by the most devout	
Coffee/tea		Strongly discouraged		
Ritual slaughter of animals	Yes	Yes		
Moderation		Practiced		Practiced
Partial or total fasting	Practiced	Practiced	Practiced	Practiced

Source: Minority Nurse. (2013b). *Hindu dietary practices: Feeding the body, mind and soul*. https://minoritynurse.com/?s=Hindu+dietary; Minority Nurse. (2013a). *Meeting Jewish and Muslim patient's dietary needs*. http://minoritynurse.com/?s=Jewish+dietary+practices; Minority Nurse. (2013c). *Understanding Buddhist patient's dietary needs*. https://minoritynurse.com/?s=Hindu+dietary

- Most Seventh-Day Adventists are lacto-ovo vegetarians; those who do eat meat avoid pork. Overeating is avoided, and coffee, tea, and alcohol are prohibited. An interval of 5 to 6 hours between meals is recommended, with no snacking between meals. Water is consumed before and after meals. Strong seasonings, such as pepper and mustard, are avoided.

Judaism

Orthodox, Conservative, and Reform are the three main denominations of the Jewish faith in the United States. Hasidic Judaism is a sect within the Orthodox. These groups differ in their interpretation of the precepts of Judaism.

- Orthodox Jewish people believe that the laws are the direct commandments of God, so they adhere strictly to dietary laws called the *kashrut* (or *kashruth*) (Box 11.10). The laws are rigid, so Orthodox Jewish people rarely eat outside the home except at homes or restaurants with kosher kitchens.
- The laws focus on three major issues:
  - Kosher animals are allowed.
  - Blood is not allowed.
  - Milk and meat are never combined.
- Reform Jewish people follow the moral law, but they may selectively follow other laws; for instance, they may not follow any religious dietary laws.
- Conservative Jewish people fall between the other two groups in their beliefs and adherence to the laws. They may follow the Jewish dietary laws at home but take a more liberal attitude on social occasions.

BOX 11.10 Kosher Dietary Laws

Kosher describes foods that are fit for consumption by Jewish people. Certain species of animals (and their eggs and milk) are allowed while others are forbidden.

- A mammal is kosher if it has split hooves and chews its cud: cows, sheep, goats, and deer.
- Kosher birds are domestic varieties of chicken, turkey, goose, pigeons, and ducks.
- Only fish and seafood that have fins and scales are kosher, such as salmon, tuna, and herring.
- Fruits, vegetables, and grains are kosher but must be insect free.
- Milk and eggs (without blood spots) are kosher only if they come from kosher animals.
- Wine and grape juice must be certified kosher.
- Kosher foods are labeled with a logo of the kosher-certifying agency, of which there are well over 100 in the United States alone. Other people who often purchase kosher foods include Muslims, Seventh-Day Adventists, vegetarians, and people with allergies (e.g., shellfish) or intolerances (e.g., milk).

Kosher foods are categorized as meat, dairy, or pareve (contains neither meat nor dairy ingredients).

- Meat cannot be consumed at the same meal as dairy.
- Dairy products are not allowed within 1 to 6 hours after eating meat, depending on the individual's ethnic tradition.
- Meat cannot be eaten for 30 minutes after dairy products have been consumed.
- Pareve foods can be mixed and eaten with either meat or dairy: kosher eggs, fruits, vegetables, grains, margarine-labeled pareve, nondairy creamers, and oils.

Certain foods and practices, such as the following, are forbidden:

- Non-kosher animals: carnivorous animals (e.g., lions), birds of prey, pork, fish without scales or fins (e.g., shrimp, lobster, swordfish, catfish, water mammals), reptiles, amphibians, worms, insects, rabbits, squirrels, bears, dogs, cats, camels, and horses.
- Blood. Meat from allowed animals must be slaughtered under the supervision of a rabbi or another authorized person to ensure blood is properly removed. The animal's throat is quickly, precisely, and painlessly cut with a sharp knife.
- Food preparation on the Sabbath. Religious holidays are celebrated with certain foods. For example, only unleavened bread is eaten during Passover, and a 24-hour fast is observed on Yom Kippur.

Source: Chabad.org. *What is kosher?* https://www.chabad.org/library/article_cdo/aid/113424/jewish/Kosher.htm

Islam

Muslim people eat as a matter of faith and for good health. Basic guidance concerning food laws is revealed in the Quran (the divine book) from Allah (the Creator) to Muhammad (the Prophet). For Muslim people, health and food are considered acts of worship for which Allah must be thanked (Minority Nurse, 2013a). Many halal laws are similar to the food laws of Judaism. Halal foods are also identified with symbols. Islam also stresses certain hygienic practices, such as washing hands before and after eating and frequent teeth cleaning.

Halal
refers to Islamic dietary standards of *lawful* or *permitted* when used to describe food.

Haram
refers to Islamic dietary standards of *prohibited* or *unlawful* when used to describe food.

There are 11 generally accepted rules pertaining to **halal** (permitted) and **haram** (prohibited) foods. The five major areas addressed by the halal are as follows:

- Kosher and halal animals are allowed. Pork, carnivorous animals with fangs (lions, wolves, dogs, etc.), birds with sharp claws (falcons, eagles, owls, etc.), land animals without ears (frog, snakes, etc.), shark, and products containing gelatin made from the horns or hooves of cattle are not allowed.
- Blood is not allowed.
- Proper methods must be used for slaughtering.
- Carrion (decaying carcass) is not allowed.
- Intoxicants are forbidden, including pure vanilla containing alcohol and wine vinegar.

Hinduism

A love of nature and desire to live a simple natural life are ideas that form the basis of Hinduism (Minority Nurse, 2013b). A number of health beliefs and dietary practices stem from the idea of living in harmony with nature and having mercy and respect for all of God's creations.

- Generally, Hindu people avoid all foods that are believed to inhibit physical and spiritual development.
- Eating meat is not explicitly prohibited, but many Hindu people are vegetarian because they adhere to the concept of **ahimsa**.
- Some foods, such as dairy products (e.g., milk, yogurt, ghee), are considered to enhance spiritual purity. Pure foods can improve the purity of impure foods when prepared together.
- Some foods, such as beef or alcohol, are innately polluted and can never be made pure.
- Jainism, a branch of Hinduism, also promotes the nonviolent doctrine of ahimsa. People who are devout Jains are complete vegetarians and may avoid blood-colored foods like tomatoes and root vegetables because harvesting them may cause the death of insects.

Ahimsa
nonviolence as applicable to foods.

Buddhism

The Buddhist code of morality is set forth in the Five Moral Precepts:

- Do not kill or harm living things.
- Do not steal.
- Do not engage in sexual misconduct.
- Do not lie.
- Do not consume intoxicants (such as alcohol, tobacco, or mind-altering drugs).

Believing that thoughtful food decisions can contribute to spiritual enlightenment, a Buddhist asks themselves these questions (ElGindy, 2013):

- What food is this? This question evaluates the origin of the food and how it reached the individual.
- Where does it come from? This question considers the amount of work necessary to grow the food, prepare it, cook it, and bring it to the table.

- Why am I eating it? This question reflects on whether the individual deserves or is worthy of the food.
- When should I eat and benefit from this food? This question is based on the idea that food is a necessity and a healing agent and people are subjected to illness without food.
- How should I eat it? This question considers the premise that food is received and eaten only for the purpose of realizing the proper way to reach enlightenment.

In Buddhism, life revolves around nature with its two opposing energy systems of yin and yang (ElGindy, 2013). Examples of these opposing energy systems are heat/cold, light/darkness, good/evil, and sickness/health. Illnesses may result from an imbalance of yin and yang. Most Buddhist people subscribe to the concept of ahimsa (not killing or harming), so many are vegetarians. Buddhist dietary practices vary widely depending on the sect and country.

How Do You Respond?

Are meal kit delivery services as good as traditionally prepared home-cooked meals? Meal kits tend to get favorable reviews for taste, variety, freshness, and convenience and eliminate waste from leftovers. They are an attractive alternative to traditionally prepared meals for people who do not have the time for, or interest in, meal planning and food shopping, and they enable people to try new cuisines without investing in exotic ingredients, such as a bottle of a spice when only a fraction of a teaspoon is needed. The downside is that they are more expensive than traditionally prepared meals, and the sodium content tends to be high. The amount of food sent is for a specified number of people, so there are usually no leftovers. This can be a positive or a negative.

Is prepared food from grocery stores healthier than other food outlets? The trend in buying prepared foods from the grocery store began with the desire for convenience. Its growth is fueled by consumer perception that prepared food is fresher and healthier than takeout dinners or convenience foods from the frozen food aisle. However, the fresh food may not actually be made on premises, sodium content is often high, serving sizes are not suggested (so it is easy to overbuy and overeat), and items are generally much more expensive than making them at home. Whether or not grocery-store-prepared foods are healthier than food from other outlets depends on the items chosen, the amounts consumed, and the methods of preparation.

REVIEW CASE STUDY

Elizabeth moved to the Midwest at the age of 26 from her native country, Iceland, where she ate seafood almost every evening for dinner. She ate fruit and vegetables daily, but the variety was limited. In her new home, she complains that good seafood is hard to find—that it is not as fresh as it is at home, it tastes different, and it is more expensive. She also misses the dark brown and black breads she is accustomed to; she is willing to try American breads but is unsure what variety is good. American fast food is well known to her, but she does not want to rely on that to satisfy her need for familiar foods. She wants to eat foods that are healthy, tasty, and affordable.

- What questions would you ask Elizabeth before coming up with suggestions about foods she could try?
- What would you say to her about her frustration with the seafood available locally? What suggestions would you make to her?
- What would you tell her about healthy breads? What fruits would you recommend as healthy, tasty, and affordable? What vegetables?

STUDY QUESTIONS

1 Which of the following religions does not encourage a vegetarian diet?
   a. Buddhism
   b. Judaism
   c. Seventh-Day Adventist
   d. Hinduism

2 What is a descriptive word that indicates a low-fat cooking technique?
   a. *au gratin*
   b. breaded
   c. roasted
   d. battered

3 What are the characteristics of a traditional Chinese diet? Select all that apply.
   a. rich in dairy products
   b. low in fat
   c. high in sodium
   d. vegetables used extensively

4 What are the characteristics of a traditional Mexican diet? Select all that apply.
   a. low in fat
   b. high in fiber
   c. rich in complex carbohydrates
   d. rich in vegetable protein

5 What are the nutritional characteristics of a traditional soul food diet? Select all that apply.
   a. high in fat
   b. high in sodium
   c. high in potassium
   d. high in cholesterol

6 Which of the following foods is not pareve?
   a. fruit
   b. vegetables
   c. kosher eggs
   d. milk

7 Which approach would be best when developing a teaching plan for an overweight woman from Mexico?
   a. Tell the client she will look better if she loses some of the extra weight she is carrying around.
   b. Encourage more nutritious food choices.
   c. Advise the client that healthy eating will help her shed inches.
   d. Provide a low-calorie diet and encourage her to eat low-calorie American foods, such as artificially sweetened soda and low-fat ice cream.

8 Muslims are prohibited from consuming
   a. alcohol.
   b. eggs.
   c. beef.
   d. shellfish.

CHAPTER SUMMARY CULTURAL AND RELIGIOUS INFLUENCES ON FOOD AND NUTRITION

American Cuisine

American cuisine has evolved from a melting pot of food, flavors, and cooking techniques contributed by immigrants over the course of U.S. history. Today, FAFH provides approximately one third of total calorie intake.

The Effect of Culture

Culture defines what is edible: how food is handled, prepared, and consumed; what foods are appropriate for particular groups within the culture; the meaning of food and eating; attitudes toward body size; and the relationship between food and health.

Acculturation

- Generally, first-generation Americans adhere more closely to cultural food patterns; second-generation Americans may eat traditional food only on special occasions.
- Acculturation is linked to an increased risk of chronic disease and obesity, although not all dietary changes are negative. Dietary counseling should encourage retention of healthy food practices, adoption of healthy new food behaviors, and avoidance of less healthy American food patterns.

Cultural Subgroups in the U.S.

Although generalizations can be made about traditional eating practices and changes related to acculturation, actual food choices vary with nationality, geographic location, socioeconomic status, and individual preferences.

African American Diet. Soul food describes traditional Southern African American foods and cooking techniques that evolved from West African, slave, and post-abolition cuisine.

(continued)

CHAPTER SUMMARY CULTURAL AND RELIGIOUS INFLUENCES ON FOOD AND NUTRITION (continued)

- Traditional soul foods tend to be high in fat, cholesterol, and sodium and low in protective nutrients, such as potassium, fiber, and calcium.
- Staples: corn and corn products (grits, cornmeal), rice, biscuits, legumes, catfish, breaded and fried beef, pork, poultry, variety meats (oxtail, pig's feet), pork rinds, "greens."
- Intakes of total vegetables, whole grains, milk, fiber, potassium, and calcium are lower among Black Americans than White Americans, and intakes of sugar-sweetened beverages and added sugars are higher.
- Nutrition-related health concerns among Black Americans are obesity and high rates of morbidity and mortality from hypertension, heart disease, and stroke.

Mexican American Diet. The traditional diet is generally a low-fat, high-fiber diet rich in complex carbohydrates and vegetable proteins, with an emphasis on corn, corn products, beans, and rice.

- Staples: tomatoes, squash, avocado, cocoa, vanilla, grains (bread, rice, tacos, tortillas), beans, rice, sweet potato, poultry fish, chorizo, and cheeses.
- Acculturation is associated with undesirable changes in the intake of vegetables, fruits, sodium, and empty calories. The intake of fast foods, pizza, non-homemade meals, and meals at sit-down restaurants increases.
- Nutrition-related health concerns are obesity and type 2 diabetes. Inactivity is high; life expectancy is longer for Hispanics than White Americans.

Chinese American Diet. The traditional diet of Chinese people is low in fat and dairy products and high in complex carbohydrates and sodium.

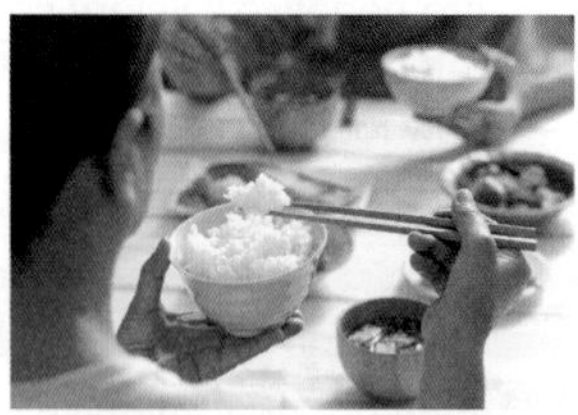

- Staples: rice (southern China), wheat products (northern China), vegetables, sea vegetables, nuts, seeds, beans, soy foods, a variety of meats, and tea.
- With acculturation, the diet becomes higher in fat, protein, sugar, and cholesterol. The intake of raw vegetables, meat, ethnic foods, and fast food increases.
- Nutrition-related health concerns are the risk of type 2 diabetes at a lower BMI for Chinese Americans than for other groups; at any BMI level, men and women who are Chinese Americans have a higher percentage of body fat than White Americans. Chinese Americans have the lowest percentage of people in fair or poor health and the lowest prevalence of obesity.

Food and Religion

Religion tends to have a greater impact on food choices than nationality or culture.

Christianity

- Dietary practices vary from none to explicit.
- Roman Catholics: This group does not eat meat on Ash Wednesday or on Fridays of Lent and food; beverages are avoided for 1 hour before communion is taken. Devout Catholics observe several fast days during the year.
- Eastern Orthodox Christians observe numerous feast and fast days throughout the year.
- Members of the Church of Jesus Christ of Latter-day Saints do not use coffee, tea, or alcohol; limiting meat intake is encouraged.
- Seventh-Day Adventists: Lacto-ovo vegetarianism is common. Overeating is avoided.

Judaism

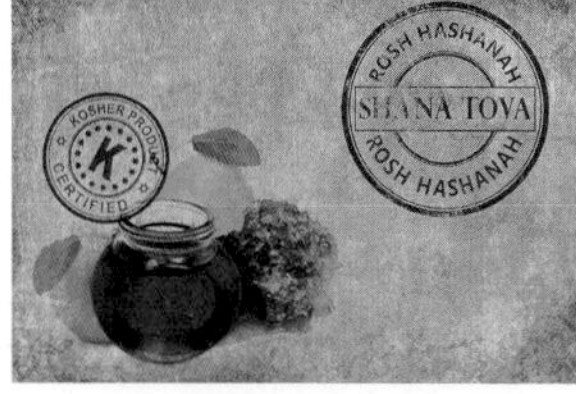

- Dietary restrictions vary among denominations.
- Kashrut is a list of dietary laws. The main principles are that animals must be kosher, blood is not allowed, and milk and meat must not mix.

Islam

- Health and food are considered acts of worship.
- Halal foods are permitted; haram foods are prohibited.
- Kosher and halal animals are allowed, blood is not allowed, slaughter must use proper methods, decaying carcasses are not allowed, and intoxicants are forbidden.

Hinduism

- Dietary practices stem from the idea of living in harmony with nature and having mercy for all of God's creations.
- Many Hindu people are vegetarian, even though meat is not explicitly forbidden.
- Foods considered pure foods enhance spiritual purity.

Buddhism

- The five moral precepts are to not kill or harm living things, steal, engage in sexual misconduct, lie, and consume intoxicants.
- Food decisions should contribute to spiritual enlightenment.

Figure sources: *shutterstock.com/Antwon McMullen, shutterstock.com/kazoka, and shutterstock.com/Protasov AN*

Student Resources on thePoint®
For additional learning materials, activate the code in the front of this book at https://thePoint.lww.com/activate

Websites

Cultural/Ethnic Food Guide Pyramids, USDA National Agricultural Library at http://fnic.nal.usda.gov/dietary-guidance/myplatefood-pyramid-resources/ethniccultural-food-pyramids

Ethnic medicine information including nutrition information: Harborview Medical Center, University of Washington at www.ethnomed.org

Office of Minority Health at http://minorityhealth.hhs.gov/

Traditional diets at Oldways Preservation & Exchange Trust at www.oldwayspt.org

Website for information on fast food and eating out: Center for Science in the Public Interest at www.cspinet.org

References

Binkley, J., & Liu, Y. (2019). Food at home and away from home: Commodity composition, nutrition differences, and differences in consumers. *Agricultural and Resource Economics Review, 48*(2), 221–252. https://www.cambridge.org/core/services/aop-cambridge-core/content/view/FD229E025ACD524B31C6D1DA48AFD2DF/S1068280519000017a.pdf/div-class-title-food-at-home-and-away-from-home-commodity-composition-nutrition-differences-and-differences-in-consumers-div.pdf

Brown, A., Houser, R., Mattei, J., Rehn, C. D., Mozaffarian, D., Lichtenstein, A. H., & Folta, S. C. (2018). Diet quality among U.S.-born and foreign-born non-Hispanic blacks: NHANES 2003–2012 data. *American Journal of Clinical Nutrition, 107*(5), 695–706. https://doi.org/10.1093/ajcn/nqy021

Carr, C. (2012). Minority ethnic groups with type 2 diabetes: The importance of effective dietary advice. *Journal of Diabetes Nursing, 16*(3), 88–96.

Centers for Disease Control and Prevention. (2019, September 15). *Hispanic/Latino Americans and type 2 diabetes.* https://www.cdc.gov/diabetes/library/features/hispanic-diabetes.html

Colby, S. L., & Ortman, J. M. (2015). *Projections of the size and composition of the U.S. population: 2014–2060.* United States Census Bureau. https://www.census.gov/library/publications/2015/demo/p25-1143.html

ElGindy, G. (2013, March 30). *Understanding Buddhist patient's dietary needs.* https://minoritynurse.com/?s=Buddhist+dietary

Federal Register. (2019, February 1). *Indian entities recognized by and eligible to receive services from the United States Bureau of Indian Affairs.* https://www.federalregister.gov/documents/2019/02/01/2019-00897/indian-entities-recognized-by-and-eligible-to-receive-services-from-the-united-states-bureau-of

Hagan, J. F., Shaw, J. S., & Duncan, P. M. (Eds.). (2017). *Bright futures: Guidelines for health supervision of infants, children, and adolescents.* American Academy of Pediatrics.

Hiza, H., Casavale, K., Guenther, P., & Davis, C. (2013). Diet quality of Americans differs by age, sex, race/ethnicity, income, and education level. *Journal of the Academy of Nutrition and Dietetics, 113*(2), 297–306. https://doi.org/10.1016/j.jand.2012.08.011

Kagawa-Singer, M., Dadia, A., Yu, M., & Surbone, A. (2010). Cancer, culture, and health disparities: Time to chart a new course? *CA: A Cancer Journal for Clinicians, 60*(1), 12–39. https://doi.org/10.3322/caac.20051

King, G., McNeely, M., Thorpe, L., Mau, M. L. M., Ko, J., Liu, L. L., Sun, A., Hsu, W. C., & Chow, E. A. (2012). Understanding and addressing unique needs of diabetes in Asian Americans, Native Hawaiians, and Pacific Islanders. *Diabetes Care, 35*(5), 1181–1188. https://doi.org/10.2337/dc12-0210

Kittler, P., Sucher, K., & Nahikian-Nelms, M. (2012). *Food and culture.* Wadsworth Cengage Learning.

Kulkarni, K. (2004). Food, culture, and diabetes in the United States. *Clinical Diabetes, 22*(4), 190–192. https://doi.org/10.2337/diaclin.22.4.190

Langellier, B. A., Glik, D., Ortega, A. N., & Prelip, M. L. (2015a). Trends in racial/ethnic disparities in overweight self-perception among U.S. adults, 1988–1994 and 1999–2008. *Public Health Nutrition, 18*(12), 2115–2125. https://doi.org/10.1017/S1368980014002560

Langellier, B., Brookmeyer, R., Wang, M., & Glik, D. (2015b). Language use affects food behaviours and food values among Mexican-origin adults in the USA. *Public Health Nutrition, 18*(2), 264–274. https://doi.org/10.1017/S1368980014000287

Lesser, L., Gasevic, D., & Lear, S. (2014). The association between acculturation and dietary patterns of south Asian immigrants. *PloS One, 9*(2), e88495. https://doi.org/10.1371/journal.pone.0088495

Mills, S., Brown, H., Wrieden, W., White, M., & Adams, J. (2017). Frequency of eating home cooked meals and potential benefits for diet and health: Cross-sectional analysis of a population-based cohort study. *International Journal of Behavioral Nutrition and Physical Activity. 14*, 109. https://doi.org/10.1186/s12966-017-0567-y

Minority Nurse. (2013a). *Meeting Jewish and Muslim patient's dietary needs.* https://minoritynurse.com/?s=Jewish+dietary

Minority Nurse. (2013b). *Hindu dietary practices: Feeding the body, mind and soul.* https://minoritynurse.com/?s=Hindu+dietary

Murphy, S., Xu, J., Kochaneck, K., & Arias, E. (2018, November 29). *Mortality in the United States, 2017.* NCHS Data Brief, no 328. National Center for Health Statistics. https://www.cdc.gov/nchs/products/databriefs/db328.htm

National Institutes of Health. (2018, January 9). *Factors contributing to higher incidence of diabetes for black Americans.* National Institutes of Health. https://www.nih.gov/news-events/nih-research-matters/factors-contributing-higher-incidence-diabetes-black-americans

Nguyen, B., & Powell, L. (2014). The impact of restaurant consumption among U.S. adults: Effects on energy and nutrient intakes. *Public Health Nutrition, 17*(11), 2445–2452. https://doi.org/10.1017/S1368980014001153

Office of Minority Health. (2019a, August 22). *Profile: Black/African Americans.* https://minorityhealth.hhs.gov/omh/browse.aspx?lvl=3&lvlid=61

Office of Minority Health. (2019b, August 22). *Profile: Hispanic/Latino Americans.* http://minorityhealth.hhs.gov/omh/browse.aspx?lvl=3&lvlid=64

Office of Minority Health. (2019c, August 22). *Profile: Asian Americans.* https://minorityhealth.hhs.gov/omh/browse.aspx?lvl=3&lvlid=63

Pew Research Center. (2019, May 22). *Six origin groups make up 85% of all Asian Americans.* https://www.pewresearch.org/fact-tank/2019/05/22/key-facts-about-asian-origin-groups-in-the-u-s/ft_19-05-23_asianamericans_sixorigingroupsmakeup85

Reininger, B., Lee, M., Jennings, R., & Evans, A. (2017). Healthy eating patterns associated with acculturation, sex and BMI among Mexican Americans. *Public Health Nutrition, 20*(7), 1267–1278. https://doi.org/10.1017/S1368980016003311

Satia, J. (2009). Diet-related disparities: Understanding the problem and accelerating solutions. *Journal of the American Dietetic Association, 109*(4), 610–615. https://dx.doi.org/10.1016%2Fj.jada.2008.12.019

U.S. Census Bureau. (2019, July 1). *QuickFacts*. https://www.census.gov/quickfacts/fact/table/US/AGE775218#AGE775218

U.S. Census Bureau. (2020, April 21). *About*. https://www.census.gov/topics/population/race/about.html#:~:text=OMB%20requires%20five%20minimum%20categories,Hawaiian%20or%20Other%20Pacific%20Islander

U.S. Department of Agriculture Agricultural Research Service. (2018). *Percentages of selected nutrition contributed by food and beverages consumed away from home, by gender and age, in the United States, 2015–2016.* https://www.ars.usda.gov/ARSUserFiles/80400530/pdf/1516/Table_9_AWY_GEN_15.pdf

Valerino-Perea, S., Lara-Castor, L., Armstrong, M. E. G., & Papadaki, A. (2019). Definition of the traditional Mexican diet and its role in health: A systematic review. *Nutrients, 11*(11), 2803. https://doi.org/10.3390/nu11112803

Yoshida, Y., Scribner, R., Chen, L., Broyles, S., Phillippi, S., & Tseng, T.-S. (2017). Role of age and acculturation in diet quality among Mexican Americans—Findings from the National Health and Nutrition Examination Survey, 1999–2012. *Preventing Chronic Disease, 14*, 14:E59. https://doi.org/10.5888/ pcd14.170004

Chapter 12

Healthy Eating for Healthy Babies

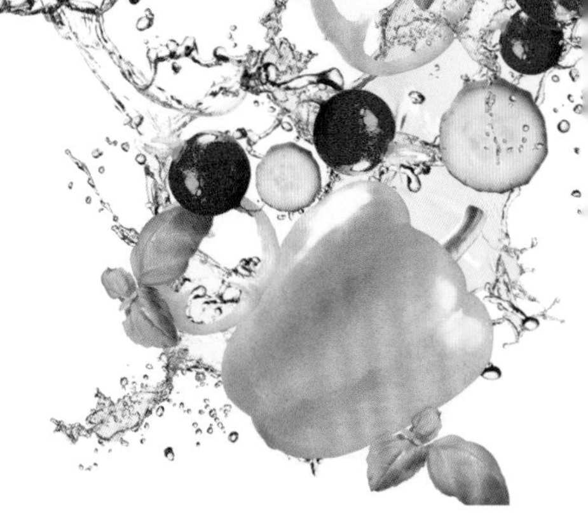

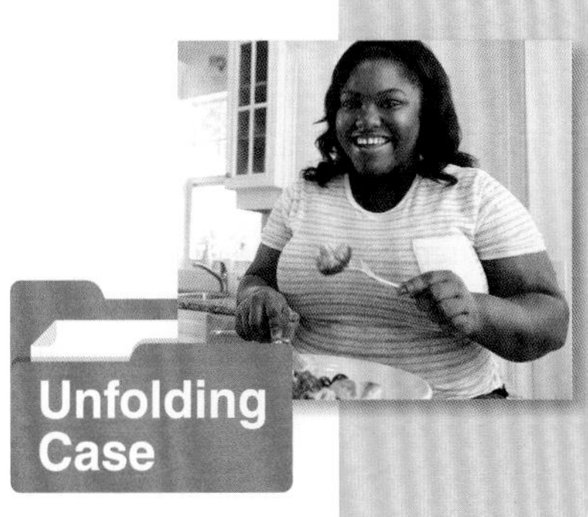

Unfolding Case

Rachel Stevens

Rachel is 27 years old and was diagnosed with polycystic ovary syndrome (PCOS) at age 18 years. She and her husband want to start a family, but she has irregular periods and fears she will have a hard time getting pregnant. She is 5 ft 5 in. and weighs 183 pounds, which gives her a body mass index (BMI) of 30.5. She has noticed that her PCOS symptoms get worse the more weight she gains. She would also like to lose some weight and "get healthy" before getting pregnant.

Learning Objectives

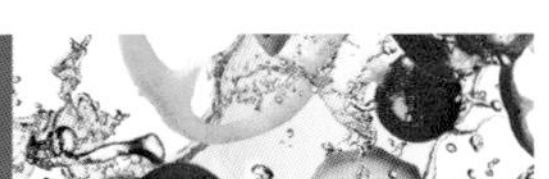

Upon completion of this chapter, you will be able to:

1. Discuss prepregnancy nutrition considerations.
2. Evaluate a woman's pattern and amount of weight gain during pregnancy based on her prepregnancy body mass index.
3. Assess whether a woman may benefit from a multivitamin and mineral supplement during pregnancy.
4. Describe characteristics of a healthy eating pattern during pregnancy.
5. Discuss the following lifestyle and dietary concerns during pregnancy: alcohol, caffeine, nonnutritive sweeteners, fish, and foodborne illness.
6. Give examples of nutrition interventions used for nausea, constipation, and heartburn during pregnancy.
7. List common risk factors for diabetes and hypertension during pregnancy.
8. Discuss how lactation affects calorie and nutrient needs.
9. List benefits of breastfeeding for mother and infant.

Nutrition plays a vital role before, during, and after pregnancy and lactation for both mother and child. Women who are healthy at the time of conception are more likely to have a successful pregnancy and a healthy infant. Being well nourished and within a healthy weight range prior to conception provides an environment conducive to normal fetal growth and development during the critical first trimester of pregnancy. During pregnancy, the fetus cannot meet its genetic potential for development if the supply of energy and nutrients is inadequate. Conversely, excessive weight gain during pregnancy is strongly associated with maternal and fetal complications, including obesity for both later in life. A healthy eating pattern provides enough but not excessive amounts of calories and nutrients to optimize maternal and fetal health.

This chapter discusses nutrition guidance for women before, during, and after pregnancy, including weight gain recommendations, common problems of pregnancy, and nutrition interventions for maternal health conditions. Nutrition for lactation is discussed.

PREPREGNANCY NUTRITION

Studies show a strong link between prepregnancy health and nutritional status and maternal and child health outcomes, with consequences that span generations (Stephenson et al., 2018). For instance:

- Overweight and obese women need a longer time to conceive and are at higher risk of infertility (Silvestris et al., 2018).
- A low folate status prior to conception increases the risk of neural tube defects (U.S. Preventive Services Task Force, 2017).
- High body mass index (BMI) increases the risk for maternal complications such as gestational hypertension, preeclampsia, gestational diabetes, and cesarean section delivery (Stang & Huffman, 2016).
- High BMI also increases the risk of poor fetal outcomes, including preterm birth, macrosomia, shoulder dystocia, select birth defects, and stillbirth (Stang et al., 2016).
- Prepregnancy overweight and obesity increase the risk childhood obesity in the infant (Liu et al., 2016).
- Prepregnancy underweight increases the risk for small-for-gestational-age births (Liu et al., 2016).

The preconception period may be a critical time to promote a healthy lifestyle to reduce the risk of undesirable birth outcomes. Stephenson et al. (2018) have shown that when initiated *during* pregnancy:

- Dietary interventions can reduce weight gain and adiposity in obese women but have little impact on pregnancy outcomes.
- Multiple micronutrient supplementation appears to be "too little, too late" to fundamentally improve child health outcomes.

Fortunately, a change in preconception eating patterns can improve prepregnancy BMI (Mohammadi et al., 2018). Likewise, adequate nutrient intakes prior to pregnancy helps ensure adequate micronutrient stores help meet the needs of a growing embryo (Dahly et al., 2018). Improvements in lifestyle should occur before conception to improve maternal and child health (Stephenson et al., 2018).

Attain and Maintain Healthy Weight

Current estimates indicate that approximately half of women of childbearing age are classified as overweight (BMI 25–29.9) or obese (BMI ≥ 30) (U.S. Department of Agriculture [USDA] & U.S. Department of Health and Human Services [USDHHS], 2020). Some of the risks to mother and infant related to entering pregnancy with a high BMI are stated earlier. Another risk is that women who are overweight or obese frequently exceed gestational weight gain (GWG) recommendations during pregnancy, which increases the risk of postpartum weight retention (USDA & USDHHS, 2020).

Healthy Weight
BMI of 18.5 to 24.9.

- Because achieving healthy weight can take months to years to accomplish, the ideal time to attain **healthy weight** may be during adolescence when most women are not planning pregnancy (Stephenson et al., 2018).
- All women who are contemplating pregnancy should be screened during the preconception period to determine their weight status.
- All women with a BMI of 25 or higher should be counseled about the risks of unhealthy weight to maternal health and future pregnancies and given guidance to help them attain and maintain healthy body weight.

Healthy Eating Patterns

The basic principles of healthy eating for the general U.S. population are also appropriate during pregnancy and lactation:

- Consume a calorie-appropriate, nutrient-dense eating pattern that includes plenty of fruits and vegetables of various kinds and colors, whole grains in place of refined grains, a variety of lean protein foods, low-fat or fat-free dairy products, and healthy oils in moderation.
- Limit solid fats, added sugars, sodium, and refined grains.
- Meet nutrient needs primarily through food and beverages, not supplements.
- Healthy eating patterns include the Healthy U.S.-style eating pattern (similar to the Dietary Approaches to Stop Hypertension [DASH] diet) and Mediterranean-style eating pattern. The Healthy Vegetarian Eating Pattern can also be used during pregnancy with careful attention to certain nutrients.

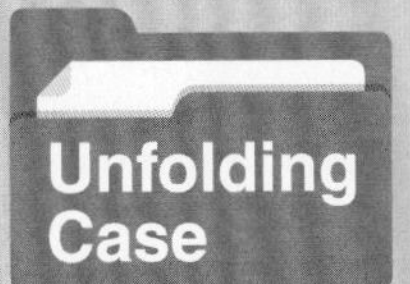

Recall Rachel. Weight loss and exercise can improve her PCOS symptoms, improve her chance of becoming pregnant, and lower her risk of adverse pregnancy outcomes. How is Rachel's BMI classified? What would be appropriate calorie and weight goals for Rachel? What type of healthy eating pattern would you recommend? What tools would you recommend she use to help her eat healthy while working toward a healthier weight?

Folic Acid

Folate
natural form of the B vitamin involved in the synthesis of DNA; only one-half is available to the body as synthetic folic acid.

Neural Tube Defects
major central nervous system birth defects, such as anencephaly (underdeveloped brain and an incomplete skull) and spina bifida (incomplete closure of the spinal cord) that occur early in pregnancy due to improper closure of the embryonic neural tube.

Folic Acid
synthetic form of folate found in multivitamins, fortified breakfast cereals, and enriched grain products.

The U.S. Preventive Services Task Force, along with many other health-related organizations, recommends that all women who are planning pregnancy or capable of becoming pregnant take a daily multivitamin supplement containing 400 to 800 mcg of folic acid based on high certainty that the net benefit in preventing neural tube defects in the developing fetus is substantial (U.S. Preventive Services Task Force, 2017). Most women do not obtain the recommended daily intake of folate from food alone.

- The critical period for supplementation begins at least 1 month before conception and continues through the first 2 to 3 months of pregnancy (U.S. Preventive Services Task Force, 2017). Because half of all pregnancies are unplanned, all women who are capable of becoming pregnant should be advised to take folic acid supplements.
- Synthetic folic acid in supplements and fortified food is better absorbed and has greater availability than natural folate in food.
- Folic acid–fortified foods and food sources of natural **folate** are encouraged in addition to using either a multivitamin or an individual folic acid supplement (Box 12.1).
- Obese women, who are at increased risk of neural tube defects, may benefit from a supplement containing 800 mcg of folic acid. Other risk factors for **neural tube defects** include maternal diabetes and mutations in folate-related enzymes.
- Obese and overweight women with a history of birth defects may benefit from consuming up to 4 mg of **folic acid** supplements before and between pregnancies (Stang et al., 2016).

Other Healthy Lifestyle Practices

Lifestyle factors are among the several factors that influence whether a pregnancy is considered high risk (Box 12.2). Healthy lifestyle practices are recommended in the preconception period to prepare women for pregnancy.

- Be physically active.
- Do not smoke, drink alcohol, or use drugs.
- Avoid herbal supplements unless approved by a physician.
- Manage existing medical conditions such as diabetes and hypertension.

BOX 12.1 Food Sources of Important Nutrients before and during Pregnancy

Folate

Folic acid (fortified foods and supplements) is better absorbed than natural folate in foods

- **Natural sources:** leafy green vegetables (e.g., spinach), asparagus, and avocado; dried peas and beans, such as lentils, soybeans, and pinto beans; and organ meats
- **Fortified foods:** 100% fortified ready-to-eat breakfast cereals; enriched bread, rolls, pasta, and cereal

Iron

Heme iron is better absorbed than nonheme iron.

- **Heme sources:** beef liver, clams, mussels, oysters, red meats, fish, and poultry
- **Nonheme sources:** beans, peas, lentils, dark green vegetables, and iron-enriched or fortified foods, such as many whole wheat breads, fortified breakfast cereals, and products made with enriched flour (e.g., white bread, pasta, rolls)

Iodine

- **Natural sources:** eggs, seafood, seaweed (e.g., kelp, nori, and kombu)
- **Fortified source:** iodized salt. Milk and dairy products are incidentally fortified with iodine via the use of iodine feed supplements and iodine-containing disinfectants used to sanitize udders, milking machines, and milk tanks

Calcium

- **Natural sources:** milk, yogurt, hard natural cheese, pasteurized processed American cheese, bok choy, broccoli, Chinese/Napa cabbage, collards, kale, okra, turnip greens, legumes, and almonds
- **Fortified foods:** fortified breakfast cereals, fortified orange juice, fortified brands of nondairy milks (almond, soy, rice, coconut)

Vitamin D

- **Natural sources:** fatty fish (salmon, tuna, sardines, swordfish), beef liver, cod liver oil, and egg yolks
- **Fortified foods:** milk (dairy and nondairy), breakfast cereals, and orange juice

BOX 12.2 Factors That May Contribute to a High-Risk Pregnancy

Maternal Age of <17 or >35

Preexisting Maternal Health Conditions

- Obesity, overweight, underweight
- Hypertension
- Diabetes
- PCOS
- Kidney disease
- Respiratory disease
- Autoimmune disease

Lifestyle Risks

- Alcohol use
- Tobacco use
- Drug use

Conditions of Pregnancy

- Multiple gestation
- Gestational diabetes
- Preeclampsia and eclampsia
- Previous preterm birth or stillbirth
- History of giving birth to an infant with birth defects

NUTRITION AND LIFESTYLE DURING PREGNANCY

Many women are motivated during pregnancy to adopt healthy lifestyle changes, which have the potential to make a long-lasting impact on the health of mother and infant. The following sections cover nutrition-related considerations during pregnancy.

Recommended Amount of Weight Gain

The weight of the infant, products of conception, and increases in maternal organs, tissues, and fluids contribute to weight gain during pregnancy (Box 12.3). Current recommendations by the Institute of Medicine (2009) for weight gain during pregnancy are based on prepregnancy BMI

BOX 12.3 Weight Gain Distribution in Normal Pregnancy (Pounds)

Birth weight of baby	7.5
Placenta	1.5
Increase in maternal blood volume	4
Increase in maternal fluid volume	4
Increase in uterus	2
Increase in breast tissue	2
Amniotic fluid	2
Maternal fat tissue	7
Total	30

(see Table 12.1). These weight gain recommendations were based on observational data, so they should be viewed as a guide, not an absolute requirement.

- Underweight: 28 to 40 pounds
- Normal/healthy BMI: 25 to 35 pounds
- Overweight BMI: 15 to 25 pounds
- Obese: 11 to 20 pounds

Weight Gain in Obese Women

Due to limited data, the weight gain guidelines do not recommend different weight gain targets based on the severity of obesity, which are Class 1 (BMI of 30–34.9), Class 2 (BMI of 35–39.9), and Class 3 (BMI of ≥40). The optimal amount of weight severely obese women should gain during pregnancy is a subject of debate (Hutcheon et al., 2015).

- No evidence exists that encouraging increased weight gain to conform to the IOM guidelines will improve maternal or fetal outcomes for obese pregnant women who are gaining less weight than recommended but have a fetus that is growing appropriately (American College of Obstetricians and Gynecologists Committee on Obstetrics, 2013, reaffirmed 2016).
- Individualized care and clinical judgment are necessary to balance the risks of a large for gestational age (LGA) fetus and small for gestational age fetus, obstetric complications, and maternal weight retention after pregnancy (American College of Obstetricians and Gynecologists Committee on Obstetric Practice, 2013, reaffirmed 2016).

Table 12.1 Recommended Weight Gain Ranges Based on Maternal Prepregnancy Body Mass Index

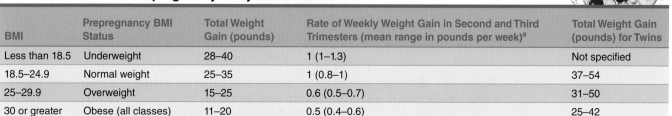

BMI	Prepregnancy BMI Status	Total Weight Gain (pounds)	Rate of Weekly Weight Gain in Second and Third Trimesters (mean range in pounds per week)[a]	Total Weight Gain (pounds) for Twins
Less than 18.5	Underweight	28–40	1 (1–1.3)	Not specified
18.5–24.9	Normal weight	25–35	1 (0.8–1)	37–54
25–29.9	Overweight	15–25	0.6 (0.5–0.7)	31–50
30 or greater	Obese (all classes)	11–20	0.5 (0.4–0.6)	25–42

[a]Calculations assume 1.1- to 4.4-pound weight gain in the first trimester.
Source: National Research Council. (2009). *Weight gain during pregnancy: Reexamining the guidelines*. The National Academies Press.

Recommended Pattern of Weight Gain

The Institute of Medicine (2009) recommends all women gain 1 to 4 pounds in the first trimester. Thereafter, recommended weekly weight gain is based on prepregnancy BMI (see Table 12.1).

- Normal-weight women are urged to gain approximately 1 pound/week during the second and third trimesters; recommended amounts of weekly gain for underweight, overweight, and obese women are slightly different.
- To monitor the amount and pattern of weight gain throughout pregnancy, weight gain is plotted on the appropriate grid based on maternal prepregnancy weight status (Figs. 12.1–12.4).
- Although slightly higher or lower rates of weight gain can be considered normal, obvious or persistent deviations warrant further investigation.

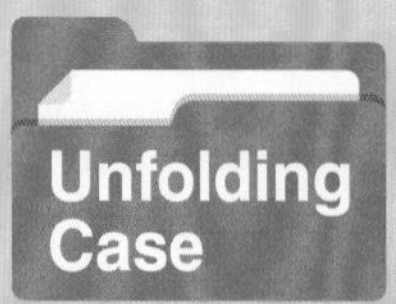

Consider Rachel. She was able to lose 10 pounds with exercise and healthy eating. After months of trying to conceive, her physician prescribed clomiphene (Clomid) to stimulate ovulation and she is now 4 weeks pregnant. How should she modify her eating pattern? What would you tell her about weight gain in the first trimester?

Increased Calorie Needs

Additional calories are needed to support growth of the fetus and maternal tissues, but the increase is relatively small. Regardless of maternal weight status, the Institute of Medicine (2009) recommends the following:

- 1st trimester: no extra calories
- 2nd trimester: +340 cal/day
- 3rd trimester: +452 cal/day

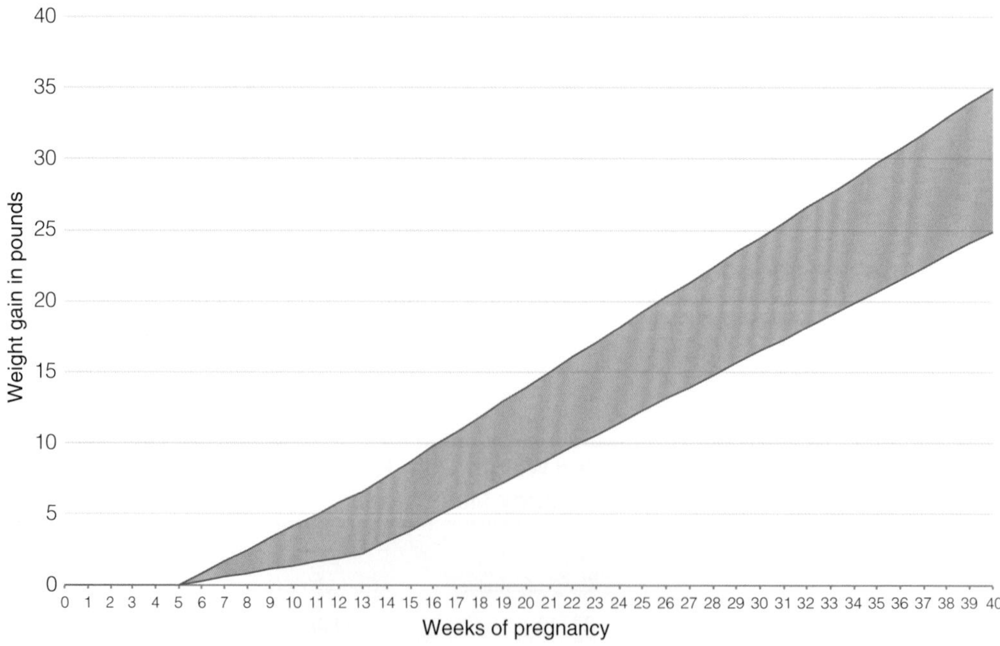

Figure 12.1 ▲ Weight gain chart for women who begin pregnancy at a normal weight: If your weight gain is within the shaded area, you're on track! (*Source:* Centers for Disease Control and Prevention. [2019, January 17]. *Tracking your weight for women who begin pregnancy at a normal weight.* https://www.cdc.gov/reproductivehealth/pdfs/maternal-infant-health/pregnancy-weight-gain/tracker/single/Normal_Weight_Tracker_508Tagged.pdf)

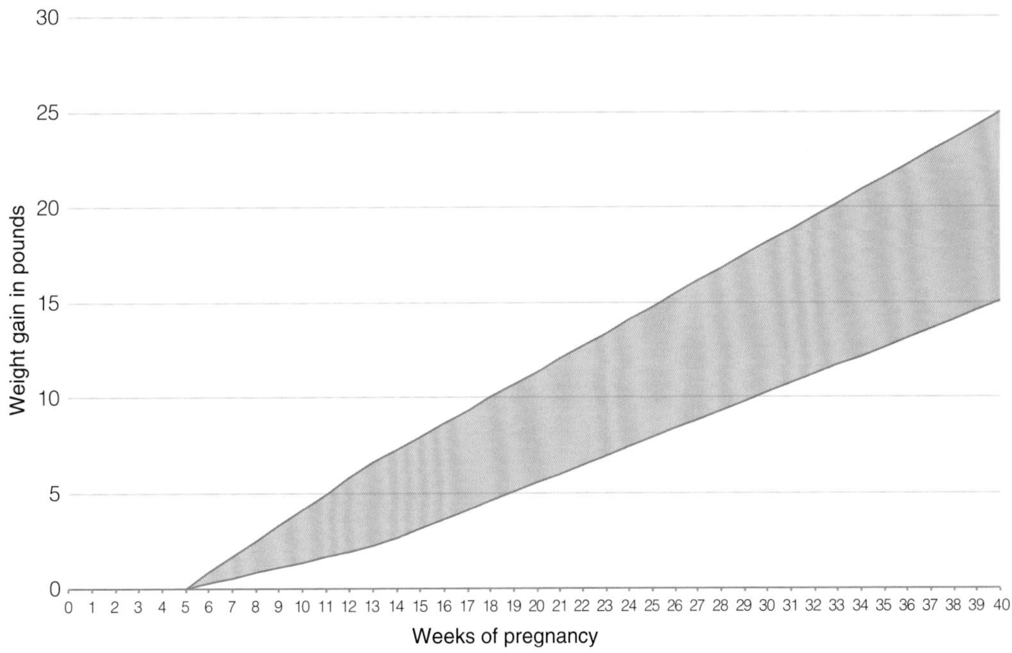

Figure 12.2 ▲ Weight gain chart for women who begin pregnancy overweight: If your weight gain is within the shaded area, you're on track! (*Source:* Centers for Disease Control and Prevention. [2019, January 17]. *Tracking your weight for women who begin pregnancy overweight.* https://www.cdc.gov/reproductivehealth/pdfs/maternal-infant-health/pregnancy-weight-gain/tracker/single/Overweight_Tracker_508Tagged.pdf)

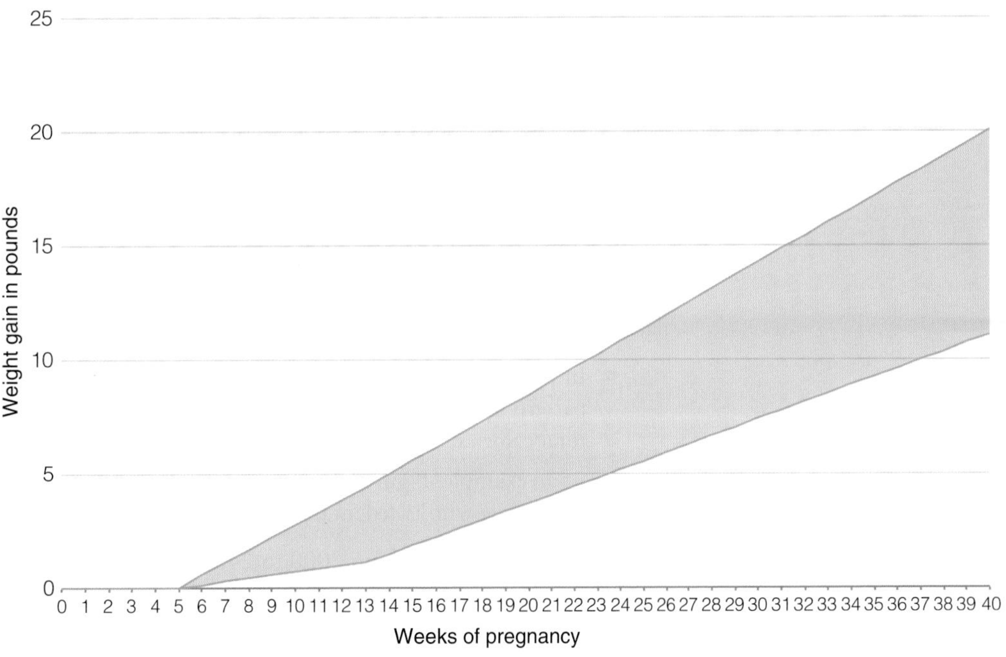

Figure 12.3 ▲ Weight gain chart for women who begin pregnancy with obesity: If your weight gain is within the shaded area, you're on track! (*Source:* Centers for Disease Control and Prevention. [2019, January 17]. *Tracking your weight for women who begin pregnancy with obesity.* https://www.cdc.gov/reproductivehealth/pdfs/maternal-infant-health/pregnancy-weight-gain/tracker/single/Obese_Weight_Tracker_508Tagged.pdf)

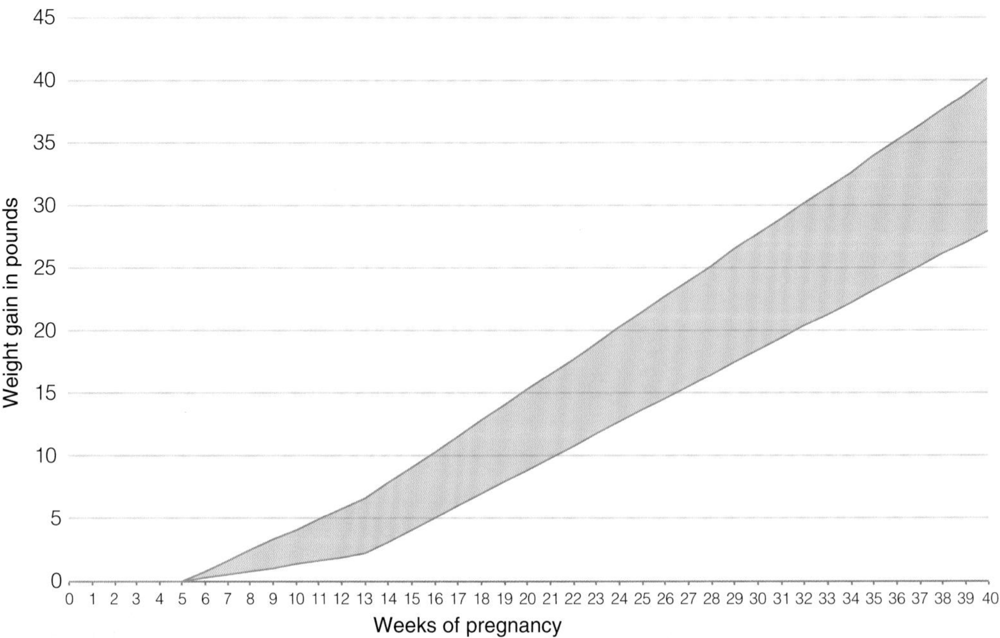

Figure 12.4 ▲ Weight gain chart for women who begin pregnancy underweight: If your weight gain is within the shaded area, you're on track! (*Source:* Centers for Disease Control and Prevention. [2019, January 17]. *Tracking your weight for women who begin pregnancy underweight.* https://www.cdc.gov/reproductivehealth/pdfs/maternal-infant-health/pregnancy-weight-gain/tracker/single/Underweight_Tracker_508Tagged.pdf)

Controversy exists over the appropriate amount of calories for pregnant women who are obese.

- Recently, and for the first time ever, researchers have provided evidence-based recommendations for calorie intake in pregnant women with obesity (U.S. Department of Health and Human Services, 2019).
- Study findings suggest that pregnant women with obesity should not consume extra calories during the first, second, and third trimesters because increased need for calories can be met by mobilizing maternal fat stores (Most et al., 2019).

Calories and Eating Patterns

The calorie levels of healthy eating patterns that are most relevant to women who are pregnant or lactating are 1800, 2000, 2200, 2400, 2600, and 2800 (USDA & USDHHS, 2020).

- In practice, women are not encouraged to actually "count" calories but to use an eating pattern approach that specifies amounts of food from each food group to approximate total calories.
- As an example, Figure 12.5 illustrates 3 calorie levels using a 5'6"-tall, 130-pound, 25-year-old female who is sedentary.
    - Calories range from 2000 to 2400 from before pregnancy through the 3rd trimester.
    - Notice how small the increase in food intake is from 2000 to 2400 calories: ½ c vegetables, 2 oz grains, and 1 oz protein foods.
    - The difference in incremental increases are not exactly 340 calories as recommended for the second trimester or 452 calories as recommended for the third trimester but are approximations.
    - All eating patterns rely on averages and approximations because actual calorie intake varies with individual foods chosen and the amount consumed.

Food Groups and Serving Sizes		Daily Amounts		
		2000 calories Nonpregnant and 1st trimester	**2200 calories** 2nd trimester	**2400 calories** 3rd trimester
Fruits	*1 cup from the Fruit Group counts as* • 1 cup raw, frozen, or cooked/canned fruit; or • ½ cup dried fruit; or • 1 cup 100% fruit juice	2 c	2 c	2 c
Vegetables	*1 cup from the Vegetable Group counts as* • 1 cup raw or cooked/canned vegetables; or • 2 cups leafy salad greens; or • 1 cup 100% vegetable juice	2 ½ c	3 c	3 c
Grains	*1 ounce from the Grains Group counts as* • 1 slice bread; or • 1 ounce ready-to-eat cereal; or • ½ cup cooked rice, pasta, or cereal	6 oz	7 oz	8 oz
Protein	*1 ounce from the Protein Foods Group counts as* • 1 ounce seafood, lean meat, or poultry; or • 1 egg; or • 1 tbsp peanut butter; or • ¼ cup cooked beans, peas, or lentils; or • ½ ounce nuts or seeds	5 ½ oz	6 oz	6 ½ oz
Dairy	*1 cup from the Dairy Group counts as* • 1 cup dairy milk or yogurt; or • 1 cup lactose-free dairy milk or yogurt; or • 1 cup fortified soy milk or yogurt; or • 1 ½ ounces hard cheese	3 c	3 c	3 c
Limit	Limit the intake of • Added sugars to less than 10% of total calories per day • Saturated fat to less than 10% of total calories per day • Sodium to less than 2300mg per day			

Figure 12.5 ▲ Examples of calorie levels that may be appropriate before and during pregnancy. (*Source:* Adapted from U.S. Department of Agriculture. [n.d.]. *MyPlate.* https://www.myplate.gov)

Current Intake of Pregnant and Lactating Women

On average, women who are pregnant or lactating have a higher-quality diet (as measured by the Healthy Eating Index-2015 score) than adult women in general (USDA & USDHHS, 2020). However, intakes are still not optimal. On average,

- intake of total vegetables, fruits, dairy, and whole grains is below recommended amounts;
- total protein foods intake is adequate but seafood intake is low; and
- limits for added sugars, saturated fat, and sodium are exceeded.

Vitamin and Mineral Requirements

The Dietary Reference Intakes (DRIs) for most nutrients increase during pregnancy. Figure 12.6 illustrates the percent change during pregnancy of selected nutrients compared to the DRIs for nonpregnant women aged 19 to 30 years. Vitamin D, vitamin K, and calcium do not appear in the figure because their requirements do not change during pregnancy.

- Nutrient needs are not actually constant throughout the course of pregnancy. Nutrient needs generally change little during the first trimester (folic acid is an exception) and are at their highest during the last trimester.

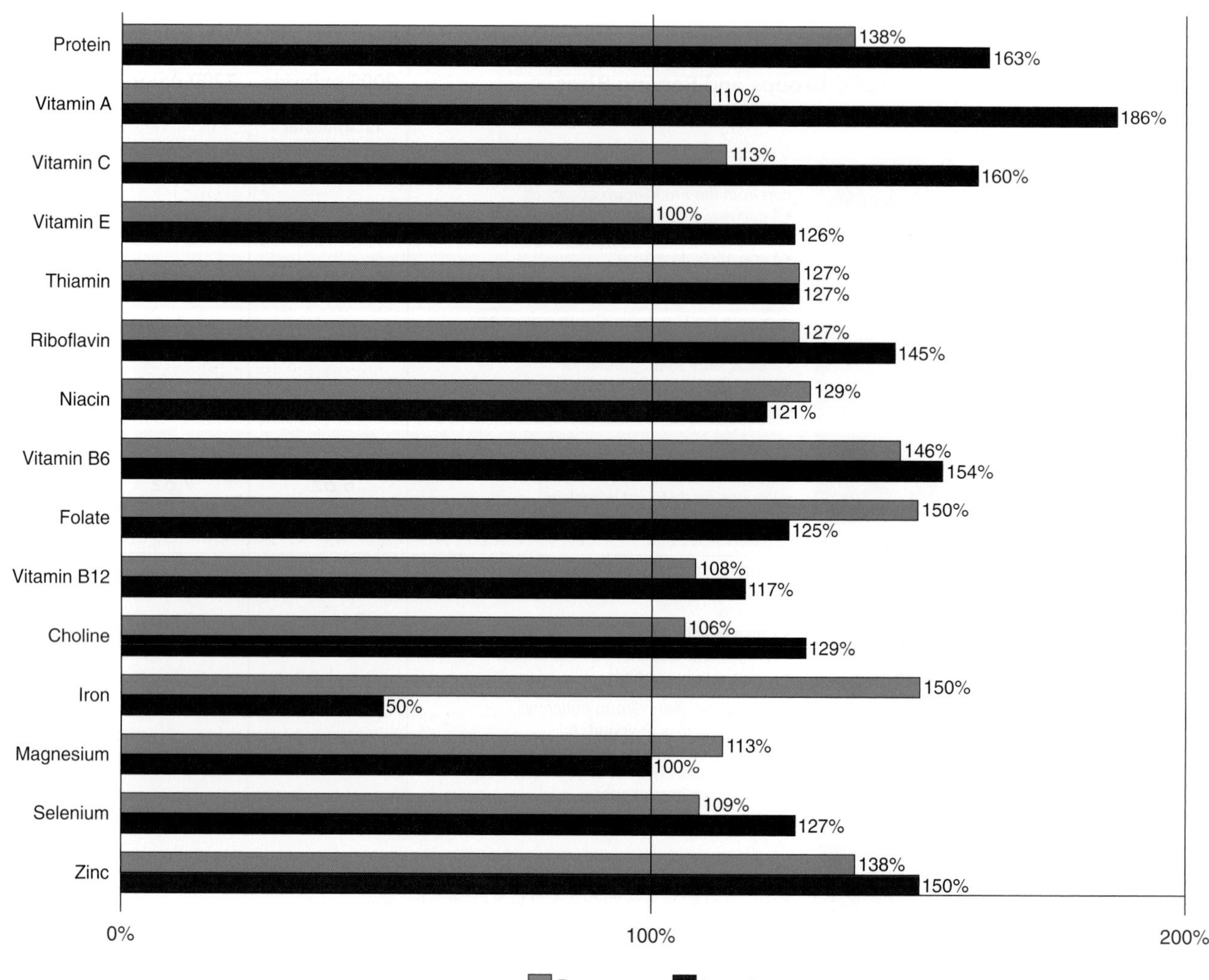

Figure 12.6 ▲ Percent change in selected nutrient recommendations during pregnancy and lactation compared to the DRIs for nonpregnant women ages 19–30 years. The recommendations for nonpregnant women are represented as 100%. (*Source:* Data from Institute of Medicine of the National Academies. [2006]. *Dietary reference intakes: The essential guide to nutrient requirements.* The National Academies Press.)

- Nutrient needs do not increase proportionately. For instance, the need for iron increases by 50% during pregnancy, yet the requirement for vitamin B_{12} increases by only about 10%. Actual requirements during pregnancy vary among individuals and are influenced by previous nutritional status and health history including chronic illnesses, multiple pregnancies, and closely spaced pregnancies.
- The requirement for one nutrient may be altered by the intake of another. For instance, women who do not meet their calorie requirements need higher amounts of protein.
- The intake of more food to meet increased calorie requirements and the increase in absorption and efficiency of nutrient use that occurs in pregnancy are generally enough to meet nutrient needs when nutrient-dense food choices are made. Exceptions are discussed in the following section.

Folic Acid

Folic acid has a vital role in DNA synthesis and thus is essential for the synthesis of new cells and transmission of inherited characteristics.

It is recommended that during pregnancy, women consume a total of 600 mcg of folic acid daily from all sources, such as 400 mcg from prenatal vitamins and the remainder from folic acid–fortified food and foods containing natural folate (Box 12.1).

Iron

The Recommended Dietary Allowance (RDA) for iron increases from 18 to 27 mg/day during pregnancy to support the increase in maternal blood volume and to provide iron for fetal liver storage, which sustains the infant for the first 4 to 6 months of life. Even with careful selections, women are not likely to consume adequate amounts of iron during pregnancy from food alone (Box 12.1). However, both dietary iron absorption and the mobilization of iron from maternal stores increase during pregnancy (Fisher & Nemeth, 2017).

- Iron deficiency affects about 1 in 10 women who are pregnant and 1 in 4 women during their third trimester (USDA & USDHHS, 2020).
- Iron supplementation is commonly recommended during pregnancy because iron deficiency and iron deficiency anemia during pregnancy have been associated with adverse maternal and child outcomes (Fisher & Nemeth, 2017).

Iodine

Iodine requirement increases substantially during pregnancy to support fetal neurocognitive development. Although iodine intake is generally adequate in women of childbearing age, those who do not use iodized salt or consume other sources of iodine may not consume enough iodine during pregnancy (Box 12.1) (USDA & USDHHS, 2020).

- Women should not be encouraged to increase their salt intake but instead should ensure the salt they use in cooking and at the table is iodized.
- Not all prenatal supplements contain iodine, so women who need a supplement should be sure to read the label.

Calcium and Vitamin D

Calcium and vitamin D are among the nutrients of public health concern for the general U.S. population, including women who are pregnant (USDA & USDHHS, 2020). These nutrients may need to be supplemented during pregnancy not because they cannot be consumed in adequate amounts but because they may not be depending on actual food choices (Box 12.1).

- The RDA for calcium does not increase during pregnancy because the rate of absorption and retention increases dramatically.
  - Three cups of milk or the equivalent provides approximately 900 mg of calcium, close to the RDA of 1000 mg.
  - Most multivitamins and prenatal vitamins have only 200 to 300 mg calcium, so an additional supplement may be needed if dietary intake is inadequate.
- The RDA for vitamin D does not increase during pregnancy.
  - Women who consume adequate amounts of vitamin D–fortified milk and have regular exposure to sunlight will probably not need supplemental vitamin D.
  - Supplements are recommended for women who consume <600 IU.

Prenatal Supplements

Aside from iron and folic acid, women who consume a varied, nutrient-dense eating pattern will probably meet vitamin and mineral needs during pregnancy.

- One exception is that pregnant women who consume little or no animal products should take a supplement of vitamin B_{12} if a reliable dietary source (vitamin B_{12}–fortified foods) is not consumed.
- Despite the likely nutrient adequacy of a varied, calorie-appropriate eating pattern, prenatal vitamin and mineral supplements are routinely recommended by physicians as insurance against less than optimal food choices.
- Prenatal vitamins have higher amounts of iron, folic acid, and calcium than regular multivitamin and mineral supplements.
- Although prenatal vitamins may not be needed, they are not likely to be harmful.

Lifestyle and Dietary Concerns

Alcohol

Fetal Alcohol Syndrome
a condition characterized by varying degrees of physical and mental growth failure and birth defects caused by maternal intake of alcohol.

Teratogen
anything that causes abnormal fetal development and birth defects.

Alcohol use during pregnancy can cause physical and neurodevelopmental problems, such as mental retardation, learning disabilities, and **fetal alcohol syndrome**.

- However, current data suggest small amounts of alcohol during pregnancy may not be harmful to the fetus (Fox, 2018).
- Yet because alcohol is a potent **teratogen** and a "safe" level of consumption is not known, women are advised to completely avoid alcohol before and during pregnancy.

Caffeine

Data do not suggest an increased risk of adverse effects on pregnancy, fertility, or fetal neurodevelopment with caffeine intake of 300 mg/day or less (Morgan et al., 2013).

- It is not known if higher caffeine intake is correlated to miscarriage (American College of Obstetricians and Gynecologists Committee on Obstetric Practice, 2010, reaffirmed 2016).
- Pregnant women should limit caffeine intake to less than 300 mg/day, the approximate amount in two to three 8-oz cups of coffee (Fox, 2018).
- Table 12.2 lists the amount of caffeine in various beverages and foods.

Nonnutritive Sweeteners

The use of nonnutritive sweeteners during pregnancy has been studied extensively and still generates controversy.

- The U.S. Food and Drug Administration (FDA) has approved six nonnutritive sweeteners as food additives and two as Generally Recognized As Safe. They are deemed safe for consumption, including during pregnancy, within defined levels of intake (U.S. Food and Drug Administration, 2018).
- The American College of Obstetricians and Gynecologists states that artificial sweeteners can be used in pregnancy but that data regarding the use of saccharin are conflicting (Fox, 2018). However, intake of that sweetener is typically low and likely safe.
- Even though their safety is established, cautious use is prudent.

Seafood

The intake of omega-3 fatty acids from at least 8 oz of fish/week during pregnancy, especially docosahexaenoic acid (DHA), is associated with improved infant visual and cognitive development (Mulder et al., 2014). Nearly all fish contain trace amounts of mercury because it occurs naturally in the environment, including waterways. Mercury can cause fetal neurologic damage; however, the possible risk from mercury in fish is offset by the neurobehavioral benefits of adequate DHA intake (Hagan et al., 2017). Advice about eating fish from the FDA and EPA is as follows (FDA, 2019):

- Women who are pregnant or breastfeeding are urged to consume 8 to 12 oz of a variety of seafood/week, from choices that are lower in mercury. Two to 3 servings/week are recommended from among the best choices: anchovy, Atlantic herring, Atlantic mackerel, mussels, oysters, farmed and wild salmon, sardines, canned light tuna, snapper, and trout. See Figure 4.3 in Chapter 4 for the complete list.
- Good choices are recommended once a week and include bluefish, Chilean sea bass, grouper, halibut, mahi mahi, monkfish, snapper, and albacore/white tuna (canned, fresh, or frozen).
- The following fish have the highest mercury levels and should be avoided by pregnant women: king mackerel, marlin, orange roughy, shark, swordfish, tilefish (from the Gulf of Mexico), and bigeye tuna.
- For women who do not consume 2 to 3 servings of fish/week, there is no clear evidence that omega-3 supplements improve outcomes in children (Fox, 2018).

Table 12.2 Caffeine Content of Selected Beverages and Foods

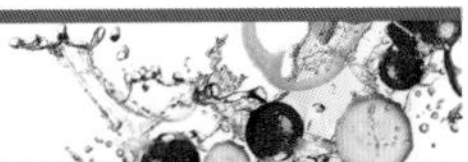

Item	Serving Size (oz)	Average Caffeine Content (mg)
Coffee		
Brewed	8	135
Instant	8	76–106
Decaffeinated instant	8	5
Starbucks coffee, blonde roast	16	360
Tea		
Brewed, average blend	8	43
Brewed, green	8	30
Instant	8	15
Brewed, herbal	8	0
Snapple Lemon Tea	16	37
Soft drinks		
Pepsi Zero Sugar	20	115
Mountain Dew, diet or regular	20	91
Dr. Pepper, diet or regular	12	41
Pepsi	12	38
Coca-Cola, Coke Zero, or diet Pepsi	16	45
Ginger ale, 7UP, Squirt, tonic water, Sprite	12	0
Energy drinks		
Bang Energy	16	300
5-hour Energy	2	200
Red Bull	8.4	80
Full Throttle	8	80
Other beverages		
Chocolate milk	8	8
Hot cocoa mix	9	5
Candy		
Dark chocolate, semisweet	1	18
Hershey's Milk Chocolate Bar	1.5	9

Source: Adapted from Government of Canada. (2012, April 13). *Caffeine in foods*. https://www.canada.ca/en/health-canada/services/food-nutrition/food-safety/food-additives/caffeine-foods.html; Center for Science and the Public Interest. (n.d.). *Caffeine chart*. https://cspinet.org/eating-healthy/ingredients-of-concern/caffeine-chart

Foodborne Illness

Due to hormonal changes that decrease cell-mediated immune function, pregnant women and their fetuses are at increased risk of developing foodborne illness. Table 12.3 outlines foods to avoid and their alternatives. Two pathogens that are of particular importance during pregnancy are *Listeria* and *Toxoplasma gondii* because they can infect the fetus without causing maternal illness.

Listeria

Listeria monocytogenes is an unusual bacterium because it can grow in refrigerated temperatures, unlike most other foodborne pathogens.

- Many animals carry this bacterium without outward symptoms.
- Listeriosis is rare except in pregnant women, newborns, older adults, and people with weakened immune systems.

Table 12.3 Potential Food Safety Risks during Pregnancy

Foods to Avoid	Potential Risks	Recommended Alternatives
Raw seafood Avoid: sushi, sashimi, raw oysters, raw clams, raw scallops, ceviche, refrigerated smoked seafood	Parasites or bacteria	Cook first to 145° F Canned smoked seafood
Unpasteurized juice, cider, and milk	*Escherichia coli* or *Listeria*	Pasteurized versions of these beverages or boil unpasteurized versions for at least 1 minute
Soft cheese made from unpasteurized milk such as Brie, feta, Camembert, Roquefort, queso blanco, queso fresco Any other cheese made from unpasteurized milk	*E. coli* or *Listeria*	Hard cheese and cheese made from pasteurized milk
Undercooked eggs such as in homemade eggnog, raw batter, homemade Caesar salad dressing, tiramisu, eggs benedict, homemade ice cream, homemade hollandaise sauce	*Salmonella*	Eggs with firm yolks Cook casseroles or other dishes containing eggs to a temperature of 160° F. Use pasteurized eggs to make foods that contain raw or undercooked eggs.
Premade deli salads (egg, pasta, chicken, etc.)	*Listeria*	Make these foods at home.
Raw sprouts such as alfalfa, clover, mung bean, and radish	*E. coli* or *Salmonella*	Cook thoroughly.
Cold hot dogs and luncheon meats	*Listeria*	Reheat to steaming hot or 165° F even if the label says "precooked."
Undercooked meat and poultry including refrigerated pâtés or meat spreads from a deli or meat counter	*E. coli*, *Salmonella*, *Campylobacter*, *Toxoplasma gondii*	Cook meat and poultry above the USDA-recommended internal temperature. Use meat spreads or pâté that do not need refrigeration (e.g., canned, jarred, sealed pouches).
Raw dough or batter	*E. coli* or *Salmonella*	Thoroughly cook.

Source: Foodsafety.gov. (2019, April 1). *People at risk: Pregnant women*. https://www.foodsafety.gov/people-at-risk/pregnant-women

- Listeriosis is usually a mild illness for pregnant women but causes severe disease in the fetus or newborn and may result in miscarriage, stillbirth, preterm labor, or newborn death (Centers for Disease Control and Prevention [CDC], 2016).
- Pregnant women are 10 times more likely to get listeriosis than other healthy adults (FoodSafety.gov, 2019).

Toxoplasma gondii

Healthy people infected by the parasite *Toxoplasma gondii* may be asymptomatic or may have flu-like symptoms. During pregnancy, the consequences are more serious.

- Toxoplasmosis passed to the fetus can cause mental disability or blindness, and hearing loss, which may not develop until later in life.
- Occasionally infected newborns have serious eye or brain damage at birth.
- In addition to the precautions outlined in Table 12.3, pregnant women should also avoid changing cat litter (cats pass an environmentally resistant form of the organism in their feces). If no one else can change the litter, women should be advised to wear disposable gloves and to thoroughly wash their hands in warm soapy water afterward. Litter should be changed daily because the parasite does not become infectious until 1 to 5 days after it is shed in the feces (CDC, 2019a).

Physical Activity

Physical activity throughout all stages of life promotes health and reduces the risk of chronic disease, such as cardiovascular disease, diabetes, and obesity.

- Because of the benefits of exercise and the data supporting its safety during pregnancy, women with uncomplicated pregnancies are urged to engage in aerobic and strength-training exercises before, during, and after pregnancy (American College of Obstetrics and Gynecologists Committee on Obstetric Practice, 2020).

BOX 12.4 Key Physical Activity Guidelines for Women during Pregnancy and the Postpartum Period

- Women should do at least 150 minutes (2 hours and 30 minutes) of moderate-intensity aerobic activity a week during pregnancy and the postpartum period. Preferably, aerobic activity should be spread throughout the week.
- Women who habitually engaged in vigorous-intensity aerobic activity or who were physically active before pregnancy can continue these activities during pregnancy and the postpartum period.
- Women who are pregnant should be under the care of a healthcare provider who can monitor the progress of the pregnancy. Women who are pregnant can consult their healthcare provider about whether or how to adjust their physical activity during pregnancy and after the baby is born.

Source: U.S. Department of Health and Human Services. (2018). *Physical activity guidelines for Americans*. U.S. Department of Health and Human Services.

- Exercise recommendations for pregnant women do not differ from those for the general public (American College of Obstetrics and Gynecologists Committee on Obstetric Practice, 2020).
- A goal of 150 minutes/week of moderate exercise is recommended (Box 12.4) (U.S. Department of Health and Human Services, 2018).
- Safe exercise should be encouraged, with attention paid to fall risk and avoiding supine positions during the second and third trimesters.

Maternal Health

Common complaints associated with pregnancy, such as nausea, heartburn, and constipation, may be prevented or alleviated by nutrition interventions (Table 12.4). Excessive weight gain, pica, diabetes mellitus, hypertension and preeclampsia, and maternal phenylketonuria (PKU) are discussed in the following sections.

Table 12.4 Common Complaints Associated with Pregnancy

Complaint	Possible Causes	Nutrition Interventions
Nausea and vomiting (common during the first trimester)	Hypoglycemia, decreased gastric motility, relaxation of the cardiac sphincter, anxiety	Eat easily digested carbohydrate foods (e.g., dry crackers, melba toast, dry cereal, hard candy) before getting out of bed in the morning. Eat frequent, small snacks of dry carbohydrates (e.g., crackers, hard candy) to prevent drop in glucose. Eat small frequent meals. Avoid liquids with meals. Limit high-fat foods because they delay gastric emptying. Eliminate individual intolerances and foods with a strong odor.
Constipation	Relaxation of gastrointestinal (GI) muscle tone and motility related to increased progesterone levels Increasing pressure on the GI tract by the fetus Decrease in physical activity Inadequate fiber and fluid intake Use of iron supplements	Increase fiber intake, especially intake of whole-grain breads and cereals. Look for breads that provide at least 2 g fiber/slice and cereals with at least 5 g fiber/serving. Drink at least eight 8-oz glasses of liquid daily. Try hot water with lemon or prune juice upon waking to help stimulate peristalsis. Participate in regular exercise.
Heartburn	Decrease in GI motility Relaxation of the cardiac sphincter Pressure of the uterus on the stomach	Eat small, frequent meals and eliminate liquids immediately before and after meals to avoid gastric distention. Avoid coffee, high-fat foods, and spices. Eliminate individual intolerances. Avoid lying down or bending over after eating.

Excessive Gestational Weight Gain

Excessive GWG, which increases the incidence of maternal and neonatal complications, is a major public health concern (Gilmore et al., 2015).

- Maternal risks of excessive GWG include increased risk of cesarean section, delivering an LGA neonate, and postpartum weight retention (Johnson et al., 2015); type 2 diabetes, cardiovascular disease, and metabolic syndrome are proposed long-term complications (Gilmore et al., 2015). Figure 12.7 illustrates long- and short-term metabolic consequences of excess GWG and postpartum weight retention.
- Risks to the infant include macrosomia and increased risk of childhood overweight or obesity (Kominiarek & Peaceman, 2017).
- In 2015, more than 48% of women who had a full-term, singleton delivery gained more weight than the recommended amount of weight (QuickStats, 2016).

Because excessive GWG early in pregnancy strongly predicts total excessive GWG, weight monitoring should begin at the onset of pregnancy. The American College of Obstetricians and Gynecologists recommends BMI be calculated at the first prenatal visit and that appropriate weight gain, eating pattern, and exercise be discussed at the first visit and periodically throughout pregnancy (American College of Obstetricians and Gynecologists, Committee on Obstetrics, 2013, reaffirmed 2016). A combination of strategies may promote appropriate GWG.

- Women need to understand that calorie needs actually increase only during the second and third trimesters and that the amount of additional food needed is relatively small.
- Women who are obese may not need to increase calories at any time during pregnancy (Most et al., 2019).
- Diet, exercise, and diet plus exercise interventions show a modest, but significant, effect on preventing excessive GWG (Muktabhant et al., 2015).

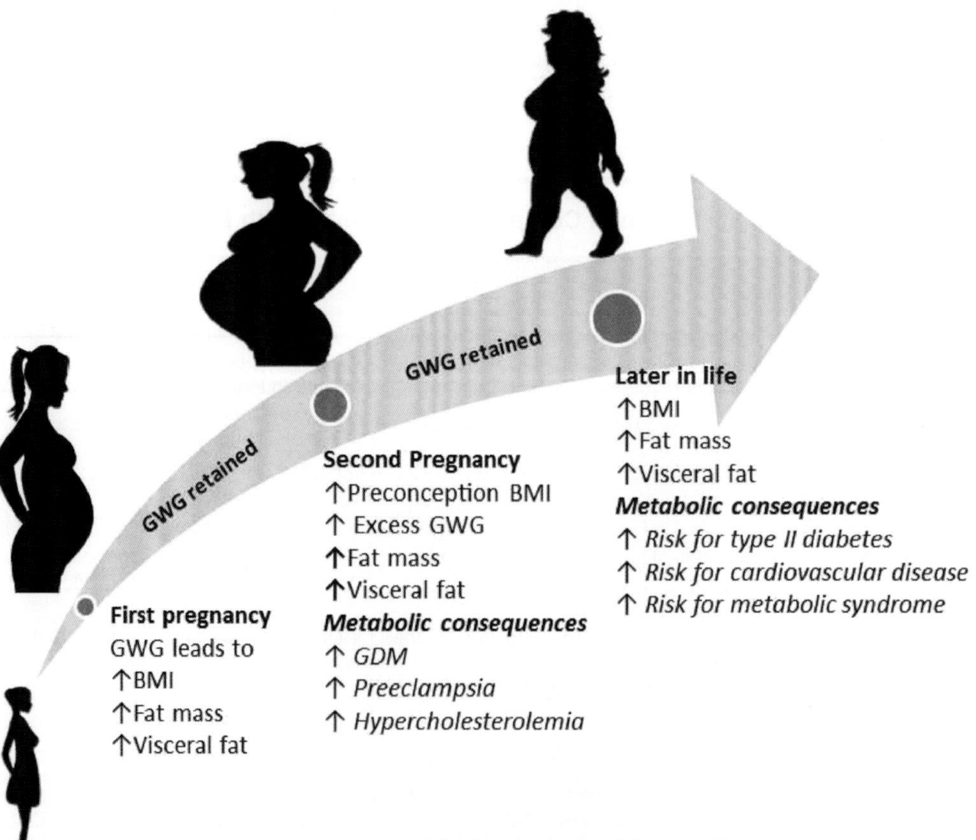

Figure 12.7 ▶ Potential complications of excessive gestational weight gain and postpartum weight retention. (*Source:* Gilmore, L. A., Klempel-Donchenko, M., & Redman, L. M. [2015]. Pregnancy as a window to future health: Excessive gestational weight gain and obesity. *Seminars in Perinatology, 39*[4], 296–303. https://doi.org/10.1053/j.semperi.2015.05.009)

- Regular self-monitoring of weight gain, such as plotting weight gain on the appropriate grid, should begin in early pregnancy and continue between prenatal visits throughout pregnancy so corrective action can be taken if necessary (Deputy et al., 2015).
- Other tools that may help women monitor behaviors include pedometers and smart phone apps to monitor intake and activity.
- Frequent provider contact beyond routine prenatal care, such as with a nurse or dietitian, may also help achieve appropriate GWG.

Remember Rachel. To help her avoid excessive weight gain, her weight is plotted against her target range at every prenatal visit. At her fourth month of pregnancy appointment, she showed a 1-month weight gain of almost double the recommended amount. What questions would you ask Rachel? What would you advise her to do?

Pica

Pica
purposeful ingestion of nonfood substances such as dirt, clay, starch, and ice.

Pica was first described by Hippocrates in 400 BCE (Miao et al., 2015). People who engage in pica may eat clay or dirt (geophagy); raw starch (amylophagy); ice and freezer frost (pagophagy); or other items, including laundry starch, soap, ashes, chalk, paint, and burnt matches (Lessen & Kavanagh, 2015). Geophagy occurs most often.

Pica has long been associated with micronutrient deficiencies, but the strength of this relationship is inconsistent (Miao et al., 2015).

- Pica may cause deficiencies by preventing the absorption of micronutrients.
- It is also possible that micronutrient deficiencies cause humans to crave and eat minerals from nonfood substances.
- Pica has been linked to a 2.4 times higher risk of anemia, a lower hemoglobin concentration, lower hematocrit, and lower plasma zinc regardless of whether the women practiced geophagy, pagophagy, or amylophagy (Miao et al., 2015).
- Screening pregnant women for pica could be a proxy for identifying risk of anemia or zinc deficiency. However, women may be reluctant to report the intake of nonfood substances.
- Counseling should focus on the potential adverse effects of pica (e.g., the effects of maternal anemia on the fetus).

Gestational Diabetes Mellitus

Gestational diabetes mellitus (GDM) is defined as glucose intolerance diagnosed during the second or third trimester of pregnancy. GDM is associated with the following:

- Increased risk of delivering an LGA infant, which in turn increases the risk of cesarean delivery, shoulder dystocia, macrosomia, birth trauma, neonatal hypoglycemia, and neonatal hyperbilirubinemia (Kampmann et al., 2015).
- Increased risk of obesity and type 2 diabetes for the offspring during childhood or adolescence.
- Increased risk of type 2 diabetes for the mother. Approximately 50% of women with GDM develop type 2 diabetes (CDC, 2019b).

More frequent prenatal medical appointments and at-home blood glucose monitoring are needed to manage gestational diabetes. A nutritional plan is based on the woman's blood glucose records, physical activity, weight gain records, and the use of medication, if any. For many women, a healthy eating pattern and regular exercise will control blood glucose levels.

Nutritional considerations are as follows:

- Excessive GWG should be avoided.
- Research does not suggest there is an optimal calorie intake for women with GDM or if their calorie needs differ from other pregnant women (Duarte-Gardea et al., 2018).
- Pregnant women with GDM have the same nutrient needs as other pregnant women.
- Evidence is lacking to determine an ideal amount (in grams or as a percentage of total calories) of carbohydrate for all women with GDM (Duarte-Gardea et al., 2018).
- For breakfast, lowering the amount of carbohydrates and emphasizing carbohydrates with low glycemic index may help achieve blood glucose targets. Individualization is based on the woman's blood glucose records.
- Smaller meals and multiple snacks may improve glucose control. Three meals with two or more snacks help reduce postprandial rises in blood glucose levels.

Preexisting Diabetes

Pregnant women with preexisting diabetes are at increased risk for a variety of adverse outcomes to herself and the infant.

- Increased risk of premature birth or stillbirth
- Birth defects, hypoglycemia, and jaundice in the newborn
- **Hydraminos**, which can lead to preterm delivery
- Macrosomia with increased risk of cesarean birth
- Diabetes complications may develop in the mother, such as retinal and kidney disease
- Mother may also develop hypertension or preeclampsia

Hydraminos
an increased amount of amniotic fluid in the amniotic sac.

Women with preexisting diabetes should achieve glycemic control before conception and maintain control throughout pregnancy.

- The nutritional considerations for gestational diabetes mentioned earlier apply to women with preexisting diabetes.
- Frequent modifications in the type and amount of antidiabetic medication and the nutritional care plan are needed as the pregnancy progresses.

Hypertensive Disorders of Pregnancy

Chronic hypertension, gestational hypertension, and preeclampsia fall under the umbrella of hypertensive disorders during pregnancy (American College of Obstetricians and Gynecologist, 2019).

- Chronic hypertension refers to elevated blood pressure that existed before pregnancy or that develops in the first 20 weeks of gestation.
  - It occurs in approximately 3% to 5% of pregnancies and is increasingly more prevalent due to increases in obesity and delaying childbirth until older age (Seely & Ecker, 2014).
  - Potential complications include preeclampsia, fetal growth restriction, placental abruption, preterm birth, and increased likelihood of cesarean delivery (Seely & Ecker, 2014).
- **Gestational hypertension** is defined as a systolic blood pressure of ≥140 mm Hg or a diastolic reading of ≥90 mm Hg with onset after 20 weeks of gestation and without proteinuria.
  - Often, gestational hypertension does not occur until 30 weeks or later.
  - Studies suggest that the chance of developing gestational hypertension is more than 6 times higher among women who begin pregnancy obese compared to women who are at normal or healthy BMI at conception (Stang & Huffman, 2016).

Gestational Hypertension
systolic blood pressure of 140 mm Hg or greater or diastolic blood pressure of 90 mm Hg or greater that develops in the second half of pregnancy and ends with childbirth.

Preeclampsia
a toxemia of pregnancy characterized by hypertension accompanied by proteinuria or edema, or both.

- **Preeclampsia** is a potentially serious syndrome involving gestational hypertension plus proteinuria, although it can occur in the absence of proteinuria but with certain other symptoms.
  - The incidence of preeclampsia has steadily increased in the United States over the last three decades, in part because of trends to delay pregnancy to a later age and the increased rate of obesity (Stevens et al., 2017).
  - Once preeclampsia is diagnosed, evidence-based interventions, namely, treatment of high blood pressure, administration of magnesium sulfate to prevent eclampsia, and inducing delivery, may reduce the risk or severity of maternal and infant health outcomes (Henderson et al., 2017).

Treating Hypertension

Early detection, classification, and treatment of hypertension with safe and effective pharmacologic therapies are critical for improving maternal and fetal outcomes (Leavitt et al., 2019). It is not known if lifestyle modification improves blood pressure control during pregnancy (Seely & Ecker, 2014)

- It is not known if initiating or continuing a DASH diet improves outcomes.
- There are no data to support limiting sodium intake to lower the risk of preeclampsia.
- Losing weight if overweight and controlling preexisting diabetes or hypertension before becoming pregnant may lower risks (American College of Obstetricians and Gynecologists, 2019).

Maternal Phenylketonuria

Phenylketonuria (PKU)
an inborn error of phenylalanine (an essential amino acid) metabolism that results in retardation and physical handicaps in newborns if they are not treated with a low-phenylalanine diet beginning shortly after birth.

Medical Foods
a food formulated to be consumed orally or administered enterally under the supervision of a physician for the specific dietary management of a disease or condition.

Phenylalanine hydroxylase deficiency, traditionally known as **phenylketonuria (PKU)**, is an inborn error of phenylalanine (an essential amino acid) metabolism, which causes severe neurologic damage when left untreated.

- Screening that detects PKU in the newborn leads to treatment that can prevent the dramatic consequences such as developmental disabilities (Vockley et al., 2014).
- As an essential amino acid, some phenylalanine is required but just enough to support growth and development. A very low-protein diet and supplements with low-phenylalanine or phenylalanine-free **medical foods** (formulas) are used to meet protein and calorie needs (Vockley et al., 2014).
- Later in childhood or adulthood when strict adherence to the diet may wane, reversible and irreversible neuropsychiatric consequences may develop. Because of that, lifelong dietary restriction and therapy are recommended to improve quality of life (American College of Obstetricians and Gynecologists, 2020).
- Frequent monitoring and dietary changes are necessary throughout life stages and health challenges.

Mothers who have PKU need to adequately control of phenylalanine levels before and throughout pregnancy to prevent fetal brain damage.

- It is recommended that low phenylalanine levels be achieved for at least 3 months prior to conception.
- Strict adherence to the diet is vital (Box 12.5).
- Pregnant women with PKU should be monitored in consultation with physicians familiar with PKU, with close follow-up with a metabolic geneticist and healthcare providers who are experienced in managing high-risk pregnancy (American College of Obstetricians and Gynecologists, 2020).
- Most infants born to mothers with PKU do not inherit PKU and cannot benefit from a low-phenylalanine diet after birth.

BOX 12.5 Diet Guidelines for Pregnant Women with Phenylketonuria

- Strict control of maternal blood phenylalanine levels is necessary to eliminate risks to the developing fetus.
- Because phenylalanine is an essential amino acid, it must be provided in the diet in limited amounts to support growth and protein synthesis.
- Low-phenylalanine diets are very low in total protein, so low-phenylalanine or phenylalanine-free medical food beverages must be consumed as a source of protein. They must be consumed in prescribed amounts to support fetal growth and prevent maternal tissue breakdown that would have the results similar to those caused by eating too much protein.
- These products have long been the mainstay of diet therapy for PKU and are designed to meet established dietary requirements. However, they may not always contain adequate amounts of essential fatty acids, vitamins, and minerals depending on individual circumstances (Vockley et al., 2014).
- Other modified low-protein foods are available to increase diet variety and provide an important source of calories. They are costly and the cost may not always be covered by third-party payers (Vockley et al., 2014).
- Diet beverages and foods sweetened with aspartame (NutraSweet) are strictly forbidden.

Adolescent Pregnancy

Low Birth Weight (LBW) a baby weighing <2500 g or 5.5 pounds.

Adolescent pregnancy increases health risks to both infant and mother. Infants born to adolescent mothers are at higher risk of **low birth weight (LBW)** and preterm delivery, especially in mothers younger than 15 years old (Althabe et al., 2015). Infants born to adolescent mothers are more likely to become teen mothers; adolescent pregnancy typically limits the mother's education and subsequent occupational opportunities. Compared with adult women, pregnant adolescents

- are more likely to be physically, emotionally, financially, and socially immature. Low socioeconomic status may be a major reason for the high incidence of LBW infants and other complications of adolescent pregnancy.
- may not have adequate nutrient stores because they need large amounts of nutrients for their own growth and development. Although adolescent growth for girls is usually complete by the age of 15 years, physical maturity is not reached until 4 years after menarche, which usually occurs by age 17 years.
- may still be growing so mother and fetus compete for nutrients.
- may give low priority to healthy eating. Dieting, erratic eating patterns, reliance on fast foods, and meal skipping are common adolescent practices.
- may have poor intake and status of certain micronutrients, such as folate, iron, and vitamin D, which increases the risk of small-for-gestational-age births in pregnant adolescents.
- may be more concerned with body image and confused about weight gain recommendations; many do not understand why they should gain more than 7 pounds, the weight of the average baby at birth.
- are more likely to smoke during pregnancy. Smoking increases the risk of premature birth.
- seek prenatal care later and have fewer total visits during pregnancy.

Nutrition Considerations

Appropriate weight gain and adequate nutrition are among the most important modifiable factors that can be used to improve birth outcomes. Optimal nutrition has the potential to decrease the incidence of LBW infants and to improve the health of infants born to adolescents.

- Adolescents within the healthy BMI range are advised to gain approximately 35 pounds to reduce the risk of delivering an LBW infant.
- MyPlate is useful both in assessing dietary strengths and weaknesses and in providing a framework for implementing dietary changes in a way the adolescent can understand.

- Adolescents living with one or more adults may have little control over what food is available to them; parents and significant others should be encouraged to attend counseling sessions.
- Women, Infants, and Children (WIC) helps pregnant women obtain adequate and nutritious food for themselves and their infants.

NUTRITION FOR LACTATION

With rare exceptions, breastfeeding is the optimal method of feeding and nurturing infants. Both the American Academy of Pediatrics (AAP) and the Academy of Nutrition and Dietetics recommend that infants be exclusively breastfed for the first 6 months of life and that breastfeeding continue with complementary foods until 1 year of age or longer (AAP, 2012; Lessen & Kavanagh, 2015). Breastfeeding is an important public health strategy for improving infant and child morbidity and mortality and improving maternal morbidity (Lessen & Kavanagh, 2015). The benefits of breastfeeding for both mother and infant are well recognized (Box 12.6).

Promoting Breastfeeding

Social support and support from healthcare professionals influence success with breastfeeding. As a learned behavior, not a physiologic response, the ability to successfully breastfeed and the duration of lactation can be positively affected by counseling.

BOX 12.6 Benefits of Breastfeeding

For the Mother

There is strong evidence that breastfeeding

- reduces the risk of postpartum hemorrhage,
- delays ovulation, and
- reduces the risk of postpartum depression.

Other potential benefits that need additional study are as follows:

- Reduced risk of hypertension, postmenopausal breast and ovarian cancer, premenopausal breast cancer, and comorbidities of excess weight (e.g., type 2 diabetes)
- Postpartum weight loss
- Improved infant bonding

For the Infant

There is strong evidence that breastfeeding reduces risks of the following:

- Nonspecific gastrointestinal infections
- Upper and lower respiratory tract infections
- Otitis media
- Sudden infant death syndrome
- Necrotizing enterocolitis among premature and low-birth-weight infants

Other potential benefits that need additional study are as follows:

- Decreased risks of atopic dermatitis, autoimmune disorders, asthma, later overweight or obesity, comorbidities related to excess weight (e.g., type 2 diabetes, heart disease)
- Promotion of cognitive development

Source: Lessen, R., & Kavanagh, K. (2015). Position of the Academy of Nutrition and Dietetics: Promoting and supporting breastfeeding. *Journal of the Academy of Nutrition and Dietetics, 115*(3), 444–449. https://doi.org/10.1016/j.jand.2014.12.014

BOX 12.7 Factors That Negatively Affect the Duration of Exclusive Breastfeeding

Delayed initiation of breastfeeding
Maternal postpartum infection
Cesarean delivery
Twin pregnancy
Infant irritability
Maternal employment
Short duration of maternity leave
Perceived breast milk insufficiency
Giving water
Use of a pacifier
History of smoking during pregnancy
Preexisting health problems
Higher maternal age
Intimate partner violence or lack of partner support

Source: Maharlouei, N., Pourhaghighi, A., Raeisi Shahraki, H., Zohoori, D., & Lankarani, K. B. (2018). Factors affecting exclusive breastfeeding, using adaptive LASSO Regression. *International Journal of Community Based Nursing and Midwifery, 6*(3), 260–271.

- Preparation for breastfeeding should begin prenatally with counseling, guidance, and support for both the woman and her partner and continue throughout the gestational period. Certified lactation consultants can help new mothers establish successful breastfeeding.
- Despite the benefits of breastfeeding, many women choose not to initiate breastfeeding, only partially breastfeed, or breastfeed for only a short duration. A variety of factors may negatively affect the duration of exclusive breastfeeding (Box 12.7).
- Even a short period of breastfeeding is better than not breastfeeding at all. Women should be encouraged to breastfeed for as long as they are able and not be made to feel guilty if they fall short of the recommendations.
- Contraindications to breastfeeding are listed in Box 12.8.

BOX 12.8 Contraindications to Breastfeeding

Mothers should not breastfeed or feed expressed breast milk if

- an infant is diagnosed with galactosemia, a rare genetic metabolic disorder
- the mother uses illegal drugs, such as PCP or cocaine
- the mother is infected with HIV
- the mother is infected with human T-cell lymphotropic virus type 1 or type 2
- the mother has suspected or confirmed Ebola virus disease

Mothers should temporarily not breastfeed and should not feed expressed milk if

- the mother is infected with untreated brucellosis (an infectious disease caused by bacteria)
- the mother takes certain medications
- the mother is undergoing diagnostic imaging with radiopharmaceuticals
- the mother has active herpes simplex virus infection with lesions on the breast

Mothers should temporarily not breastfeed but can feed expressed milk if

- the mother has untreated, active tuberculosis
- the mother has active varicella (chicken pox) infection that developed within 5 days prior to delivery to the 2 days after delivery

Source: Centers for Disease Control and Prevention. (2019, December 14). *Contraindications to breastfeeding or feeding expressed breast milk to infants*. https://www.cdc.gov/breastfeeding/breastfeeding-special-circumstances/Contraindications-to-breastfeeding.html

Nutrient Needs

Nutrient needs during lactation are based on the nutritional content of breast milk and the "cost" of producing milk. The healthy eating pattern consumed during pregnancy should continue during lactation. The higher calorie intake from nutrient-dense foods can generally meet increased nutrient needs. As illustrated in Figure 12.6, the requirements for many vitamins and minerals are higher during lactation than during pregnancy.

- The content of macronutrients and most minerals in breast milk is maintained at the expense of maternal stores if maternal intake is inadequate. For instance, if calcium intake is inadequate, the calcium content of breast milk is maintained at the expense of maternal bone density.
- Maternal intake has been reported to influence the concentrations of fatty acids and fat-soluble vitamins, namely, vitamins A, D, B_6, and B_{12} (Innis, 2014). However, most of the evidence on the relationship between maternal intake and breast milk composition is limited and weak (Bravi et al., 2016).

Calories

Well-nourished women who exclusively breastfeed need approximately 500 cal/day above their nonpregnant calorie needs to produce an adequate supply of breast milk. However, recommended daily increases in calories are less than 500 calories based on the idea that eating less than the total will mobilize calories stored as fat during pregnancy, thereby helping women regain their prepregnancy weight. Recommendations vary with the length of breastfeeding:

- An extra 330 cal/day for the first 6 months.
- An extra 400 cal/day for the second 6 months.
- Breastfeeding supplemented with formula requires a smaller increase in calorie intake.

For the sample woman used in Figure 12.5, the eating pattern recommended while she exclusively breastfeeds for the first 6 months is 2400 calories, the same number of calories recommended during the third trimester of pregnancy. This calorie level would allow her to mobilize fat accumulated during pregnancy to provide the additional calories needed to produce enough breast milk.

Adequacy of calorie intake is evaluated by changes in a woman's weight.

- Women who failed to gain enough weight during pregnancy, who have inadequate fat reserves, or who lose too much weight while breastfeeding may need to increase their calorie intake.
- Women who are not losing weight while lactating can reduce their calorie intake after lactation is established.
- Generally, intake should not fall below 1500 to 1800 cal/day because milk production may be decreased.

Fluid

A rule-of-thumb suggestion is that breastfeeding mothers drink a glass of fluid every time the baby nurses and with all meals or approximately twelve 8-oz glasses of caffeine-free fluids/day.

- Thirst is a good indicator of need except among women who live in a dry climate or who exercise in hot weather.
- Fluids consumed in excess of thirst quenching do not increase milk volume.

Vitamins and Minerals Supplements

Generally, a woman eating a varied and balanced eating pattern of the appropriate amount of calories should not need a vitamin or mineral supplement.

- One exception is iron. Iron supplements may be needed to replace depleted iron stores, not to increase the iron content of breast milk.

- Vegans who do not eat any animal products need a reliable source of vitamin B_{12}.
- Daily or intermittent high-dose vitamin D supplements enrich breast milk and can be an alternative to giving vitamin D supplements to infants (Umaretiya et al., 2017). Many mothers prefer taking supplements themselves rather than giving them to the infant.
- Vitamin and mineral supplements are usually not necessary if a balanced, varied eating pattern is consumed. However, many healthcare professionals recommend women continue to take prenatal vitamins during lactation.

Other Considerations

Other considerations concerning maternal intake and breast milk are as follows:

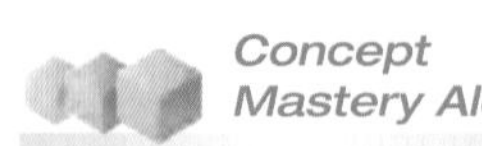

Concept Mastery Alert

It is not necessary for a mother to avoid highly flavored or spicy foods while breastfeeding unless the infant is affected.

- Highly flavored or spicy foods may have an impact on the flavor of breast milk but need only be avoided if infant feeding is affected. Infants rarely react to a food that mothers eat and the few foods that have been observed to cause reactions differ among infants (Jeong et al., 2017).
- Avoiding alcohol is the safest level of intake while breastfeeding. However, moderate intake (up to 1 drink/day) has not shown to be harmful. Because alcohol can be detected for about 2 to 3 hours/drink after consumption, mothers should wait at least 2 hours after a single drink before nursing (CDC, 2018).
- Caffeine quickly enters breast milk after maternal consumption. Insufficient high-quality data are available to make good evidence-based recommendations on safe maternal intake (Drugs and Lactation Database [LactMed], updated 2019). A daily limit of 300 mg might be a safe intake for most mothers (Table 12.2). Newborns and preterm infants are especially sensitive to caffeine.
- Lactating women are urged to follow the same guidelines for seafood consumption as pregnant women to ensure an adequate concentration of DHA in breast milk. Eight to 12 oz/week of a variety of seafood that is low in mercury is recommended because its omega-3 fatty acid content is important for neurologic development. Fish that have the highest mercury level should be avoided.

Postpartum Weight Retention

Excessive GWG increases the risk of postpartum weight retention and obesity in mothers (see Fig. 12.7) and children (Deputy et al., 2015).

- Approximately half of women retain ≥10 pounds and nearly 1 in 4 women retain 20 pounds or more at 12 months postpartum (USDA & USDHHS, 2020).
- Postpartum weight retention results in approximately 1 in 7 women moving from a healthy weight classification before pregnancy to an overweight classification postpartum (USDA & USDHHS, 2020).
- A combination of diet, regular physical activity, routine self-monitoring of weight, and frequent provider contact may be most effective at promoting postpartum weight loss (Deputy et al., 2015).

Unfolding Case

Think of Rachel. She gained 28 pounds during pregnancy—more than the 11 to 20 pounds her doctor recommended. She understands the importance of managing her weight for her own health and for future pregnancies. She has been successfully breastfeeding for 2½ months yet has not lost any weight, so she will lower her calorie intake to help promote weight loss. What would you recommend as an appropriate calorie level and goal weight? What kind of eating pattern may be healthiest for her given high risk for type 2 diabetes and hypertension?

NURSING PROCESS

Normal Pregnancy

Jana is a 33-year-old moderately active professional who is entering the second trimester of pregnancy with her first baby. Her prepregnancy BMI was 19.2. She has gained 4 pounds. She plans on returning to work 8 weeks after delivery and wants to limit her weight gain to 10 pounds so that she can fit into her clothes by the time she returns to work. She has asked you what she should eat that will be good for the baby but not cause her to get fat.

Assessment

Medical–Psychosocial History

Medical history that may have nutritional implications, such as diabetes, hypertension, lactose intolerance, PKU, or other chronic disease

- Use of medications and over-the-counter drugs
- Adequacy of sunlight exposure
- Symptoms of constipation, including frequency, interventions attempted, and results
- Any complaints related to pregnancy, such as heartburn
- Usual frequency and intensity of physical activity
- Attitude about pregnancy; knowledge about normal amount and pattern of weight gain during pregnancy
- Attitude/plan regarding breastfeeding
- Level of family/social support

Anthropometric Assessment

Height, prepregnancy weight, pattern of 4-pound weight gain during pregnancy

Biochemical and Physical Assessment

- Check hemoglobin to screen for iron deficiency anemia. (Many laboratory values change during pregnancy related to normal changes in maternal physiology and so cannot be validly compared with nonpregnancy standards.)
- Check glucose, other laboratory values as available.
- Assess blood pressure.

Dietary Assessment

- How is your appetite?
- Do you follow a balanced and varied eating pattern that includes all food groups from MyPlate in reasonable amounts?
- Do you eat at regular intervals?
- How have you modified your intake since becoming pregnant?
- Do you eat nonfoods or have nonfood cravings?
- Do you take a vitamin and/or mineral supplement?
- Do you use alcohol, tobacco, caffeine, or herbal supplements?
- What are your concerns about nutrient needs during pregnancy?
- Do you have cultural, religious, or ethnic factors that influence your food choices?

Analysis

Possible Nursing Analysis

- Insufficient understanding of the importance of adequate weight gain during pregnancy as evidenced by a desire to limit total weight gain to 10 pounds

Planning

Client Outcomes

The client will do the following:

- Consume an adequate, varied, and balanced eating pattern based on MyPlate.
- Explain the amount and pattern of recommended weight gain during pregnancy.
- Gain approximately 1 pound of weight/week during the remainder of pregnancy.

NURSING PROCESS Normal Pregnancy

Nursing Interventions

Nutrition Therapy

- Provide a 2400-calorie eating plan that includes all food groups and emphasizes ample fruits and vegetables, whole grains, lean protein, fat-free dairy, and healthy fats.

Client Teaching

Instruct the client on the following:
- The role of nutrition and weight gain in the outcome of pregnancy
- Choosing nutrient-dense foods over calorie-dense items
- Choosing a variety of foods within each major food group
- Selecting the appropriate number of servings from each major food group
- Items to avoid during pregnancy: alcohol, herbal supplements, unpasteurized juice, milk, and cheese; raw seafood, undercooked eggs and meats, premade deli salads, raw sprouts, cold hot dogs, and luncheon meats

Behavioral matters including the following:
- Abandoning the idea of limiting weight gain to fit into clothes after pregnancy
- The importance of maintaining physical activity

Where to find more information (see "Websites" at the end of this chapter)

Evaluation

Evaluate and Monitor

- Monitor amount and pattern of weight gain.
- Monitor quality and adequacy of intake based on meal plan provided.
- Suggest changes in the food plan as needed.
- Provide periodic feedback and support.

How Do You Respond?

To limit calories and weight gain, can I just take calcium supplements instead of drinking 3 cups of milk day? Milk is a rich source of calcium but it provides many other essential nutrients, such as protein, vitamin D, riboflavin, potassium, and magnesium. Calcium supplements cannot substitute for these nutrients. Also, the absorption of calcium from milk is promoted by the lactose and vitamin D content of milk whereas the absorption of calcium from supplements varies depending on the form of calcium, how well the supplement dissolves, and the dose. A better option for controlling calories is to choose nonfat milk or yogurt and choose nutrient-dense foods from all food groups.

Should pregnant women avoid eating peanuts during pregnancy to reduce the risk of peanut allergy in their children? The advice to avoid peanuts and other allergens during pregnancy has been overturned. According to the AAP, there is a lack of evidence to support maternal dietary restrictions either during pregnancy or during lactation to prevent atopic disease, such as atopic dermatitis, asthma, allergic rhinitis, and food allergy (Greer et al., 2019).

REVIEW CASE STUDY

Sarah is 28 years old and 7 months pregnant with her third child. Her other children are aged 2½ years and 1½ years. She had uncomplicated pregnancies and deliveries. Sarah is 5 ft 6 in. tall; she weighed 142 pounds at the beginning of this pregnancy, which made her prepregnancy BMI 23. She has gained 24 pounds so far. Prior to her first pregnancy, her BMI was 20 (124 pounds). She is unhappy about her weight gain, but the stress of having two young children and being a stay-at-home mom made losing weight impossible.

She went online for her MyPlate plan, which recommends she consume 2400 cal/day. She doesn't think she eats that much because she seems to have constant heartburn. She takes a prenatal supplement, so she feels pretty confident that even if her intake is not perfect, she is getting all the nutrients she needs through her supplement. A typical day's intake for her is shown on the right:

- Evaluate her prepregnancy weight and weight gain thus far. How much total weight should she gain?
- Based on the 2400-calorie meal pattern in Figure 12.5, what does Sarah need to eat more of? What is she eating in more than the recommended amounts? How would you suggest she modify her intake to minimize heartburn?
- What would you tell her about weight gain during pregnancy? What strategies would you suggest her after her baby is born that would help her achieve her healthy weight?
- Is her conclusion about the adequacy of supplements appropriate? What would you tell her about supplements?

Devise a 1-day menu for her that would provide all the food she needs in the recommended amounts and alleviate her heartburn.

Breakfast: Cornflakes with whole milk (because the children drink whole milk), orange juice
Snack: Bran muffin and whole milk
Lunch: Either a peanut butter and jelly sandwich or tuna fish sandwich with mayonnaise, snack crackers, whole milk, and pudding or cookies
Snack: Ice cream
Dinner: Macaroni and cheese, green beans, roll and butter, whole milk, and cake or ice cream for dessert
Evening: Chips and salsa

STUDY QUESTIONS

1 A woman trying to become pregnant was told by her physician to take a daily supplement containing 400 mg of folic acid. She asks why a supplement is better than eating natural sources of folate through food. Which statement is the nurse's best response?
   a. "There are few natural sources of folate in food."
   b. "Synthetic folic acid in supplements and fortified foods is better absorbed, more available, and a more reliable source than the folate found naturally in food."
   c. "Folate in food is equally as good as folic acid in supplements. It is just easier to take it in pill form and then you don't have to worry about how much you're getting in food."
   d. "If you are sure that you eat at least five servings of fruits and vegetables every day, you don't really need to take a supplement of folic acid."

2 A woman who was at her healthy weight when she got pregnant is distraught by her 4-pound weight gain between 20 and 24 weeks of gestation. Her weight gain up to 20 weeks was on target. What is the nurse's best response?
   a. "A 4-pound-per-month weight gain at this point in your pregnancy is normal."
   b. "Although it is considerably less than the recommended amount, it is not a cause for concern. Just be sure to follow your meal plan next month so you get enough calories and nutrients."
   c. "I recommend you write down everything you eat for a few days so we can identify where the problem lies."
   d. "A 4-pound weight gain in 1 month at this point in your pregnancy may be a sign that you are at risk of preeclampsia. You should cut back on the 'extras' in your eating pattern to limit your weight gain for next month."

3 The nurse knows her instructions on healthy eating during pregnancy have been effective when the woman verbalizes she should
   a. avoid seafood because of its mercury content.
   b. limit alcohol to 2 drinks/day.
   c. increase her intake of milk to 4 cups/day.
   d. eliminate hot dogs and deli meats unless heated to steaming hot immediately before eating.

4 At her first prenatal visit, an overweight woman asks how much weight she should gain during the course of her pregnancy. What is the nurse's best response?
   a. "You should not gain any weight during your pregnancy. You have adequate calorie reserves to meet all the energy demands of pregnancy without gaining additional weight."
   b. "You should try to gain less than 15 pounds."
   c. "Aim for a 15- to 25-pound weight gain."
   d. "The recommended weight gain for your weight is 25 to 35 pounds."

5 Which of the following statements indicates that the pregnant woman understands the recommendations about caffeine intake during pregnancy?
  a. "I have to give up drinking coffee and cola."
  b. "I will limit my intake of coffee to about 2–3 cups a day and avoid other sources of caffeine."
  c. "As long as I don't drink coffee, I can eat other sources of caffeine because they don't contain enough to cause any problems."
  d. "Caffeine is harmless during pregnancy, so I am allowed to consume as much as I want."

6 What nutrient is not likely to be consumed in adequate amounts during pregnancy so a supplement may be needed?
  a. Iron
  b. Vitamin A
  c. Vitamin B_{12}
  d. Vitamin C

7 A woman at 5 weeks of gestation is complaining of nausea throughout the day. What should the nurse recommend?
  a. Small, frequent meals of easily digested carbohydrates
  b. Small, frequent meals that are high in protein
  c. A liquid diet until the nausea subsides
  d. Increasing fluids with all meals and snacks

8 Which of the following statements is true?
  a. "Women who breastfeed almost always achieve their prepregnancy weight at 6 weeks postpartum."
  b. "Weight loss during lactation is not recommended because it lowers the quantity and quality of breast milk produced."
  c. "Most breastfeeding women do not have to increase their intake by the full amount of calories it 'costs' to produce milk because they can mobilize fat stored during pregnancy for some of the extra energy required."
  d. "Women do not need to increase their calorie intake at all for the first 6 months of breastfeeding because they can use calories stored in fat to produce milk."

CHAPTER SUMMARY HEALTHY EATING FOR HEALTHY BABIES

Women who are healthy at the time of conception are more likely to have a successful pregnancy and a healthy infant.

Preconception Nutrition

The preconception period may be a critical time to promote a healthy lifestyle to reduce the risk of undesirable maternal and child health outcomes. Before conception, women should:

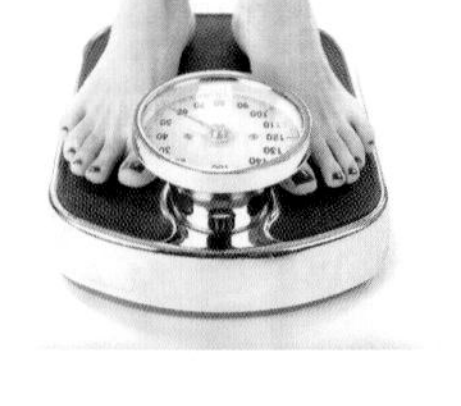

- Attain and maintain a healthy BMI of 25 or less
- Consume an appropriate amount of calories with an emphasis on fruits, vegetables, whole grains, lean proteins, and low-fat or fat-free dairy; they should also consume healthy fats and limit added sugars, solid fats, and sodium
- Take 400 to 800 mcg of folic acid to reduce the risk of neural tube defects
- Be physically active
- Not smoke, drink alcohol, or use drugs
- Avoid herbal supplements unless approved by a physician
- Manage existing medical conditions such as diabetes and hypertension

Nutrition and Lifestyle during Pregnancy

The same healthy nutrition and lifestyle recommendations for the prepregnancy period continue throughout pregnancy. Additional considerations are as follows:

- Keep the pattern and amount of weight gain within recommended levels. Women with a normal BMI should gain a total 25 to 35 pounds with 1 to 4 pounds gained in the first trimester and slightly less than 1 pound/week thereafter.
- Increase calories modestly. No increase is necessary in the first trimester. Approximately 340 and 420 extra calories/day, respectively, are needed during the second and third trimesters.
- The increased need for folic acid continues. Iron supplements are routinely recommended. If food choices are less than optimal, supplemental iodine, vitamin D, and calcium may be appropriate. Prenatal vitamins and minerals are routinely recommended as a safeguard.

Numerous environmental concerns need attention during pregnancy.

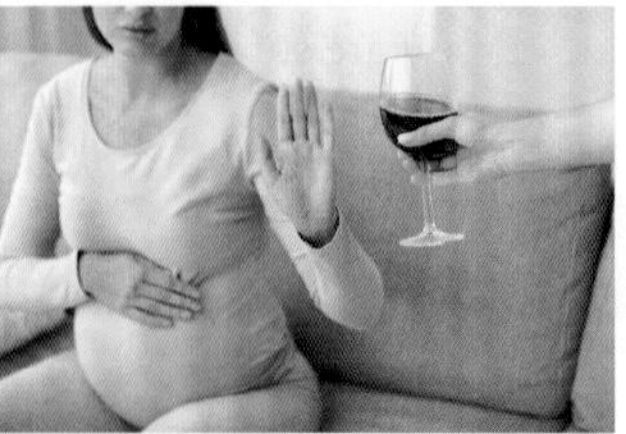

- **Alcohol:** There is not an established safe level of intake, although occasional limited use may not be harmful.

CHAPTER SUMMARY HEALTHY EATING FOR HEALTHY BABIES (continued)

- **Caffeine:** Amounts up to 300 mg/day, or approximately 2 to 3 cups of brewed coffee, are assumed to be safe.
- **Nonnutritive sweeteners:** Approved sweeteners are safe during pregnancy but cautious use is prudent.
- **Seafood:** 8 to 12 oz/week of fish with low mercury content is advised to promote normal fetal growth and development while limiting mercury exposure.
- **Foodborne illness:** Pregnant women are more susceptible to foodborne illness due to hormonal changes. In addition to normal food safety precautions, foods to avoid include unpasteurized milk and juices, raw or undercooked meat, poultry, seafood, and eggs; refrigerated smoked seafood, pâtés, and meat spreads; and unpasteurized soft cheese, hot dogs, and deli meats unless heated to steaming hot.
- **Physical activity:** Women should do at least 150 minutes (2 hours and 30 minutes) of moderate-intensity aerobic activity a week during pregnancy and the postpartum period

Maternal Health

- **Common complaints of pregnancy:** Nausea, vomiting, constipation, and heartburn may be alleviated by nutrition interventions.
- **Excessive weight gain:** Women should learn their BMI and weight gain goals at the first prenatal visit. At prenatal appointments throughout pregnancy, weight, diet, and exercise should be discussed. Women should self-monitor weight gain, intake, and activity.
- **Pica:** The ingestion of nonfood stuffs is linked to micronutrient deficiencies and anemia. Counseling should address the potential risks.
- **Gestational diabetes:** Excessive weight gain should be avoided. Diet and exercise may control blood glucose levels for many. Blood glucose monitoring provides data to adjust the meal plan as necessary. Small frequent meals and snacks and breakfasts that provide less carbohydrate of low glycemic index foods may aid blood glucose control.
- **Preexisting diabetes:** Frequent blood glucose monitoring and adjustments in diet and exercise are needed to promote glycemic control.
- **Hypertensive disorders of pregnancy:** Chronic hypertension, gestational hypertension, and preeclampsia fall under this umbrella term. Medications are used to control blood pressure. It is not known if lifestyle modification improves blood pressure control during pregnancy
- **Maternal PKU:** Women should achieve low phenylalanine levels before conception to reduce the risk of fetal mental impairments. A strict low-protein diet with low-phenylalanine medical formulas is necessary to control phenylalanine intake while achieving adequate calorie intake. Close monitoring is needed.

Adolescent Pregnancy

- Adolescent pregnancy increases health risks to both infant and mother.
- Adolescents within the healthy BMI range should gain approximately 35 pounds to reduce the risk of delivering an LBW infant.

Nutrition for Lactation

Breastfeeding is an important public health strategy for improving infant and child morbidity and mortality and improving maternal morbidity. Many nutrients are needed in higher amounts during lactation than during pregnancy.

- **Calories:** Exclusive breastfeeding requires approximately 500 calories extra/day, approximately 300 to 400 calories from food and the rest from mobilized fat stores to help women return to prepregnancy weight.
- **Fluid:** Women are encouraged to drink 8 oz of fluid with meals and each time they breastfeed.

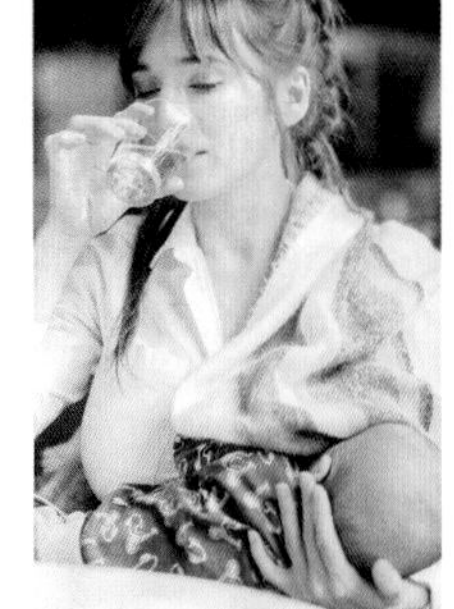

- **Vitamin and mineral supplements:** Are usually not necessary if a balanced, varied eating pattern is consumed. However, many healthcare professionals recommend women continue to take prenatal vitamins during lactation.
- **Alcohol:** Women should not drink within 2 hours before nursing to minimize concentration in breast milk.
- **Caffeine:** A daily limit of 300 mg might be a safe intake for most mothers
- **Fish consumption:** Lactating women should follow the same guidelines as during pregnancy are recommended, which is 8 to 12oz/week of lower mercury fish.
- **Postpartum weight retention:** Is common and a risk factor for obesity. Diet and exercise combined with self-monitoring are recommended.

Figure sources: *shutterstock.com/Kzenon, shutterstock.com/Prostock-studio, shutterstock.com/Iryna Inshyna*

Student Resources on thePoint®
For additional learning materials, activate the code in the front of this book at https://thePoint.lww.com/activate

Websites

Academy of Nutrition and Dietetics at www.eatright.org
American Academy of Pediatrics at www.aap.org
American College of Obstetricians and Gynecologists at www.acog.org
La Lèche League International at www.lalecheleague.org
March of Dimes at www.marchofdimes.org
MyPlate for Pregnancy and Breastfeeding at www.choosemyplate.gov
Nutrition.gov at www.nutrition.gov
Supplemental Nutrition Program for Women, Infants, and Children (WIC) at http://www.fns.usda.gov/wic/women-infants-and-children-wic

References

Althabe, F., Moore, J. L., Gibbons, L., Berrueta, M., Goudar, S. S., Chomba, E., Derman, R. J., Patel, A., Saleem, S., Pasha, O., Esamai, F., Garces, A., Leichty, E. A., Hambidge, K. M., Krebs, N. F., Hibberd, P. L. Goldenberg, R. L., Koso-Thomas, M., Carlo, W. A., … McClure, E. M. (2015). Adverse maternal and perinatal outcomes in adolescent pregnancies: The Global Network's Maternal Newborn Health Registry study. *Reproductive Health, 12,* S8. https://doi.org/10.1186/1742-4755-12-S2-S8

American Academy of Pediatrics. (2012). Breastfeeding and the use of human milk: Policy statement. *Pediatrics, 129*(3), e827–e841. http://pediatrics.aappublications.org/content/pediatrics/129/3/e827.full.pdf

American College of Obstetricians and Gynecologists. (2019). Preeclampsia and high blood pressure during pregnancy. Frequently asked questions. https://www.acog.org/patient-resources/faqs/pregnancy/preeclampsia-and-high-blood-pressure-during-pregnancy

American College of Obstetricians and Gynecologists Committee on Genetics. (2020). Committee Opinion Number 802: Management of women with phenylalanine hydroxylase deficiency (phenylketonuria). *Obstetrics and Gynecology, 135*(4), e167–e170. https://www.acog.org/-/media/project/acog/acogorg/clinical/files/committee-opinion/articles/2020/04/management-of-women-with-phenylalanine-hydroxylase-deficiency.pdf

American College of Obstetricians and Gynecologists Committee on Obstetric Practice. (2010, reaffirmed 2016). Moderate caffeine consumption during pregnancy. Committee Opinion Number. 462. *Obstetrics and Gynecology, 116,* 467–468. https://www.acog.org/-/media/project/acog/acogorg/clinical/files/committee-opinion/articles/2010/08/moderate-caffeine-consumption-during-pregnancy.pdf

American College of Obstetricians and Gynecologists Committee on Obstetrics. (2013, reaffirmed 2016). Weight gain during pregnancy. Committee Opinion No. 548. *Obstetrics and Gynecology, 121,* 210–212. https://www.acog.org/-/media/project/acog/acogorg/clinical/files/committee-opinion/articles/2013/01/weight-gain-during-pregnancy.pdf

American College of Obstetrics and Gynecologists Committee on Obstetric Practice with the assistance of Birsner, M. L., & Gyamfi-Bannerman, C. (2020). Committee Opinion Number 804: Physical activity and exercise during pregnancy and the postpartum period. *Obstetrics and Gynecology, 135*(4), e178–e188. https://www.acog.org/clinical/clinical-guidance/committee-opinion/articles/2020/04/physical-activity-and-exercise-during-pregnancy-and-the-postpartum-period

Bravi, F., Wiens, F., Decarli, A., Dal Pont, A., Agostoni, C., & Ferraroni, M. (2016). Impact of maternal nutrition on breast-milk composition: A systematic review. *American Journal of Clinical Nutrition, 104*(3), 646–662. https://doi.org/10.3945/ajcn.115.120881

Centers for Disease Control and Prevention. (2016, December 12). *Listeria (Listeriosis). People at risk—pregnant women and newborns.* https://www.cdc.gov/listeria/risk-groups/pregnant-women.html

Centers for Disease Control and Prevention. (2018). *Breastfeeding: Alcohol.* https://www.cdc.gov/breastfeeding/breastfeeding-special-circumstances/vaccinations-medications-drugs/alcohol.html

Centers for Disease Control and Prevention. (2019a, June 26). *Parasites-toxoplasmosis. Pregnant women.* https://www.cdc.gov/parasites/toxoplasmosis/gen_info/pregnant.html

Centers for Disease Control and Prevention. (2019b, May 30). *Gestational diabetes.* https://www.cdc.gov/diabetes/basics/gestational.html

Dahly, D., Li, X., Smith, H., Khashan, A. S., Murray, D. M., Kiely, M., O'B Hourihand, J., McCarthy, F. P., Kenny, L. C., Kearney, P. M., & the SCOPE Ireland cohort study and the Cork BASELINE birth cohort study. (2018). Associations between maternal life-style factors and neonatal body composition in the Screening for Pregnancy Endpoints (Cork) cohort study. *International Journal of Epidemiology, 47*(1), 131–145. https://doi.org/10.1093/ije/dyx221

Deputy, N., Sharma, A., & Kim, S. (2015). Gestational weight gain—United States, 2012 and 2013. *Morbidity and Mortality Weekly Report, 64*(43), 1215–1220. https://doi.org/10.15585/mmwr.mm6443a3

Drugs and Lactation Database (LactMed) [Internet]. Bethesda (MD): National Library of Medicine (U.S.); 2006-. Caffeine. [Updated June 30, 2019]. https://www.ncbi.nlm.nih.gov/books/NBK501467/

Duarte-Gardea, M., Gonzales-Pacheco, D. M., Reader, D. M., Thomas, A. M., Wang, S. R., Gregory, R. P., Piemonte, T. A., Thompson, K. L., & Moloney, L. (2018). Academy of Nutrition and Dietetics gestational diabetes evidence-based nutrition practice guideline. *Journal of the Academy of Nutrition and Dietetics, 118*(9), 1719–1742. https://doi.org/10.1016/j.jand.2018.03.014

Fisher, A. L., & Nemeth, E. (2017). Iron homeostasis during pregnancy. *The American Journal of Clinical Nutrition, 106*(suppl 6), 1567S–1574S. https://doi.org/10.3945/ajcn.117.155812

FoodSafety.gov. (2019, April 1). *People at risk: Pregnant women.* https://www.foodsafety.gov/people-at-risk/pregnant-women

Fox, N. S. (2018). Dos and don'ts in pregnancy: Truths and myths. *Obstetrics and Gynecology, 131*(4), 713–721. https://doi.org/10.1097/AOG.0000000000002517

Gilmore, L. A., Klempel-Donchenko, M., & Redman, L. M. (2015). Pregnancy as a window to future health: Excessive gestational weight gain and obesity. *Seminars in Perinatology, 39*(4), 296–303. https://doi.org/10.1053/j.semperi.2015.05.009

Greer, F., Sicherer, S., Burks, A., & Committee on Nutrition and Section on Allergy and Immunology. (2019). The effects of early nutritional interventions on the development of atopic disease in infants and children: The role of maternal dietary restriction, breastfeeding, hydrolyzed formulas, and timing of introduction of allergenic complementary foods. *Pediatrics, 143*(4), e20190281. https://doi.org/10.1542/peds.2019-0281

Hagan, J. F., Shaw, J. S., & Duncan, P. M. (Eds.). (2017). *Bright futures: Guidelines for health supervision of infants, children, and adolescents.* American Academy of Pediatrics. https://ebooks.aappublications.org/content/bright-futures-guidelines-for-health-supervision-of-infants-children-and-adolescents-4th-ed

Henderson, J., Thompson, J., Burda, B., & Cantor, A. (2017). Preeclampsia screening. Evidence report and systematic review for the U.S. Preventive Services Task Force. *Journal of the American Medical Association, 317*(16), 1668–1683. https://doi.org/10.1001/jama.2016.18315

Hutcheon, J. A., Platt, R. W., Abrams, B., Himes, K. P., Simhan, H. N., & Bodnar, L. M. (2015). Pregnancy weight gain charts for obese and overweight women. *Obesity, 23*(3), 532–535. https://doi.org/10.1002/oby.21011

Innis, S. M. (2014). Impact of maternal diet on human milk composition and neurological development of infants. *American Journal of Clinical Nutrition, 99*(3), 734S–741S. https://doi.org/10.3945/ajcn.113.072595

Institute of Medicine. (2009). *Weight gain during pregnancy: Reexamining the guidelines*. The National Academies Press.

Jeong, G., Park, S. W., Lee, Y. K., Ko, S. Y., & Shin, S. M. (2017). Maternal food restrictions during breastfeeding. *Korean Journal of Pediatrics, 60*(3), 70–76. https://doi.org/10.3345/kjp.2017.60.3.70

Johnson, J. L., Farr, S. L., Dietz, P. M., Sharma, A. J., Barfield, W. D., & Robbins, C. L. (2015). Trends in gestational weight gain: The Pregnancy Risk Assessment Monitoring System, 2000–2009. *American Journal of Obstetrics and Gynecology, 212*(6), 806.e1–806.e8. https://doi.org/10.1016/j.ajog.2015.01.030

Kampmann, U., Madsen, L. R., Skajaa, G. O., Iversen, D. S., Moeller, N., & Ovesen, P. (2015). Gestational diabetes: A clinical update. *World Journal of Diabetes, 6*(8), 1065–1072. https://doi.org/10.4239/wjd.v6.i8.1065

Kominiarek, M. A., & Peaceman, A. M. (2017). Gestational weight gain. *American Journal of Obstetrics and Gynecology, 217*(6), 642–651. https://doi.org/10.1016/j.ajog.2017.05.040

Leavitt, K., Obican, S., & Yankowitz, J. (2019). Treatment and prevention of hypertensive disorders during pregnancy. *Clinics in Perinatology, 46*(2), 173–185. https://doi.org/10.1016/j.clp.2019.02.002

Lessen, R., & Kavanagh, K. (2015). Position of the Academy of Nutrition and Dietetics: Promoting and supporting breastfeeding. *Journal of the Academy of Nutrition and Dietetics, 115*(3), 444–449. https://doi.org/10.1016/j.jand.2014.12.014

Liu, P., Xu, L., Wang, Y., Zhang, Y., Du, Y., Sun, Y., & Wang, Z. (2016). Association between perinatal outcomes and maternal prepregnancy body mass index. *Obesity Reviews, 17*(11), 1091–1102. https://doi.org/10.1111/obr.12455

Miao, D., Young, S., & Golden, C. (2015). A meta-analysis of pica and micronutrient status. *American Journal of Human Biology, 27*(1), 84–93. https://doi.org/10.1002/ajhb.22598

Mohammadi, M., Maroufizadeh, S., Omani-Samani, R., Almasi-Hashiani, A., & Amini, P. (2018). The effect of prepregnancy body mass index on birth weight, preterm birth, cesarean section, and preeclampsia in pregnant women. *Journal of Maternal- Fetal & Neonatal Medicine, 32*(22), 3813–3823. https://doi.org/10.1080/14767058.2018.1473366

Morgan, S., Koren, G., & Bozzo, P. (2013). Is caffeine consumption safe during pregnancy? *Canadian Family Physician, 59*(4), 361–362.

Most, J., St. Amant, M., Hsia, D. S., Altazan, A. D., Thomas, D. M., Gilmore, L. A., Vallo, P. M., Beyl, R. A., Ravussin, E., & Redman, L. M. (2019). Evidence-based recommendations for energy intake in pregnant women with obesity. *Journal of Clinical Investigation, 129*(11), 4682–4690. https://doi.org/10.1172/JCI130341

Muktabhant, B., Lawrie, T., Lumbiganon, P., & Laopaiboon, M. (2015). Diet or exercise, or both, for preventing excessive weight gain in pregnancy. *Cochrane Database of Systematic Reviews, 6*, CD0071457. https://doi.org/10.1002/14651858.CD007145.pub3

Mulder, K. A., King, D. J., & Innis, S. M. (2014). Omega-3 fatty acid deficiency in infants before birth identified using a randomized trial of maternal DHA supplementation in pregnancy. *PloS One, 9*(1), e83764. https://doi.org/10.1371/journal.pone.0083764

QuickStats. (2016). Gestational weight gain among women with full-term, singleton births, compared with recommendations—48 states and the District of Columbia, 2015. *Morbidity and Mortality Weekly Report, 65*(40), 1121. http://dx.doi.org/10.15585/mmwr.mm6540a10

Seely, E., & Ecker, J. (2014). Chronic hypertension in pregnancy. *Circulation, 129*(11), 1254–1261. https://doi.org/10.1161/CIRCULATIONAHA.113.003904

Silvestris, E., dePergola, G., Rosania, R., & Loverro, G. (2018). Obesity as disruptor of the female fertility. *Reproductive Biology and Endocrinology, 16*, Article 22. https://doi.org/10.1186/s12958-018-0336-z

Stang, J., & Huffman, L. G. (2016). Position of the Academy of Nutrition and Dietetics: Obesity, reproduction, and pregnancy outcomes. *Journal of the Academy of Nutrition and Dietetics, 116*(4), 677–691. https://doi.org/10.1016/j.jand.2016.01.008

Stephenson, J., Heslehurst, N., Hall, J., Schoenaker, D. A. J. M., Hutchinson, J., Cade, J. E., Poston, L., Barrett, G., Crozier, S. R., Barker, M., Kumaran, K., Yajnik, C. S., Baird, J., & Mishra, G. D. (2018). Before the beginning: Nutrition and lifestyle in the preconception period and its importance for future health. *Lancet, 391*(10132), 1830–1841. https://doi.org/10.1016/S0140-6736(18)30311-8

Stevens, W., Shih, T., Incerti, D., Ton, T. G. N., Lee, H. C., Peneva, D., Macones, G. A., Sibai, B., & Jena, A. B. (2017). Short-term costs of preeclampsia to the United States health care system. *American Journal of Obstetrics and Gynecology, 217*(3), 237–248. https://doi.org/10.1016/j.ajog.2017.04.032

Umaretiya, P. J., Oberhelman, S. S., Cozine, E. W., Maxon, J. A., Quigg, S. M., & Thacher, T. D. (2017). Maternal preferences for vitamin D supplementation in breastfed infants. *Annals of Family Medicine, 15*(1), 68–70. https://doi.org/10.1370/afm.2016

U.S. Department of Agriculture & U.S. Department of Health and Human Services. (2020, December). *Dietary guidelines for Americans, 2020–2025*. https://www.dietaryguidelines.gov

U.S. Department of Health and Human Services. (2018). *Physical activity guidelines for Americans*. U.S. Department of Health and Human Services.

U.S. Department of Health and Human Services. (2019, October 23). *New evidence-based recommendations for calorie intake in pregnant women with obesity*. https://www.niddk.nih.gov/news/archive/2020/new-evidence-based-recommendations-calorie-intake-pregnant-women-obesity

U.S. Food and Drug Administration. (2018, February 8). *Additional information about high-intensity sweeteners permitted for use in food in the United States*. https://www.fda.gov/food/food-additives-petitions/additional-information-about-high-intensity-sweeteners-permitted-use-food-united-states#Steviol_glycosides

U.S. Food and Drug Administration. (2019, July 2). *Advice about eating fish. For women who are or might become pregnant, breastfeeding mothers, and young children*. https://www.fda.gov/food/consumers/advice-about-eating-fish

U.S. Preventive Services Task Force. (2017). *Folic acid for the prevention of neural tube defects: Preventive medication*. https://www.uspreventiveservicestaskforce.org/Page/Document/UpdateSummaryFinal/folic-acid-for-the-prevention-of-neural-tube-defects-preventive-medication?ds=1&s=folic%20acid%20pregnancy

Vockley, J., Andersson, H., Antshel, K., Braverman, N. D., Burton, B. K., Frazier, D. M., Mitchell, J., Smith, W. E., Thompson, B. H., & Berry, S. A., for the American College of Medical Genetics and Genomics Therapeutics Committee. (2014). Phenylalanine hydroxylase deficiency: Diagnosis and management guideline. *Genetics in Medicine, 16*(2), 188–200. https://doi.org/10.1038/gim.2013.157

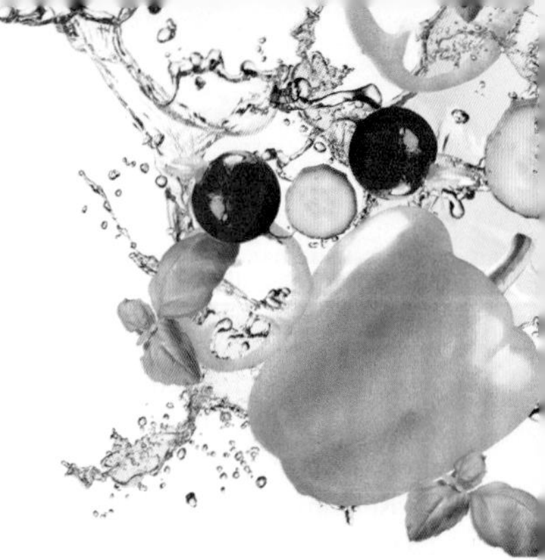

Chapter 13 Nutrition for Infants, Children, and Adolescents

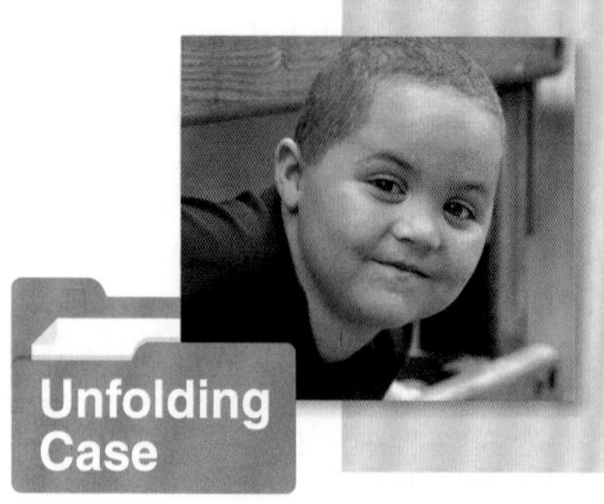

Luis Guzman

Luis is a 7-year-old boy who is 48 in. tall and weighs 90 pounds. He is the only child of a single mother who worries that his weight is out of control. She admits she lets him eat whatever he wants, even though she knows he is eating inappropriately. His grandmother is his primary caregiver before school starts, and when school is not in session, and she also gives him whatever he wants, including fast food twice a week.

Learning Objectives

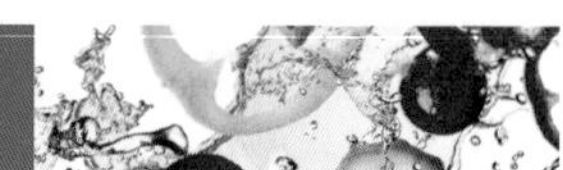

Upon completion of this chapter, you will be able to:

1 Discuss breastfeeding teaching points.
2 Describe key points about introducing solid foods into the diet.
3 Explain fluid and food recommendations for feeding infants.
4 Summarize eating characteristics and recommendations during early childhood.
5 Discuss calorie needs during middle childhood and adolescence.
6 Identify food groups most likely to be underconsumed by youth ages 5 to 18.
7 Name nutrients most likely to be underconsumed by adolescents.
8 Define overweight and obesity in youth.
9 Describe the stages of obesity treatment in youth.
10 Give examples of obesity prevention strategies from pregnancy through adolescence.

The goals of nutrition and physical activity for children are to promote optimal physical and cognitive development, a healthy weight, an enjoyment of food, and a decreased risk of chronic disease (Ogata & Hayes, 2014). Actual nutrient requirements vary according to health status, activity pattern, and growth rate. The greater the rate of growth, the more intense the nutritional needs.

The health trends of American children are mixed. Although deficiency diseases are rare and infant mortality has declined over recent decades, the prevalence of overweight and obesity is a public health concern. Today, nearly 1 out of 5 American children are obese, placing them at risk for chronic diseases that were once only diagnosed in adults, such as coronary artery disease, type 2 diabetes, hypertension, metabolic syndrome, and sleep apnea. Today's children may experience shorter life expectancies related to young-onset obesity.

This chapter presents nutrition from birth through adolescence, including calorie and nutrient needs and eating practices. Nutrition concerns during childhood and adolescence—namely, poor diet quality and overweight and obesity—are discussed.

INFANCY (BIRTH TO 1 YEAR)

Excluding fetal growth, growth in the first year of life is more rapid than at any other time in the life cycle. Birth weight doubles in the first 6 months (Box 13.1). From 6 to 12 months, rapid growth continues but at a slower pace. The Centers for Disease Control and Prevention (CDC) (2010) recommends that growth be monitored from birth to 2 years of age by using the World Health Organization (WHO) growth charts. WHO growth charts are based on growth of a population of healthy breastfed infants, whereas the CDC growth charts from birth to 2 years are based on observational data from overweight populations and include a large number of formula-fed infants (Hagan et al., 2017). The WHO growth charts can be accessed at www.cdc.gov/growthcharts/who_charts.htm#. Infants who are growing appropriately are consuming adequate nutrition.

Over the course of the first year of life, significant change occurs in the infant's size, development, nutrient needs, and feeding patterns. As the infant becomes more skillful in signaling hunger and satiety, the ability to self-feed, and language, parents learn how to identify and assess infant cues and gain a sense of confidence (Hagan et al., 2017).

Nutrient Needs

Adequate calories and nutrients are needed to support the unprecedented rate of growth that occurs during the first year of life. Recommendations for the amount of calories and nutrients infants should consume are approximations based on estimated average intakes of healthy full-term newborns that are exclusively breastfed by well-nourished mothers—even though the content of breast milk varies and it is impossible to measure how much an infant consumes.

Although the total amount of calories and nutrients is generally far less than what adults need, proportionately infants require more calories and nutrients than adults. Fat provides 40% to 50% of calories in breast milk and infant formulas. This is a contrast to the recommendation that adults consume 20% to 35% of their total calories from fat. Infants need calorically dense fat to meet the demands of growth within the constraints of small stomach capacity.

Because infants are born with low amounts of vitamin K stored in the body and a decreased ability to utilize vitamin K, infants are given a single intramuscular dose of vitamin K at birth to protect them from hemorrhagic disease of the newborn. With few exceptions noted in the following section, all other vitamin and mineral needs are met with breast milk or properly prepared formula.

BOX 13.1 Average Growth in the First Year of Life

First week of life

- May lose up to 10% of birth weight

By 14 days of age

- Birth weight regained

Between 4 and 6 months of age

- Birth weight doubles
- Usual weekly gain is 4 to 7 oz

From 6 months to 1 year

- Usual weekly gain of 2 to 3 oz in breastfed infants, 3 to 5 oz in formula-fed infants

At 1 year

- Birth weight triples
- Length increases by 50%

Source: Hagan, J. F., Shaw, J. S., & Duncan, P. M. (Eds.). (2017). *Bright futures: Guidelines for health supervision of infants, children, and adolescents*. American Academy of Pediatrics.

BOX 13.2 Composition of Breast Milk

Protein

- Amount is adequate to support growth without contributing to an excessive renal solute load.
- Most of the protein is easy to digest whey.
- The concentration of potentially harmful amino acids (e.g., phenylalanine) is low and there are high levels of amino acids that infants cannot synthesize (e.g., taurine).

Fat

- High content of linoleic acid (an essential fatty acid).
- High cholesterol content may help infants develop enzyme systems capable of handling cholesterol later in life.

Minerals

The minerals are mostly protein bound and balanced to enhance bioavailability. For instance, the rate of iron absorption from breast milk is approximately 50% compared with about 4% for iron-fortified formulas. Zinc absorption is better from breast milk than from either cow's milk or formula.

Enzymes

- Contains amylase to promote carbohydrate digestion when pancreatic amylase levels are low.
- Contains lipases to promote fat digestion.

Renal Solute Load

- Minerals and protein in adequate, but not excessive, amounts keep renal solute load suited to the immature kidneys' inability to concentrate urine.
- Contains antibodies and anti-infective factors. Although higher in colostrum, breast milk contains antibodies.
- Bifidus factor promotes the growth of normal GI flora (e.g., *Lactobacillus bifidus*) that protect the infant against harmful GI bacteria.

Breast Milk

Breast milk is specifically designed to support optimal growth and development in the newborn, and its composition makes it uniquely superior for infant feeding (Box 13.2). Breastfeeding is recommended for at least the first year of life with exclusive breastfeeding for the first 6 months of life (U.S. Department of Agriculture [USDA] & U.S. Department of Health and Human Services [USDHHS], 2020).

- Some of the potential health benefits for the infant include reduced risk of diarrhea and respiratory tract infection; possible protective effect against inflammatory bowel disease, leukemias, and certain types of type 1 diabetes; lowered risk of obesity in some populations; lower risk of atopic illness; and close mother–infant bonding (Hagan et al., 2017).
- All infants who are exclusively breastfed or who receive breast milk and formula need a vitamin D supplement of 400 IU/day beginning soon after birth (USDA & USDHHS, 2020).

Infant Formula

Infant formulas may be used in place of breastfeeding, as an occasional supplement to breastfeeding, or when exclusively breastfed infants are weaned before 12 months of age.

- The Infant Formula Act regulates the levels of nutrients in formulas, specifying both minimum and maximum amounts of each essential nutrient.
- Almost all formula used in the United States is iron fortified, a practice that has greatly reduced the risk of iron deficiency in older infants.
- Because the minimum recommended amount of each nutrient is more than the amount provided in breast milk, nutrient supplements are unnecessary for the first 6 months of life.
- Infant formula companies in the United States market directly to consumers and release new formulas with or without slightly different compositions on a regular basis, such as formulas with added DHA or lutein to "support eye health."
- There is debate over the associations between some formula ingredients and health outcomes, such as the unknown effects of adding prebiotics and probiotics to infant formulas (Rossen et al., 2016). The U.S. Food and Drug Administration (FDA) does not "approve" new formulas but rather reviews the proposed formula composition and background

information provided by the formula manufacturer. The FDA is more empowered to evaluate safety than efficacy of infant formulas (Abrams, 2015).

- Categories of infant formulas for full-term and preterm infants include the following (American Academy of Pediatrics, 2020; Rossen et al., 2016):
  - Cow's milk–based formulas account for 69% of formulas used; most are iron fortified.
  - Soy formulas. According to AAP, there are few circumstances for choosing soy formula over cow's milk–based formula.
  - Hydrolyzed formulas are intended for infants with cow's milk and soy protein allergies.
  - Specialized formulas are specifically altered to be lacking or deficient in one or more nutrients (e.g., phenylalanine) so are not suitable for healthy infants.
  - Preterm formulas are designed to promote "catch-up growth." They are higher than routine formulas in calories, protein, and certain minerals.
  - Premature infant discharge formulas are less calorically dense than preterm formulas but higher in calories than term formulas. They are used to supplement breastfed preterm infants

Infant Feedings

Successful infant feeding requires parents to recognize verbal and nonverbal feeding cues (Hagan et al., 2017).

- Newborns signal hunger by rooting, sucking, and hand movements. Hunger cues in an older infant may include hand-to-mouth movements, lip smacking, crying, excited arm and leg movements, opening the mouth, and moving toward a spoon as it comes near.
- Depending on the infant's age, satiety cues include fussiness during feedings, slowing the pace of eating, turning away from the nipple, stopping sucking, spitting out/refusing the nipple, falling asleep, or spitting up milk.

Frequency of Breastfeeding

- In the first months of life, breastfed infants are fed a minimum of 8 to 12 times/24 hours, or approximately every 2 to 3 hours.
- Feedings become less frequent as the infant grows.
- Teaching points for breastfeeding are listed in Box 13.3.

BOX 13.3 Teaching Points for Breastfeeding

- The infant should be allowed to nurse for 5 minutes on each breast on the first day to achieve letdown and milk ejection. By the end of the first week, the infant should be nursing up to 15 minutes/breast.
- Mothers should offer the breast whenever the infant shows early signs of hunger. The first breast offered should be alternated with every feeding so both breasts receive equal stimulation and draining.
- Even though the infant will be able to virtually empty the breast within 5 to 10 minutes once the milk supply is established, the infant needs to nurse beyond that point to satisfy the need to suck and to receive emotional and physical comfort.
- The supply of milk is equal to the demand—the more the infant sucks or the more frequently milk is manually expressed, the more milk is produced. Infants age 6 weeks or 12 weeks who suck more are probably experiencing a growth spurt and so need more milk.
- Early substitution of formula or introduction of solid foods may decrease the chance of maintaining lactation.
- Breast milk can be pumped, placed in a sanitary bottle, and immediately refrigerated or frozen for later use. Milk should be used within 24 hours if refrigerated or within 3 months if stored in the freezer compartment of the refrigerator.

BOX 13.4 Teaching Points for Formula Feeding

- Never force the infant to finish a bottle or to take more than they want.
- Discourage the misconception that "a fat baby = a healthy baby = good parents."
- Each feeding should last 20 to 30 minutes.
- Formula may be given at room temperature, slightly warmed, or directly from the refrigerator; however, always give formula at approximately the same temperature.
- Spitting up of a small amount of formula during or after a feeding is normal. Feed the infant more slowly and burp more frequently to help alleviate spitting up.
- Hold the infant closely and securely. Position the infant so that the head is higher than the rest of the body.
- Avoid jiggling the bottle and making extra movements that could distract the infant from feeding.
- Bottles should never be propped for independent feeding.
- Check the flow of formula by holding the bottle upside down. A steady drip from the nipple should be observed. If the flow is too rapid because of a too large nipple opening, the infant may overfeed and develop indigestion. If the flow rate is too slow because of a too small nipple opening, the infant may tire and fall asleep without taking enough formula. Discard any nipples with holes that are too large, and enlarge holes that are too small with a sterilized needle.
- Reassure caregivers that there is no danger of "spoiling" an infant by feeding them when they cry for a feeding.
- Burp the infant halfway through the feeding, at the end of the feeding, and more often if necessary to help get rid of air swallowed during feeding. Burping can be accomplished gently rubbing or patting the infant's back as they are held on the shoulder, lie on their stomach over the caregiver's lap, or sit in an upright position.
- After the teeth erupt, the baby should be given only plain water for a bedtime bottle-feeding.

Formula Feeding

The recommendations for formula feeding listed in the following are based on meeting the infant's total calorie and fluid needs, not for the maximum volumes per feeding (Hagan et al., 2017). During growth spurts, infants temporarily increase the volume of formula consumed. Teaching points for formula feeding are listed in Box 13.4.

- In the first weeks of life,
  - offer 2 oz every 2 to 3 hours; a newborn in the 50th percentile for weight consumes an average of 20 oz formula/day with a range of 16 to 24 oz/day;
  - more formula should be offered if the infant still appears hungry.
- Infants around the age of 2 months need 6 to 8 feedings/24 hours.
- A 4-month-old consumes an average of 31 oz/day (range of 26–36 oz/day) without complementary foods.
- At 6 months and older, formula intake is 24 to 32 oz/day in addition to complementary foods. As solid food intake increases, the volume of formula consumed decreases.
- To avoid nursing bottle caries, infants should not be put to bed with a bottle of formula or other liquids that contain sugar (Fig. 13.1).

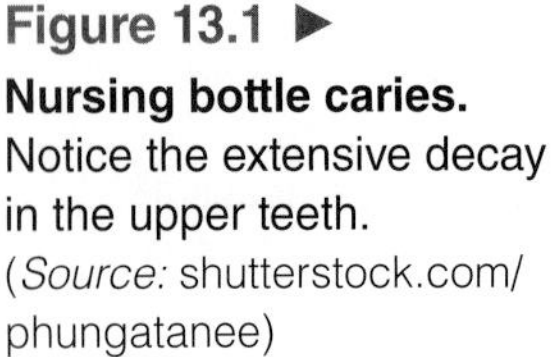
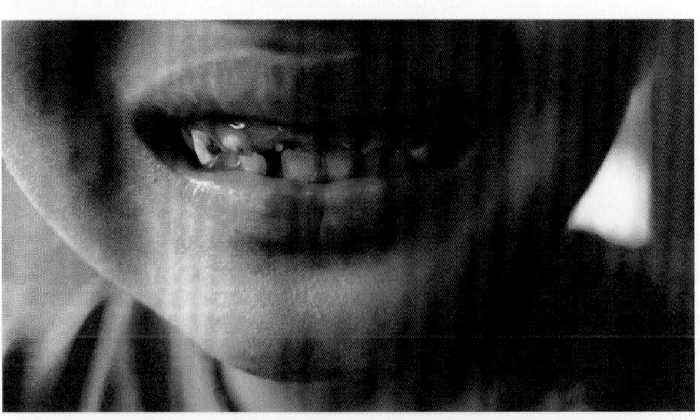

Figure 13.1 ▶ Nursing bottle caries. Notice the extensive decay in the upper teeth. (*Source:* shutterstock.com/phungatanee)

Complementary Foods

Complementary foods, also known as solids, are added to the infant's diet at about 6 months of age and when the infant is developmentally ready (USDA & USDHHS, 2020).

Nutrient Needs

Around 6 months of age, breast milk or formulas are not adequate as the sole source of nutrition and nutrient-dense, developmentally appropriate complementary foods become necessary.

- Infant iron stores are usually adequate for about the first 6 months of life so the first solids offered should be iron-rich foods, such as meats, seafood, and iron-fortified infant cereals.
- Iron-rich foods should continue through 11 months to maintain adequate stores (USDA & USDHHS, 2020). Formula-fed infants should continue to use iron-fortified formula.
- To support adequate zinc status, zinc-rich complementary foods, such as meats, beans, and zinc-fortified cereals, are important from age 6 months onward (USDA & USDHHS, 2020).
- At 6 months of age, exclusively breastfed infants and infants who receive ready-to-use infant formula need supplemental fluoride.
- Infants who consume formula that is prepared with local water need supplemental fluoride only if the water contains less than 0.3 ppm of fluoride.

Introducing Solids

Initially, small amounts of pureed foods are offered. As the infant's mouth patterns, hand and body skills, and feeding skills develop, the amount and texture of food offered progresses (Table 13.1).

- Iron-fortified cereal or pureed foods are usually recommended as first foods; there is no evidence to support any particular order or rate for introducing other solids.

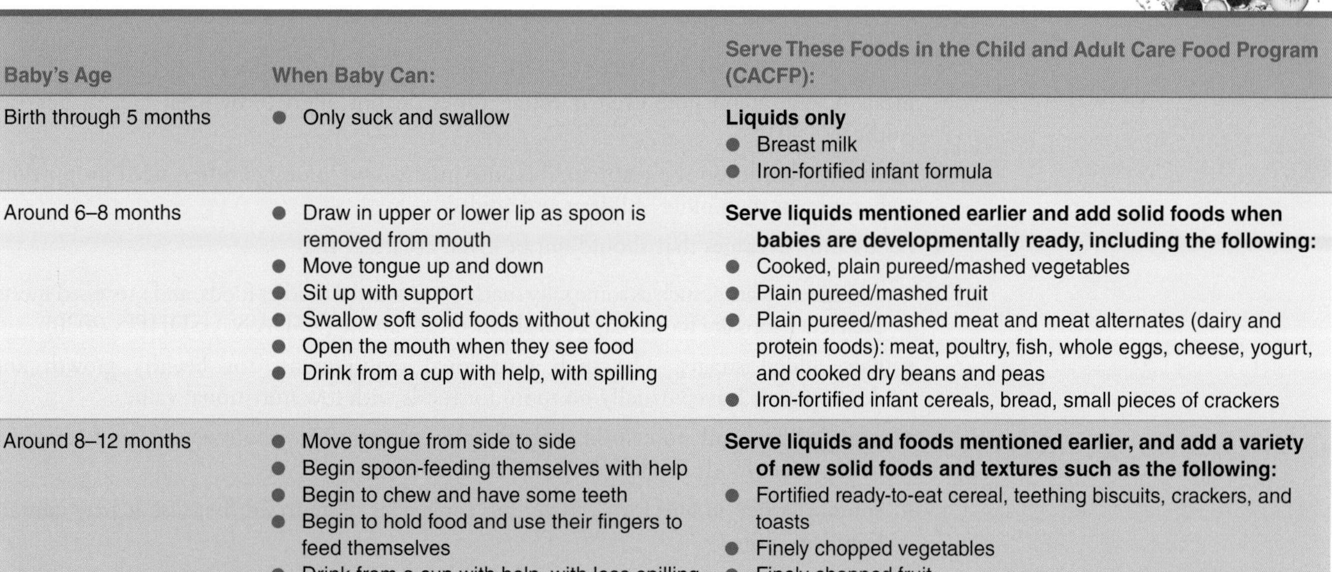

Table 13.1 For Child Care Providers: Feeding Babies in Their First Year

Baby's Age	When Baby Can:	Serve These Foods in the Child and Adult Care Food Program (CACFP):
Birth through 5 months	• Only suck and swallow	**Liquids only** • Breast milk • Iron-fortified infant formula
Around 6–8 months	• Draw in upper or lower lip as spoon is removed from mouth • Move tongue up and down • Sit up with support • Swallow soft solid foods without choking • Open the mouth when they see food • Drink from a cup with help, with spilling	**Serve liquids mentioned earlier and add solid foods when babies are developmentally ready, including the following:** • Cooked, plain pureed/mashed vegetables • Plain pureed/mashed fruit • Plain pureed/mashed meat and meat alternates (dairy and protein foods): meat, poultry, fish, whole eggs, cheese, yogurt, and cooked dry beans and peas • Iron-fortified infant cereals, bread, small pieces of crackers
Around 8–12 months	• Move tongue from side to side • Begin spoon-feeding themselves with help • Begin to chew and have some teeth • Begin to hold food and use their fingers to feed themselves • Drink from a cup with help, with less spilling	**Serve liquids and foods mentioned earlier, and add a variety of new solid foods and textures such as the following:** • Fortified ready-to-eat cereal, teething biscuits, crackers, and toasts • Finely chopped vegetables • Finely chopped fruit • Finely chopped meat and meat alternates (dairy and protein foods): meat, poultry, fish, whole eggs, cheese, yogurt, and cooked dry beans and peas

Source: U.S. Department of Agriculture Food and Nutrition Service. (2019). Feeding infants in the child and adult care food program. FNS 786. https://fns-prod.azureedge.net/sites/default/files/resource-files/FI_FullGuide-a.pdf

- Generally, single-ingredient foods are introduced one at a time so that allergic reactions, such as rashes, vomiting, or diarrhea, can be identified.
- The amount of solid food taken at a feeding may vary from 1 to 2 tsp initially to ¼ to ½ cup as the infant gets older. To increase the likelihood of acceptance, it may be beneficial to give a small amount of formula or breast milk to take the edge off hunger before introducing the first solid.
- After 3 days of apparent tolerance, another new food is introduced.
- Solids may be given 2 to 3 times/day with the infant deciding how much to eat.
- Within a few months, the infant is eating texture-appropriate meats, cereal, fruits, and vegetables in addition to breast milk and/or formula.
- To limit the likelihood that infants will become picky eaters, a variety of colors, flavors, and textures should be offered.
- It may take as many as 8 to 10 exposures over several months before an infant "likes" a particular food.
- Establishing regular meal times and snack times instead of continuous grazing will help prevent overweight and obesity (Hagan et al., 2017).

Feeding Guidelines

Parents decide what infants (and children) are offered, whereas infants (and children) always decide whether to eat and how much to eat (Satter, 2016). Parents need to trust their child's natural ability to eat the amount of food they need. By 12 months of age, infants should be eating a variety of table foods and various textures.

Fluids

- Breast milk and/or iron-fortified formula are consumed until the infant reaches the age of 12 months. Breastfeeding may continue longer, if desired.
- Plain cow milk is avoided until 12 months of age because it lacks adequate iron and has excessive amounts of sodium, potassium, and protein compared to formula or breast milk (Rossen et al., 2016).

Food

- Three to 5 solid feedings/day are appropriate. Infants should be included in family meals whenever possible even if eating times do not align (Provincial Health Services Authority, 2016).
- Fat intake should not be restricted because infants and young children need proportionately more fat than older children and adults.
- Foods and beverages that should not be given are those that
  - are higher sodium, such as some salty snacks, commercial toddler foods, and processed meats. Preference for salty foods may be established early in life (USDA & USDHHS, 2020).
  - have added sugars. The high nutritional requirements for healthy growth and development leave virtually no room for foods with low nutritional value.
  - contain low- and no-calorie sweeteners so as to not promote a taste preference for overly sweet foods (USDA & USDHHS, 2020).
  - contain honey in any form, including cooked or pasteurized, because it may contain botulism spores.
  - are unpasteurized, such as unpasteurized juices, milk, yogurt, or cheeses because they may contain harmful bacteria (USDA & USDHHS, 2020).
  - may cause choking (Box 13.5).

BOX 13.5 Foods That May Cause Choking in Small Children

Round slices of hot dogs and sausages
Hard candy
Cough drops
Peanuts and other whole nuts
Whole grapes and cherries
Raw carrot sticks
Whole cherry or grape tomatoes
Large pieces of raw vegetables or fruit
Olives with pits
Tough meat
Celery
Popcorn
Dried fruit
Marshmallows
Potato and corn chips and similar snack foods
Chewing gum

Food Allergies

According to the American Academy of Pediatrics (Greer et al., 2019)

- there is no evidence that delaying the introduction of allergenic foods, including peanuts, eggs, and fish, beyond 4 to 6 months of age prevents atopic disease
- evidence now shows that early introduction of infant-safe forms of peanuts (e.g., small amounts of thinned peanut butter mixed in infant cereal or yogurt) reduces the risk for peanut allergies.
    - High-risk infants should be introduced to peanuts as early as 4 to 6 months of age.
    - Infants with mild-to-moderate risk (e.g., mild-to-moderate eczema) should be introduced to peanuts around 6 months of age.
    - Low-risk infants (no eczema or any food allergy) should be given peanut-containing food when age appropriate (e.g., after 6 months of age if exclusively breastfed).

NUTRITION DURING EARLY CHILDHOOD (1–5 YEARS)

Adequate nutrition during early childhood focuses on promoting normal growth through the appropriate amount and types of foods within an environment that allows the child to self-regulate (Hagan et al., 2017). Beginning at age 2 years, CDC growth charts are used to monitor size and growth patterns by plotting body mass index (BMI) for age (Figs. 13.2 and 13.3). Weight status outside the definition of normal or healthy (Table 13.2) and deviations in a child's percentile channel warrant further attention.

Physical activity is intertwined with nutrition in promoting growth and development and overall health. Key physical activity guidelines for preschool-aged children state that children ages 3 to 5 should be physically active throughout the day and that adult caregivers should encourage active play that includes a variety of activity types (USDHHS, 2018).

Parental Influences on Eating Habits

Early parental influence is associated with the development of a child's relationship with food later in life (Ogata & Hayes, 2014). Young children are especially dependent on parents and caregivers as to which foods are available, the portion sizes offered, how often eating occurs, and the social context of eating. For instance, eating all food on the plate, dessert used as a reward, and eating

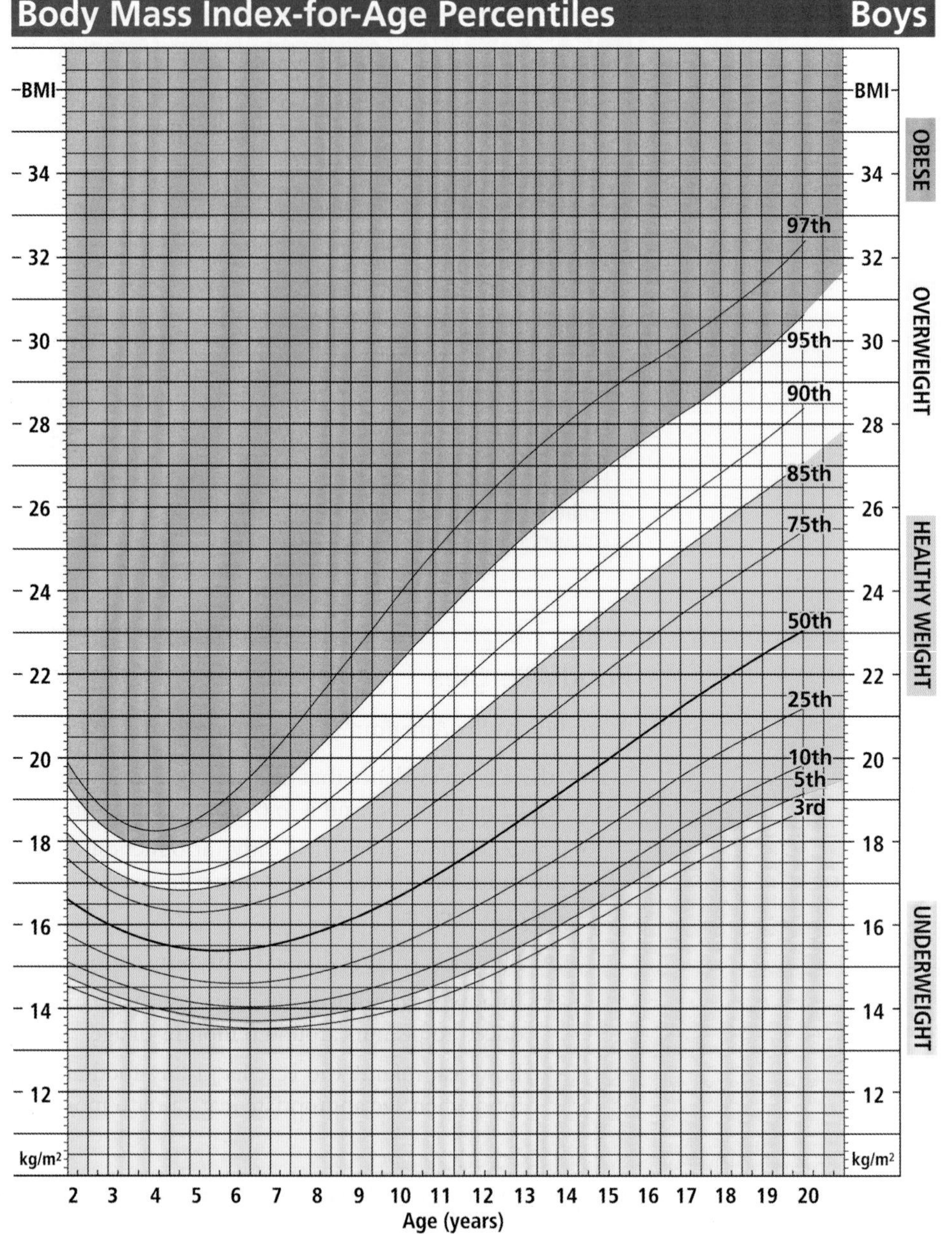

Figure 13.2 ▶ **Body mass index-for-age percentiles for boys.** (*Source:* Adapted from the CDC. [2010]. Growth charts. National Center for Health Statistics. https://www.cdc.gov/growthcharts/)

regularly scheduled meals are behaviors that may be instilled in children by their parents. Parents who offer large food portions (especially of calorie-dense, sweet, or salty foods), pressure their child to eat or restrict the child's eating, and model excessive eating undermine the child's ability to self-regulate food intake (Ogata & Hayes, 2014).

As the infant becomes a toddler, parents determine what food is served, when food is served, and where it is served. Dividing feeding responsibilities into parental tasks and child tasks helps children become competent eaters who are able to self-regulate intake, thereby decreasing the risk of overweight/obesity and disordered eating (Box 13.6) (Satter, 2016).

Developmental Milestones Related to Eating

The dramatic decrease in growth rate that occurs after the first year of life is reflected in a decrease in appetite and unpredictable food intake as calorie needs per kilogram of body weight decrease. At age 1 year, the child should be drinking from a cup. By the age of 2, the toddler should eat most of the same foods as the rest of the family with precautions taken to avoid choking.

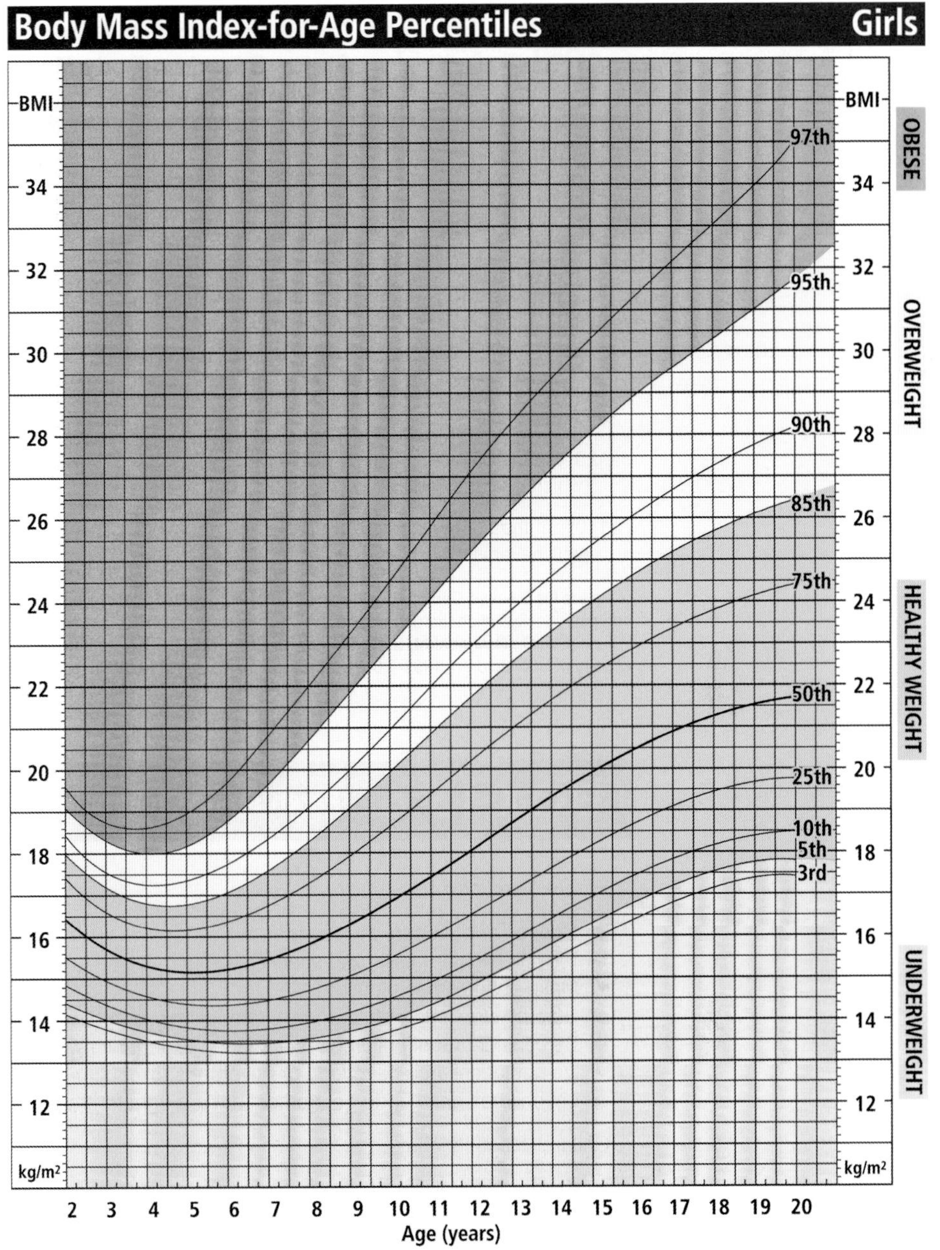

Figure 13.3 ▶ Body mass index-for-age percentiles for girls. (*Source:* Adapted from the CDC. [2010]. Growth charts. National Center for Health Statistics. https://www.cdc.gov/growthcharts/)

The typical daily pattern is 3 meals and 2 to 3 snacks. By 24 months of age, toddlers should be able to use utensils and spill little of their food.

Eating characteristics from age 2 to 5 or 6 are as follows (Provincial Health Services Authority, 2016):

- Young children continue to be at risk of choking until around the age of 4 years.
- Beginning around 15 months of age, a child may develop food jags as a normal expression of autonomy as the child develops a sense of independence.
- By the end of the second year, children can completely self-feed and can seek food independently.
- Picky eating is a normal behavior.
- Adult role modeling is important.

Table 13.2 Childhood and Adolescent Weight Status Based on Body Mass Index Percentile Categories

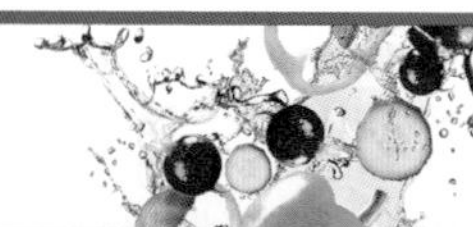

BMI Percentile Range[a]	Weight Status Category
<5th	Underweight
≥5th–84th	Normal or healthy weight
≥85th–94th	Overweight
≥95th	Obese
Classification of Severe Obesity[b]	
≥95th percentile	Class 1 Obesity
≥120% of the 95th percentile or a BMI ≥ 35 (whichever is lower)	Class 2 Obesity
≥140% of the 95th percentile or a BMI ≥ 4 0 (whichever is lower)	Class 3 Obesity

[a]Centers for Disease Control and Prevention. (2018, July 3). Defining childhood obesity. *Overweight & Obesity*. https://www.cdc.gov/obesity/childhood/defining.html
[b]Skinner, A. C., Ravanbakht, S. N., Skelton, J. A., Perrin, E. M., & Armstrong, S. C. (2018). Prevalence of obesity and severe obesity in U.S. children, 1999–2016. *Pediatrics*, *141*(3), e20173459. https://doi.org/10.1542/peds.2017-3459

BOX 13.6 Parents' and Children's Responsibilities in Feeding

Parents' feeding jobs:

- Choose and prepare the food.
- Provide regular meals and snacks.
- Make eating times pleasant.
- Step-by-step, show children by example how to behave at family mealtime.
- Be considerate of children's lack of food experience without catering to likes and dislikes.
- Do not let children have food or beverages (except for water) between meal and snack times.
- Let children grow up to get bodies that are right for them.

Children's eating jobs:

- Children will eat.
- They will eat the amount they need.
- They will learn to eat the food their parents eat.
- They will grow predictably.
- They will learn to behave well at mealtime.

Source: Satter, S. (2016). *Ellyn Satter's division of responsibility in feeding*. https://www.ellynsatterinstitute.org/wp-content/uploads/2016/11/handout-dor-tasks-cap-2016.pdf

Calories and Nutrient Needs

Daily calorie needs for ages 12 to 23 months range from 800 to 1000 for both girls and boys (USDA & USDHHS, 2020). Two- to 5-year-old children need 1000 to 1600 cal/day depending on activity (Table 13.3).

- Estimated calorie needs were based on reference median length or height and reference weight (healthy) (USDA & USDHHS, 2020). Actual needs may vary.

Table 13.3 Estimated Calorie Needs per Day by Age, Sex, and Physical Activity Level, Ages 2 to 18

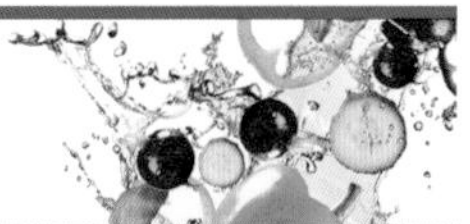

	Boys				Girls		
	Sedentary[a]	Moderately Active[b]	Active[c]		Sedentary[a]	Moderately Active[b]	Active[c]
Age				**Age**			
2	1000	1000	1000	2	1000	1000	1000
3	1000	1400	1400	3	1000	1200	1400
4	1200	1400	1600	4	1200	1400	1400
5	1200	1400	1600	5	1200	1400	1600
6	1400	1600	1800	6	1200	1400	1600
7	1400	1600	1800	7	1200	1600	1800
8	1400	1600	2000	8	1400	1600	1800
9	1600	1800	2000	9	1400	1600	1800
10	1600	1800	2200	10	1400	1800	2000
11	1800	2200	2200	11	1600	1800	2000
12	1800	2200	2400	12	1600	2000	2200
13	2000	2200	2600	13	1600	2000	2200
14	2000	2400	2800	14	1800	2000	2400
15	2200	2600	3000	15	1800	2000	2400
16–18	2400	2800	3200	16	1800	2000	2400

[a]Sedentary means a lifestyle that includes only the physical activity of independent living.
[b]Moderately active means a lifestyle that includes physical activity equivalent to walking about 1.5 to 3 miles/day at 3 to 4 miles/hour, in addition to the activities of independent living.
[c]Active means a lifestyle that includes physical activity equivalent to walking more than 3 miles/day at 3 to 4 miles/hour, in addition to the activities of independent living.
Source: Institute of Medicine. (2002). *Dietary reference intakes for energy, carbohydrate, fiber, fat, fatty acids, cholesterol, protein, and amino acids*. The National Academies Press; U.S. Department of Agriculture and U.S. Department of Health and Human Services. (2020, December). *Dietary guidelines for Americans, 2020–2025*. https://dietaryguidelines.gov

- All foods within the eating patterns are to be in nutrient-dense forms and made with minimal added sugars, refined starch, or sodium. The exception is that whole milk, reduced-fat plain yogurt, and reduced-fat cheese are recommended until the age of 2.
- Under the age of 2, there is no room for calories for other uses (e.g., added sugars, saturated fat, or more than recommended amounts of any food group).
- If consuming up to 2 oz of seafood/week, children should only be fed cooked varieties of seafood that have low amounts of mercury, such as catfish, cod, flounder, salmon, and haddock. See Chapter 4 for more on seafood.

Feeding Guidelines

The Dietary Guidelines for Americans recommends a healthy eating pattern be followed from 12 months of age through adulthood (USDA & USDHHS, 2020). Healthy eating patterns are adequate to meet nutrient needs, help achieve a healthy body weight, and reduce the risk of chronic disease.

Table 13.4 outlines the Healthy U.S.-Style eating pattern for ages 12 to 23 months; Table 13.5 outlines eating patterns appropriate from the age 2 to 18. General considerations regarding fluid and food intake are summarized in the following sections.

Table 13.4 Healthy U.S.-Style Eating Pattern for Toddlers Ages 12 to 23 Months Who Are No Longer Receiving Human Milk or Infant Formula, with Daily or Weekly Amounts from Food Groups and Components

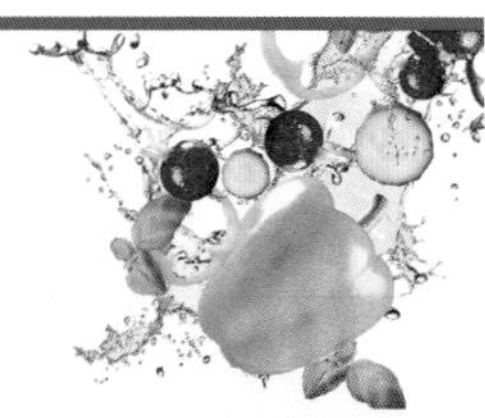

Calorie Level of Pattern[a]	700	800	900	1000
Food Group[b]	**Daily Amount of Food from Each Group**			
Vegetables (cup-eq/day)	⅔	¾	1	1
Fruits (cup-eq/day)	½	¾	1	1
Grains (oz-eq/day)	1¾	2¼	2½	3
Dairy (cup-eq/day)	1⅔	1¾	2	2
Protein Foods (oz-eq/day)	2	2	2	2
Oils (grams/day)	9	9	8	13
Limit on calories for other uses				

[a]Calorie level ranges: Energy levels are calculated based on median length and body weight reference individuals. Calorie needs vary based on many factors. The DRI Calculator for Healthcare Professionals available at nal.usda.gov/fnic/dri-calculator/ can be used to estimate calorie needs based on age, sex, and weight.
[b]All foods are assumed to be in nutrient-dense forms and prepared with minimal added sugars, refined starches (which are a source of calories but few or no other nutrients), or sodium. Foods are also lean or in low-fat forms with the exception of dairy, which includes whole-fat fluid milk, reduced-fat plain yogurts, and reduced-fat cheese. There are no calories available for additional added sugars, for saturated fat, or to eat more than the recommended amount of food in a food group.
Source: U.S. Department of Agriculture & U.S. Department of Health and Human Services. (2020, December). *Dietary guidelines for Americans, 2020–2025*. https://www.dietaryguidelsines.gov

Table 13.5 Healthy U.S.-Style Eating Pattern: Recommended Amounts of Food from Each Food Group from 1400 Calories to 3200 Calories Levels

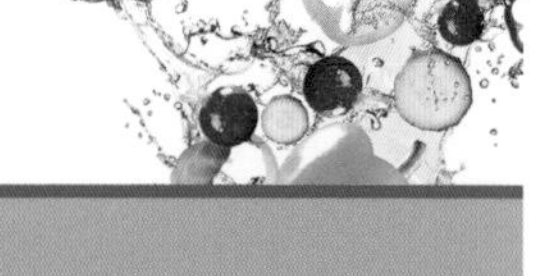

	Amounts Recommended/Day/Calorie Level											
Food Groups	**1000**	**1200**	**1400**	**1600**	**1800**	**2000**	**2200**	**2400**	**2600**	**2800**	**3000**	**3200**
Vegetables (cup-eq)	1	1.5	1.5	2	2.5	2.5	3	3	3.5	3.5	4	4
Fruits (cup-eq)	1	1	1.5	1.5	1.5	2	2	2	2	2.5	2.5	2.5
Grains (oz-eq)	3	4	5	5	6	6	7	8	9	10	10	10
Dairy (cup-eq)	2	2.5	2.5	3	3	3	3	3	3	3	3	3
Protein Foods (oz-eq)	2	3	4	5	5	5.5	6	6.5	6.5	7	7	7
Oils (g)	15	17	17	22	24	27	29	31	34	36	44	51
Limit on calories for other uses	130	80	110	130	170	270	280	350	380	400	470	610

Source: U.S. Department of Agriculture and U.S. Department of Health and Human Services. (2020, December). *Dietary guidelines for Americans, 2020–2025*. https://www.dietaryguidelines.gov

Milk Anemia
an iron deficiency anemia related to excessive milk intake, which displaces the intake of iron-rich foods from the diet.

Fluid

From 12 to 23 months

- Whole milk becomes a major source of nutrients, including fat; children between the ages of 1 and 2 years have a relatively higher need for fat to support growth and development. Milk intake should not exceed 2 to 3 cups/day (Muth, 2019) because, in greater amounts, it may displace the intake of iron-rich foods from the diet and promote **milk anemia**.

- The child may consume 1 to 4 cups of water/day. Only water should be allowed between meals and snacks and water should be offered when the child is thirsty.
- Children should not be given sugar-sweetened beverages, such as regular soda, sports, drinks, and flavored water, as well as caffeinated beverages.

From ages 2 to 5

- Children should drink 2 to 2½ cups/day of low-fat or nonfat milk and 1 to 5 cups of water daily (Muth, 2019).
- Because young children introduced to sweet drinks at a young age develop a strong preference for them, 100% fruit juice should be offered only when whole fruit is not available (Muth, 2019). Recommended daily limits for 100% fruit juice are no more than 4 oz for children aged 2 to 3 and 4 to 6 oz for 4- to 5-year-olds.

Food

- A variety of nutrient-dense foods from all food groups should be offered.
- The MyPlate graphic illustrates the concept of balance (Fig. 13.4)
- A regular schedule of 3 meals and 2 to 3 nutrient-dense snacks should be established.
- Although the food children need is the same as adults, the portion sizes are not. A rule-of-thumb guideline to determine age-appropriate serving sizes is to provide 1 tbsp of food/year of age (e.g., the serving size for a 3-year-old is 3 tbsp). By age 4 to 6, serving size may be close to adult size.
- To decrease the risk of choking, foods that are difficult to chew and swallow should be avoided until around the age of 4 (see Box 13.5).
    - Meals and snacks should be supervised.
    - Foods should be prepared in forms that are easy to chew and swallow (e.g., cut grapes into smaller pieces and spread peanut butter thinly).
    - Infants should not be allowed to eat or drink from a cup while lying down, playing, or strapped in a car seat.

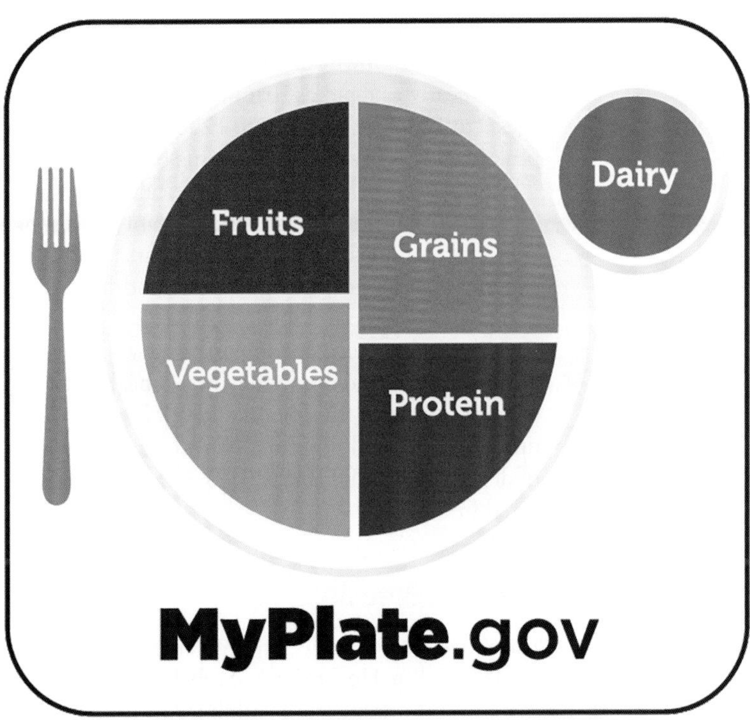

Figure 13.4 ▶ MyPlate graphic. (*Source:* U.S. Department of Agriculture. [n.d.]. MyPlate graphics. https://www.myplate.gov)

Promoting Healthy Habits

Healthy child-feeding practices are critical for helping children develop healthy eating habits later in life (Provincial Health Services Authority, 2016).

- Toys, books, and/or screens should not be used during mealtime to avoid distracted eating.
- Children should not be pressured or cajoled into eating more.
- Avoid empty calorie foods. Hot dogs, burgers, pizza, cookies, cakes, and candy are only occasional treats.
- Sweet drinks, such as flavored milk, plant-based milks (except for soymilk), artificially sweetened drinks, sugar-sweetened beverages, and caffeinated drinks, should be avoided.
- Portions offered should be small. Allow the child to ask for more.
- Give children the opportunity to improve self-feeding skills, even though it may be messy.
- Toddlers and preschoolers are often ready to leave the table after 15 to 20 minutes. Food should be removed from the table at that time.
- Eating with the family is associated with better diet quality and lower rates of overweight/obesity and less disordered eating (Provincial Health Services Authority, 2016).
- Behaviors in young children that may indicate nutrition risk include the following:
  - Poor appetite
  - Inadequate intake from any food group
  - Frequent intake of fast food
  - Consumption of sugar-sweetened or artificially sweetened beverages
  - Persistent bottle feeding
  - Child does not eat with the family
  - Growth or weight concerns

NUTRITION FOR CHILDREN (6–10 YEARS) AND ADOLESCENTS (11–18 YEARS)

Physical growth rate during childhood is slow and steady. Annually, children gain an average of 7 pounds and 2.5 in in height. Body fat increases in preparation for the adolescent growth spurt.

The slow growth of childhood abruptly and dramatically increases with pubescence until the rate is nearly as rapid as that of early infancy. On average, the growth spurt and puberty begin at ages 9 to 11 for girls and 10 to 12 for boys (Hagan et al., 2017). Because peak weight occurs before peak height, many girls and parents become concerned about what appears to be excess weight.

Adolescence is a period of physical, emotional, social, and sexual maturation. Approximately 15% to 20% of adult height and 50% of adult weight are gained during adolescence. Fat distribution shifts and sexual maturation occurs. Sex differences are obvious. For instance, girls generally experience peak growth at 12 years and boys usually peak at 14 years. Stature growth ceases at a median age of approximately 21 years. Nutritional needs increase later for boys than for girls.

Physical activity encompassing a variety of age-appropriate, enjoyable activities should be a regular part of daily living for all healthy Americans. Health benefits attributed to physical activity in middle childhood and adolescence include improved bone health, weight status, cardiorespiratory and muscular fitness, cardiometabolic health, and cognition, as well as lower risk of depression (USDHHS, 2018). Key physical activity guidelines for children and adolescents are listed in Box 13.7.

Calorie Needs

Estimated daily calorie requirements for children and adolescents are included in Table 13.3. Table 13.5 lists Healthy U.S.-Style Eating Pattern recommendations for the range of calorie levels that are appropriate from childhood through adolescence. Generalizations are summarized in the following section.

BOX 13.7 Key Physical Activity Guidelines for Children and Adolescents

It is important to provide young people opportunities and encouragement to participate in physical activities that are appropriate for their age, are enjoyable, and offer variety.

Children and adolescents ages 6 to 17 years should do at least 60 minutes (1 hour) of moderate-to-vigorous physical activity daily:

Aerobic: Most of the 60 minutes or more/day should be either moderate- or vigorous-intensity aerobic physical activity and should include vigorous-intensity physical activity on at least 3 days a week.

Muscle strengthening: As part of their 60 minutes or more of daily physical activity, children and adolescents should include muscle-strengthening physical activity on at least 3 days a week.

Bone strengthening: As part of their 60 minutes or more of daily physical activity, children and adolescents should include bone-strengthening physical activity on at least 3 days a week.

Source: U.S. Department of Health and Human Services. (2018). *Physical activity guidelines for Americans* (2nd ed.). https://health.gov/sites/default/files/2019-09/Physical_Activity_Guidelines_2nd_edition.pdf

During Middle Childhood (6–10 Years of Age)

- Total calorie needs steadily increase, although calories per kilogram of body weight progressively fall.
- Sedentary boys need an average intake of 1400 to 1600 cal/day and sedentary girls need 1200 to 1400 cal/day.
- An additional 200 cal/day are recommended for children who are moderately active, and another increase of 200 cal/day may be needed for those who are active.
- These are calorie estimates, not prescriptions, and counting calories is not appropriate.
- The challenge in childhood is to meet nutrient requirements without exceeding calorie needs.

During Adolescence

- Calorie needs and appetite increase to support the rapid rate of growth, but exactly when those increases occur depends on the timing and duration of the growth spurt.
- Due to wide variations in the timing of the growth spurt among individuals, chronological age is a poor indicator of physiologic maturity and nutritional needs.
- Girls require fewer calories than boys because they have proportionally more fat tissue and less muscle mass from the effects of estrogen. Girls also experience less bone growth than boys.

Nutrient Needs

The Dietary Reference Intakes category of children is divided into two age groups: 1- to 3-year-olds and 4- to 8-year-olds. Thereafter, age groups are further divided by sex: For both girls and boys, the age groups through adolescence are 9- to 13-year-olds and 14- to 18-year-olds. Generally, nutrient needs increase with each age grouping and reach adult levels at the 14- to 18-year-old age group.

Promoting Healthy Habits

During childhood, parents continue to have the greatest influence on children's behaviors and attitudes regarding food, although outside influences such as friends and media become increasingly significant. School, friend houses, childcare centers, and social events present opportunities for children to make their own choices beyond parental supervision.

BOX 13.8 Healthy Snacks

Unsweetened whole-grain cereal with or without milk
Lean meat or cheese on whole-grain bread or crackers
Graham crackers and fig bars
Whole-grain cookies or muffins made with oatmeal, dried fruit, or iron-fortified cereal
Raw vegetables and vegetable juices
Fresh fruit or canned fruit without sugar
Low-fat yogurt with or without fresh fruit added
Nuts (when age appropriate)
Air-popped popcorn (not before age 4 years)
Peanut butter on bread, whole grain crackers, celery, and apple slices
Nonfat or 1% milk (after age 2 years)
Low-fat cheese and low-fat cottage cheese
Popcorn cakes

As adolescents become increasingly independent, more self-selected meals and snacks are purchased and eaten outside the home. The influence of peer pressure on food choices increases. A natural increase in appetite and a decrease in physical activity increase the risk of overeating.

- Parents should decide what nutritious food is served and when; children should decide how much to eat.
- Have family meals as frequently as possible. Children and adolescents who have a high frequency of eating family meals tend to have better quality eating patterns as evidenced by higher intakes of fruits, vegetables, grains, and calcium-rich foods and lower intakes of carbonated beverages (Golden et al., 2016). A higher-quality eating pattern also leads to a more appropriate intake of calories, protein, iron, folate, fiber, and vitamins A, C, D, and B_6.
- Family meals should be a pleasant social interaction experience without the distraction of electronic devices.
- Parents should continue to model healthy eating behaviors by providing and consuming nutrient-dense meals and snacks (Box 13.8).
- Encourage adolescents to make healthy food choices when eating away from home.
- Avoid or limit calorie-dense foods, such as fried foods, sugar-sweetened beverages, most fast foods, chips, and fatty meats.
- The MyPlate graphic (see Fig. 13.4) illustrates the concept of balance and proportion that is appropriate for all people over the age of 2 years.

Diet Quality during Middle Childhood and Adolescence

Analysis shows that from an early age, eating patterns are not aligned with the Dietary Guidelines (USDA & USDHHS, 2020). During 2015 to 2016, the Healthy Eating Index-2015 score for children ages 2 to 4 was 61 out of 100, indicating poor quality. Scores deteriorated throughout the childhood age groupings to a score of 51 among ages 14 to 18.

- Across the 5- to 8-year-old, 9- to 13-year-old, and 14- to 8-year-old age groupings (USDA & USDHHS, 2020)
  - consumption of total vegetables, all vegetable subgroups, fruit, dairy, whole grains, and seafood was below recommended levels of intake.
  - consumption of refined grains, added sugar, saturated fat, and sodium was above recommended levels of intake.
- For both girls and boys, average intake is inadequate in fiber, choline, vitamin C, vitamin D, vitamin E, potassium, and magnesium (U.S. Department of Agriculture [USDA] & Agricultural Research Service [ARS], 2018).
- Additionally, girls have inadequate intakes of vitamin A, calcium, and iron (USDA & ARS, 2018). Nutrients of particular concern for adolescents are highlighted in Box 13.9.

BOX 13.9 Nutrients of Particular Concern during Adolescence

Calcium

- Approximately half of adult bone mass is accrued during adolescence; optimizing calcium intake during adolescence increases bone mineralization and may decrease the risk of fracture and osteoporosis later in life.
- For boys and girls from age 9 to 18 years, the Recommended Dietary Allowance (RDA) for calcium is 1300 mg—higher than at any other time in the life cycle. The RDA drops to 1000 mg/day for young adults aged 19 to 21.
- Low intakes of calcium are related to underconsumption of dairy.
- Nondairy sources of calcium include the following:
  - Calcium-fortified orange juice, soy milk, and breakfast cereals
  - Certain greens such as bok choy, collard greens, kale, and turnip greens

Iron

- Adolescents have increased needs for iron related to an expanding blood volume, the rise in hemoglobin concentration, and the growth of muscle mass.
- In boys, peak iron requirement occurs between 14 and 18 years of age as muscle mass expands. Their RDA is 11 mg iron/day.
- The requirement for iron in adolescent girls increases to 15 mg/day at 14 to 18 years of age to account for menstrual losses.
- Girls tend to develop an iron deficiency slowly after puberty, particularly if menstrual losses are compounded by poor eating habits or chronic fad dieting.
- Heme iron, found in meats, is better absorbed than nonheme iron, which is found in plants, such as iron-fortified cereals and enriched bread.
- Nonheme iron absorption increases when a source of vitamin C, such as orange juice or tomatoes, is consumed at the same time.

Folic Acid (in young women)

- All young women capable of becoming pregnant are advised to consume 400 mcg of synthetic folic acid daily, from either supplements or fortified foods, in addition to folate naturally present in food, to reduce the risk of neural tube defects.
- Natural folate is found in certain foods, such as legumes, organ meats, and dark green leafy vegetables. It is not as well absorbed as synthetic folic acid.

NURSING PROCESS Well Child

Amanda is a 24-month-old girl who is seen regularly in the well-baby clinic for her checkups and immunizations. At this visit, you discover that her height and weight are in the 25th percentile for her age. Records indicate that previously, she had consistently ranked in the 75th percentile for weight and 50th percentile for height. The change has occurred over the last 6 months. Her mother complains that Amanda is "fussy" and has lost interest in eating.

Assessment

Medical–psychosocial history

- Medical history including prenatal, perinatal, and birth history; specifically assess for gastrointestinal (GI) problems such as slow gastric emptying, constipation, diarrhea, and allergies.
- Use of medications that can cause side effects such as delayed gastric emptying, diarrhea, constipation, or decreased appetite
- Level of development for age
- Elimination and reflux patterns, if applicable
- Caregiver's ability to understand; attitude toward health and nutrition and readiness to learn
- Psychosocial and economic issues such as the living situation, who does the shopping and cooking, adequacy of food budget, need for food assistance, and level of family and social support
- Use of vitamins, minerals, and nutritional supplements: what, how much, and why they are given

Anthropometric assessment

- Obtain height and weight to calculate BMI; determine BMI-for-age percentile.
- Head circumference for age
- Pattern of weight gain and growth

Biochemical and physical assessment

- Laboratory values, including hemoglobin and hematocrit, and the significance of any other values that are abnormal

NURSING PROCESS Well Child (continued)

Dietary Assessment

- Food records, if available
- Interview the primary caregiver to assess the following:
  - What does Amanda usually eat in a 24-hour period, including types and amounts of food, frequency and pattern of eating, and texture of foods eaten?
  - How does her intake compare to a 1000-calorie (the calorie level appropriate for 2-year-olds) MyPlate intake pattern?
  - What food groups is she consuming less than recommended amounts of?
  - Are self-feeding skills appropriate for Amanda's age?
  - Is the mealtime environment positive?
  - What is the caregiver's attitude about Amanda's current weight, recent weight loss, and eating behaviors?
  - Are the caregiver's expectations about how much Amanda should eat reasonable and appropriate? What is the problem according to the caregiver?
  - Are there cultural, religious, and ethnic influences on the family's eating habits?

Analysis

Possible Nursing Analysis

Malnutrition risk related to loss of interest in eating as evidenced by a decrease of two percentile channels in growth charts.

Planning

Client Outcomes

The client will do the following:
- Experience appropriate growth in height and weight.
- Consume, on average, an intake consistent with MyPlate recommendations for a 1000-calorie eating pattern by eating a variety of foods within each food group.
- Achieve or progress toward age-appropriate feeding skills.

Nursing Interventions

Nutrition Therapy

Promote MyPlate food plan of 1000 calories, which is appropriate for her age.

Client Teaching

Instruct the caregiver on the following:
- The role of nutrition in maintaining health and promoting adequate growth and development, including the importance of adequate calories and protein
- Eating plan essentials, including the importance of the following:
  - Choosing a varied diet to help ensure an adequate intake
  - Providing foods of appropriate texture for age
  - Providing three meals plus three or more planned snacks to maximize intake
  - Providing liquids after meals, instead of with meals, to avoid displacing food intake
  - Avoiding low-nutrient-dense foods (e.g., fruit drinks, carbonated beverages, sweetened cereals) because they displace the intake of more nutritious foods
  - The need to modify the diet, as appropriate, to improve elimination patterns

Address behavioral matters, such as the following:
- Providing a positive mealtime environment (e.g., limiting distractions, having the child well rested before mealtime)
- Not using food to punish, reward, or bribe the child
- Promoting eating behaviors and skills appropriate for the age
- Keeping accurate food records
- Modifying foods to increase their nutrient density, such as by fortifying milk with skim milk powder; using milk in place of water in recipes; melting cheese on potatoes, rice, or noodles

Evaluation

Evaluate and Monitor

- Monitor growth in height and weight.
- Evaluate food records to assess adequacy of intake according to a 1000-calorie MyPlate plan.
- Progress toward age-appropriate feeding skills.

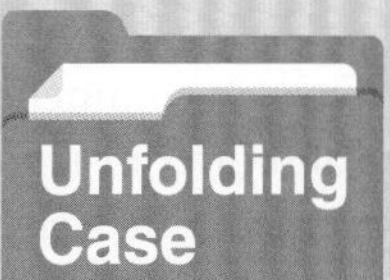

Think of Luis. His calorie intake is excessive as evidenced by his weight, and his essentially self-selected diet is of poor quality. Luis's doctor has warned his mother that his diastolic blood pressure is high and that he is overweight. His mother evades answering questions about Luis's typical eating pattern. How do you proceed with helping them achieve a healthier intake without knowing what his usual intake is?

OVERWEIGHT AND OBESITY

Maintaining healthy weight during childhood and adolescence is crucial for overall health and well-being during these periods and into adulthood. Although a variety of factors affect body weight (e.g., heredity, metabolism, health), nutrition and physical activity are the two most important behavioral determinants (Hagan et al., 2017). A healthy, nutrient-dense eating pattern and regular physical activity are vital to preventing overweight and obesity.

Weight status in children and adolescents is defined by BMI percentiles specific for age and sex (Table 13.2). Standards for defining severe obesity are included in that table. During late adolescence, adult cutoffs for overweight (BMI ≥ 25) and obesity (BMI ≥ 30) can be used when doing so would define overweight and obesity at weights lower than the 84th and 95th percentile channels, respectively. For instance, a 17-year-old girl with a BMI of 25.2 is slightly below the 85th percentile (healthy weight), yet by adult standards she is overweight (Hagan et al., 2017).

Overweight and Obesity Prevalence

The prevalence of overweight and obesity has been increasing in the United States for 4 decades (Skinner et al., 2018). Currently, 41% of children and adolescents are overweight or obese, and the prevalence is higher among Hispanic and non-Hispanic Black children and adolescents than non-Hispanic Asians and Whites (USDA & USDHHS, 2020).

Risks Associated with Obesity in Youth

Youth who are obese are at risk of becoming obese adults; the higher the degree of excess weight, the more likely obesity will persist into adulthood (Singh et al., 2008). Chronic conditions related to obesity previously seen only in adults, such as type 2 diabetes, hypertension, dyslipidemia, nonalcoholic fatty liver disease, obstructive sleep apnea, and cardiovascular disease, are now affecting an increasing number of adolescents and even children (Hagan et al., 2017). Children and adolescents with obesity are also more likely to experience psychological concerns (e.g., anxiety, depression) and social concerns (bullying, stigmatization) (USDA & USDHHS, 2020).

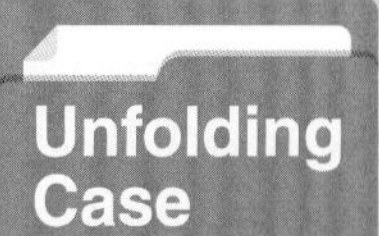

Recall Luis. At 48 in. tall and 90 pounds, his BMI is approximately 27.5. His mother is obese and claims she gained 40 pounds during pregnancy, which is excessive. Although his mom says they rarely eat red meat or fried food, she admits he eats at will, often asking for sugar-sweetened and low-fiber cereal within 15 minutes of eating dinner. His favorite dinner is breaded chicken fingers, baked french fries, and a sweetened beverage. What recommendations would you make for improving the quality of his favorite dinner? How would you advise Luis's mother to respond to his request for more food so soon after eating dinner?

Obesity Screening

The United States Preventive Services Task Force recommends that clinicians screen for obesity in children and adolescents aged 6 and older and offer or refer them to comprehensive, intensive behavioral interventions to promote improvements in weight status (U.S. Preventive Services Task Force, 2017).

- Among young children, maternal diabetes, maternal smoking, high gestational weight gain, rapid infant growth, and short sleep duration are risk factors for obesity (O'Connor et al., 2016).
- Although all children and adolescents are at risk for obesity, certain specific risk factors have been identified, namely (O'Connor et al., 2016)
  - parental obesity
  - poor diet (e.g., consumption of sugar-sweetened beverages and calorie-dense foods)
  - low levels of physical activity
  - inadequate sleep
  - sedentary behaviors, such as high amounts of screen time
  - low family income
- The racial/ethnic differences in obesity prevalence are related to differences in both non-genetic and genetic risk factors, with socioeconomic status as one of the strongest factors. Other factors may include the intake of sugar-sweetened beverages, intake of fast food, and having a television in the bedroom (O'Connor et al., 2016).

In addition to calculating and plotting BMI at least once a year, other actions are recommended to screen and assess all children for obesity prevention or early intervention with counseling.

- Assess family history (e.g., parents, siblings, grandparents) for type 2 diabetes and cardiovascular disease risk factors, such as hypertension.
- Conduct a medical history and physical examination to identify any existing obesity-related comorbidities.
- Assess dietary intake, such as the usual foods and beverages consumed and pattern of intake.
- Assess frequency, duration, and intensity of moderate and vigorous physical activity, in both structured and unstructured settings.
- Determine hours of screen time.
- Assess family attitudes about weight and physical activity.
- Assess for socioeconomic stressors.
- Assess willingness to change.

Obesity Prevention Strategies

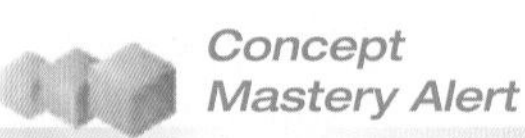
Concept Mastery Alert

Formula-fed infants consume more protein per kilogram of body weight than do breastfed infants. This may predispose the formula-fed infant to obesity later in life.

The low success in treating obesity makes prevention crucial. Early prevention strategies include (Hagan et al., 2017) the following:

- Encouraging women to attain healthy BMI before becoming pregnant and gaining the recommended amount of weight during pregnancy
- Smoking cessation prior to pregnancy
- Exclusive breastfeeding for the first 6 months of life
- Continuation of breastfeeding is at least until the age of 1 in combination with complementary foods

Prevention strategies for toddlers include the following:

- A transition to nutrient-dense foods with weaning
- Eliminating sedentary entertainment
- Active play for physical activity
- Parental role modeling of healthy eating and physical activity behaviors

Obesity prevention strategies for children and adolescents with a healthy BMI include permanent lifestyle modifications (Box 13.10) aimed at the following:

- Consuming a nutrient-dense healthy eating pattern
- Decreasing sedentary behaviors
- Increasing physical activity
- Obtaining adequate sleep

Treatment Strategies for Obesity in Youth

The goals of obesity treatment are to improve long-term physical and psychosocial health by establishing permanent healthy lifestyle behaviors and changes to the environment where the child or adolescent lives (Hagan et al., 2017). Stages of obesity treatment are outlined in Box 13.11.

BOX 13.10 Lifestyle Modification Obesity Prevention Strategies

Healthier Nutrition

Healthy Eating Behaviors

- Eat family meals as often as possible with parents role modeling healthy eating.
- Eat more home-prepared meals.
- Use other things instead of food or screen time as rewards.
- Limit eating out.
- Eat breakfast daily.
- Keep healthy foods and beverages available and in plain sight, such as water pitchers, fruits, vegetables, and other low-calorie snacks.
- Decrease the size of serving spoons, plates, bowls, and glasses.
- Limit before bed snacks.

Healthy Choices

- Promote a healthy eating pattern that emphasizes nutrient-dense foods such as fruits, vegetables, whole grains, low-fat or nonfat dairy, lean meats, legumes, and seafood.
- Limit sugar-sweetened beverages and those containing artificial sweeteners.
- Limit foods containing refined carbohydrates.
- Limit calorie-dense foods, such as fried foods, baked goods, and pizza.
- If high-calorie snacks and sweets are purchased for a special occasion, buy them immediately before the event and remove them immediately afterward.

Reduce Sedentary Behaviors

- Avoid screen time in infants and toddlers younger than 18 months of age.
- Limit screen time in children 18 months to 4 years to no more than 1 hour/day (American Academy of Pediatrics Council on Communications and Media, 2016).
- Limit total entertainment screen time to less than 2 hours/day for older children and adolescents (Golden et al., 2016).
- Do not allow a television in bedrooms.
- Turn off the TV and other screens during mealtimes.

Increase Physical Activity

Meet national physical activity guideline of at least 60 minutes of physical activity each day with most of it in moderate-to-vigorous aerobic activity (see Box 13.8).

Adequate Sleep

Counsel parents on age-appropriate sleep durations based on age.

Source: Daniels, S. R., Hassink, S. G., & Committee on Nutrition. (2015). The role of the pediatrician in primary prevention of obesity. *Pediatrics, 136*(1), e275–e292. https://doi.org/10.1542/peds.2015-1558; Golden, N. H., Schneider, M., Wood, C., & Committee on Nutrition, Committee on Adolescence and Section on Obesity. (2016). Preventing obesity and eating disorders in adolescents. *Pediatrics*, *138*(3), e20161649. https://doi.org/10.1542/peds.2016-1649

BOX 13.11 Staged Approach for Obesity Treatment in Childhood and Adolescence

Stage 1: Prevention Plus

- For youth with overweight or obesity.
- Existing healthy eating behaviors are continued and reinforced.
- Lifestyle modifications focus on basic specific goals, such as at least 5 fruits and vegetables a day, less than 1 hour of screen time/day, at least 1 hours of moderate-to-vigorous physical activity/day, elimination of sugar-sweetened beverages, practicing healthy eating behaviors (e.g., 3 daily meals, family meals).
- Goal is to improve BMI status.
- Office-based visits.
- Brief motivational interviewing on selected behaviors (e.g., more fruits and vegetables) to motivate the youth and family.
- Advance to Stage 2 if lack of improvement after 3 to 6 months.

Stage 2: Structured Weight Management

- Continued focus on lifestyle modifications.
- Monthly office-based visits with youth and family (e.g., physician, nurse, or dietitian).
- More structured timing and content of daily meals and snacks for the whole family.
- Reduce nonacademic screen time to less than 1 hour/day.
- Increase amount of moderate and vigorous physical activity.
- Self-monitoring, such as logging screen time, physical activity, and intake.
- Progress to Stage 3 if no improvement in BMI (e.g., maintenance or decrease) after 3 to 6 months.

Stage 3: Comprehensive Multidisciplinary Intervention

- A dedicated pediatric multidisciplinary structured behavioral program that includes more structured physical activity, diet, and behavior modification.
- Use dedicated pediatric weight management program with weekly visits for 8 to 12 weeks followed by monthly follow-up.
- Strong family involvement is encouraged especially for children less than 12 years.
- Only advance to Stage 4 after considering patient's maturity and ability to understand risks and willingness to maintain physical activity and appropriate diet and behavioral monitoring.

Stage 4: Tertiary Care Intervention

- Intended for overweight or obese youth with comorbidities or for severely obese youth.
- Comprehensive multidisciplinary program is conducted under medical supervision at a pediatric weight-management center with a focus on resolving or improving comorbidities.
- Treatments options may include very-low-calorie diets (less than 1000 cal/day) or meal replacements, pharmacologic treatment, or bariatric surgery.

Source: Barlow, S. E., & the Expert Committee. (2007). Expert committee recommendations regarding the prevention, assessment, and treatment of child and adolescent overweight and obesity: Summary report. *Pediatrics*, *120*(Suppl 4), S164–S192. https://doi.org/10.1542/peds.2007-2329C; Hagan, J. F., Shaw, J. S., & Duncan, P. M. (Eds.). (2017). *Bright futures: Guidelines for health supervision of infants, children, and adolescents*. American Academy of Pediatrics.

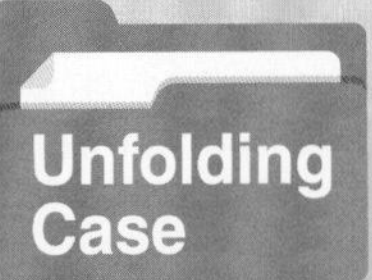

Consider Luis. He and his mother enroll in a 12-week-long weight management program at their community center. The program began by stressing healthy behaviors, including types of food to eat. What eating strategies would you encourage them to adopt? What recommendations would you make about exercise, physical activity, and sedentary activity?

The Parent's Role

Parental role modeling of a healthy lifestyle is vital to initiating and sustaining changes in eating and physical activity behaviors.

- Parents often recognize that they need to set an example for their children but lack the time to do so.
- Parents who are overweight may feel they cannot set a good example because they do not practice what they preach.
- Other barriers to parents taking action are (1) a belief that children will outgrow their excess weight, (2) a lack of knowledge about how to help children control their weight, and (3) a fear they will cause eating disorders in their children.
- Parents should be encouraged to not talk about weight but rather about healthy eating and healthy physical activity (Golden et al., 2016).

Family involvement in the treatment of obesity has been shown to be more effective than an adolescent-only approach (Golden et al., 2016).

Motivational Interviewing a goal-oriented, client-centered counseling style that facilitates and engages intrinsic motivation to change behavior.

- Family-centered **motivational interviewing** can be effective technique to promote healthy behaviors by inspiring parents to serve as role models by serving healthy meals, eating with their children, avoiding talk about weight, engaging in regular physical activity, and limiting their own sedentary behaviors.
- Even in adolescence, parents are still the primary role models for eating and physical activity behaviors and have a direct impact on the adolescent's food and activity environment (Daniels & Hassink, 2015).
- Parents and other family members should be encouraged to implement the same changes as the child.
- Dieting is a risk factor for both obesity and eating disorders, so emphasis should be on healthy lifestyle, not restrictive eating.

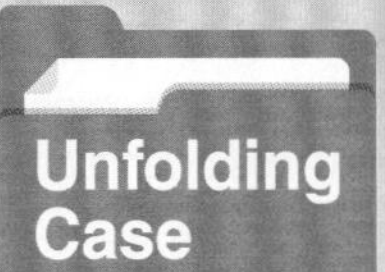

Recall Luis. He has not lost weight but has grown taller, so there has been some improvement in his BMI. His mom continues counseling to improve her parenting skills, which she now admits influenced her son's overeating. She has had a hard time eating vegetables herself and tends to graze, although they are eating family dinners almost every day. How would you respond to her question of how long this "diet thing" needs to continue?

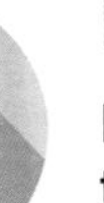

How Do You Respond?

Does early introduction of solid foods help infants sleep through the night? A frequently given reason for introducing solids before 4 months of age is the unsupported belief that it will help infants to sleep through the night. A major objection to the early introduction of solids is that it may interfere with establishing sound eating habits and may contribute to overfeeding because infants less than 4 months old are unable to communicate satiety by turning away and leaning back.

Does diet contribute to acne prevalence? Although the pathogenesis of acne is complex and not completely understood, several dietary components are being investigated. In a study based on self-reported acne among young adults, participants with moderate-to-severe acne reported a higher dietary glycemic index and higher intakes of total sugar, added sugar, fruit/fruit juice, number of milk servings/day, saturated fat, and trans fats than participants with no or mild acne (Burris et al., 2014). Studies have found an association between vitamin D deficiency and acne and that vitamin D supplementation reduces acne inflammation (Stewart & Bazergy, 2018). Studies on the association between increased BMI and acne are mixed (DiLandro et al., 2012; Halvorsen et al., 2012; Stewart & Bazergy, 2018). Further research is needed to clarify the link between diet and acne and determine if nutrition therapy can play a role in acne treatment.

REVIEW CASE STUDY

Andrew is 16 years old and sedentary. He is 5 ft 8 in. tall, weighs 218 pounds, and has a BMI of 33. He has been overweight for most of his life, as is most of his extended paternal family. His mother has tried "everything" over the years to get him to lose weight, from putting him on her own weight loss diet to hiding foods he shouldn't have, such as soft drinks and chips, to limit his access. He has a part-time job in a fast-food restaurant and is able to leave the school property at lunchtime to have lunch where he works. He is not good at sports but loves to play video games and watch movies. He hates that he's so big but feels hopeless about changing. His normal day's intake is shown on the right:

- Using the BMI-for-age percentile for boys, what is Andrew's weight status? Is it an appropriate approach to limit Andrew's calories to outgrow his current weight status?
- How many calories should Andrew consume daily? Based on the MyPlate intake levels, which food groups is he consuming the appropriate amounts of? Which groups is he overeating? Which groups is he not eating enough of? What are the sources of empty calories in his diet?
- What specific goals would you encourage Andrew to set regarding his intake, activity, and weight?
- What would you suggest his mother do to support better eating habits and a healthier weight?

Breakfast: Two doughnuts and a large glass of apple juice
Lunch: A double cheeseburger, large fries, and a large shake
Snacks: Frozen mini pizzas, a large soft drink, and a handful of cookies
Dinner: The same as lunch on nights he works; if he's home, he eats whatever is available, often pizza or sandwiches and chips, ice cream, and a soft drink
Snacks: Chips and salsa and a soft drink

STUDY QUESTIONS

1 Which statement indicates the mother understands the nurse's instructions about breastfeeding?
  a. "Breastfeeding should only last 5 minutes on each breast."
  b. "Sometimes, babies cry just because they are thirsty, so a bottle of water should be offered before breastfeeding begins to see if the infant is just thirsty."
  c. "The longer the baby sucks, the less milk I will have for the next feeding."
  d. "The first breast offered should be alternated with each feeding."

2 A mother asks why toddlers shouldn't drink all the milk they want. Which of the following is the nurse's best response?
  a. "Consuming more than the recommended amount of milk can displace the intake of iron-rich foods from the diet and increase the toddler's risk of iron deficiency anemia."
  b. "Consuming more than the recommended amount of milk increases the risk of milk allergy."
  c. "Too much milk can lead to overhydration."
  d. "Consuming more than the recommended amount of milk will provide too much calcium."

3 The nurse knows her instructions about introducing solids into the infant's diet have been effective when the mother states,
  a. "Babies should be introduced to solid foods at 1 to 3 months of age."
  b. "New foods should be given for at least 3 days so that allergic responses can be easily identified."
  c. "Infants are more likely to accept infant cereal for the first time if it is mixed with breast milk or formula and given from a bottle."
  d. "The appropriate initial serving size for solids is 1 to 2 tbsp."

4 Which of the following would be the best snack for a 2-year-old?
  a. Popcorn
  b. Banana slices
  c. Fresh cherries
  d. Raw celery

5 Which foods are youth ages 5 to 18 most likely to eat in inadequate amounts? Select all that apply.
  a. Whole grains
  b. Vegetables
  c. Fruits
  d. Meat

6 The client asks if her 10-year-old daughter needs a weight loss diet. Which of the following would be the nurse's best response?
  a. "Rather than a diet at this age, you should just forbid her to eat sweets and empty calories."
  b. "Because prevention of overweight is more effective than treatment, you should start to limit her calorie intake by only serving low-fat and artificially sweetened foods."
  c. "Ten-year-old girls are about to enter the growth spurt of puberty, and it is natural for her to gain weight before she grows taller. Diets are not recommended for children, although healthy eating and moderation are always appropriate."
  d. "She needs extra calories for the upcoming growth spurt, so you should be encouraging her to eat more than she normally does."

7 Calorie requirements during adolescence
  a. are higher than during adulthood because of growth and developmental changes.
  b. peak early (e.g., ages 12 and 13) and then fall until adulthood is reached.
  c. are lower than during childhood.
  d. do not change from middle childhood.

8 Which is a nutrient of concern particularly for adolescent girls?
  a. Vitamin A
  b. Protein
  c. Zinc
  d. Folic acid

CHAPTER SUMMARY NUTRITION FOR INFANTS, CHILDREN, AND ADOLESCENTS

The goals of nutrition and physical activity for children are to promote optimal physical and cognitive development, a healthy weight, an enjoyment of food, and a decreased risk of chronic disease. Nutritional requirements are less precise for youth than they are for adults due to variations in growth and activity.

Infancy: Birth to 1 year

Excluding fetal growth, growth in the first year of life is more rapid than at any other time in the life cycle.

- **Nutrient needs:** Proportionately infants require more calories and nutrients than adults. Adequate growth means the infant is consuming adequate nutrition.
- **Breast feeding:** Exclusive breastfeeding is recommended for the first 6 months and should continue through the first year or longer if desired.
- **Infant formula:** Most are made from cow milk to resemble breast milk.
- **Complementary foods:** Complementary foods are added when the infant is developmentally ready, usually around 6 months of age.
  - Foods that provide iron should be added first, such as iron-fortified infant cereals or pureed meats.
  - New foods are added one at a time for about 3 days so that any allergic reaction can be identified.
  - There is no evidence that delaying the introduction of allergenic foods such as peanuts, eggs, and fish beyond 6 months of age prevents allergies.
  - By 12 months of age, infants should be eating a variety of table foods and various textures.

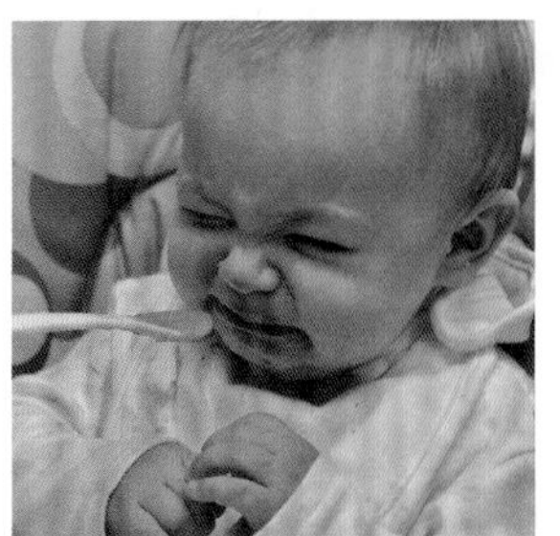

Nutrition during Early Childhood

Adequate nutrition during early childhood focuses on promoting normal growth through the appropriate amount and types of foods within an environment that allows the child to self-regulate.

- **Parental influence:** Parents are the primary gatekeepers of their children's nutritional intake. They should make healthy foods available and not introduce foods into their children's diet that have no value other than calories.
- **Developmental milestones:** The dramatic decrease in growth rate that occurs after the first year of life causes a decrease in appetite and unpredictable food intake. Picky eating is normal. Adult role modeling is important.
- **Calorie and nutrient needs:** Daily calorie need for ages 12 to 23 months range from 800 to 1000. From 2 to 5 years of age, total daily calories range from 1000 to 1600 depending on activity.
- **Feeding guidelines:** Calorie-appropriate, nutrient-dense eating patterns are recommended across the life span.
  - Beverages used at 12 months are whole milk and water. Sweet and caffeinated beverages should not be offered.
  - A variety of nutrient-dense foods should be consumed in 3 meals and 2 to 3 nutrient-dense snacks/day.
  - Healthy child-feeding practices are critical for helping children develop healthy eating habits later in life.

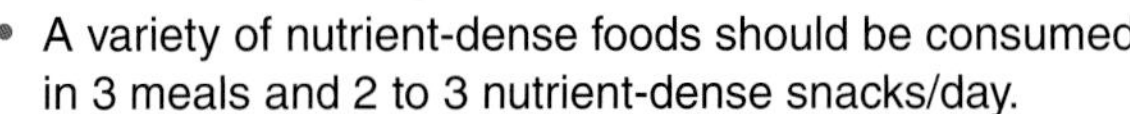

Nutrition for Children (6–10 years) and Adolescents (11–18 years)

Childhood growth rate is slow and steady. It abruptly and dramatically increases with pubescence until the rate is nearly as rapid as that of early infancy.

- **Calorie needs:** They increase during adolescence to support the rapid rate of growth. Timing and duration of the growth spurt vary among individuals.
- **Nutrient needs:** They reach adult levels at the 14- to 18-year-old age group.
- **Promoting healthy habits:** Parental influence on eating behaviors is still important but waning. Eating family dinners is strongly encouraged.

(continued)

CHAPTER SUMMARY NUTRITION FOR INFANTS, CHILDREN, AND ADOLESCENTS (continued)

- **Diet quality:** The unhealthy eating pattern of youth causes diet quality to be low. Youth underconsume fruit, vegetables, whole grains, seafood, and dairy, resulting in inadequate intakes of fiber, vitamin C, vitamin D, vitamin E, potassium, and magnesium. Additional nutrients of concern for adolescent girls are calcium, iron, and folic acid. Youth overconsume refined grains, saturated fat, added sugars, and sodium.

Overweight and Obesity

Maintaining healthy weight during childhood and adolescence is crucial for overall health and well-being during these periods and into adulthood:

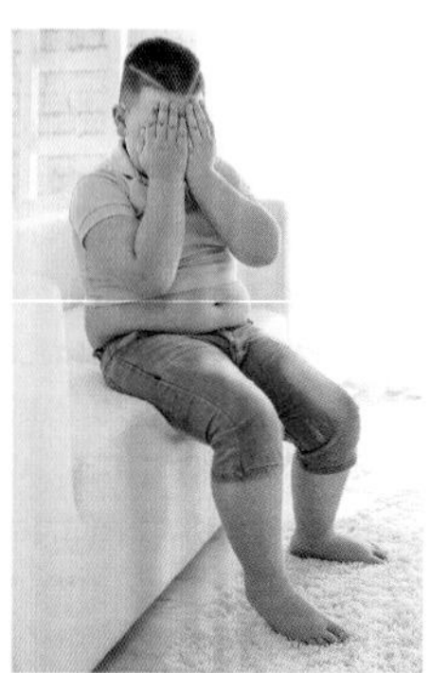

- Prevalence of overweight and obesity has been increasing for 4 decades.
- Chronic conditions related to obesity previously seen only in adults are now affecting an increasingly number of adolescents and even children. Obesity also impairs quality of life.
- All youth should be screened for obesity beginning at age 6 using BMI for age percentiles.
- The low success in treating obesity makes prevention crucial. Early prevention strategies include preventing excessive weight gain during pregnancy, exclusive breastfeeding for the first 6 months of life, allowing children to self-regulate how much they consume, and parental role modeling of healthy eating and physical activity.
- Primary prevention in youth who have a healthy weight focuses on maintaining weight to prevent overweight and obesity. A healthy eating pattern, limiting screen time, promoting adequate physical activity, and ensuring adequate sleep are stressed.
- Treatment strategies for overweight and obese youth are staged and range from a more structured lifestyle approach to intense intervention that may include a very low-calorie diet, pharmacologic treatment, or bariatric surgery.
- Family involvement in treatment of obesity may be more effective than an adolescent-only approach.

Figure sources: *shutterstock.com/Marcel Jancovic, shutterstock.com/Monkey Business Images, and shutterstock.com/Nina Buday*

Student Resources on thePoint®
For additional learning materials, activate the code in the front of this book at https://thePoint.lww.com/activate

Websites

Academy of Nutrition and Dietetics: Kids Eat Right provides science-based resources for families at www.eatright.org/kids

American Academy of Pediatrics Bright Futures, Promoting Healthy Nutrition at https://brightfutures.aap.org/Bright%20Futures%20Documents/BF4_HealthyNutrition.pdf

American Academy of Pediatrics Institute for Healthy Childhood Weight at https://ihcw.aap.org provides obesity prevention and management and treatment resources

Children's Nutrition Research Center at Baylor College of Medicine at www.bcm.edu/cnrc/

Dietary Guidelines for Americans, 2020–2025 at https://dietaryguidelines.gov

Ellyn Satter Institute for information on ways to make feeding a positive and joyful experience at https://www.ellynsatterinstitute.org/

Healthychildren.org for dietary recommendations, parenting skills advice, etc. at https://www.healthychildren.org

KidsHealth at www.kidshealth.org

Let's Move provides links to many government and private efforts to raise a healthier generation of children at www.letsmove.gov

MyPlate Kid's Place provides a variety of activities and resources at www.myplate.gov/kids

National Institutes of Health, National Heart, Lung, and Blood Institute: We Can! contains dietary recommendations, physical activity recommendations, and monitoring tools at http://www.nhlbi.nih.gov/health/educational/wecan/

Nutri-eSTEP nutrition screen designed to screen toddlers 18 to 35 months and preschoolers 3 to 5 years at www.nutritionscreen.ca

References

Abrams, S. (2015). Is it time to put a moratorium on new infant formulas that are not adequately investigated? *The Journal of Pediatrics, 166*, 756–760. https://doi.org/10.1016/j.jpeds.2014.11.003

American Academy of Pediatrics. (2020, September 16). *Choosing an infant formula.* The AAP Parenting Website. https://www.healthychildren.org/English/ages-stages/baby/formula-feeding/Pages/Choosing-an-Infant-Formula.aspx

American Academy of Pediatrics Council on Communications and Media. (2016). Media and young minds. *Pediatrics, 138*(5), e20162591. https://doi.org/10.1542/peds.2016-2591

Burris, J., Rietkerk, W., & Woolf, K. (2014). Relationships of self-reported dietary factors and perceived acne severity in a cohort of New York young adults. *Journal of the Academy of Nutrition and Dietetics, 114*, 384–392. https://doi.org/10.1016/j.jand.2013.11.010

Centers for Disease Control and Prevention. (2010). Growth charts. National Center for Health Statistics. https://www.cdc.gov/growthcharts/

Daniels, S. R., & Hassink, S. G. (2015). The role of the pediatrician in primary prevention of obesity. *Pediatrics, 136*(1), e275–e292. https://doi.org/10.1542/peds.2015-1558

DiLandro, A., Cazzaniga, S., Parazzini. F., Ingordo, V., Cusano, F., Atzori, L., Cutri, F., Musumeci, M., Zinetti, C., Pezzarossa, E., Bettoli, V., Caproni, M., Lo Scocco, G., Bonci, A., Bencini, P., Naldi, L., & GISED Acne Study Group. (2012). Family history, body mass index, selected dietary factors, menstrual history, and risk of moderate to severe acne in adolescents and young adults. *Journal of the American Academy of Dermatology, 67*(6), 1129–1135. https://doi.org/10.1016/j.jaad.2012.02.018

Federal Interagency Forum on Child and Family Statistics. (2019). *America's children: Key national indicators of well-being, 2019.* U.S. Government Printing Office.

Golden, N., Schneider, M., Wood, C., & AAP Committee on Nutrition. (2016). Preventing obesity and eating disorders in adolescents. *Pediatrics, 138*(3), e20161649. https://doi.org/10.1542/peds.2016-1649

Greer, F. R., Sicherer, S. H., Burks, A. W., AAP Committee on Nutrition, & AAP Section on Allergy and Immunology. (2019). The effects of early nutritional interventions on the development of atopic disease in infants and children: The role of maternal dietary restriction, breastfeeding, hydrolyzed formulas, and timing of introduction of allergenic complementary foods. *Pediatrics, 143*(4), e20190281. https://doi.org/10.1542/peds.2019-0281

Hagan, J. F., Shaw, J. S., & Duncan, P. M. (Eds.). (2017). *Bright futures: Guidelines for health supervision of infants, children, and adolescents.* American Academy of Pediatrics.

Halvorsen, J., Vleugels, R., Bjertness, E., & Lien, L. (2012). A population-based study of acne and body mass index in adolescents. *Archives of Dermatology, 148*(1), 131–132. https://doi.org/10.1001/archderm.148.1.131

Muth, N. (2019, September 19). *Recommended drinks for young children ages 0–5.* The American Academy of Pediatrics AP Parenting Website. https://www.healthychildren.org/English/healthy-living/nutrition/Pages/Recommended-Drinks-for-Young-Children-Ages-0-5.aspx

O'Connor, E. A., Evans, C. V., Burda, B. U., Walsh, E. S., Eder, M., & Lozano, P. (2016). Screening for obesity and intervention for weight management in children and adolescents: A systematic evidence review for the U.S. Preventive Services Task Force. Evidence Synthesis No. 150. Agency for Healthcare Research and Quality AHRQ Publication No. 15-05219-EF-1.

Ogata, B., & Hayes, D. (2014). Position of the Academy of Nutrition and Dietetics: Nutrition guidance for healthy children ages 2 to 11 years. *Journal of the Academy of Nutrition and Dietetics, 114*(8), 1257–1276. https://doi.org/10.1016/j.jand.2014.06.001

Provincial Health Services Authority. (2016, November). *Pediatric Nutrition Guidelines (Six Months to Six Years).* https://www.health.gov.bc.ca/library/publications/year/2017/pediatric-nutrition-guidelines.pdf

Rossen, L. M., Simon, A. E., & Herrick, K. A. (2016). Types of infant formulas consumed in the United States. *Clinical Pediatrics, 55*(3), 278–285. https://doi.org/10.1177/0009922815591881

Satter, E. (2016). Ellyn Satter's division of responsibility in feeding. The Ellen Satter Institute. https://www.ellynsatterinstitute.org/wp-content/uploads/2016/11/handout-dor-tasks-cap-2016.pdf

Singh, A., Mulder, C., Twisk, J., van Mechelen, W., & Chinapaw, J. (2008). Tracking of childhood overweight into adulthood: A systematic review of the literature. *Obesity Reviews, 9*(5), 474–488. https://doi.org/10.1111/j.1467-789X.2008.00475.x

Skinner, A. C., Ravanbakht, S. N., Skelton, J. A., Perrin, E. M., & Armstrong, S. C. (2018). Prevalence of obesity and severe obesity in U.S. children, 1999–2016. *Pediatrics, 141*(3), e20173459. https://doi.org/10.1542/peds.2017-3459

Stewart, T., & Bazergy, C. (2018). Hormonal and dietary factors in acne vulgaris versus controls. *Dermato-Endocrinology, 10*(1), e1442160. https://doi.org/10.1080/19381980.2018.1442160

U.S. Department of Agriculture & Agricultural Research Service. (2018). Nutrient intakes from food and beverages: Mean amounts consumed per individual, by gender and age. What We Eat in America, NHANES 2015–2016. www.ars.usda.gov/nea/bhnrc/fsrg

U.S. Department of Agriculture & U.S. Department of Health and Human Services. (2020, December). *Dietary Guidelines for Americans, 2020–2025.* https://dietaryguidelines.gov

U.S. Department of Health and Human Services. (2018). *Physical activity guidelines for Americans* (2nd ed.). https://health.gov/sites/default/files/2019-09/Physical_Activity_Guidelines_2nd_edition.pdf

U.S. Preventive Services Task Force. (2017). Screening for obesity in children and Adolescents. U.S. Preventive Services Task Force Recommendation Statement. *Journal of the American Medical Association, 317*(23), 2417–2426. https://doi.org/10.1001/jama.2017.6803

Chapter 14

Nutrition for Older Adults

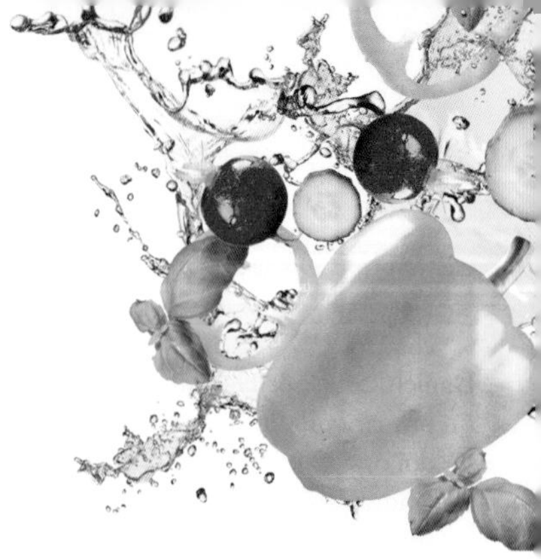

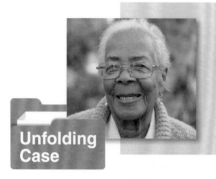

Unfolding Case

Clara Wellington

Clara, 74 years old, lives alone in her own home. She is relatively healthy and has a home health aide come 2 hours per week to help her with light housekeeping. Her only medication is an occasional antacid for gastroesophageal reflux disease. She is 5 ft 5 in., and for all of her adult life, she has weighed 135 pounds. At her most recent doctor visit, she was down 7 pounds from the previous visit 6 months ago.

Learning Objectives

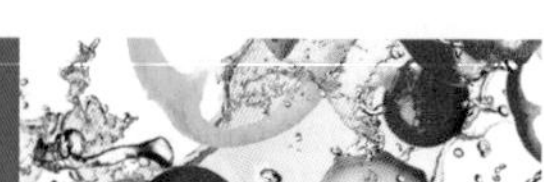

Upon completion of this chapter, you will be able to:

1 Give examples of physiologic changes that occur with aging and that have an impact on nutrition.
2 Discuss why older adults may need more protein than younger adults.
3 Explain why older adults may need supplements of calcium, vitamin D, and vitamin B_{12}.
4 Describe the characteristics of the Mediterranean diet and why it may promote healthy aging.
5 Describe the characteristics of the MIND diet and how it differs from the MedDiet.
6 Discuss criteria that may be used to screen for malnutrition in older adults.
7 Debate the benefits of using a liberal diet in long-term care facilities.
8 Propose strategies for enhancing food intake in long-term care residents.
9 Explain the effects Alzheimer's disease may have on nutritional status.

Approximately 1 out of 7 Americans, or 15.2% of the population, is 65 years or older (U.S. Department of Health and Human Services [USDHHS] & Administration on Aging [AOA], 2018). The older population is not only increasing, it is also getting increasingly older. In 2016, nearly 82,000 adults were over the age of 100 years (USDHHS & AOA, 2018). Despite the misconceptions and stereotypes people have of older adults, they are a heterogeneous group that varies in age, marital status, social background, financial status, health status, and living arrangements.

With the exception of Chapter 12 (pregnancy and lactation) and Chapter 13 (infants, children, and adolescents), this book implicitly addresses nutrition as it pertains to adults. Yet adulthood represents a wide age range, from young adults at 18 years to the "oldest old." Adults over 50 years, and especially those over 70 years, have different nutritional needs and concerns than do younger adults. This chapter focuses on how aging affects nutrition for older adults.

AGING AND OLDER ADULTS

Aging is a gradual, inevitable, complex process of progressive physiologic, cellular, cultural, and psychosocial changes that begin at conception and end at death. As cells age, they undergo degenerative changes in structure and function that eventually lead to impairment of organs, tissues, and body functioning. Table 14.1 outlines changes related to aging and their association with nutrition.

Table 14.1 Changes Related to Aging and Their Nutritional Implications

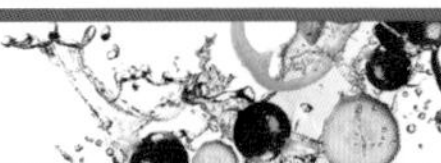

Changes Related to Aging	Association with Nutrition
Changes in physiology and function	
Loss of bone density.	Increases risk of osteoporosis; increased need for calcium.
Loss of muscle mass, strength, and physical function; increased risk of sarcopenia.	Loss of muscle mass and strength becomes evident in the early 60s; 20%–40% of muscle strength may be lost by age 70. Lowers body mass index (BMI) and calorie requirements, making it more difficult to meet micronutrient requirements. Sarcopenia and frailty increase risk of malnutrition.
Increase in body fat related to decreased physical activity.	Lowered need for calories.
Changes in body fat distribution related to hormonal changes.	Increased deposition of abdominal fat increases the risk of metabolic syndrome, which increases the risk of heart disease and diabetes.
Digestive system changes	
Difficulty chewing related to loss of teeth and periodontal disease. Jaw bone deterioration may be related to osteoporosis	If intake is limited to soft, easy-to-chew foods, some essential nutrients may be deficient. Meat intake is most commonly affected when chewing is impaired.
Decrease in gastric acid secretion	Less gastric acid can impair iron and vitamin B_{12} absorption.
Decreases in digestive enzyme secretion, GI motility, and organ function	Increased risk of digestive disorders including constipation
Appetite and thirst dysregulation occurs	Decreased awareness of hunger; decreased sense of thirst increases risk of dehydration.
Delayed gastric emptying	Feeling of fullness persists longer after eating, slowing the return of hunger.
Changes in the nervous system and cognition	
Increased risk of cognitive decline	Independence and quality of life are affected. Decreased ability to prepare food, forgetting to eat, and inability to access food are the earliest signs of mild cognitive impairment or pre-Alzheimer's disease.
Changes in immune system functioning	
Immune response dysfunction with increased susceptibility to infection and chronic inflammation	Infections increase metabolism, calorie needs, and nutrient requirements; malnutrition can occur, which further impairs immune function.
Changes in kidney function	
Decreased kidney function related to decrease in kidney mass, blood flow, and glomerular filtration rate	Impaired kidney function may alter vitamin D metabolism, lower vitamin D levels, and contribute to osteoporosis.
Sensory changes	
Increased risk of nutrition deficiencies because:	
Hearing loss	Impaired socialization can impair appetite and intake in older adults.
Vision loss	Food purchasing, preparation, and eating are more difficult.
Diminished senses of taste and smell	Eating becomes less appealing.
Changes in income	
Fixed income related to retirement	Food budget may decrease.
Changes in health	
Older adults have a high prevalence of cardiovascular disease, type 2 diabetes, hypertension, bone and joint problems, and neurodegenerative conditions, which increase the risk of fragility and disability	Nutrient requirements, intake, digestion, metabolism, or excretion may be altered, increasing the risk of malnutrition. Disability conditions may impair food purchasing, preparation, or eating.
Reliance on medication	Medications may affect appetite, ability to smell or taste, or the digestion, absorption, metabolism, and excretion of nutrients.
Alcohol abuse; alcohol may be used to relieve boredom, loneliness, depression, or pain.	Alcohol abuse can cause impairments in nutrient intake, absorption, metabolism, and excretion.
Psychosocial changes	
Social isolation related to death of a spouse, death of friends, living alone, impaired mobility	Loneliness can lead to disinterest in living and eating and may lead to malnutrition.
Poor self-esteem related to change in body image, lack of purpose, feelings of aimlessness.	May lead to poor intake.
Move to a health care facility	Health care facility residents are at increased risk of malnutrition.

Source: Amarya, S., Singh, K., & Sabharwal, M. (2015). Changes during aging and their association with malnutrition. *Journal of Clinical Gerontology and Geriatrics*, *6*(3), 78–84. https://doi.org/10.1016/j.jcgg.2015.05.003

NUTRITIONAL NEEDS OF OLDER ADULTS

Age-related changes in metabolism, body composition, and nutrient absorption are among the factors that alter calorie needs and nutrient requirements among older adults. Dietary Reference Intake (DRI) references separate older adulthood into two categories: ages 51 to 70 years and older than 70. Generally, most DRIs remain constant throughout adulthood. However, because health status, physiologic functioning, physical activity, and nutritional status may vary more among older adults (especially those older than 70) than among individuals in any other age group, recommendations may not be appropriate for all older individuals at all times.

Calories

Estimated calorie needs per day decrease with age (Fig. 14.1). The decrease results from a decrease in energy spent on all three components of energy expenditure, namely, basal metabolic rate (BMR), physical activity, and the thermic effect of processing food (Institute of Medicine, 2005).

Lean Body Mass
all body components except stored fat; the fat-free mass of the body.

- BMR represents the largest component of total energy expenditure and is closely correlated to the amount of **lean body mass.** The progressive loss of muscle mass that occurs with aging lowers BMR.
- Calories spent on physical activity may decrease due to changes in health or functional limitations. Individual variations exist.
- Although calorie needs decrease in older adults, most nutrient requirements do not change, making the concept of nutrient density even more important.

Protein

For more than 70 years, the Recommended Dietary Allowance (RDA) for protein has been set at 0.8 g/kg/day for healthy adults aged 19 years and older (Institute of Medicine, 2005). This level of intake is an estimate of the minimum amount of protein that must be consumed to avoid loss of body nitrogen. However, the data were gathered almost entirely in college-aged men, which are likely not applicable to older adults (Traylor et al., 2018). Furthermore, critics cite numerous shortcomings in nitrogen balance techniques to estimate protein need, such as the difficulty in accurately measuring all sources of nitrogen excretion (Wolfe et al., 2017). It is recommended that nitrogen balance no longer be used as the gold standard for assessing adequacy of protein intake (Institute of Medicine, 2005).

A body of data from studies using isotope tracers supports recommending protein intakes greater than the RDA for older people (Traylor et al., 2018).

- Observational studies also show that higher protein intakes are associated with greater muscle mass and better muscle function with aging (Houston et al., 2008; Isanejad et al., 2016).
- One reason why older adults need more protein than younger adults is that they have a declining anabolic response to protein intake; that is, their threshold for the amount of protein needed to stimulate protein synthesis is higher.

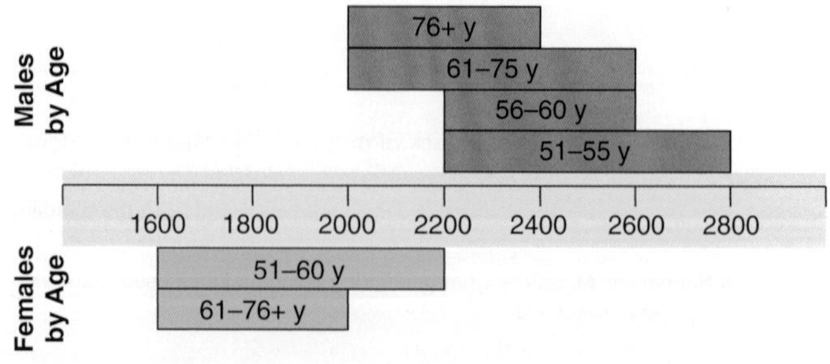

FIGURE 14.1 ▶ Estimated calorie needs per day for men and women ages 51 to 76 years and older.

- Protein need may also be higher due to inflammatory and catabolic effects of chronic and acute diseases that commonly occur with aging.
- In addition to the total amount of protein consumed per day, other aspects of protein intake may also affect muscle mass and strength during aging, such as the distribution over the day, the amount per meal, and protein quality.

The PROT-AGE Study Group, composed of an international panel of experts, developed evidence-based recommendations for optimal protein intake for older adults (Bauer et al., 2013). They recommend the following:

- A higher protein intake is needed than the current RDA and higher amounts are needed when health is compromised:
  - healthy older adults: 1.0 to 1.2 g/kg protein/day
  - older adults with an acute or chronic disease: 1.2 to 1.5 g/kg/day
  - older adults with severe illness or injury or with marked malnutrition: as much as 2.0 g/kg/day
- Protein should be evenly distributed throughout the day (e.g., 25–30 g protein per meal, the equivalent of 3–4 oz of protein foods), to maximally stimulate muscle protein synthesis.
- At least 2.5 g of leucine per meal is recommended for healthy older adults. Leucine is an essential amino acid that plays a key role in stimulating skeletal muscle synthesis. The best sources of leucine are eggs, dairy, meat, poultry, and fish.
- Protein quality may also be an important factor in the maintenance of muscle mass. Current evidence suggests that plant proteins (e.g., in soy and wheat) result in lower muscle protein synthesis than animal proteins, possibly because of the relative lack of leucine in plants compared to animal-based proteins (Gingrich et al., 2019).

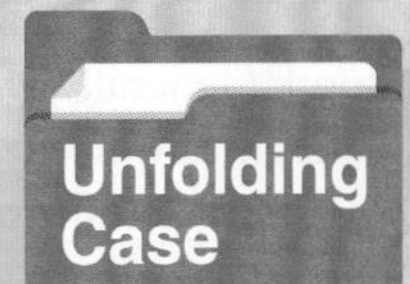

Recall Clara. She currently weighs 128 pounds. How much protein should she have per day? She complains that meats are too difficult to chew. What sources of protein may be easier for Clara to consume? Which sources of protein are most economical and easiest to prepare for someone living alone? If she is willing to eat in between meal snacks, what would you recommend?

More research is needed to determine protein and leucine thresholds, the causes of anabolic resistance to low protein intakes in older adults, and who best benefits from protein interventions to prevent or manage sarcopenia (Rodriguez, 2015). Researchers are also considering whether increasing protein intake earlier in life, such as during middle age, will promote long-term muscle health.

Fiber

The recommendation for fiber decreases for adults age 50 years and older because the Adequate Intake (AI) for fiber is based on total calorie intake.

- At age 51, the AI for fiber decreases to 30 g/day for men and 21 g/day for women.
- The AI is based on median intake levels observed to protect against coronary heart disease (CHD) (Institute of Medicine, 2005).
- However, fiber also helps prevent constipation, a condition older adults are more prone to due to decreased abdominal muscle tone, a decrease in physical activity, or as a side effect of drug therapy. Older adults may benefit from increasing their fiber intake despite the lower AI for their age group.
- Fiber sources that promote laxation include wheat bran, whole grains, nuts, and the skins and seeds of fruits and vegetables.

Micronutrients

The most notable changes in DRIs for older adults are for vitamin D, calcium, vitamin B_{12}, and iron.

Vitamin D

After age 70, the RDA for vitamin D increases from 15 mcg/day (600 IU) to 20 mcg/day (800 IU) for both men and women. Vitamin D is well known for its role in maintaining skeletal health. Epidemiologic evidence suggests that low vitamin D levels may be involved in age-related diseases, such as cognitive decline, depression, osteoporosis, cardiovascular disease, hypertension, type 2 diabetes, and cancer (Meehan & Penckofer, 2014).

- Various risk factors place older adults at increased risk for vitamin D deficiency, such as inadequate intake, limited sun exposure, decreased ability to synthesize vitamin D on the skin, and impaired activation by the liver and kidneys.
- There are few dietary sources of vitamin D: fortified milk and other vitamin D–fortified foods, egg yolks, fatty fish, and beef liver.
- Supplements of vitamin D may be necessary to achieve adequacy. The Endocrine Society recommends that adults consume at least the RDA of vitamin D for their age and states that 1500 to 2000 IU/day may be required to achieve serum levels >30 ng/mL of vitamin D, the level they believe is optimal to prevent deficiency and maximize bone health (Holick et al., 2011).

Calcium

Consuming adequate amounts of calcium, vitamin D, and other nutrients is critical for optimum bone health. Low bone mineral density and osteoporosis are common in the United States, especially in older adults, and can lead to fractures and increased risk of morbidity and mortality.

- After age 70, the RDA for calcium increases for men from 1000 to 1200 mg/day. For women, the increase to 1200 mg/day occurs at age 51.
- Calcium is preferably obtained from food. Generally, three daily servings of milk, yogurt, or cheese plus nondairy sources of calcium are needed to ensure an adequate calcium intake. Nondairy sources of calcium include calcium-fortified orange juice, soy milk, and breakfast cereals and certain greens (bok choy, collard greens, kale, turnip greens).
- People who are unwilling or unable to consume adequate calcium through food sources need calcium supplements.

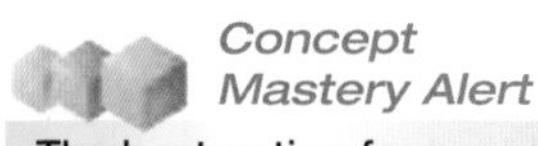
Concept Mastery Alert

The best option for a client concerned about an osteoporosis diagnosis after fracturing their hip is medication to treat osteoporosis. Once bone loss has occurred, medications are necessary.

Vitamin B_{12}

Vitamin B_{12} holds the distinction of being the only vitamin not found in plants; naturally, it occurs only in animal products such as meat, fish, poultry, eggs, milk, and milk products. Although the RDA for vitamin B_{12} does not change with aging, the recommended source does: Adults over the age of 50 are advised to meet their B_{12} requirement mostly from fortified foods (e.g., fortified ready-to-eat cereal) or supplements (Institute of Medicine, 1998). Vitamin B_{12} status tends to decline with age, possibly due to a decrease in gastric acidity, which impairs the freeing of vitamin B_{12} bound to protein in foods, a necessary step in the process of absorption.

Iron

The recommendation for iron for men does not change with aging. In women, the requirement for iron decreases after menopause due to the cessation of monthly blood loss. However, iron deficiency may occur in older adults secondary to low stomach acid, the use of antacids, or chronic blood loss from diseases or medications. Iron intake may be low in adults who do not regularly eat red meat.

Vitamin and Mineral Supplements

In theory, older adults should be able to obtain adequate amounts of all essential micronutrients through well-chosen foods. However, according to 2015 to 2016 data, mean intakes of vitamin A, vitamin D, vitamin E, calcium, magnesium, and potassium fall below recommended amounts for adults age 50 years and older (U.S. Department of Agriculture [USDA] & Agricultural Research Service [ARS], 2018).

- Supplement use is high among older adults. A 2017 study showed that 70% of adults age 60 and older used one or more dietary supplements in the previous 30 days, with multivitamin or mineral the most common supplement used (Gahche et al., 2017).
- As noted earlier, supplements of vitamin D, calcium, and vitamin B_{12} may be necessary for older adults.
- Low-dose multivitamin and mineral supplements can help achieve adequate micronutrient intakes, especially when food selection is limited.

HEALTHY AGING

Genetic and environmental "life advantages"—such as genetic potential for longevity, intelligence, motivation, curiosity, good socialization, religious affiliation, marriage and family, avoidance of substance abuse, availability of health care, adequate sleep, and sufficient rest and relaxation—have positive effects on both length and quality of life. Although there is no universally agreed upon definition of healthy or successful aging, criteria often cited include no major chronic diseases, no cognitive impairment, no physical disabilities, and no mental health limitations (Sun et al., 2009).

The goal of healthy aging is not only to prolong life but more importantly to extend healthy active years (Shlisky et al., 2017). Unfortunately, chronic diseases become more prevalent with age and are often considered an inevitable consequence of aging. The fact that many chronic diseases are occurring at younger ages points to a cause other than aging, namely, nutrition and lifestyle factors. According to the World Health Organization (WHO), at least 80% of all heart disease, stroke, and type 2 diabetes as well as over 40% of all cancer would be prevented through a healthy diet, regular physical activity, and avoidance of tobacco (World Health Organization, 2005).

Healthy Eating

Across the human life span, healthy eating patterns and diet quality are linked to health promotion and disease prevention. A healthy eating pattern

- provides the appropriate amount of calories from a variety of foods across food groups,
- emphasizes nutrient-dense foods: fruit, vegetables, whole grains, seafood, eggs, legumes, nuts, low-fat and fat-free dairy, and lean meats and poultry, and
- limits saturated fats, sodium, refined starches, and added sugars.

Healthy Eating Index

The Healthy Eating Index (HEI-2015), the tool used to measure how closely intake aligns with the *Dietary Guidelines for Americans* recommendations, shows that adults aged 60 and older have the highest diet quality among all age groups, scoring 63 out of a possible 100 points (U.S. Department of Agriculture [USDA] & U.S. Department of Health and Human Services [USDHHS], 2020). However, this score is still low and indicates that older adults are not meeting the recommendations for food group and nutrient intakes. Older adults can improve their intake by

- consuming more vegetables, fruits, dairy, whole grains, and seafood (USDA & USDHHS, 2020).
- consuming less added sugars, saturated fat, and sodium.

Healthy Eating Patterns

The healthy eating patterns featured in the *Dietary Guidelines*, namely, the Healthy U.S.-Style, Healthy Mediterranean-Style, and Healthy Vegetarian Eating Patterns, are all appropriate across the life span. Healthy eating patterns that have been investigated for specifically promoting healthy aging include the Mediterranean diet (MedDiet) and the Mediterranean–DASH Intervention for Neurodegenerative Delay (MIND) diet. Both diets have been independently associated with better cognitive function and lower risk of cognitive impairment (McEvoy et al., 2017). Both are rich in plants and have features that overlap. Table 14.2 compares the general guidelines for each eating pattern.

The Mediterranean Diet

The Mediterranean diet (MedDiet) describes the traditional eating habits of people living in the olive-growing areas of the Mediterranean region before the mid-1960s (Trichopoulou et al., 2014). Historically, Mediterranean countries have been among the healthiest countries in the world, with relatively low rates of cardiovascular diseases and cancer and greater longevity (Trichopoulou et al., 2014). Interest in the traditional MedDiet began in the late 1950s, when it was proposed that the low incidence of coronary heart disease (CHD) in Mediterranean countries may be linked to the low saturated fat content of the MedDiet. Compared to other healthy eating patterns, the MedDiet

- is relatively high in total fat (e.g., 40% of total calories), with a high ratio of monounsaturated fat to saturated fat coming primarily from virgin olive oil, nuts, and fatty fish.
- includes a moderate intake of red wine consumed during meals.

Table 14.2 A Comparison of the Mediterranean Diet and MIND Diet

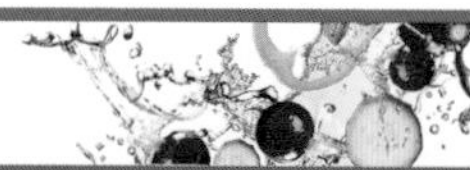

Mediterranean Diet	MIND Diet

Consists primarily of minimally processed foods, such as whole grains, legumes, vegetables, fruit, nuts, and fish
Relatively high fat intake (e.g., 40% of total calories) with a high ratio of monounsaturated fat to saturated fat due to the liberal use of olive oil
 	
Main meals contain the following:
• 1–2 servings of grains, preferably whole grains
• 2 or more servings of vegetables, at least one of which is raw
• 1–2 servings of fruit
 	
Daily
• 2 servings of low-fat yogurt, cheese, and other fermented daily products
• Use olive oil as the principal source of fat
• Add a variety with spices, herbs, garlic, and onions
• A reasonable intake of olives, nuts, and seeds as healthy snacks
• Moderate consumption of wine during meals
 	
Weekly
• Eat a variety of plant and animal proteins
  • 2 or more servings of fish
  • 2 servings of white meat
  • 2–4 eggs
• Less than 2 servings of lean red meat
• Less than 1 serving processed meat
 	
Occasionally
Sweets in small amounts and only for special occasions
	Composed of specific foods that provide nutrients that may help delay neuron aging, such as vitamin E, DHA, B vitamins, vitamin C, and vitamin D
	
	10 "brain healthy" food components to emphasize:
	• Green leafy vegetables: at least 1 serving/day
	• All other vegetables: at least 1 serving/day
	• Berries: at least 2 servings/week
	• Nuts: 5 or more servings/week
	• Olive oil: use as main cooking oil
	• Whole grains: at least 3 servings/day
	• Fish: at least 1 serving/week
	• Beans: at least 4 servings/week
	• Poultry: 2 or more servings/week
	• Wine: no more than 1 glass/day
	
	5 unhealthy groups to avoid or limit:
	• Butter/margarine: less than 1 tbsp/day
	• Cheese: less than 1 ounce/week
	• Red meat: no more than 3 servings/week
	• Fried food/fast food: less than once/week
	• Pastries and sweets: no more than 4 times/week

Source: Bach-Faig, A., Berry, E., Lairon, D., et al. (2011). Mediterranean diet pyramid today. Science and cultural updates. *Public Health Nutrition, 14*(12A), 2274–2284. https://doi.org/10.1017/S1368980011002515; Di Fiore, N. (2015, March 16). *Diet may help prevent Alzheimer's: MIND diet rich in vegetables, berries, whole grains, nuts*. Rush University Medical Center. https://www.rush.edu/news/diet-may-help-prevent-alzheimers">https://www.rush.edu/news/diet-may-help-prevent-alzheimers

Potential Age-Related Benefits

Increasing evidence suggests that high adherence to a MedDiet promotes good health during aging (Assmann et al., 2018). For instance, studies link close adherence to a MedDiet to:

- lower the risk of mild cognitive impairment and Alzheimer's disease (AD) (Shlisky et al., 2017),
- less age-related brain shrinkage (Luciano et al., 2017),
- prolonged survival (study participants who most closely followed a MedDiet were significantly less likely to die over the 8-year study period [Bonaccio et al., 2018]),
- reduced risk of frailty, even among very old elderly (Rahi et al., 2018),
- greater chance of living beyond 70 years with greater health and well-being (Samieri et al., 2013).

Components Attributed to Benefits

The EPIC study credited a high intake of plants, moderate alcohol intake, low meat intake, and liberal use of olive oil with reducing total mortality among a prospective cohort consuming the MedDiet (Trichopoulou et al., 2009). The benefits of the MedDiet may be related to its high alpha-linolenic acid content, high antioxidant content, high fiber content, low glycemic load, or some other components or combination of components (Trichopoulou et al., 2014).

MIND Diet

The Mediterranean-DASH Intervention for Neurodegenerative Delay or MIND diet is a combination of the MedDiet and DASH diets, which are two diets shown to lower blood pressure and reduce the risk of cardiovascular disease and diabetes. The goal of the MIND diet is to specifically reduce the risk of dementia and decline in brain health that usually occurs with aging (Pike, 2019). Fifteen foods are specifically named, with 10 that are encouraged and 5 that should be limited. The MIND diet differs from the MedDiet in that (Hosking et al., 2019):

- it recommends daily and weekly servings of specific foods and food groups rather than an eating pattern.
- it specifies berry intake but not other fruits. Both the MedDiet and the DASH diet recommend a high intake of fruit in general but not berries specifically.
- green leafy vegetables comprise a separate category due to their high content of nutrients that are thought to lower the risk of cardiovascular disease and cognitive decline. Other vegetables are also recommended daily but grouped into one category. The MedDiet and DASH diet encourage a liberal intake of fruit and vegetables of all varieties.

Potential Age-Related Benefits

Created in 2015, the MIND diet is relatively new. The handful of study results indicate:

- The diet substantially slows cognitive decline with age (Morris et al., 2015a).
- Greater adherence to the MIND diet has been linked to a 53% decrease in the rate of Alzheimer's disease (AD) (Morris et al., 2015b). Even modest adherence to the MIND diet may have substantial benefits for the prevention of AD.

Components Attributed to Benefits

A diet that promotes vascular health is inherently protective against vascular dementia. In addition to those benefits, certain foods and food components emphasized in the MIND diet have been directly linked to improved neurological function or reduced AD markers in the brain (Mosconi et al., 2014). The MIND diet is high in vitamin E, DHA, B vitamins, vitamin C, and vitamin D, all of which have been found to help delay neuron aging (Mohajeri et al., 2015).

BOX 14.1 Key Physical Activity Guidelines for Older Adults

These guidelines are the same for adults and older adults:

- Adults should move more and sit less throughout the day. Some physical activity is better than none. Adults who sit less and do any amount of moderate to vigorous physical activity gain some health benefits.
- For substantial health benefits, adults should do at least 150 minutes (2 hours and 30 minutes) to 300 minutes (5 hours) a week of moderate-intensity aerobic physical activity or 75 minutes (1 hour and 15 minutes) to 150 minutes (2 hours and 30 minutes) a week of vigorous-intensity aerobic physical activity or an equivalent combination of moderate- and vigorous-intensity aerobic activity. Preferably, aerobic activity should be spread throughout the week.
- Additional health benefits are gained by engaging in physical activity beyond the equivalent of 300 minutes (5 hours) of moderate-intensity physical activity a week.
- Adults should also do muscle-strengthening activities of moderate or greater intensity that involve all major muscle groups on 2 or more days a week, as these activities provide additional health benefits.

Guidelines only for older adults:

- As part of their weekly physical activity, older adults should do multicomponent physical activity that includes balance training as well as aerobic and muscle-strengthening activities.
- Older adults should determine their level of effort for physical activity relative to their level of fitness.
- Older adults with chronic conditions should understand whether and how their conditions affect their ability to do regular physical activity safely.
- When older adults cannot do 150 minutes of moderate-intensity aerobic activity a week because of chronic conditions, they should be as physically active as their abilities and conditions allow.

Source: U.S. Department of Health and Human Services. (2018). *Physical Activity Guidelines for Americans* (2nd ed.). https://health.gov/sites/default/files/2019-09/Physical_Activity_Guidelines_2nd_edition.pdf

Physical Activity

Older adults are urged to follow the same physical activity guidelines as those for younger adults in order to reap similar health benefits (Box 14.1). Regular physical activity also reduces the risk of falls and fall-related injuries in older adults. Other benefits include (U.S. Department of Health and Human Services [USDHHS], 2018)

- lower risk of all-cause mortality, cardiovascular disease, hypertension, type 2 diabetes, dyslipidemia, certain cancers, and dementia.
- delayed progression of certain chronic illnesses, hypertension, and type 2 diabetes,
- weight loss, particularly when combined with a lower calorie intake, and improved weight maintenance,
- improvements in cognition, quality of life, sleep, bone health, and physical function,
- reduced risk of anxiety and depression.

NUTRITION AND HEALTH CONCERNS OF OLDER ADULTS

How people rank their own health is an important indicator of overall health and a significant predictor of mortality (United Health Foundation, 2019). In 2017, 45% of community-dwelling adults aged 65 and older ranked their health as excellent or very good yet most older adults have at least one chronic health condition (USDHHS & AOA, 2018).

Malnutrition

Although older adults generally perceive themselves as healthy, many are at risk of malnutrition. A recent meta-analysis revealed an overall malnutrition prevalence of 2.3% and risk of malnutrition prevalence of 19% in community-dwelling older adults (Verlaan et al., 2017). The quality and quantity of food intake, food insecurity, and acute or chronic physical or mental health conditions may be contributing factors (Saffel-Shrier et al., 2019). Loss of appetite, which may arise from physiologic, psychosocial, and medical factors, is a key predictor of malnutrition in older adults.

Malnutrition impairs quality of life and is a strong predictor of short-term mortality in older adults (Gentile et al., 2013). Common symptoms of malnutrition, such as confusion, fatigue, and weakness, are often attributed to other conditions and are misdiagnosed or unrecognized as malnutrition (Marshall et al., 2016). Selected risk factors for malnutrition in older adults are shown in Box 14.2.

Nutrition Screening for Malnutrition

Nutrition screening, a simple process to quickly identify the risk of malnutrition, is appropriate in any setting where older adults receive services or care, as in hospitals, long-term care facilities, community-based care, home health, and physician office. Although there are many screening tools that can be used to screen for malnutrition in older adults, the Academy of Nutrition and Dietetics recommends the Malnutrition Screening Tool (MST) be used to screen adults for malnutrition (undernutrition) regardless of age, medical history, or setting (Skipper et al., 2020).

The MST asks only three questions:

- Have you lost weight without trying?
- If yes, how much weight have you lost?
- Have you been eating poorly because of a decreased appetite?

BOX 14.2 Selected Risk Factors to Assess for Malnutrition in Older Adults

Physical and Medical Conditions

- Chronic diseases that directly or indirectly affect intake by leading to:
  - Decreased appetite
  - Impaired taste
  - Impaired ability to eat, prepare, or purchase food
  - Restrictive diets
  - Dysphagia
- Acute or chronic diseases that cause:
  - Increased nutrient needs through inflammation
  - Altered nutrient digestion (e.g., chronic pancreatitis) or absorption (e.g., celiac disease)
  - Impaired nutrient utilization (e.g., uncontrolled diabetes) or excretion (e.g., chronic kidney disease)
  - Geriatric syndromes, such as pressure ulcers, falls, functional decline, delirium, incontinence, sleeping problems, dizziness, and self-neglect

Physical Assessment

- Loss of subcutaneous fat
- Muscle loss
- Oral impairments, such as loss of teeth, ill-fitting dentures, or dry mouth
- Dysphagia
- Impaired sense of taste or smell
- Constipation or diarrhea

Nutrition Assessment Findings

- Unintentional weight loss
- Inadequate intake as per diet history, although food recall may be inaccurate, especially in adults with cognitive impairment
- Nutrition risk identified through:
  - Nutrition screening
  - Use of multiple medications, including prescriptions, over-the-counter medications, vitamins, and supplements; assess for side effects that affect appetite or intake

Mental Health Status

- Cognition and dementia
- Mood and anxiety disorders
- Depression

Functioning

- Gait, strength, and balance
- Ability to perform ADLs and IADLs

Social Domain

- Social networks
- Financial constraints
- Living arrangements

Environment

- Housing, such as ability to use stairs to gain access to the outside
- Adequacy of transportation to purchase food
- Accessibility to grocery stores

Source: DiMaria-Ghalili, R. (2014). Integrating nutrition in the comprehensive geriatric assessment. *Nutrition in Clinical Practice*, *29*, 420–427. https://doi.org/10.1177/0884533614537076

Criterion is scored to determine malnutrition risk.

- An individual who is eating well with little or no weight loss is deemed not at a nutritional risk.
- An individual who is eating poorly and/or has recent weight loss is determined to be at nutritional risk.
- The MST has been shown to have a moderate degree of validity, agreement, and inter-rater reliability in identifying malnutrition. The strength of evidence for the MST is good/strong with good generalizability.
- See Chapter 15 for the actual MST tool.

Interventions to Improve Intake and Weight

Regardless of living situation, ongoing screening that identifies risk of actual or potential malnutrition should be followed by a nutrition assessment that leads to an individualized plan to improve overall intake.

- One option is to increase the nutrient density of foods eaten by adding ingredients that provide calories and/or protein (Box 14.3). The effect is to increase the nutritional value while the volume of food served remains the same.
- Homemade or commercial oral nutrition supplements are an effective option to increase overall nutrient intake for nursing home residents as well as for community-dwelling older adults.
  - Smoothies, milk shakes, and protein powder–based milk drinks can be consumed between meals. Liquids leave the stomach more quickly than solids and are less likely to interfere with the next meal.
  - Commercial supplements offer convenience but are more expensive.
  - Taste fatigue may occur over time. Consider altering the amount, timing, flavors, or types to maintain acceptance.
  - Monitor overall intake to ensure that supplements are adding to instead of replacing food intake.

Additional Considerations for Community-Dwelling Adults

Among community-dwelling adults, eating with others may help improve the intake and nutritional status of those who live alone. Efforts should be made to eat with friends and relatives whenever possible. Federally funded nutrition programs, such as congregate meals and Meals on Wheels, are also options.

- These programs are designed to provide low-cost, nutritious, hot meals; education about food and nutrition; opportunities for socialization and recreation; and information on other health and social assistance programs.
- The congregate meal program provides a hot, balanced, midday meal and the opportunity to socialize in senior citizen centers and other public or private facilities. Those who choose to pay may do so; otherwise, the meal is free.

BOX 14.3 Examples of Foods Made More Nutrient/Calorie Dense

- Mashed potatoes made with extra butter, whole milk, and/or cheese
- Milk fortified with nonfat dry milk powder to make "double strength" milk that can be used in cereal, soups, milk-based desserts, milk shakes
- Casseroles, soups, rice, noodles, or sandwiches with added cheese or chopped fine hard-cooked eggs
- Fruit, plain cake, or other desserts topped with vanilla Greek yogurt
- Oatmeal made with added butter, nonfat dry milk, and sugar
- Coffee with half and half, whole milk, and/or honey
- Scrambled eggs with added cheese

- Meals on Wheels is a home-delivered meal program for older adults who are unable to get to congregate meal centers because they live in an isolated area or have a chronic illness or physical limitations. Usually, a hot meal is delivered before midday with a bagged lunch to be eaten as the evening meal. Modified diets, such as carbohydrate-controlled diets and low-sodium diets, are provided as needed.

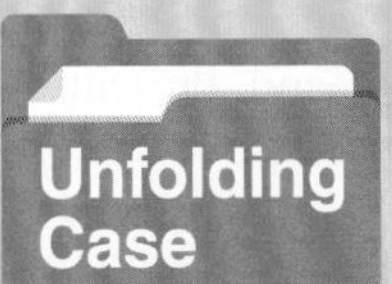

Think of Clara. Clara agreed to go to the senior center for noon-time meals but stopped going after a few days because she got lost driving there and fears she may be developing dementia. She is now receiving Meals on Wheels but eats only 50% of each meal. Her weight continues to decline. Could she be considered at risk for malnutrition? What other options or strategies may help improve Clara's intake?

Additional Considerations for Long-Term Care Residents

Preventing malnutrition is a quality-of-life issue. To meet the needs of individual residents, a holistic approach is advocated that includes the individual's personal goals, overall prognosis, risk–benefit ratio, and quality of life.

- Mealtime should be made as enjoyable as possible. Noise and distractions in the dining room should be minimized.
- Family involvement increases resident intake.
- Honor individual food preferences whenever possible.
- Encourage independence in eating and supervise dining areas so that proper feeding techniques are used when residents are assisted or fed by certified nursing assistants.
- For residents with functional or cognitive impairments, specialized utensils and dishes, finger foods, and tactile prompts may facilitate independence.
- A liberalized eating pattern, which is a healthy diet of nutrient-dense foods that contains neither excessive nor restrictive amounts of cholesterol, sodium, and added sugar, may help improve intake and lower the risk of weight loss (Box 14.4)
- The liberal diet can be modified to meet the requirements of residents with increased needs, such as those who have pressure ulcers. Using foods that are made more nutrient dense or adding extra meat and/or milk will provide increased amounts of calories, protein, and fluid.
- Restrictive diets should be used only when a significant improvement in health can be expected, as in the case of ascites or constipation.
- Consistently and accurately record food intake. Intakes less than 75% and weight loss of 5% in 30 days warrant investigation.

BOX 14.4 Sample Liberal Eating Pattern for Older Adults

Breakfast

- Orange juice
- Oatmeal
- One soft-cooked egg
- One slice buttered whole wheat toast
- Low-fat milk
- Coffee/tea

Lunch

- Turkey sandwich made with two slices whole-wheat bread, tomato, romaine lettuce, and low-fat salad dressing
- Vegetable soup
- Sliced strawberries over angel food cake
- One cup low-fat milk
- Coffee/tea

Dinner

- Roast pork
- Oven-roasted potatoes
- Baked acorn squash
- Fresh-fruit salad
- Ice cream
- Coffee/tea

Snack

- One cup low-fat yogurt

Obesity

For adults of any age, underweight is defined as a BMI less than 18.5, overweight at BMI of 25 to 29.9, and obesity at BMI of 30 or more.

- Only 0.9% of community-dwelling adults aged 60 and older are estimated to be underweight (Fryar et al., 2018).
- In contrast, an estimated 40.2% of men and 43.5% of women aged 65 to 74 years are obese (Centers for Disease Control and Prevention [CDC], 2017). Obesity exacerbates most chronic health conditions, such as sarcopenia, frailty, disability, and diabetes (Saffel-Shrier et al., 2019).

Certainly, obesity is not unique to older adults. The question of what is appropriate obesity treatment for older adults is where controversy lies.

- Loss of weight is not synonymous with—nor does it have the same benefit as—loss of fat.
- Intentional weight loss causes loss of muscle—even when the goal is fat loss. In fact, calorie restriction or diet-alone-induced weight loss contributes to the development of sarcopenia and bone loss and thus to a higher risk of functional impairment and disability (Batis et al., 2015).
- Other challenges include the difficulty of changing behavior with advancing age.
  - Many older people may not feel a need to make changes at this point in life.
  - Active participation in physical activity may be difficult because of medical problems, financial limitations, or impaired hearing or vision.
  - Diminished sense of taste, living alone, depression, and a limited food budget may impede changes in intake.
  - Because of these challenges, there has been no consensus on optimal therapy, including the use of high-protein diets, which do not ensure preservation of muscle during weight loss in older adults (Coker & Wolfe, 2017).

Sarcopenia

Sarcopenia
age-related progressive loss of lean mass and muscle strength associated with morbidity, reduced quality of life, frailty, disability, and increased rates of mortality.

Sarcopenia is a progressive and generalized skeletal muscle disorder characterized by accelerated loss of muscle mass and insidious functional decline (Cruz-Jentoft & Sayer, 2019).

- Adverse outcomes include physical disability, frailty, falls, fractures, poor quality of life, and death (Cruz-Jentof et al., 2014). It has become one of the most important challenges to healthy aging (Chen et al., 2016).
- Estimates of sarcopenia prevalence in community-dwelling older adults range from 9.9% to 40.4% depending on the definition used (Mayhew et al., 2019).
- Sarcopenia should be considered in all older adults with observed declines in physical function, strength, or overall health and especially in older adults who are bedridden, who cannot rise independently from a chair, or who have a slow gait (Evans, 2010).
- In part, sarcopenia may be caused by nutritional deficiencies, such as an inadequate intake of protein (Cruz-Jentof et al., 2014). It is not known whether protein and/or amino acid supplementation are effective treatment interventions. High-quality clinical trials are needed to identify effective prevention and treatment strategies.
- Sarcopenic obesity refers to obesity with low skeletal muscle function and mass. There is no consensus on its definition and diagnostic criteria and effective prevention and treatment strategies remain inadequate. Optimal dietary options and medical nutritional support to preserve muscle mass in obese people remain largely undefined (Barazzoni et al., 2018).

Frailty

An international definition of frailty is as follows: *a medical syndrome with multiple causes and contributors that is characterized by diminished strength, endurance, and reduced physiological function that increases an individual's vulnerability for dependency and/or death* (Saffel-Shrier et al., 2019).

- Frailty has a prevalence of nearly 10% among community-dwelling older adults, is more common in women than men, and increases sharply with age (Collard et al., 2012).
- Multiple factors contribute to frailty, including malnutrition, chronic diseases, and psychological factors. Although sarcopenia may be a component of frailty, frailty is more multidimensional than sarcopenia alone (Fielding et al., 2011).
- Criteria used to identify frailty include weight loss and loss of muscle mass, weakness, poor endurance, exhaustion, slowness, and low activity. Three or more positive findings may indicate the presence of frailty (Fried et al., 2001).
- Although there are numerous screening tools to identify frailty, there is no international standard measurement (Dent et al., 2016).
- Several simple validated screening tools are available to enable physicians to quickly identify adults with physical frailty syndrome who are in need of a more in-depth assessment. One example is the simple FRAIL questionnaire screening tool (Fig. 14.2).
- Frailty screening is recommended for all adults age 70 years and older and anyone with significant weight loss (5% or more over the last year) due to chronic illness (Morley et al., 2013).

Nutrition Therapy for Frailty

Nutrition therapy recommendations for frailty varies with weight status.

- Frailty related to weight loss can be partially prevented or treated with protein–calorie supplementation (Morley et al., 2013).
- Frailty associated with obesity may be lessened with intentional weight loss (Porter Starr et al., 2016).
- Vitamin D supplements for older adults who are deficient in vitamin D may reduce the risk of falls, hip fractures, and mortality and may improve muscle function (Morley et al., 2013).

Fatigue:	Are you fatigued?	
Resistance:	Cannot walk up 1 flight of stairs?	
Aerobic:	Cannot walk 1 block?	
Illness:	Do you have more than 5 illnesses?	
Loss of weight:	Have you lost more than 5% of your weight in the past 6 months?	
	3 or greater = frailty *1 or 2 = prefrail*	

FIGURE 14.2 ▲ The FRAIL questionnaire. (*Source:* Morley, J., Vellas, B., van Kan, G., Anker, S. D., Bauer, J. M., Bernabei, R., Cesari, M., Chumlea, W., Doehner, W., Evans, J., Fried, L., Guralnik, J., Katz, P., Malmstrom, T., McCarter, R., Robledo, L., Rockwood, K., von Haehling, S., Vanewoude, M., & Walston, J. (2013). Frailty consensus: A call to action. *Journal of the American Medical Directors Association, 14*(6), 392–397. https://doi.org/10.1016/j.jamda.2013.03.022).

Alzheimer's Disease

Several of the leading causes of death among adults aged 45 to 64 are also the leading causes of death among adults aged 65 and older, such as heart disease, cancer, chronic lower respiratory diseases, and diabetes. A leading cause of death among adults aged 65 and older that is not one of the 10 leading causes of death among people aged 64 and younger is Alzheimer's Disease (AD). AD ranks as the fifth leading cause of death among adults aged 65 and older and the third leading cause among adults aged 85 and older (Heron, 2019).

AD is an irreversible, progressive brain disorder that gradually destroys memory and cognition. It appears to result from a complex series of events in the brain that occur over decades. Disruptions in nerve cell communication, metabolism, and repair eventually cause many nerve cells to stop functioning, lose connections with other nerve cells, and die, resulting in gradual atrophy of the brain. Like CHD, AD is at least partially a vascular problem, but plaques and tau tangles that form with AD are filled with beta-amyloid, an indissoluble protein, not fat and cholesterol.

The cause of early-onset AD is usually a genetic mutation. Suspected causes of late-onset AD include a combination of genetic, environmental, and lifestyle factors (National Institute on Aging [NIA] & National Institutes of Health [NIH], 2019). Increased age and family history of AD are known risk factors for AD; cardiovascular disease, stroke, hypertension, and diabetes may also increase the risk (NIA, NIH, 2019). As stated previously, the MedDiet and MIND diet may decrease the risk of cognitive impairment and AD (McEvoy et al., 2017; Morris et al., 2015b; Shlisky et al., 2017). However, it is a multifactorial disease, and a cure does not exist.

Effect on Nutritional Status

AD can have a devastating impact on an individual's nutritional status.

- Compared with healthy older adults, older adults diagnosed with cognitive impairment or AD may have lower intakes of all nutrients (Bernstein & Munoz, 2012).
- Early in the disease, impairments in memory and judgment may make shopping, storing, and cooking food difficult. The client may forget to eat or may forget that they have already eaten and consequently may eat again.
- Changes in the sense of smell may develop, a preference for sweet and salty foods may occur, and unusual food choices are not uncommon.
- Agitation and fidgeting increases energy expenditure, and weight loss is common.
- Choking may occur if the client forgets to chew food sufficiently before swallowing or hoards food in the mouth.
- Eating of nonfood items may occur, and eventually self-feeding ability is lost.
- Clients in the latter stage of AD no longer know what to do when food is placed in the mouth. When this occurs, a decision regarding the use of other means of nutritional support (e.g., nasogastric or percutaneous endoscopic gastrostomy tube feedings) must be made.

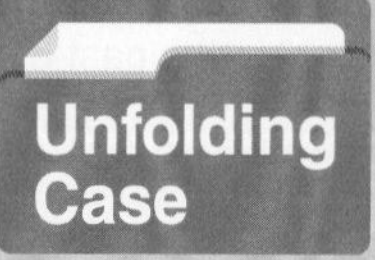

Recall Clara. Clara is admitted to a memory care facility. What symptoms did she display that are characteristic of the progressive decline in function seen in adults with AD? Her intake continues to be approximately 50% at each meal. She pushes food around her plate and hides it under the plate. She also prefers wandering the halls to sitting. She has a health care proxy who explicitly states that she does not want artificial food or fluids should there be no hope of recovery. How can you best care for Clara?

NURSING PROCESS Older Adult

Harold Hausman is a regular participant of the monthly congregational nursing program sponsored at his church. He is a sedentary 82-year-old widower who lives alone. You have noticed that he has lost weight over the past several months. He has asked you to answer a few questions he has about the low-sodium, low-cholesterol diet his doctor recommended.

Assessment

Medical–Psychosocial History

- medical history that may have nutritional implications, such as hyperlipidemia, hypertension, cardiovascular disease, or GI complaints
- ability to understand, attitude toward health and nutrition, and readiness to learn
- attitude about his present weight and recent weight loss
- usual activity patterns
- medications that may affect nutrition
- use of prescribed and over-the-counter drugs
- functional limitations such as impaired ability to shop, cook, and eat
- psychosocial and economic issues such as who does the shopping and cooking, adequacy of food budget, need for food assistance, and level of family and social support

Anthropometric Assessment

- height, current and usual weight
- percentage of weight change
- determine BMI

Biochemical and Physical Assessment

- cholesterol level, if available
- blood pressure
- dentition and ability to swallow

Dietary Assessment

- Why did your doctor give you this low-sodium, low-cholesterol eating plan?
- How many daily meals and snacks do you usually eat?
- What is a normal day's intake for you?
- What changes have you made in implementing this eating plan? For instance, did you stop using the saltshaker at the table or are you reading labels for sodium content? Did you change the type of butter/margarine you use? The type of salad dressing?
- Do you prepare food with added fat, or do you bake, broil, steam, or boil your food?
- Do any cultural, religious, or ethnic considerations influence your eating habits?
- Do you use vitamins, minerals, or nutritional supplements? If so, which ones, how much, and why are they taken?
- Do you use alcohol, tobacco, and caffeine?
- How is your appetite?

Analysis

Possible Nursing Analysis

Malnutrition risk related to restrictive diet and eating alone as evidenced by weight loss.

Planning

Client Outcomes

The client will

- attain/maintain a "healthy" weight
- consume, on average, a varied and balanced eating pattern that meets the recommended number of servings from the 2000-calorie MyPlate meal plan
- implement healthy low-sodium, low-cholesterol changes to his usual intake without compromising nutritional or caloric adequacy

NURSING PROCESS Older Adult (continued)

Nursing Interventions

Nutrition Therapy

Encourage a varied and balanced eating pattern that meets the recommended number of servings from each of the major MyPlate food groups for a 2000-calorie eating pattern.

Client Teaching

Instruct the client on:

- The role of nutrition in maintaining health and quality of life, including the following:
  - A balanced eating pattern consisting of a variety of nutrient-dense foods helps maximize the quality of life.
  - Avoiding excess salt is prudent for all people. Recommendations on sodium intake should be made on an individual basis according to the client's cardiac and renal status, appetite, and use of medications.
  - Although it is wise to avoid high-fat, nutrient-poor foods such as most cakes, cookies, pastries, pies, chips, full-fat dairy products, and fried foods, observing too severe fat restriction compromises calorie intake and may result in undesirable weight loss.
- Eating plan essentials, including the importance of
  - choosing a variety of foods to help ensure an average adequate intake (limiting food choices or skipping a food group increases the risk of both nutrient deficiencies and excesses)
  - eating enough food to avoid unfavorable weight loss
  - eating enough high-fiber foods such as whole-grain breads and cereals, dried peas and beans, and fresh fruits and vegetables
  - drinking adequate fluid regularly throughout the day
- Behavioral matters, including
  - the importance of discussing the rationale for the low-sodium, low-cholesterol diet with his physician, particularly because he has had an unfavorable weight loss
  - how to read labels to identify low-sodium foods
- Physical activity goals that may help improve appetite and intake

Evaluation

Evaluate and Monitor

- Monitor weight and blood pressure.
- Provide periodic feedback and reinforcement on food intake and questions about the eating plan.

How Do You Respond?

Can diet help alleviate osteoarthritis pain? The most compelling link between diet and osteoarthritis (OA) is body weight. Currently, weight loss and increased physical activity are the strongest evidence-based lifestyle modifications for arthritis (Thomas et al., 2018). Obesity not only increases the load on weight-bearing joints (Messier et al., 2014); it also leads to low-grade systemic inflammation, which can exacerbate symptoms (Hauner, 2005). Although a 10% weight loss may be enough to reduce pain and improve physical functioning and mobility, the ultimate goal should be to attain and maintain normal BMI (Thomas et al., 2018). While observational studies suggest that consuming omega-3 fatty acids from fish, using monounsaturated oils in place of polyunsaturated oils, and consuming adequate amounts of vitamins D, A, C, and E may help alleviate arthritis symptoms, the evidence is limited (Thomas et al., 2018). However, even if those strategies do not directly improve arthritis symptoms, they may improve overall intake and health.

REVIEW CASE STUDY

Annie is an 80-year-old widow who lives alone. She has a long history of hypertension and diabetes and suffers from the complications of CHD and neuropathy. She has diabetic retinopathy, which has left her legally blind. She has never been compliant with a diabetic eating plan but takes insulin as directed. She is 5 ft 5 in. tall and weighs 170 pounds, down from her usual weight of 184 pounds 5 months ago.

Annie reluctantly agreed to receive Meals on Wheels, so she does not have to prepare lunch and dinner except on weekends. Her daughter buys groceries for Annie every week, and her grocery list generally consists of milk, oatmeal, two cans of soup, two bananas, a bag of chocolate candy, a layer cake, two doughnuts, and mixed nuts. Her weekend meals consist of whatever she has available to eat.

- What is Annie's BMI? How would you assess her weight status?
- Is her recent weight loss significant? Is it better for her to lose weight, maintain her present weight, or try to regain what she has lost?
- What would you recommend Annie eat for breakfast? For snacks? For weekend meals? Would you discourage her from eating sweets?
- What arguments would you make for her to eat better?

STUDY QUESTIONS

1 A 68-year-old man who has steadily gained excess weight over the years complains that it is too late for him to make any changes in diet or exercise regimen that would effectively improve his health, particularly the arthritis in his knees. Which of the following would be the nurse's best response?
   a. "Unfortunately, you're right. You cannot benefit from a change in diet and exercise now."
   b. "It is too hard for older people to change their habits. You should just continue what you've been doing and know that it's a quality of life issue to enjoy your food."
   c. "It may not help to change your intake and exercise, but it certainly wouldn't hurt. Why don't you give it a try and see what happens?"
   d. "It is not too late to make changes, and losing weight through diet and exercising are the best lifestyle interventions for osteoarthritis."

2 The nurse knows their instructions about vitamin B_{12} are effective when a 65-year-old client verbalizes they will
   a. consume more meat.
   b. consume more fruits and vegetables.
   c. eat vitamin B_{12}–fortified cereal.
   d. drink more milk.

3 A client complains that she is not eating any more than she did when she was 30 years old and yet she keeps gaining weight. Which of the following would be the nurse's best response?
   a. "As people get older, they lose muscle mass, which lowers their calorie requirements, and physical activity often decreases too. You can increase the number of calories you burn by building muscle with resistance exercises and increasing your activity."
   b. "You may not think you are eating more calories but you probably are because the only way to gain weight is to eat more calories than you burn."
   c. "Weight gain is an inevitable consequence of getting older that is related to changes in your body composition. Do not worry about it because older people are healthier when they are heavier."
   d. "Weight gain among older adults is inevitable and untreatable. Concentrate on eating a healthy eating pattern and do not focus on weight."

4 Which mineral is likely to be consumed in inadequate amounts by older adults?
   a. iron
   b. calcium
   c. iodine
   d. sodium

5 The MedDiet differs from other healthy eating plans in that it
   a. prohibits dairy intake.
   b. is higher in fat content, primarily from olive oil, nuts, and fatty fish.
   c. does not include fruit.
   d. does not limit sweets.

6 Why are older adults at increased risk of vitamin D deficiency? Select all that apply.
   a. inadequate intake
   b. impaired activation by the liver and kidneys
   c. decreased ability to synthesize vitamin D on the skin
   d. decreased GI absorption

7 What is a source of leucine that may help stimulate protein synthesis?
   a. milk
   b. nuts
   c. legumes
   d. grains

8 The MIND diet differs from the MedDiet in that it
   a. prohibits the intake of alcohol.
   b. prohibits the intake of red meat.
   c. does not make a recommendation regarding fish intake.
   d. lists green leafy vegetables as a separate recommendation from other vegetables.

CHAPTER SUMMARY NUTRITION FOR OLDER ADULTS

The population of older adults is increasing and is getting older. Older adults represent a heterogeneous group that varies in health, activity, and nutritional status.

Aging and Older Adults

Aging causes changes numerous changes in physiology and function, digestion, nervous system functioning, kidney function, senses, income, health, and psychosocial status. These changes can alter nutrient intake, digestion, metabolism, excretion, or nutrient requirements.

Nutritional Needs of Older Adults

- **Calories:** Requirements decrease because fewer calories are expended on basal metabolic rate and on physical activity. Nutrient density becomes more important.
- **Protein:** The RDA for protein appears to be too low for older adults to maintain muscle mass. Need may increase to at least 1.0 to 1.2 g/kg/day for healthy older adults.

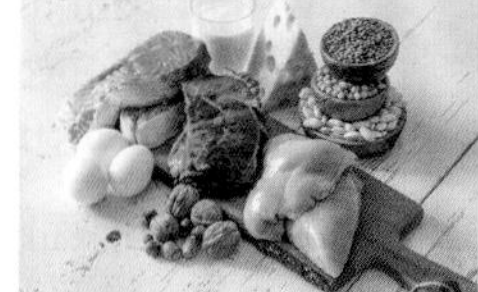

- **Fiber:** Although the AI decreases due to a decrease in calorie intake, older adults may benefit from increasing fiber to maintain regularity.
- **Micronutrients:** Most micronutrient needs remain constant throughout adulthood except that:
  - Vitamin D and calcium requirements increase.
  - Vitamin B_{12} should be consumed from fortified foods or supplements.
  - Iron requirement decreases for women after menopause.
- **Vitamin and mineral supplements:** A healthy eating pattern should provide adequate amounts of micronutrients, but numerous micronutrients are under-consumed by older adults. A multivitamin and mineral supplement can help meet micronutrient requirements.

Healthy Aging

Healthy aging is generally considered as being free of major chronic diseases, cognitive impairment, physical disabilities, and mental health limitations. Healthy eating, physical activity, and not smoking greatly influence aging.

- **Healthy eating:** Healthy eating means consuming the appropriate amount of calories; consuming a mostly plant-based, nutrient-dense eating pattern; and limiting the intake of added sugars, solid fats, and sodium.
- **Healthy eating index:** Older adults eat healthier than other age groups yet underconsume vegetables, fruits, whole grains, seafood, and dairy products. Older women also consume less protein foods than recommended. Average intakes of refined grains, added sugars, saturated fat, and sodium exceed recommendations.
- **Healthy eating patterns:** Certain eating patterns may be associated with better cognitive function and lower risk of cognitive impairment.
  - The MedDiet is a plant-based diet that is high in fat from olive oil, nuts, and fish. Alcohol, in the form of red wine, is consumed in moderate amounts with meals.
  - The MIND diet, a hybrid of the MedDiet and the DASH diet, was specifically designed to reduce the risk of dementia and the decline in brain health that usually occurs with aging. It features 10 foods to emphasize and 5 to avoid.
- **Physical activity:** Older adults receive the same benefits as younger adults from regular physical activity; in addition, it may reduce the risk of falls. Adaptations may be necessary based on physical functioning.

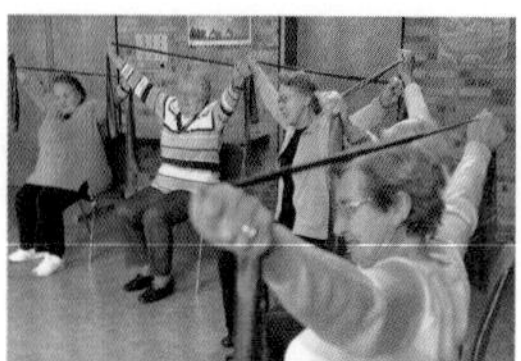

Nutrition and Health Concerns of Older Adults

Older adults generally consider themselves to be healthy even though most have at least one chronic disease.

Malnutrition

Older adults are at disproportionate risk for inadequate intake and protein–calorie malnutrition.

- Unintentional weight loss and loss of appetite may be used to screen for malnutrition.
- Nutrition interventions that may improve intake and weight are: eating with others, increasing the nutrient density of foods consumed, and oral nutrition supplements between meals.

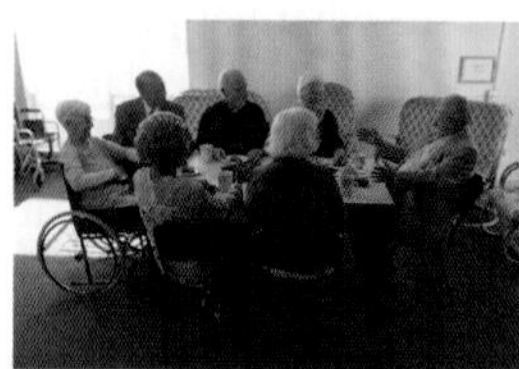

- Additional nutrition interventions for community dwelling adults: Congregate meals and Meals on Wheels provide low-cost, nutritious hot meals and opportunities for socialization.
- Additional nutrition interventions for long-term care residents: making mealtimes enjoyable, promoting independence in eating, using appropriate feeding strategies, and providing a liberal diet with few dietary restrictions may help prevent malnutrition and improve quality of life.
- **Obesity**: Obesity is a more prevalent weight issue than underweight. The appropriate obesity treatment for older adults is controversial.
- **Sarcopenia**: A progressive and generalized skeletal muscle disorder characterized by accelerated loss of muscle mass and insidious functional decline.

CHAPTER SUMMARY NUTRITION FOR OLDER ADULTS (continued)

- In part, sarcopenia may be caused by nutritional deficiencies, such as an inadequate intake of protein.
- It is not known whether protein and/or amino acid supplementation can effectively treat sarcopenia.
- Sarcopenic obesity refers to obesity with low skeletal muscle function and mass.

- **Frailty:** a condition characterized by weight loss and loss of muscle mass, weakness, poor endurance, exhaustion, slowness, and low activity.
  - Frailty can occur in people who are obese.
  - Nutrition therapy varies from protein–calorie supplements, planned weight loss, and vitamin D supplementation.
- **Alzheimer's disease:** A disease that is not a leading cause of death until after age 65. It has a devastating effect on nutritional intake.

Figure sources: *shutterstock.com/Oleksandra Naumenko, shutterstock.com/rkl_foto, shutterstock.com/wavebreakmedia*

Student Resources on thePoint®
For additional learning materials, activate the code in the front of this book at https://thePoint.lww.com/activate

Websites

Administration on Aging, Administration for Community Living at https://acl.gov/about-acl/administration-aging
Alzheimer's Association at www.alz.org
American Association of Retired Persons at www.aarp.org
The American Geriatrics Society at www.americangeriatrics.org
America's Health Rankings, United Health Foundation Senior Report at https://www.americashealthrankings.org/learn/reports/2019-senior-report
Arthritis Foundation at www.arthritis.org
A guide to completing the MNA-SF at www.mna-elderly.com/forms/mna_guide_english_sf.pdf
National Institute of Aging Information Office at www.nia.nih.gov

References

Amarya, S., Singh, K., & Sabharwal, M. (2015). Changes during aging and their association with malnutrition. *Journal of Clinical Gerontology and Geriatrics*, *6*(3), 78–84. https://doi.org/10.1016/jcgg2015.05.003

Assmann, K., Adjibade, M., Adnreeva, V., Hercberg, S., Galan, P., & Kesse-Guyot, E. (2018). Association between adherence to the Mediterranean diet at midlife and healthy aging in a cohort of French adults. *The Journals of Gerontology: Series A*, *73*(3), 347–354. https://doi.org/10.1093/gerona/glx066

Barazzoni, R., Bischoff, S., Boirie, Y., Busetto, L., Cederholm, T., Dicker, D., Toplak, H., Van Gossum, A., Yumuk, V., & Bettor, R. (2018). Sarcopenic obesity: Time to meet the challenge. *Obesity Facts*, *11*(4), 294–305. https://doi.org/10.1159/000490361

Batis, J., Mackenzie, T., Lopez-Jimenez, F., & Bartels, S. (2015). Sarcopenia, sarcopenic obesity, and functional impairments in older adults: National Health and Nutrition Examination Surveys 1999–2004. *Nutrition Research*, *35*(12), 1031–1039. https://doi.org/10.1016/j.nutres.2015.09.003

Bauer, J., Biolo, G., Cederholm, T., Cesari, M., Cruz-Jentoft, A. J., Morley, J. E., Phillips, S., Sieber, C., Stehle, P., Teta, D., Visvanathan, R., Volpi, E., & Boirie, Y. (2013). Evidence-based recommendations for optimal dietary protein intake in older people: A position paper from the PROT-AGE Study Group. *Journal of the American Medical Directors Association*, *14*(8), 542–559. https://doi.org/10.1016/j.jamda.2013.05.021

Bernstein, M., & Munoz, N. (2012). Position of the Academy of Nutrition and Dietetics: Food and nutrition for older adults—Promoting health and wellness. *Journal of the Academy of Nutrition and Dietetics*, *112*(8), 1255–1277. https://doi.org/10.1016/j.jand.2012.06.015

Bonaccio, M., De Castelnuovo, A., Costanzo, S., Gialluisi, A., Perichillo, M., Cerletti, C., Donati, M., de Gaetano, G., & Iacoviello, L. (2018). Mediterranean diet and mortality in the elderly: A prospective cohort study and a meta-analysis. *British Journal of Nutrition*, *120*(8), 841–854. https://doi.org/10.1017/S0007114518002179

Centers for Disease Control and Prevention. (2017, January 19). *Older persons' health*. National Center for Health Statistics. https://www.cdc.gov/nchs/fastats/older-american-health.htm

Chen, L.-K., Lee, W.-J., Peng, L.-N., Liu, L.-K., Arai, H., Akishita, M., & Asian Working Group for Sarcopenia. (2016). Recent advances in sarcopenia research in Asia: 2016 update from the Asian Working Group for Sarcopenia. *Journal of American Medical Directors Association*, *17*(8), 767. e1-767.e7. https://doi.org/10.1016/j.jamda.2016.05.016

Coker, R., & Wolfe, R. (2017). Weight loss strategies in the elderly: A clinical conundrum. *Obesity*, *26*(1), 22–28. https://doi.org/10.1002/oby.21961

Collard, R., Boter, H., Schoevers, R., & Oude Voshaar, R. (2012). Prevalence of frailty in community-dwelling older persons: A systematic review. *Journal of the American Geriatrics Society*, *60*(8), 1487–1492. https://doi.org/10.1111/j.1532-5415.2012.04054.x

Cruz-Jentof, A., Landi, F., Schneider, S., Zuniga, C., Arai, H., Boirie, Y., Chen, L.-K., Fielding, R., Martin, F., Michel, J.-P., Sieber, C., Stout, J., Studenski, S., Vellas, B., Woo, J., Zamboni, M., & Cederholm, T. (2014). Prevalence of and interventions for sarcopenia in ageing adults: A systematic review. Report of the International Sarcopenia Initiative (EWGSOP and IWGS). *Age and Ageing*, *43*(6), 748–759. https://doi.org/10.1093/ageing/afu115

Cruz-Jentoft, A., & Sayer, A. (2019). Sarcopenia. *Lancet*, *393*(10191), 2636–2646. https://doi.org/10.1016/S0140-6736(19)31138-9

Dent, E., Kowal, P., & Hoogendijk, E. (2016). Frailty measurement in research and clinical practice: A review. *European Journal of Internal Medicine*, *31*, 3–10. https://doi.org/10.1016/j.ejim.2016.03.007

Evans, W. (2010). Skeletal muscle loss: Cachexia, sarcopenia, and inactivity. *The American Journal of Clinical Nutrition, 91*(4), 1123S–1127S. https://doi.org/10.3945/ajcn.2010.28608A

Fielding, R., Vellas, B., Evans, W., Bhasin, S., Morley, J. E., Newman, A. B., van Kan, G., Andrieu, S., Bauer, J., Breuille, D., Cederholm, T., Chandler, J., De Meynard, C., Donini, L., Harris, T., Kannt, A., Guibert, F., Onder, G., Papanicolaou, D., ... Zamboni, M. (2011). Sarcopenia: An undiagnosed condition in older adults. Current consensus definition: Prevalence, etiology, and consequences. International Working Group on Sarcopenia. *Journal of the American Medical Directors Association, 12*(4), 249–256. https://doi.org/10.1016/j.jamda.2011.01.003

Fried, L., Tangen, C., Walston, J., Newman, A., Hirsch, C., Gottdiener, J., Seeman, T., Tracy, R., Kop, W., Burke, G., & McBurnie, M. A. (2001). Frailty in older adults: Evidence for a phenotype. *Journal of Gerontology: Series A, 56*(3), M146–M157. https://doi.org/10.1093/gerona/56.3.M146

Fryar, C., Carroll, M., & Ogden, C. (2018, September). *Prevalence of underweight among adults aged 20 and over: United States, 1960–1962 through 2015–2016.* National Center for Health Statistics, Health E-Stats. https://www.cdc.gov/nchs/data/hestat/underweight_adult_15_16/underweight_adult_15_16.pdf

Gahche, J., Bailey, R., Potischman, N., & Dwyer, J. (2017). Dietary supplement use was very high among older adults in the United States in 2011–2014. *Journal of Nutrition, 147*(10), 1968–1976. https://doi.org/10.3945/jn.117.255984

Gentile, S., Lacroix, O., Durand, A., Cretel, E., Alazia, M., Sambuc, R., & Bonin-Guillaume, S. (2013). Malnutrition: A highly predictive risk factor of short-term mortality in elderly presenting to the emergency department. *The Journal of Nutrition, Health, and Aging, 17,* 290–294. https://doi.org/10.1007/s12603-012-0398-0

Gingrich, A., Spiegel, A., Gradl, J., Skurk, T., Hauner, H., Sieber, C., Volkert, D., & Kiesswetter, E. (2019). Daily and per-meal animal and plant protein intake in relation to muscle mass in healthy older adults without functional limitations: An enable study. *Aging Clinical and Experimental Research, 31,* 1271–1281. https://doi.org/10.1007/s40520-018-1081-z

Hauner, H. (2005). Secretory factors from human adipose tissue and their functional role. *Proceedings of the Nutrition Society, 64*(2), 163–169. https://doi.org/10.1079/PNS2005428

Heron, M. (2019, June 24). Deaths: Leading causes for 2017. *National Vital Statistics Reports, 68*(6), 1–77. Retrieved August 3, 2020, from https://www.cdc.gov/nchs/data/nvsr/nvsr68/nvsr68_06-508.pdf

Holick, M., Binkley, N., Bischoll-Ferrari, H., Gordon, C., Hanley, D. A., Heaney, R. P., Murad, M. H., & Weaver, C. M. (2011). Evaluation, treatment, and prevention of vitamin D deficiency: An Endocrine Society clinical practice guideline. *The Journal of Clinical Endocrinology and Metabolism, 96*(7), 1911–1930. https://doi.org/10.1210/jc.2011-0385

Hosking, D., Eramudugolla, R., Cherbuin, N., & Anstey, K. (2019). MIND not Mediterranean diet related to 12-year incidence of cognitive impairment in an Australian longitudinal cohort study. *Alzheimer's & Dementia: The Journal of the Alzheimer's Association, 15*(4), 581–589. https://doi.org/10.1016/j.jalz.2018.12.011

Houston, D. K., Nicklas, B., Ding, J., Harris, T. B., Tylavsky, F. A., Newman, A. B., Lee, J. S., Sahyoun, N., Visser, M., Kritchevsky, S. B., & Health ABC Study. (2008). Dietary protein intake is associated with lean mass change in older, community-dwelling adults: The Health, Aging, and Body Composition (Health ABC) Study. *The American Journal of Clinical Nutrition, 87*(1), 150–155. https://doi.org/10.1093/ajcn/87.1.150

Institute of Medicine. (1998). *Dietary reference intakes for thiamin, riboflavin, niacin, vitamin B_6, folate, vitamin B_{12}, pantothenic acid, biotin, and choline.* The National Academies Press.

Institute of Medicine. (2005). *Dietary reference intakes for energy, carbohydrate, fiber, fat, fatty acids, cholesterol, protein, and amino acids (macronutrients).* The National Academies Press.

Isanejad, M., Mursu, J., Sirola, J.,Kroger, H., Rikkonen, T., Tuppurainen, M., & Erkkila, A. (2016). Dietary protein intake is associated with better physical function and muscle strength among elderly women. *British Journal of Nutrition, 11*(suppl 7), 1281–1291. https://doi.org/10.1017/S000711451600012X

Luciano, M., Corley, J., Cox, S., Valdes Hernandez, M., Craig, L., Dickie, D., Karama, S., McNeill, G., Bastin, M., Wardlaw, J., & Deary, I. (2017). Mediterranean-type diet and brain structural change from 73 to 76 years in a Scottish cohort. *Neurology, 88*(5), 449–455. https://doi.org/10.1212/WNL.0000000000003559

Marshall, S., Young, A., Bauer, J., & Isenring, E. (2016). Malnutrition in geriatric rehabilitation: Prevalence, patient outcomes, and criterion validity of the Scored Patient-Generated Subjective Global Assessment and the Mini Nutritional Assessment. *Journal of the Academy of Nutrition and Dietetics, 116*(5), 785–794. https://doi.org/10.1016/j.jand.2015.06.013

Mayhew, A., Amog, K., Phillips, S., Parise, G., McNicholas, P., de Souza, R., Thabane, I., & Raina, P. (2019). The prevalence of sarcopenia in community-dwelling older adults, an exploration of differences between studies and within definitions: A systematic review and meta-analyses. *Age and Ageing, 48*(1), 48–56. https://doi.org/10.1093/ageing/afy106

McEvoy, C., Guyer, H., Langa, K., & Yaffe, K. (2017). Neuroprotective diets are associated with better cognitive function: The health and retirement study. *Journal of the American Geriatrics Society, 65*(8), 1857–1862. https://doi.org/10.1111/jgs.14922

Meehan, M., & Penckofer, S. (2014). The role of vitamin D in the aging adult. *Journal of Aging and Gerontology, 2*(2), 60–71. https://doi.org/10.12974/2309-6128.2014.02.02.1

Messier, S., Pater, M., Beavers, D., Legault, C., Loeser, R., Hunter, D., & DeVita, P. (2014). Influences of alignment and obesity on knee joint loading in osteoarthritis gait. *Osteoarthritis and Cartilage, 22*(7), 912–917. https://doi.org/10.1016/j.joca.2014.05.013

Mohajeri, M., Troesch, B., & Weber, P. (2015). Inadequate supply of vitamins and DHA in the elderly: Implications for brain aging and Alzheimer-type dementia. *Nutrition, 31*(2), 261–275. https://doi.org/10.1016/j.nut.2014.06.016

Morley, J., Vellas, B., van Kan, G., Anker, S. D., Bauer, J. M., Bernabei, R., Cesari, M., Chumlea, W., Doehner, W., Evans, J., Fried, L., Guralnik, J., Katz, P., Malmstrom, T., McCarter, R., Robledo, L., Rockwood, K., von Haehling, S., Vanewoude, M., & Walston, J. (2013). Frailty consensus: A call to action. *Journal of the American Medical Directors Association, 14*(6), 392–397. https://doi.org/10.1016/j.jamda.2013.03.022

Morris, M. C., Tangney, C. C., Wang, Y., Sacks, F. M., Barnes, L. L., Bennett, D. A., & Aggarwal, N. T. (2015a). MIND diet slows cognitive decline with aging. *Alzheimer's & Dementia: The Journal of the Alzheimer's Association, 11*(9), 1015–1022. https://doi.org/10.1016/j.jalz.2015.04.011

Morris, M. C., Tangney, C. C., Wang, Y., Sacks, F. M., Bennett, D. A., & Aggarwal, N. T. (2015b). MIND diet associated with reduced incidence of Alzheimer's disease. *Alzheimer's & Dementia: The Journal of the Alzheimer's Association, 11*(9), 1007–1014. https://doi.org/10.1016/j.jalz.2014.11.009

Mosconi, L., Murray, J., Davies, M., Davies, M., Williams, S., Pirraglia, E., Spector, N., Tsui, W., Li, Y., Butler, T., Osorio, R., Glodzik, L., Vallabhajosula, S., McHugh, P., Marmar, C., & de Leon, M. (2014). Nutrient intake and brain biomarkers of Alzheimer's disease in at-risk cognitively normal individuals: A cross-sectional neuroimaging pilot study. *British Medical Journal Open, 4*(6), e004850. https://doi.org/10.1136/bmjopen-2014-004850

National Institute on Aging & National Institutes of Health. (2019, December 24). *What causes Alzheimer's disease?* https://www.nia.nih.gov/health/what-causes-alzheimers-disease#genetics

Pike, A. (2019, January 15). *What is the MIND diet?* International Food Information Council Foundation. https://foodinsight.org/what-is-the-mind-diet/

Porter Starr, K. N., McDonald, S. R., Weidner, J. A., & Bales, C. W. (2016). Challenges in the management of geriatric obesity in high risk populations. *Nutrients, 8*(5), 262. https://doi.org/10.3390/nu8050262

Rahi, B., Ajana, S., & Tabue-Teguo, M. (2018). High adherence to a Mediterranean diet and lower risk of frailty among French older adults community-dwellers: Results from the Three-City-Bordeaux Study. *Clinical Nutrition, 37*(4), 1293–1298. https://doi.org/10.1016/j.clnu.2017.05.020

Rodriguez, N. (2015). Introduction of Protein Summit 2.0: Continued exploration of the impact of high-quality protein on optimal health. *The American Journal of Clinical Nutrition, 101*(6), 1317S–1319S. https://doi.org/10.39445/ajcn.114.083980

Saffel-Shrier, S., Johnson, M. A., & Francis, S. (2019). Position of the Academy of Nutrition and Dietetics and the Society for Nutrition Education and Behavior: Food and nutrition programs for community-residing older adults. *Journal of the Academy of Nutrition and Dietetics, 119*(7), 1188–1204. https://doi.org/10.1016/j.jand.2019.03.011

Samieri, C., Sun, Q., Townsend, M., Chiuve, S. E., Okereke, O. I., Willett, W. C., Stampfer, M., & Grodstein, F. (2013). The association between dietary patterns at midlife and health in aging: An observational study. *Annals of Internal Medicine, 159*(9), 584–591. https://doi.org/10.7326/0003-4819-159-9-201311050-00004

Shlisky, J., Bloom, D. E., Beaudreault, A. R., Tucker, K. L., Keller, H. H., Freund-Levi, Y., Fielding, R. A., Cheng, F. W., Jensen, G. L., Wu, D., & Meydani, S. N. (2017). Nutritional considerations for healthy aging and reduction in age-related chronic disease. *Advances in Nutrition* (Bethesda, Md.), *8*(1), 17–26. https://doi.org/10.3945/an.116.013474

Skipper, A., Coltman, A., Tomesko, J., Charney, P., Porcari, J., Piemonte, T., Handu, D., & Cheng, F. (2020). Position of the Academy of Nutrition and Dietetics: Malnutrition (undernutrition) screening tools for all adults. *Journal of the Academy of Nutrition and Dietetics, 120*(4), 709–713. https://doi.org/10.1016/j.jand.2019.09.011

Sun, Q., Townsend, M., Okereke, O., Franco, O. H., Hu, F. B., & Grodstein, F. (2009). Adiposity and weight change in mid-life in relation to healthy survival after age 70 in women: Prospective cohort study. *British Medical Journal, 339*, b3796. https://doi.org/10.1136/bmj.b3796

Thomas, S., Browne, H., Mobasheri, A., & Rayman, M. (2018). What is the evidence for a role for diet and nutrition in osteoarthritis? *Rheumatology, 57*(supple 4), iv61–iv74. https://doi.org/10.1093/rheumatology/key011

Traylor, D., Gorissen, S., & Phillips, S. (2018). Perspective: Protein requirements and optimal intakes in aging—Are we ready to recommend more than the Recommended Daily Allowance? *Advances in Nutrition, 9*(13), 171–182. https://doi.org/10.1093/advances/nmy003

Trichopoulou, A., Bamia, C., & Trichopoulos, D. (2009). Anatomy of health effects of Mediterranean diet: Greek EPIC prospective cohort study. *British Medical Journal, 338*, b2337. https://doi.org/10.1136/bmj.b2337

Trichopoulou, A., Martínez-González, M., Tong, T., Forouhi, N., Khandelwal, S., Prabhakaran, D., Mozaffarian, D., & de Lorgeril, M. (2014). Definitions and potential health benefits of the Mediterranean diet: Views from experts around the world. *BioMed Central Medicine, 12*, 112. https://doi.org/10.1186/1741-7015-12-112

United Health Foundation. (2019). 2019 senior report. https://www.americashealthrankings.org/learn/reports/2019-senior-report

United States Department of Agriculture & U.S. Department of Health and Human Services. (2020, December). *Dietary guidelines for Americans, 2020–2025*. https://www.dietaryguidelines.gov

U.S. Department of Agriculture. (2019, January 31). *HEI scores for Americans*. Food and Nutrition Service. https://www.fns.usda.gov/hei-scores-americans

U.S. Department of Agriculture & Agricultural Research Service. (2018). Nutrient intakes from food and beverages: Mean amounts consumed per individual, by gender and age. What we eat in America, NHANES 2015–2016. https://www.ars.usda.gov/ARSUserFiles/80400530/pdf/1516/Table_1_NIN_GEN_15.pdf

U.S. Department of Health and Human Services. (2018). *Physical activity guidelines for Americans* (2nd ed.). https://health.gov/sites/default/files/2019-09/Physical_Activity_Guidelines_2nd_edition.pdf

U.S. Department of Health and Human Services. (2019, December 24). *What causes Alzheimer's disease?* National Institute on Aging. https://www.nia.nih.gov/health/what-causes-alzheimers-disease#genetics

U.S. Department of Health and Human Services & Administration on Aging. (2018). 2017 Profile of older Americans. https://acl.gov/sites/default/files/Aging%20and%20Disability%20in%20America/2017OlderAmericansProfile.pdf

Verlaan, S., Ligthart-Melis, G., Wijers, S., Cederholm, T., Maier, A., & van der Schueren, M. (2017). High prevalence of physical frailty among community-dwelling malnourished older adults: A systematic review and meta-analysis. *Journal of Post-Acute and Long-Term Care Medicine, 18*(5), 374–382. https://doi.org/10.1016/j.jamda.2016.12.074

White, J., Guenter, P., Jensen, G., Malone, A., Schofield, M., Academy of Nutrition and Dietetics Malnutrition Work Group; ASPEN Malnutrition Task Force, and the ASPEN Board of Directors. (2012). Consensus statement of the Academy of Nutrition and Dietetics and American Society for Parenteral and Enteral Nutrition: Characteristics recommended for the identification and documentation of adult malnutrition (undernutrition). *Journal of Parenteral and Enteral Nutrition, 36*(3), 275–283. https://doi.org/10.1177/0148607112440285

Wolfe, R., Cifelli, A., Kostas, G., & Kim, I.-L. (2017). Optimizing protein intake in adults: Interpretation and application of the Recommended Dietary Allowance compared with the Acceptable Macronutrient Distribution Range. *Advances in Nutrition, 8*(2), 266–274. https://doi.org/10.3945/an.116.013821

World Health Organization. (2005). *Preventing Chronic Diseases a vital investment*. https://www.who.int/chp/chronic_disease_report/contents/part1.pdf.

UNIT THREE

Nutrition in Clinical Practice

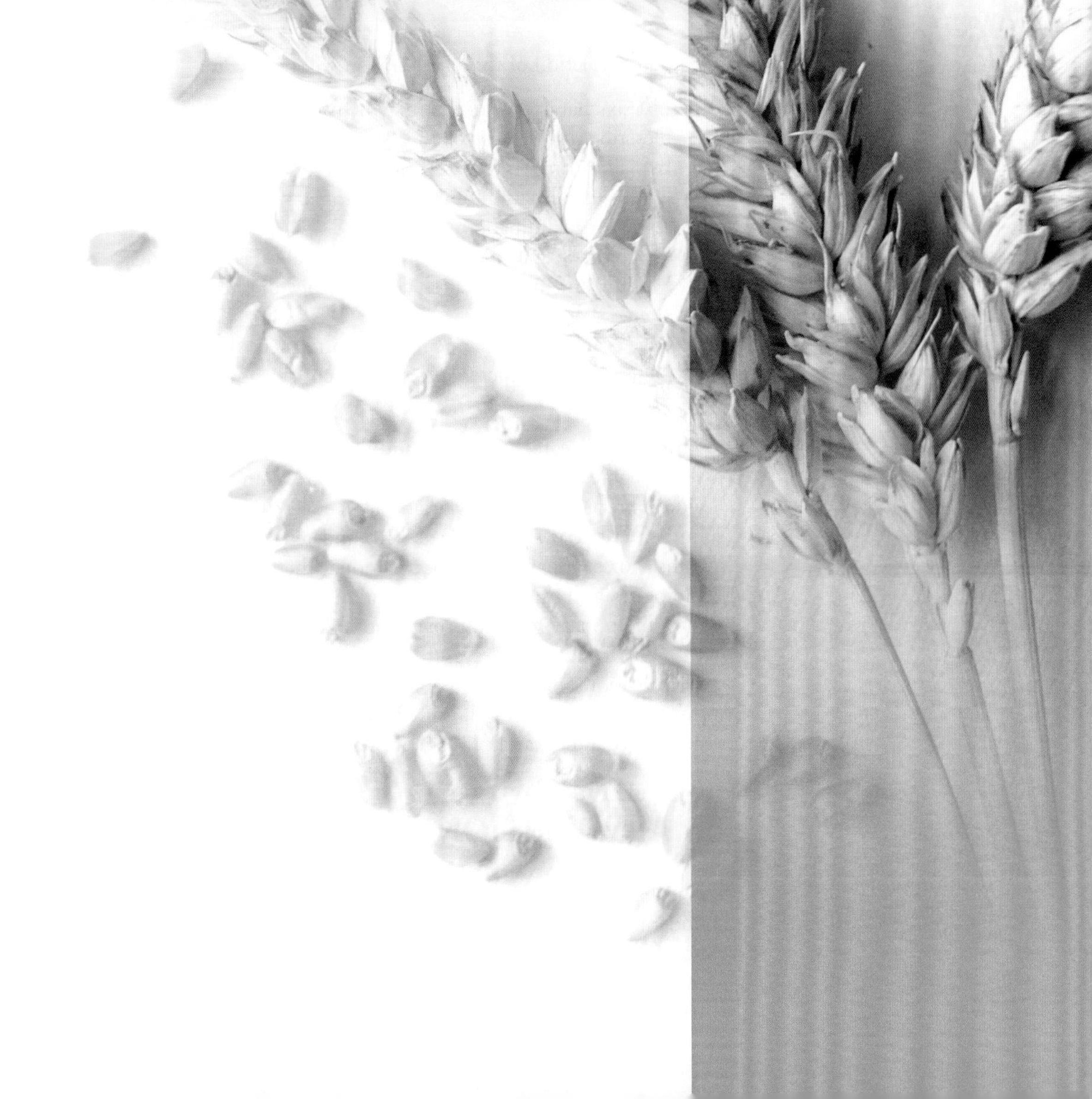

Chapter 15

Hospital Nutrition: Identifying Nutrition Risk and Feeding Clients

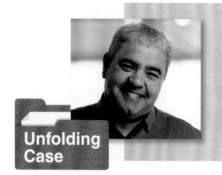

Miguel Hernandez

Miguel Hernandez is a 46-year-old man admitted to the hospital for a laminectomy. Over the past month, he has experienced considerable pain to the point where he restricts his activity and has lost his appetite. He is 5 ft 10 in. tall and weighs 193 pounds, down from his usual weight of 209 pounds. He has a history of type 2 diabetes. The plan is for him to be discharged the day after surgery to ensure his blood glucose levels are controlled.

Learning Objectives

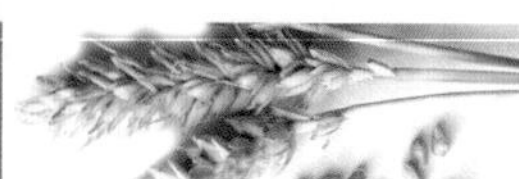

Upon completion of this chapter, you will be able to:

1 List six characteristics that may be used to diagnose malnutrition.
2 Describe the purpose of a nutrition screen.
3 Explain nutrition therapy guidelines for clients at nutrition risk.
4 Discuss information obtained during a nursing history and physical that can be used to assess for malnutrition.
5 Suggest strategies to promote an optimal intake in clients.
6 Modify a menu to an altered consistency diet (e.g., clear liquid, pureed diet, mechanically altered diet).
7 Give examples of therapeutic diets and their uses.
8 Describe the characteristics of different categories of oral nutrition supplements.

Through all degrees of health and illness, understanding and applying nutrition knowledge and skills enable all members of the health care team to effectively evaluate nutrition status and provide appropriate care (DiMaria-Ghalili et al., 2014). Client care is improved when evidence-based nutrition care is synchronized with and reinforced by all health professionals, including physicians, nurses, pharmacists, occupational therapists, physical therapists, speech and language pathologists, and psychologists. Although the dietitian is the primary nutrition authority, it takes an interdisciplinary team to provide optimal nutrition care.

This chapter serves as the introduction to clinical nutrition, covering the prevalence of malnutrition among hospitalized clients and how it is identified and treated, how nutrition is integrated throughout the nursing care process, and the optimal approach for feeding clients, namely, oral diets and oral nutritional supplements (ONS).

MALNUTRITION

Malnutrition
literally, bad nutrition. In practice, malnutrition refers specifically to protein–calorie undernutrition.

The primary focus of clinical nutrition is to prevent or treat malnutrition (or protein–calorie undernutrition in this context). **Malnutrition** is a common and often unrecognized problem among hospitalized clients. Whether clients are admitted with malnutrition or it develops during the course of hospitalization, malnutrition is estimated to affect 20% to 50% of adult hospitalized clients in the United States (Jensen et al., 2013). Among clients undergoing surgery, an estimated 24% to 65%

are at nutrition risk (Wischmeyer et al., 2018). In practice, as few as 5% to 8% of clients receive a documented or coded diagnosis of malnutrition during their hospitalization (Tobert et al., 2018).

Malnutrition is a major contributor to morbidity and mortality, impaired function, decreased quality of life, increased frequency and length of hospital stay, and higher health care costs (White et al., 2012). Suboptimal nutritional status is also a strong independent predictor of poor postoperative outcomes (Wischmeyer et al., 2018). The deleterious effect of malnutrition not only affects virtually all organ systems but can also impair cognitive ability, leaving clients unable to make independent, informed consent when they are in a severely compromised nutritional state (Russo et al., 2016).

Diagnosis of Malnutrition

The Academy of Nutrition and Dietetics and the American Society of Parenteral and Enteral Nutrition (ASPEN) have proposed that clients who have at least two of the following six criteria are malnourished (White et al., 2012):

- inadequate calorie intake
- unintentional weight loss
- loss of muscle mass
- loss of subcutaneous fat
- localized or generalized fluid accumulation that may mask weight loss
- diminished functional status as measured by handgrip strength

Malnutrition is classified as severe or non-severe (moderate) based on specific thresholds and/or descriptions for each of the above criteria.

The etiology-based approach for defining malnutrition involves assessing the client for the presence of inflammation, a potent contributor to disease-related malnutrition (Fig. 15.1) (Malone & Hamilton, 2013).

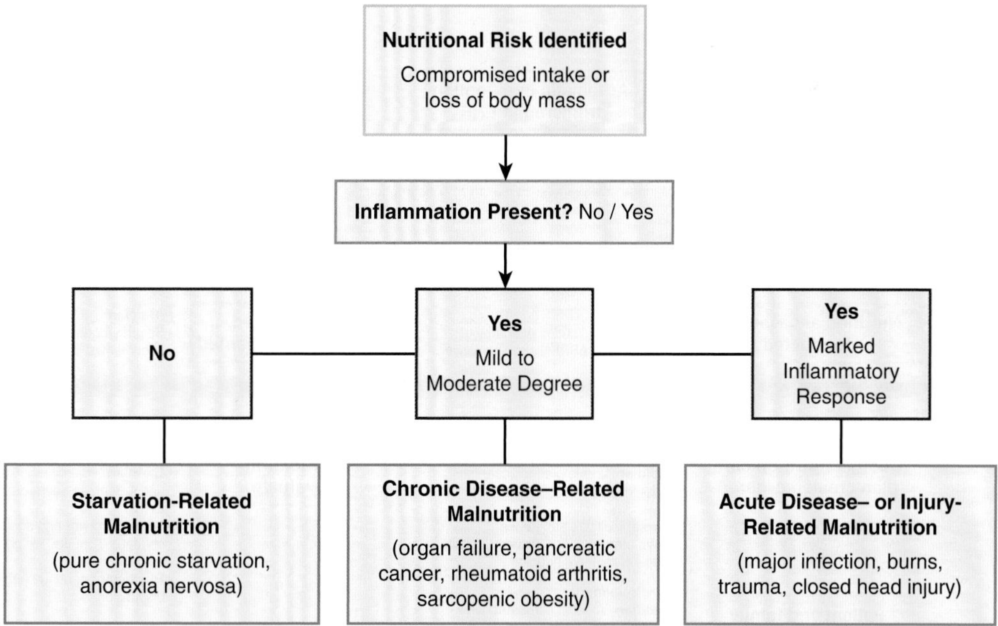

Figure 15.1 ▲ Etiology-based malnutrition definitions. (*Source:* White, J., Guenter, P., Jensen, G., Malone, A., & Schofield, M., Academy of Nutrition and Dietetics Malnutrition Work Group, ASPEN Malnutrition Task Force, and the ASPEN Board of Directors. [2012]. Consensus statement of the Academy of Nutrition and Dietetics and American Society for Parenteral and Enteral Nutrition: Characteristics recommended for the identification and documentation of adult malnutrition (undernutrition). *Journal of the Academy of Nutrition and Dietetics, 112*[5], 730–738. https://doi.org/10.1016/j.jand.2012.03.012)

- **Starvation-related** malnutrition occurs when food is not available due to environmental or social circumstances. Inflammation is absent. It usually develops slowly and may be caused by abuse, neglect, famine, poverty, or disordered eating (Skipper, 2012).
- **Chronic disease–related** malnutrition may occur in clients with diseases such as congestive heart failure or chronic obstructive pulmonary disease. A mild to moderate degree of inflammation impedes appetite, intake, or nutrient utilization.
- **Acute disease–related or injury-related** malnutrition may occur in clients with critical illness, multi-trauma, or major infection due to a marked inflammatory response. These clients may be adequately nourished upon admission but are at high risk for malnutrition due to the nature of their illness.

Timely identification and treatment of malnutrition is critical to improving client outcomes (Field & Hand, 2015). The process of identification begins with nutrition screening and continues with a nutrition assessment and individualized nutrition care plan as needed. Figure 15.2 illustrates the interdisciplinary approach to nutrition care.

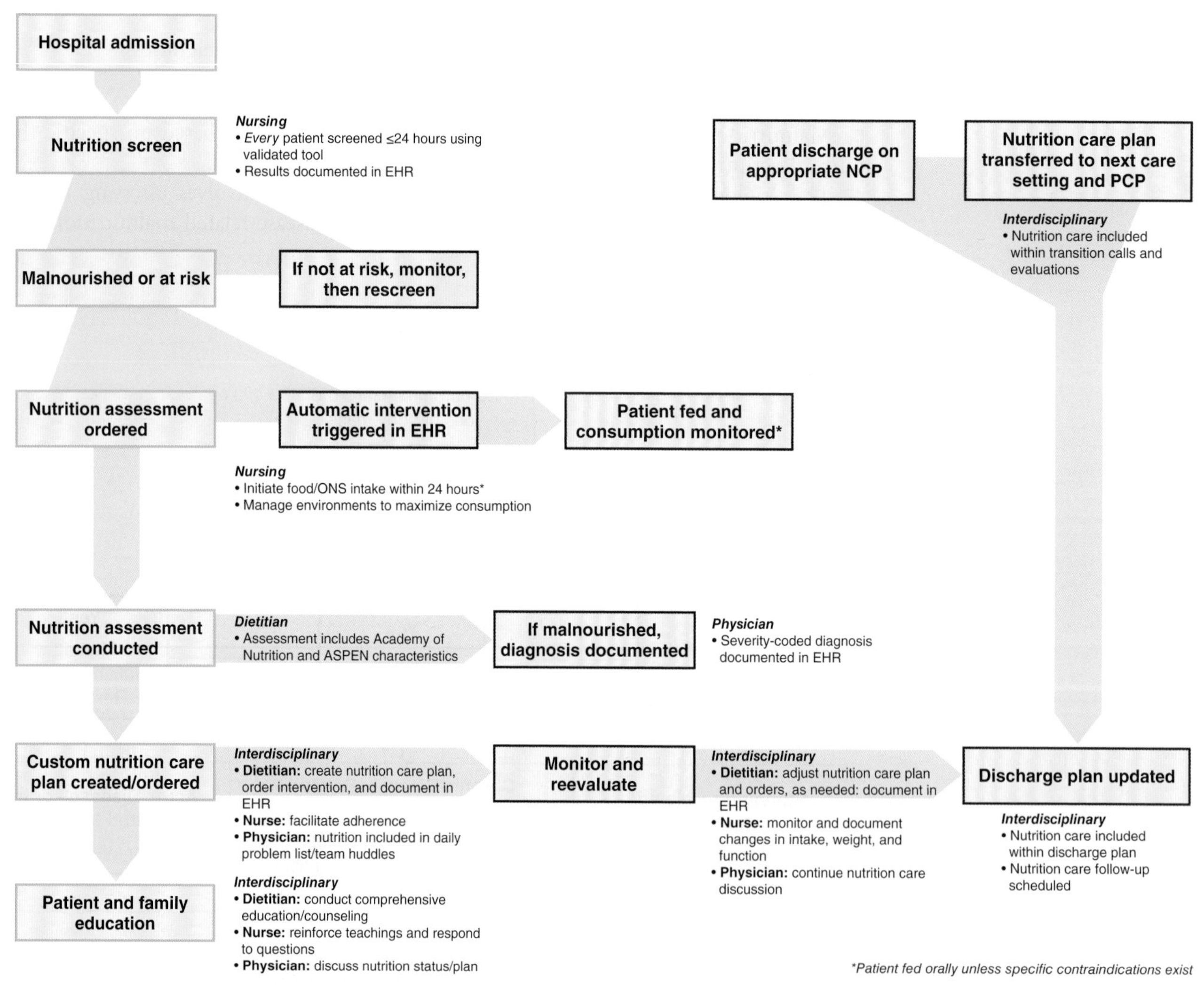

Figure 15.2 ▲ The Alliance to Advance Patient Nutrition approach to interdisciplinary nutrition care. (*Source:* Tappenden, K. A., Quatrara, B., Parkhurst, M. L., Malone, A. M., Fanjiang, G., & Ziegler, T. R. [2013]. Critical role of nutrition in improving quality of care: An interdisciplinary call to action to address adult hospital malnutrition. *Journal of the Academy of Nutrition and Dietetics, 113*[9], 1219–1237. https://doi.org/10.1016/j.jand.2013.05.015)

Nutrition Screening

Nutrition Screening
a quick look at a few variables to judge a client's relative risk for nutritional problems. Nutrition screening can be general for malnutrition or custom designed for a particular population (e.g., pregnant women).

Nutrition screening is used to identify clients at risk for malnutrition and those who are likely to benefit from further assessment and intervention. Note that when a client is found *not* to be at risk for malnutrition, it does not mean the client is without health risks. For instance, a client admitted with symptoms of a myocardial infarction may not have malnutrition but may still be at high risk for morbidity and mortality related to the admitting diagnosis.

Screening Protocol

The Joint Commission, a nonprofit organization that sets health care standards and accredits health care facilities that meet those standards, specifies that nutrition screening must be conducted within 24 hours after admission to a hospital or other health care facility.

- Because the standard applies 24 hours a day, seven days a week, staff nurses are usually responsible for completing the screen as part of the admission process.
- Each facility is able to determine the criteria it uses for screening, who completes nutrition screening, and when rescreening is required.
- Clients identified as at risk for malnutrition are referred to a dietitian for further nutrition assessment, diagnosis, and intervention.
- Clients determined to be at low risk are rescreened within a specified time frame to identify if changes in risk have developed (Field & Hand, 2015).

Screening Tools

A number of screening tools are available.

- Tools vary in their intended population (e.g., adults or older adults), intended setting (e.g., hospital or community settings), levels of agreement, reliability, generalizability, complexity, and validity (Skipper et al., 2020).
- To be useful, screening tools should be quick, simple, valid (sensitive and specific), and reliable and done regularly to identify changes in risk (Field & Hand, 2015).
- Criteria that often comprise a screening tool are recent weight loss, recent food intake, and current body mass index (BMI); disease severity may also be included (Rasmussen et al., 2010).
- An example of a widely used validated tool for screening adults, including older adults, in inpatient and outpatient settings is the Malnutrition Screening Tool (MST) (Fig. 15.3). It consists of only two criteria that are scored to determine at risk status.

Figure 15.3 ▶ Malnutrition Screening Tool. (*Source:* Ferguson, M., Capra, S., Bauer, J., & Banks, M. [1998, August 30]. Development of a valid and reliable malnutrition screening tool for adult acute hospital patients. *Nutrition, 15*[6]. 458–464. https://doi.org/10.1016/S0899-9007(99)00084-2)

MALNUTRITION SCREENING TOOL	
Have you lost weight recently without trying?	
No	0
Unsure	2
If yes, how much weight (kilograms) have you lost?	
1–5	1
6–10	2
11–15	3
>15	4
Unsure	2
Have you been eating poorly because of a decreased appetite?	
No	0
Yes	1
Total	

Score of 2 or more = patient at risk of malnutrition.

- The Academy of Nutrition and Dietetics recommends the MST as the single tool to screen adults for malnutrition (undernutrition) regardless of their age, medical history, or the setting (Skipper et al., 2020).

Think of Miguel. Based on findings from his health assessment, is he at nutrition risk according to the MST (Fig. 15.3)?

NUTRITION ASSESSMENT

Clients found to be at risk for malnutrition through screening are referred to a dietitian for a comprehensive nutritional assessment to identify specific risks or confirm the existence of malnutrition. **Nutrition assessment** encompasses the nutrition care process and its four steps (Fig. 15.4). While nurses use the same problem-solving model to develop nursing or multidisciplinary care plans that may integrate nutrition, the nutritional care plan created by dietitians is specific for nutrition problems. Box 15.1 identifies activities of the dietitian.

Nutrition Assessment
an in-depth analysis of a person's nutritional status. In the clinical setting, nutritional assessments focus on at-risk clients with suspected or confirmed protein–energy malnutrition.

Nutrition Therapy for Clients at Nutritional Risk

An adequate intake of calories and protein is the focus of nutrition therapy for clients at nutritional risk. When protein intake is inadequate, loss of lean body mass occurs and recovery and quality of life are impaired. Calories are essential for sparing protein from being used for energy, yet glucose without protein (e.g., simple IV solutions of dextrose and water) cannot promote anabolism (Wischmeyer et al., 2018). Both calories and protein are needed to maintain lean body mass and weight.

Dietitians may use the following general guidelines to calculate a nutrition prescription that is then individualized according to the client's nutritional status and response to feedings:

- **Calories:** A simple method of estimating calorie needs is to multiply a person's weight in kilograms by a factor appropriate for the medical condition. A range frequently used is 25 to 30 cal/kg/day. Calories per kilogram are adjusted upward or downward as appropriate for the client's condition or response to nutrition therapy.
  - Other predictive equations are available to estimate resting energy expenditure (REE) such as the Mifflin-St Jeor equation (see Chapter 8). REE is then multiplied by factors to account for activity and degree of physiologic stress.
  - Indirect calorimetry, which measures oxygen consumption and carbon dioxide production, is the reference standard for determining calorie expenditure in critically ill patients and in patients who fail to respond to presumed adequate nutrition support (Mtaweh et al., 2018). It provides a more accurate estimate of energy needs than predictive equations, but it is not always available, necessary, or feasible.
- **Protein:** Ensure adequate protein intake.
  - Actual protein need varies with the client's medical condition. For instance, clients with cancer may need 1.2 to 1.5 g protein/kg/day to help maintain or restore lean body mass (Arends et al., 2017) and postsurgical clients may need 1.5 to 2.0 g/kg/day (Wischmeyer et al., 2018). Protein is more of a priority for postsurgical clients than is total calorie intake.
  - To achieve an adequate protein intake, high-protein ONS may be recommended 2 to 3 times/day.
- **Feeding method:** Clients who are unable to consume at least 50% of their protein and calorie goals orally may require enteral nutrition support.
  - Parenteral nutrition is considered only if the oral and enteral routes are inadequate or unavailable.

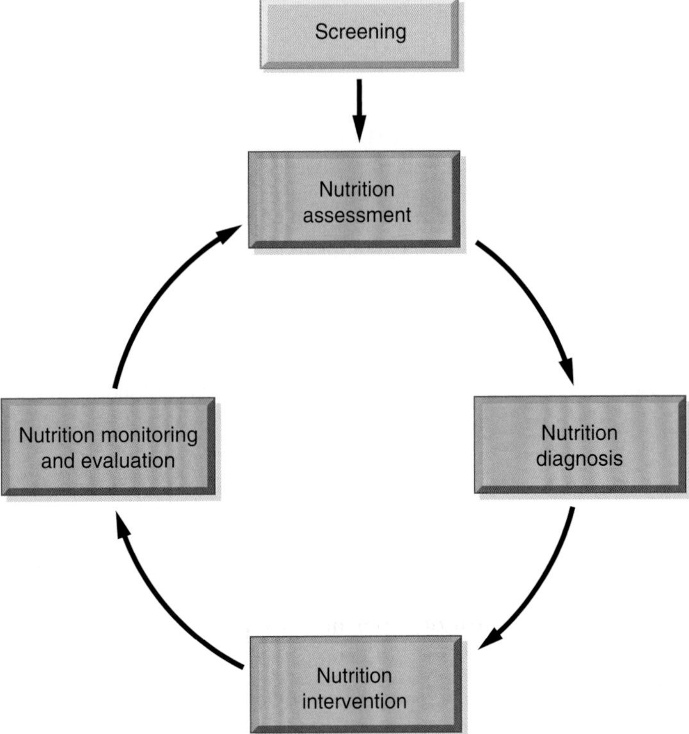

Figure 15.4 ▶
The nutrition care process. Like the nursing process, the nutrition care process is a problem-solving method used to evaluate and treat nutrition-related problems.

BOX 15.1 Activities of the Dietitian

- Dietitians interview clients and/or families to obtain a nutrition history which can help differentiate nutrition problems caused by inadequate intake from those related to disease.
  - A nutrition history may include information on
    - current dietary habits,
    - recent changes in intake or appetite,
    - usual snack and meal pattern,
    - alcohol intake,
    - food allergies and intolerances,
    - ethnic, cultural, or religious diet influences, and
    - nutrition knowledge and beliefs.
- They calculate estimated calorie and protein requirements based on the assessment data and determine whether the diet ordered is adequate and appropriate for the client.
- They determine nutrition diagnoses that define the nutritional problem, etiology, and signs and symptoms. While a nursing analysis statement may be malnutrition risk a nutrition diagnosis would be more specific, such as, "inadequate protein-energy intake."
- Dietitians determine the appropriate malnutrition diagnosis code for the client for hospital reimbursement purposes.
- They determine the appropriate nutrition intervention, such as a nutrition prescription detailing specific recommendation regarding diet, calorie intake, or feeding method, nutrition education, and coordination of nutrition care.

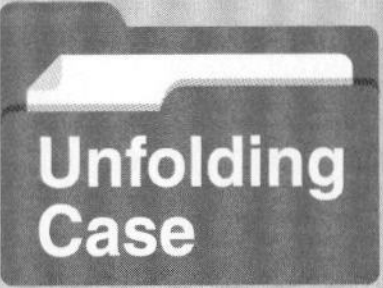

Think of Miguel. Using the general guidelines, how many calories does he need? How much protein? Does a regular oral diet provide Miguel with all the protein he needs? Is he a good candidate for ONS?

NURSING PROCESS Malnutrition

Neil Stein is 42 years old, 5 ft 11 in. tall, and has weighed 185 pounds for most of his adult life. He was diagnosed with acute myelogenous leukemia 7 weeks ago and spent 31 days in the hospital for the first round of chemotherapy. He is admitted to the hospital for a week of chemotherapy that starts with his admission. His admitting weight is 162 pounds. He appears thin and fatigued. He complains of nausea, anxiety, taste changes, and poor appetite. His weight loss and loss of appetite qualify him for a diagnosis of malnutrition.

Assessment

Medical–Psychosocial History
- Medical history that may have nutritional implications, such as diabetes or GI disorders
- Medications that may affect nutrition
- Current treatment plan
- Other symptoms Neil is experiencing related to leukemia or its treatment

Anthropometric Assessment
- Current BMI
- Percent weight loss

Biochemical and Physical Assessment
- Check abnormal laboratory values for their nutritional significance.
- Assess body fat, muscle mass, handgrip.
- Assess blood pressure.

Dietary Assessment
- How many meals do you consume daily?
- Do you avoid any foods?
- What foods do you eat most often?
- Do you feel hungry?
- Do you use ONS?
- How do you compensate for taste alterations?
- Does he understand the importance of eating an adequate intake?
- Did you have any dietary restrictions before being diagnosed with leukemia?

Analysis

Possible Nursing Analysis

Malnutrition risk related to poor intake and other side effects from cancer and cancer treatment as evidenced by weight loss

Planning

Client Outcomes

The client will
- maintain his weight,
- consume three meals each day,
- consume three ONS each day, and
- verbalize the importance of consuming an adequate calorie and protein intake.

Nursing Interventions

Nutrition Therapy
- Provide a regular diet as prescribed.
- Encourage alternate selections when the menu does not offer desirable foods.
- Encourage consumption of the ONS.

Client Teaching
- Instruct the client on the following:
- Eating plan essentials:
  - The importance of eating an adequate intake to maintain weight
  - The importance of consuming adequate protein to restore lean body mass
  - The importance of consuming the ONS
- Behavioral matters:
  - Relying entirely on ONS, which can provide complete nutrition, if unable to consume solid foods
  - Thinking of food as medicine, not as a pleasurable option

NURSING PROCESS

Malnutrition (continued)

Evaluation

Evaluate and Monitor

- Monitor weight and intake.
- Assess tolerance to regular diet.
- Monitor tolerance to ONS.
- Need for additional nutrition counseling.

NUTRITION IN THE NURSING PROCESS

Nutrition has been an integral component of nursing care since Florence Nightingale noted nutrition as the second most important area for nursing (Nightingale, 1992). Until the dietetics profession was founded, nurses were responsible for preparing and serving food to the sick. Today, nurses play a vital role in creating a culture that values nutrition and in achieving successful nutrition-related client outcomes (Tappenden et al., 2013). Nurses are often responsible for nutrition screening, integrate nutrition into nursing care plans, and obtain assessment data that dietitians use in completing nutrition assessments. The following sections are intended to help nurses provide quality nursing care that includes basic nutrition, rather than help nurses become dietitians.

Nursing Assessment

Dietitians may obtain much of their preliminary assessment data about the client from the nursing history and physical examination, such as skin integrity, problems chewing, swallowing, or self-feeding, use of supplements and over-the-counter medications, and living situation. Dietitians rely on nurses for ongoing monitoring and documentation of changes in intake, weight, and function.

Medical–Psychosocial History

The chief complaint and medical history may reveal disease-related risks for malnutrition and the presence of inflammation (see Fig. 15.1).

- Medical conditions often associated with malnutrition include AIDS, alcoholism, cancer, cardiovascular disease, celiac disease, chronic kidney disease, diabetes, liver disease, and dementia and other mental illness.
- Among surgical clients, the risk of malnutrition is often most significant after major gastrointestinal (GI) and oncologic surgery (Wischmeyer et al., 2018).
- Box 15.2 lists psychosocial factors that may affect intake or requirements and may help identify nutrition counseling needs.

Body Mass Index (BMI) an index of weight in relation to height that is calculated mathematically by dividing weight in kilograms by the square of height in meters. BMI interpretations are as follows:

<18.5	Underweight
18.5–24.9	Healthy weight
25–29.9	Overweight
≥30	Obese

Height, Weight, and Body Mass Index

Weight status, as determined by **BMI**, is an important factor in a person's overall health and risk for disease.

- An accurate BMI is dependent upon accurate measures of height and weight. Because it is relatively quick and easy to measure height and weight and requires little skill, *actual* measures, and not *estimates*, should be used whenever possible.
- A client's *stated* height and weight should be used only when there are no other options.
- Although malnutrition can occur at any BMI, people at extremes of BMI may be at increased risk of poor nutritional status (White et al., 2012).

BOX 15.2 Psychosocial Factors That May Affect Intake, Nutritional Requirements, or Nutrition Counseling

Psychological Factors

- Depression
- Anxiety
- Eating disorders
- Psychosis

Social Factors

- Illiteracy
- Language barriers
- Limited knowledge of nutrition and food safety
- Lack of caregiver or social support system
- Social isolation
- Lack of or inadequate cooking arrangements
- Limited or low income
- Limited access to transportation to obtain food
- Advanced age (older than 80)
- Lack of or extreme physical activity
- Use of tobacco or recreational drugs
- Limited use or knowledge of community resources

Weight Loss

Unintentional weight loss is a well-validated indicator of malnutrition (White et al., 2012).

Percentage of Weight Loss a calculation where the amount of weight lost is divided by usual body weight then multiplied by 100.

(amount of weight loss/ usual body weigh) × 100 = percentage of weight loss

- The significance of weight change is determined after the **percentage of weight loss** in a given period of time is calculated (Table 15.1).
- The client's weight can be unreliable or invalid due to hydration status. Edema, anasarca, fluid resuscitation, heart failure, and chronic liver or kidney disease can falsely inflate weight.

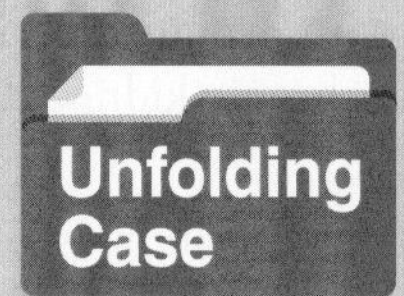

Remember Miguel. What is his percent weight loss? How would you classify it? What is his BMI? Does his BMI indicate a risk of malnutrition? Do the screening findings support a diagnosis of malnutrition?

Table 15.1 Interpretation of Weight Loss by Malnutrition Etiology

Etiology of Malnutrition	Moderate Malnutrition	Severe Malnutrition
Starvation or chronic disease	5%/1 month 7.5%/3 months 10%/6 months 20%/1 year	>5%/1 month >7.5%/3 months >10%/6 months >20%/1 year
Acute disease or injury	1%–2%/1 week 5%/1 month 7.5%/3 months	>2%/1 week >5%/1 month >7.5%/3 months

Source: Malone, A., & Hamilton, C. (2013). The Academy of Nutrition and Dietetics/The American Society for Parenteral and Enteral Nutrition consensus malnutrition characteristics: Application in practice. *Nutrition in Clinical Practice*, *28*(6), 639–650. https://doi.org/10.1177/0884533613508435

Dietary Intake

An intake of food that is less than estimated requirements is a characteristic of malnutrition. However, like other data, a food intake history obtained from the client or caregiver may not be reliable.

- Simply asking a client "How is your appetite?" will not provide sufficient information regarding their dietary intake. A better question is, "Has the type or amount of food you usually eat changed recently?" with a follow-up question to explain their answer ("How did it change?" or "Why do you think it has changed?" are examples).
- Another question to avoid while obtaining a nursing history is, "Are you on a diet?" To most people, the word *diet* is synonymous with *weight loss*. They may fail to mention that they use nutrition therapy to limit sodium, modify fat, or count carbohydrates. A better question is, "Do you avoid any particular foods?" or "Do you watch what you eat in any way?"
- Depending on the circumstances, valuable information may be gained by asking the client what concerns they have about what or how they eat, how illness has affected their choice or tolerance of food, and if they have enough food to eat.

Physical Findings

Physical findings occur only with overt malnutrition, not with subclinical malnutrition, and can vary among population groups because of genetic and environmental differences. Physical findings that may indicate risk for malnutrition include the following:

- loss of subcutaneous fat, such as in the orbital region, upper arm, and thoracic regions
- loss of muscle mass, such as in the quadriceps, trapezium, and deltoid muscles
- localized or generalized fluid retention in the lower and upper extremities, face and eyes, and/or scrotal area
  - Fluid accumulation may also be caused by other conditions like congestive heart failure or chronic kidney disease.
- diminished handgrip strength as measured by a dynamometer
- other physical findings as listed in Box 15.3
  - Most findings cannot be considered diagnostic because the evaluation of normal versus abnormal findings is subjective, and the signs of malnutrition may be nonspecific. For instance, dull, dry hair may be related to severe protein deficiency, overexposure to the sun, or the use of harsh hair products.

Laboratory Data

Currently, there is no universally agreed-upon biochemical indicators to diagnose malnutrition.

- While albumin has traditionally been used as an indicator of malnutrition, it is neither specific nor sensitive enough to be a marker for malnutrition (Nelson et al., 2015).

BOX 15.3 Physical Findings Suggestive of Malnutrition

- Hair that is dull, brittle, dry, or falls out easily
- Swollen glands of the neck and cheeks
- Dry, rough, or spotty skin that may have a sandpaper feel
- Poor or delayed healing of wounds or sores
- Depressed mood
- Abnormal heart rate, heart rhythm, or blood pressure
- Enlarged liver or spleen
- Loss of balance and coordination

- The major cause of low albumin and other visceral proteins is inflammation, not malnutrition (Cederholm et al., 2015). Inflammation is considered an etiologic factor of malnutrition, not a diagnostic feature.
- However, albumin is often part of a nutrition screen because it is a good indicator of disease severity and outcome and a strong predictor of surgical risk and mortality (Wischmeyer et al., 2018).

Nursing Analysis

Nursing analyses relate directly to nutrition when the pattern of nutrition and metabolism is the problem. For example, *risk of malnutrition related to poor intake as evidenced by weight loss* is a nursing analysis. Other nursing analyses may not be as specific for nutrition but may involve nutrition as part of the nursing care plan, such as teaching the client how to increase fiber intake to relieve constipation.

Nutrition-Related Client Outcomes

Whenever possible, the client should actively participate in goal setting, even if the client's perception of need differs from yours. In matters that do not involve life or death, it is best to first address the client's concerns. For example, your primary consideration for a client who has undergone six months of chemotherapy may be their significant weight loss, whereas the client's major concern may be fatigue. The two concerns are undoubtedly related, but your effectiveness as a change agent is greater if you approach the problem from the client's perspective. Commitment to achieving the goal is greatly increased when the client believes they own the goal.

- The goal for all clients is to consume adequate calories, protein, and nutrients using foods they like and tolerate, as appropriate.
- If possible, additional short-term goals may be set to alleviate symptoms or side effects of disease or treatments and to prevent complications or recurrences if appropriate.
- After short-term goals are met, attention can expand to promoting healthy eating to reduce the risk of chronic-diet-related diseases such as obesity, diabetes, hypertension, and heart disease.

Nutrition Interventions

Nutrition care plans include a nutrition prescription based on the client's nutrition diagnoses and estimated needs. Specific nutrition intervention strategies focus on the etiology of the problem. The nurse is involved in implementing nutrition interventions, basic nutrition education/reinforcing nutrition teaching, and communicating with other members of the health care team.

Implementation

The nutrition prescription may detail recommendations regarding calories, protein, other nutrients, specific foods, or the method of feeding. The nurse's role may be to

- ensure that dietitian-prescribed interventions occur in a timely manner,
- facilitate nursing interventions to treat clients who have or are at risk of malnutrition,
- ensure clients receive automated nutrition intervention (e.g., food, oral supplements) if there is a delay between nutrition screening and nutrition assessment,
- promote optimal intake of food and ONS (Box 15.4).

Educate and Reinforce

Include nutrition in all discussions with clients and their family members.

- Reinforce the importance of obtaining adequate nutrition.
- Review basic principles of the eating plan and avoid the term *diet*.

BOX 15.4 Strategies to Promote an Optimal Intake

- Avoid disconnecting enteral or parenteral nutrition for client repositioning, ambulation, procedures, etc.
- Advocate discontinuation of intravenous therapy as soon as feasible.
- Advocate aggressively for diet progressions.
- Replace meals withheld for diagnostic tests.
- Promote congregate dining, if appropriate.
- Question diet orders that appear inappropriate.
- Display a positive attitude when serving food or discussing nutrition.
- Help the client select appropriate foods. Offer standby choices for clients who do not like menu selections.
- Gently motivate the client to eat.
- Encourage clients who feel full quickly to eat the most nutrient-dense items first: meat and milk rather than juice, soup, or coffee, etc.
- Order snacks and ONS.
- Request assistance with feeding or meal setup.
- Get the client out of bed to eat, if possible.
- Encourage good oral hygiene.
- Screen the client from offensive sights and remove unpleasant odors from the room.
- Downgrade the consistency of the diet (e.g., provide a soft diet) if the client has difficulty chewing or swallowing.

- Counsel the client about drug–nutrient interactions.
- Emphasize things "to do" instead of things "*not* to do."
- Keep the message simple.
- Respond to questions.
- Review written handouts with the client.
- Advise the client to avoid foods that are not tolerated.

Communicate

Dietitians rely on nurses for their observations and feedback.

- Communicate concerns regarding eating, nutrition, or client knowledge.
- Communicate changes in the client's condition that may indicate nutrition risk.
- Include nutrition discussions into handoff of care and nursing care plans.

Nutrition-Related Monitoring

Monitoring the client's acceptance and tolerance to the nutrition prescription allows for timely revision of the plan as needed. Nurses are in an ideal position to monitor the client's nutrition because of their close, ongoing contact with the client and their family.

- Observe intake of food and supplements whenever possible.
- Document appetite and take action when the client does not eat.
- Order supplements if intake is low or needs are high.
- Initiate calorie counts.
- Request a nutritional consult.
- Assess tolerance (i.e., absence of side effects).
- Monitor weight.
- Monitor progression of nothing by mouth status and restrictive diets.
- Monitor the client's grasp of the information and motivation to change.
- Rescreen clients within established time frame.

FEEDING HOSPITALIZED CLIENTS

The goal of nutrition intervention for all hospitalized clients, whether or not they have been diagnosed with malnutrition, is to provide sufficient calories and nutrients to meet the client's estimated needs in a form the client can tolerate and utilize.

Private and government regulatory agencies stipulate meal timing, frequency, and nutritional content and require that hospital menus be supervised by a qualified dietitian. Many hospital food service departments offer a room service, cook-to-order menu. Compared to more traditional food service menus, a restaurant-style service gives clients greater control over what and when they eat. Restaurant-style service has also been shown to improve calorie and protein intake, reduce plate waste, and improve client satisfaction (McCray et al., 2018).

Oral Diets

Oral diets are the easiest and most preferred method of providing nutrition. In most facilities, clients choose what they want to eat from a menu representing the diet ordered by the physician. Oral diets may be categorized as regular, modified consistency, or therapeutic. Often, combination diets are ordered, such as a pureed, low-sodium diet or a high-protein, soft diet. The actual foods allowed on a diet varies among institutions and the diet manual in use.

Although hospital diets provide adequate amounts of calories and protein, most clients do not consume complete meals. A recent study found that 32.1% of adult hospitalized clients ate a quarter of their meal or less (Sauer et al., 2019).

- Appetite may be impaired by fear, pain, or anxiety.
- Hospital food may be refused because it is unfamiliar, tasteless (e.g., cooked without salt), inappropriate in texture (e.g., pureed meat), religiously or culturally unacceptable, or served at times when the client is unaccustomed to eating.
- Clients may underestimate the importance of nutrition in their recovery process.

Regular Diet

Regular diets are used to achieve or maintain optimal nutritional status in clients who do not have impaired ability to eat or tolerate an oral intake or altered nutritional needs. No foods are excluded, and portion sizes are not limited. The nutritional value of the diet varies significantly with the actual foods chosen by the client.

Regular diets are adjusted to meet age-specific needs throughout the life cycle. For instance, a regular diet for a child differs from that of an adult. Regular diets are also altered to meet specifications for vegetarian or kosher eating.

Sometimes, physicians order a *diet as tolerated* (DAT) on admission or after surgery. This order is interpreted according to the client's appetite and ability to eat and tolerate food. The nurse has the authority to advance the DAT.

Remember Miguel. He is ordered on a regular diet for his first meal postoperatively. Why wasn't he ordered on a carbohydrate-controlled diet due to his history of type 2 diabetes? When his tray arrives, Miguel doesn't want to eat it, stating that his throat is sore and the foods provided are not items he normally eats. What steps would you take to encourage Miguel to eat?

Modified Consistency Diets

Modified consistency diets include clear liquid and mechanically altered diets (Table 15.2). Clear liquid diets are most commonly used in preparation for colonoscopy.

- Traditionally, a clear liquid diet was ordered as the first postoperative meal based on the rationale that a gradual progression from a clear liquid diet to a regular diet maximized tolerance when eating resumed.

Table 15.2 Characteristics of Modified Consistency Diets

Diet Characteristics	Foods Allowed	Indications
Clear liquid A short-term, highly restrictive diet composed only of fluids or foods that are transparent and liquid at body temperature (e.g., gelatin). It requires minimal digestion and leaves a minimum of residue. Inadequate in calories and all nutrients except vitamin C if vitamin C–fortified juices are used.	• Clear broth or bouillon • Coffee, tea, and carbonated beverages, as allowed and as tolerated • Fruit juices: clear (apple, cranberry, grape) and strained (orange, lemonade, grapefruit) • Fruit ice made from clear fruit juice • Gelatin • Popsicles • Sugar, honey, hard candy • Commercially prepared clear liquid supplements	• In preparation for bowel surgery or colonoscopy • Acute gastrointestinal disorders • Transitional feeding after parenteral nutrition • Routine use of a clear liquid diet after surgery is not recommended (Wischmeyer et al., 2018).
Pureed diet A diet composed of foods that are blended, whipped, or mashed to pudding-like consistency. All foods should be smooth, not sticky, and free of lumps. Requires minimal chewing ability. Most foods can be liquefied by combining equal parts of solids and liquids; fruits and vegetables need less liquid. Broth, gravy, cream soups, cheese, tomato sauce, milk, and fruit juice are preferable to water for blenderizing due to their higher calorie and nutritional value. Liquids may be thickened to improve ease of swallowing.	All foods are allowed, but consistency is changed to liquid.	• Used after oral or facial surgery • For wired jaws • Chewing and swallowing problems
Mechanically altered diet A regular diet modified in texture only and excludes most raw fruits and vegetables and foods containing seeds, nuts, and dried fruit. Gravies, sauces, milk, and water are used to soften foods that are chopped, ground, mashed, or cooked soft. Sticky foods such as peanut butter are avoided.	• Milk • Yogurt • Pudding • Cottage cheese • Mashed, soft ripened fruit (peaches, pears, bananas) • Cooked, mashed soft vegetables (peas, carrots, yams) • Ground meats • Soft casseroles • Smooth cooked cereals • Soft bite-sized pasta • Bread products made into a slurry with the addition of gravy or syrup	Used for clients who have limited chewing ability such as clients who • are edentulous • have ill-fitting dentures • have undergone surgery to the head, neck, or mouth
Soft diet A regular diet that features soft-textured foods that are easy to chew and swallow. Hard, sticky, dry, or crunchy foods are excluded.	• Soft-cooked vegetables • Shredded lettuce • Canned fruit • Soft, peeled fresh fruit • Well-moistened, thin-sliced, tender, or ground meats; poultry; or fish • Eggs • Milk • Yogurt • Mashed potatoes • White rice • Well-cooked pasta • Well-moistened cereals without dried fruits or nuts	• Used to limit gastrointestinal irritation and minimize gut activity for healing purposes • Not intended for long-term use because it can cause constipation

- It is now known that early resumption of oral feeding after major surgery, including GI surgery, is associated with a decrease in postoperative complications, length of stay, and mortality (Warren et al., 2011).
- It is recommended that clear liquid diets not be routinely used postoperatively because they do not provide adequate nutrition or protein (Wischmeyer et al., 2018). The current recommendation is that a high-protein diet of food and/or high-protein ONS be initiated on the day of surgery in most cases (Wischmeyer et al., 2018).

Mechanically altered diets contain foods that are pureed, chopped/ground, or soft for clients who have difficulty chewing or swallowing. Dysphagia diets are another variation of modified consistency diets that are covered in Chapter 19.

Therapeutic Diets

Therapeutic diets differ from a regular diet in the amount of one or more nutrients or food components for the purpose of preventing or treating disease or illness. The number or timing of meals may also be altered. Table 15.3 outlines the characteristics and indications of selected therapeutic diets.

Oral Nutrition Supplements

Oral nutrition supplements (ONS) are often used for inadequate intake or to treat malnutrition. They provide calories, protein, and micronutrients to help limit weight loss and promote recovery of lost lean body mass (Bally et al., 2016). ONS use has been shown to reduce readmission rates and health care costs (Philipson et al., 2013).

Table 15.3 Selected Therapeutic Diets: Characteristics and Indications

Type of Diet	Characteristics	Indications
Heart healthy (cardiac)	• Limited in saturated fats (less than 7%–10% total calories), trans fats, and sodium (less than 2300 mg/day) • Encourages whole grains, fruits, vegetables, unsaturated fats, and appropriate calories to attain/maintain healthy weight	• High-serum low-density lipoprotein (LDL) cholesterol • Prevention or treatment of cardiovascular disease
Consistent carbohydrate	• Consistent total daily carbohydrate content with emphasis on heart-healthy food choices • Calories are based on attaining and maintaining healthy weight • A high fiber intake is encouraged and sodium may be limited	• Type 1 and type 2 diabetes • Gestational diabetes • Impaired glucose tolerance • Impaired fasting glucose
Fat restricted	• Limits total fat: Limitations vary from less than 25–50 g/day	• Malabsorption syndromes • Liver disease • Pancreatic disease • Chronic cholecystitis • Gastroesophageal reflux
High fiber	A general diet with low-fiber foods replaced by foods high in fiber with a goal of 25–35 g or more per day	To prevent or treat • constipation • diabetes • irritable bowel syndrome • hypercholesterolemia • obesity
Low fiber	• Limits fiber by eliminating skins, membranes, and seeds from fruits and vegetables • Allows grains with less than 2 g fiber/serving • Excludes nuts, seeds, and dried fruits • Lactose may also be restricted	• Before surgery to minimize fecal residue • During acute phases of intestinal disorders such as ulcerative colitis, Crohn's disease, and diverticulitis • Radiation therapy to the pelvis and lower bowel • Recent intestinal surgery • New colostomy or ileostomy

Table 15.3 Selected Therapeutic Diets: Characteristics and Indications (continued)

Type of Diet	Characteristics	Indications
High calorie, high protein	A diet rich in calorie-dense and/or protein-dense foods	• To meet increased nutritional requirements • Also used in clients with poor intakes
Renal	• Slightly lower in protein • Emphasizes heart-healthy fats • Adequate in calories • Sodium, potassium, and phosphorus levels adjusted depending on the stage of chronic kidney disease	Stages 1–4 chronic kidney disease
Potassium modified	Potassium may be increased or restricted by manipulating potassium-rich foods, such as • fruits • vegetables • whole grains • milk • meats • legumes	• Low-potassium diets may be used in the treatment of certain renal diseases in conjunction with certain medications or in adrenal insufficiency • High-potassium diets may be used in conjunction with certain medications and with certain renal diseases
Sodium restricted	Sodium limit may be set at 1500 mg/day or 2000 mg/day	• May be prescribed for hypertension and congestive heart failure • Acute and chronic renal disease • Liver disease
Gluten free	• Sources of gluten (a protein in wheat, rye, and barley) are eliminated from the diet • Gluten-free grains, such as corn, potato, rice, soy, and quinoa, are encouraged as sources of complex carbohydrates	• Celiac disease (celiac sprue, nontropical sprue, gluten-sensitive enteropathy) • Dermatitis herpetiformis rash
Lactose restricted	Limits foods with lactose ("milk sugar") to the amount tolerated by the individual	• Lactose intolerance • Lactase insufficiency that may occur secondary to certain inflammatory gastrointestinal disorders such as ulcerative colitis and Crohn's disease

Categories of supplements include clear liquid supplements, milk-based drinks, commercially prepared liquid supplements, specially prepared foods, and bariatric meal replacements (Table 15.4). Liquid supplements are easy to consume, are generally well accepted, and tend to leave the stomach quickly making them a good choice for snacks that are between meals.

ONS compliance in hospitalized clients has been estimated at 67% (Hubbard et al., 2012). Despite uncertain compliance, ONS have been found to provide clinical benefits (Sriram et al., 2017). Actions that help promote compliance include obtaining taste preferences, explaining the potential benefits, serving supplements cold, and rotating different types of supplements and flavors to help forestall or prevent taste fatigue that tends to occur over time. Acceptance should be closely monitored and the percentage consumed documented.

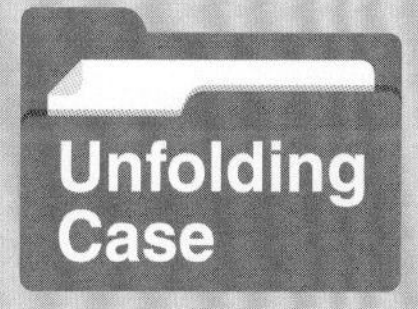

Recall Miguel. He vomited after eating. Would he be a candidate for an ONS? What category of ONS would be appropriate for him? Would an ONS be appropriate for him after discharge?

Table 15.4 Oral Nutrition Supplements

Type	Examples	Characteristics	Comments
Clear liquid	• Ensure Clear Nutrition Drink • Boost Breeze	They provide protein and carbohydrates with 0 g fat for clients on clear liquid diets	• Comes in flavors • Taste varies between brands
Milk based	• Carnation Breakfast Essentials Original and High Protein Powder Drink Mix • Resource Milk Shake Mix	• Contains nonfat milk • Powdered forms are mixed with milk • Provides significant amounts of protein and calories • Relatively inexpensive and palatable	It is not suitable for clients with lactose intolerance
Commercially prepared liquid	• Ensure products: Regular, high protein, plus, light nutrition, plant-based protein, presurgery, surgery, rapid hydration, and other varieties • Boost products: Original, high protein, plus, glucose control, very high calorie, and other varieties	• Regular varieties: 8–10 g protein, 220–250 cal/8 oz • High protein: 12–20 g protein/8 oz • Plus: 14 g protein, 360 cal/8 oz • Are lactose free	• Generally sweet and flavored • Quick, easy, varied in flavor • Often available in grocery stores • Most provide complete nutrition, so can be used as sole source of nutrition
Commercially prepared supplemental foods	• Hormel Solutions juices and custard • Ensure Original Pudding • Boost Pudding	They are specially designed to provide a concentrated source of protein and calories	They offer an alternative to sweetened drinks
Bariatric meal replacement	• Bariatric fusion meal replacement • Bariatric advantage high-protein meal replacement	• Provides 27 g high-quality protein/150–160 calorie serving • Low fat • Low carbohydrate • Provides fiber, vitamins, and minerals	It is formulated for before and after weight-loss surgery

How Do You Respond

Should I save my menus from the hospital to help me plan meals at home? This is not a bad idea if the in-house and discharge food plans are the same. The menus should serve *only* as a guide. If shrimp was not included on the hospital menu then that doesn't mean it should be avoided. Likewise, if the client hated the orange juice served every morning, they shouldn't think they need to continue drinking it. Hospital menus are more rigid than at-home eating plans by necessity.

REVIEW CASE STUDY

Mildred is an 80-year-old woman who lives independently in her own home. She was brought to the emergency department due to worsening generalized weakness that resulted in a fall with probable hip fracture. She has a history of lower GI bleeding and presents with anemia. She is alert and oriented. Her BMI is 16.8. Three months ago, she weighed 135 pounds, and she currently weighs 104 pounds. She states that she has not had an appetite for several months. Her health has been stable since her last hospital admission for GI bleeding two years ago.

- Using Figure 15.3, what is Mildred's nutrition screening score?
- What is her percent weight change?
- Mildred is admitted and ordered a regular diet. What nutrition interventions would you initiate to help maximize Mildred's intake?
- The nutrition diagnosis is underweight related to loss of appetite and poor intake as evidenced by BMI of 16.8. What criteria will you monitor that will enable the dietitian to evaluate Mildred's progress?

STUDY QUESTIONS

1 Nurses are in an ideal position to
  a. screen clients for risk of malnutrition.
  b. order therapeutic diets.
  c. conduct nutrition assessments.
  d. calculate a client's calorie and protein needs.

2 Which of the following criteria would most likely be on a nutrition screen in the hospital?
  a. prealbumin
  b. weight loss
  c. serum potassium value
  d. cultural food preferences

3 Which of the following statements regarding nutrition screening is false?
  a. A nutrition screen is completed only when a client is suspected of having a nutritional problem.
  b. A nutrition screen must be completed within 24 hours after admission to a hospital or other health care facility.
  c. The purpose of nutrition screening is to detect the risk of malnutrition.
  d. Health care facilities are free to choose their own screening criteria and to determine how quickly a client must be rescreened.

4 Which of the following statements is accurate regarding the physical signs and symptoms of malnutrition?
  a. Physical signs of malnutrition appear before changes in weight or laboratory values occur.
  b. Physical signs of malnutrition are suggestive, not definitive, for malnutrition.
  c. Physical signs have a clear threshold that identifies what is considered abnormal.
  d. All races and sexes exhibit the same intensity of physical changes in response to malnutrition.

5 Which of the following strategies may help promote an adequate oral intake in hospitalized clients? Select all that apply.
  a. Tell the client that you wouldn't want to eat the food either, but it is important for their recovery.
  b. Encourage the client to select their own menu.
  c. Offer standby alternatives when the client cannot find anything on the menu they want to eat.
  d. Advance the diet as quickly as possible, as appropriate.

6 A pureed diet is the most appropriate diet in which of the following situations?
  a. It is appropriate as an initial oral diet after surgery to establish tolerance.
  b. It is appropriate as a transition between a full liquid diet and a regular diet.
  c. It is appropriate for clients who need a low-fiber diet.
  d. It is appropriate for clients who have had their jaw wired.

7 Your client has a question about the ONS they receive twice a day. What is the best response?
  a. "Ask your doctor when they make their rounds."
  b. "What is your question? If I can't answer it, then I will get the dietitian to talk with you."
  c. "You need to drink it to get better. You can discontinue it after discharge but you need it now."
  d. "If I see the dietitian around, then I will tell them to stop by to see you."

8 Which of the following statements is true regarding albumin?
  a. Albumin is a reliable and sensitive indicator of protein status and can help diagnose malnutrition.
  b. Albumin levels rise in response to inflammation.
  c. Albumin and other visceral proteins are good indicators of disease severity and outcome but not malnutrition.
  d. An increase in albumin level means nutrition therapy is effectively treating malnutrition.

CHAPTER SUMMARY HOSPITAL NUTRITION: IDENTIFYING NUTRITION RISK AND FEEDING CLIENTS

Malnutrition

Malnutrition is common and often unrecognized among hospitalized clients. It is a major contributor to morbidity and mortality.

- **Diagnosis:** The presence of more than two of the following characteristics indicates malnutrition: inadequate calorie intake, unintentional weight loss, loss of muscle mass, loss of subcutaneous fat, localized or generalized fluid accumulation, and diminished functional status as measured by handgrip strength.
- **Nutrition screening** is used to identify people at risk for malnutrition. It is usually the responsibility of the nurse to perform a nutrition screening.

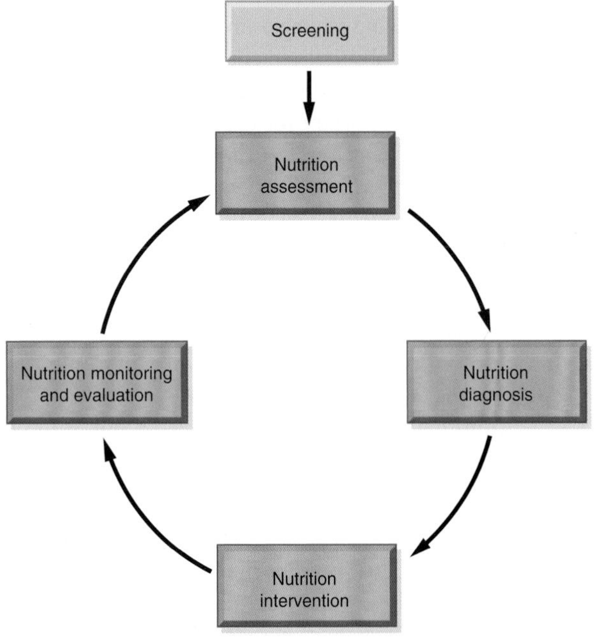

- Health care facilities determine their own screening criteria, who completes the screen, and how quickly a rescreen is required.
- Screening tools should be quick, easy, valid, and reliable. Most use weight loss, food intake, and BMI to evaluate malnutrition risk.

Nutrition Assessment

A dietitian completes a nutrition assessment on clients found to be at risk for malnutrition. Steps include assessment, diagnosis, intervention, and monitoring and evaluation. Nurses may directly or indirectly be involved in any or all steps.

- **Nutrition therapy for malnutrition:** General guidelines often suggest 25 to 30 cal/kg/day and 1.2 to 2.0 g protein/kg/day depending on the client's status and response to therapy. High-protein ONS consumed 2 to 3 times per day can help meet protein needs. If necessary, enteral nutrition is provided. Parenteral nutrition is considered only if the oral and enteral routes are inadequate or unavailable.

Nutrition in the Nursing Process

Nutrition may be integrated throughout the steps of the nursing process.

- **Nursing assessment:** Dietitians rely on nurses for much of the initial information about the client and for ongoing monitoring and documentation of changes in intake, weight, and function.
  - **Medical–Psychosocial history** can identify disease-related nutrition risks.
  - **Height, weight, BMI:** Accurate measures are vital. Risk of poor nutritional status increases at either extreme of BMI.
  - **Weight loss:** The percentage of unintentional weight loss over a specified period of time is used to diagnose malnutrition.
  - **Dietary intake:** Loss of appetite indicates risk.

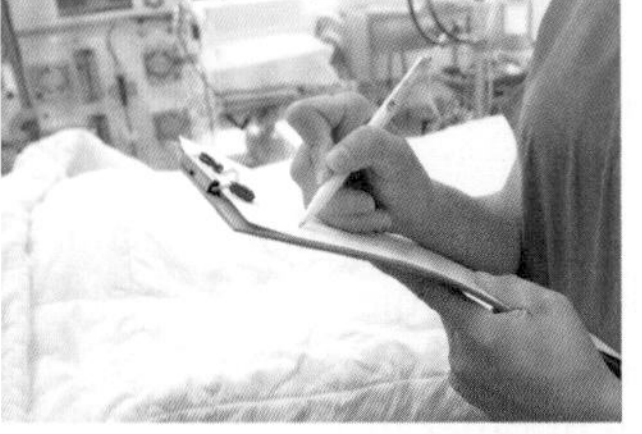

  - **Physical findings:** Loss of muscle, fat, and decreased handgrip may indicate malnutrition.
  - **Lab data:** There is no universally agreed-upon biochemical indicators to diagnose malnutrition.
- **Nursing analyses:** Nursing analyses may be specifically related to nutrition (e.g., underweight) or may include nutrition in the etiology of the problem (e.g., constipation related to lack of dietary fiber).
- **Nutrition-related client outcomes:** The goal for all clients is to consume adequate calories, protein, and nutrients using foods they like and can tolerate, as appropriate. Alleviating symptoms or side effects may be additional short-term goals.
- **Nutrition interventions:** Nurses are involved with promoting an adequate nutritional intake, providing or reinforcing basic nutrition education, and communicating with the dietitian.
- **Nutrition-related monitoring:** Nurses monitor the client's intake, weight, and tolerance to the diet.

CHAPTER SUMMARY HOSPITAL NUTRITION: IDENTIFYING NUTRITION RISK AND FEEDING CLIENTS (continued)

Feeding Hospitalized Clients

Private and government regulatory agencies stipulate meal timing, frequency, and nutritional content and require that hospital menus be supervised by a qualified dietitian.

- **Oral diets** are the preferred method of providing nutrition.
  - **Regular diets** are for clients who do not have altered nutrient needs. No foods are excluded.
  - **Modified consistency diets** include clear liquid and mechanically altered diets, such as pureed, chopped/ground, or soft diets.

- **Therapeutic diets** differ in the amount of one or more nutrients or food components for the purpose of preventing or treating disease or illness.

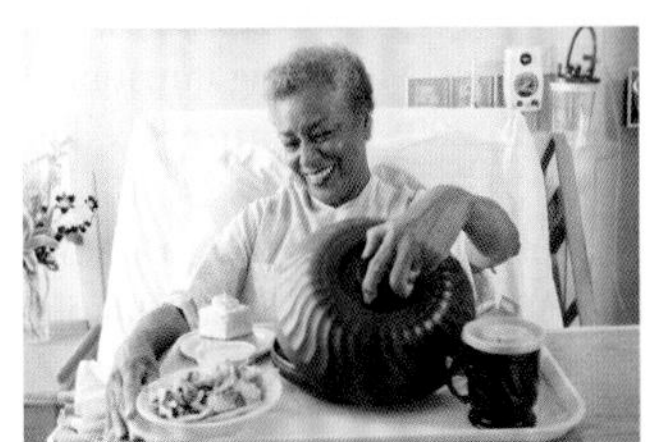

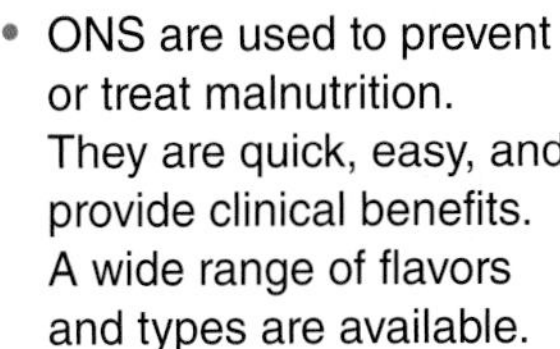

- ONS are used to prevent or treat malnutrition. They are quick, easy, and provide clinical benefits. A wide range of flavors and types are available.

Figure sources: *shutterstock.com/sfam_photo and shutterstock.com/Monkey Business Images*

Student Resources on thePoint®
For additional learning materials, activate the code in the front of this book at https://thePoint.lww.com/activate

Websites

Oral nutrition supplement product information at www.abbottnutrition.com; nestlehealthscience.us

Screening and assessment tools from the American Society for Parenteral and Enteral Nutrition at https://www.nutritioncare.org/Guidelines_and_Clinical_Resources/Toolkits/Malnutrition_Toolkit/Screening_and_Assessment_Tools/

References

Arends, J., Baracos, V., Bertz, H., Bozzetti, F., Calder, P. C., Deutz, N. E., Erickson, N., Laviano, A., Lisanti, M. P., Lobo, D. N., McMillan, D. C., Muscaritoli, M., Ockenga, J., Pirlich, M., Strasser, F., de van der Schueren, M., Van Gossum, A., Vaupel, P., & Weimann, A. (2017). ESPEN expert group recommendations for action against cancer-related malnutrition. *Clinical Nutrition, 36*, 1187–1196. https://doi.org/10.1016/j.clnu.2017.06.017

Bally, M., Blaser Yildirim, P., Bounoure, L., Gloy, V., Mueller, B., Briel, M., & Schuetz, P. (2016). Nutritional support and outcomes in malnourished medical inpatients: A systematic review and meta-analysis. *JAMA Internal Medicine, 176*(1), 43–53. https://doi.org/10.1001/jamainternmed.2015.6587

Cederholm, T., Bosaeus, I., Barazzoni, R., Bauer, J., Van Gossum, A., Klek, S., Muscaritoli, M., Nyulasi, I., Ockenga, J., Schneider, S. M., de van der Schueren, M., & Singer, P. (2015). Diagnostic criteria for malnutrition: An ESPEN consensus statement. *Clinical Nutrition, 34*(3), 335–340. https://doi.org/10.1016/j.clnu.2015.03.001

DiMaria-Ghalili, R., Mirtallo, J., Tobin, B., Hark, L., Van Horn, L., & Palmer, C. (2014). Challenges and opportunities for nutrition education and training in the health care professions: Intraprofessional and interprofessional call to action. *American Journal of Clinical Nutrition, 99*(5), 1184S–1193S. https://doi.org/10.3945/ajcn.113.073536

Field, L., & Hand, R. (2015). Differentiating malnutrition screening and assessment: A nutrition care process perspective. *Journal of the Academy of Nutrition and Dietetics, 115*(5), 824–828. https://doi.org/10.1016/j.jand.2014.11.010

Hubbard, G., Elia, M., Holdoway, A., & Stratton, R. (2012). A systematic review of compliance to oral nutritional supplements. *Clinical Nutrition, 31*(3), 293–312. https://doi.org/10.1016/j.clnu.2011.11.020

Jensen, G., Compher, C., Sullivan, D., & Mullin, G. (2013). Recognizing malnutrition in adults: Definitions and characteristics, screening, assessment, and team approach. *Journal of Parenteral and Enteral Nutrition, 37*(6), 802–807. https://doi.org/10.1177/0148607113492338

Malone, A., & Hamilton, C. (2013). The Academy of Nutrition and Dietetics/The American Society for Parenteral and Enteral Nutrition consensus malnutrition characteristics: Application in practice. *Nutrition in Clinical Practice, 28*(6), 639–650. https://doi.org/10.1177/0884533613508435

McCray, S., Maunder, K., Krikowa, R., & MacKenzie-Shalders, K. (2018). Room service improves nutritional intake and increases client satisfaction while decreasing food waste and cost. *Journal of the Academy of Nutrition and Dietetics, 118*(2), 284–293. https://doi.org/10.1016/j.jand.2017.05.014

Mtaweh, H., Tuira, L., Floh, A. A., & Parshuram, C. S. (2018). Indirect calorimetry: History, technology, and application. *Frontiers in pediatrics, 6*, 257. https://doi.org/10.3389/fped.2018.00257

Nelson, C., Elkassabany, N., Kamath, A., & Liu, J. (2015). Low albumin levels, more than morbid obesity, and are associated with complications after TKA. *Clinical Orthopaedics and Related Research, 473*, 3163–3172. https://doi.org/10.1007/s11999-015-4333-7

Nightingale, F. (1992). *Notes of nursing: What is it, and what it is not* (commemorative edition). Lippincott Williams & Wilkins.

Philipson, T., Snider, J., Lakdawalla, D., Stryckman, B., & Goldman, D. P. (2013). Impact of oral nutritional supplementation on hospital outcomes. *The American Journal of Managed Care, 19*(2), 121–128.

Rasmussen, H., Holst, M., & Kondrup, J. (2010). Measuring nutritional risk in hospitals. *Clinical Epidemiology, 2*, 209–216. https://dx.doi.org/10.2147%2FCLEP.S11265

Russo, E., Gupta, R., & Merriman, L. (2016). Implementing the care plan for patients diagnosed with malnutrition: Why do we wait? *Journal of the Academy of Nutrition and Dietetics, 116*(5), 865–867. https://doi.org/10.1016/j.jand.2016.03.005

Sauer, A., Goates, S., Malone, A., Mogensen, K., Gerwirtz, G., Sulz, I., Moick, S., Laviano, A., & Hiesmayr, M. (2019). Prevalence of malnutrition risk and the impact of nutrition risk on hospital outcomes: Results from nutrition day in the U.S. *Journal of Parenteral and Enteral Nutrition, 43*(7), 918–926. https://doi.org/10.1002/jpen.1499

Skipper, A. (2012). Agreement on defining malnutrition. *Journal of Parenteral and Enteral Nutrition, 36*(3), 261–262. https://doi.org/10.1177/0148607112441949

Skipper, A., Coltman, A., Tomesko, J., Charney, P., Porcari, J., Piemonte, T. A., Handu, D., & Cheng, F. W. (2020). Position of the Academy of Nutrition and Dietetics: Malnutrition (undernutrition) screening tools for all adults. *Journal of the Academy of Nutrition and Dietetics, 129*(4), 709–713. https://doi.org/10.1016/j.jand.2019.09.011

Sriram, K., Sulo, S., VanDerBosch, G., Partridge, J., Feldstein, J., Hegazi, R., & Summerfelt, W. (2017). A comprehensive nutrition-focused quality improvement program reduces 30-day readmissions and length of stay in hospitalized patients. *Journal of Parenteral and Enteral Nutrition, 41*(3), 384–391. https://doi.org/10.1177/0148607116681468

Tappenden, K., Quatrara, B., Parkhurst, M., Malone, A. M., Fanjiang, G., & Ziegler, T. R. (2013). Critical role of nutrition in improving quality of care: An interdisciplinary call to action to address adult hospital malnutrition. *Journal of Parenteral and Enteral Nutrition, 37*(4), 482–497. https://doi.org/10.1177/0148607113484066

Tobert, C., Mott, S., & Nepple, K. (2018). Malnutrition diagnosis during adult inpatient hospitalizations: Analysis of a multi-institutional collaborative database of academic medical centers. *Journal of the Academy of Nutrition and Dietetics, 118*(1), 125–131. https://doi.org/10.1016/j.jand.2016.12.019

Warren, J., Bhalla, V., & Cresci, G. (2011). Postoperative diet advancement: Surgical dogma vs evidence-based medicine. *Nutrition in Clinical Practice, 26*(2), 115–125. https://doi.org/10.1177/0884533611400231

White, J., Guenter, P., Jensen, G., Malone, A., & Schofield, M. Academy of Nutrition and Dietetics Malnutrition Work Group; ASPEN Malnutrition Task Force, and the ASPEN Board of Directors. (2012). Consensus statement of the Academy of Nutrition and Dietetics and American Society for Parenteral and Enteral Nutrition: Characteristics recommended for the identification and documentation of adult malnutrition (undernutrition). *Journal of Parenteral and Enteral Nutrition, 36*(3), 275–283. https://doi.org/10.1177/0148607112440285

Wischmeyer, P., Carli, F. C., Evans, D., Guilbert, S., Kozar, R., Pryor, A., Thiele, R., Everett, S., Grocott, M., Gan, T., Shaw, A., Thacker, J., Miller, T., Hedrick, T., McEvoy, M., Mythen, M., Gergamaschi, R., Gupta, R., Holubar, S., … Fiore, J., for the Perioperative Quality Initiative (POQI) 2 Workgroup. (2018). American Society for Enhanced Recovery and Perioperative Quality Initiative joint consensus statement on nutrition screening and therapy within a surgical enhanced recovery pathway. *Anesthesia & Analgesia, 126*(6), 1883–1895. https://doi.org/10.1213/ANE.0000000000002743

Chapter 16

Enteral and Parenteral Nutrition

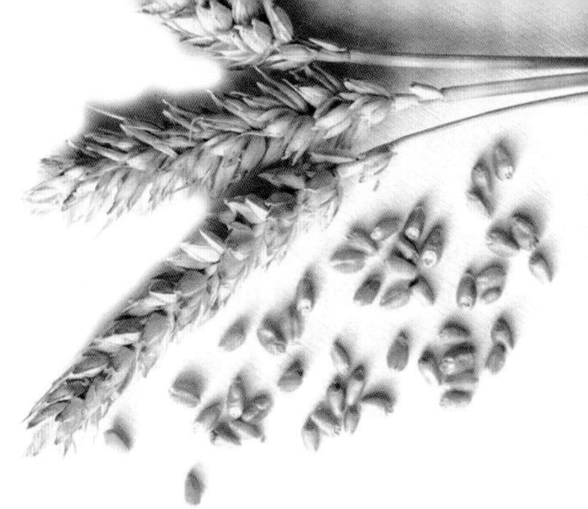

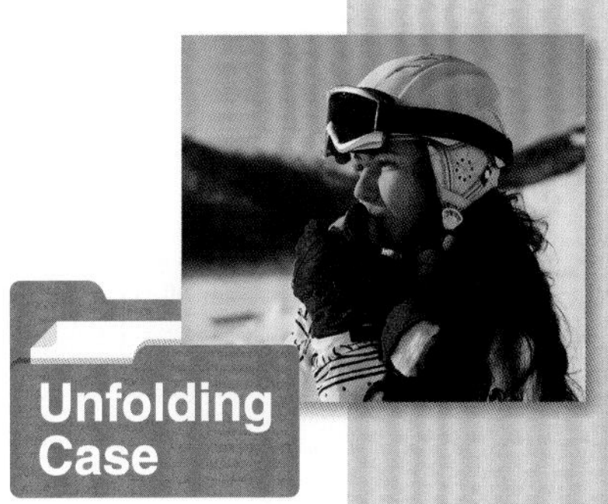

Unfolding Case

Sandy Arnold

Sandy is a 21-year-old downhill skier who is training for international competition. She has been hospitalized for the last 7 days after a skiing accident, where she sustained multiple fractures and internal injuries. She is intubated, a nasointestinal (NI) feeding tube is placed, and the enteral nutrition (EN) order is written for 2200 mL/day of a standard formula that provides 1.0 cal/mL, 44 g protein/L, and 842 g water/L. The formula is to be given over 18 hours. She has no medical history. She is 5 ft 8 in. and weighs 130 pounds upon admission.

Learning Objectives

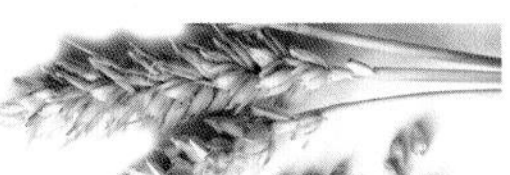

Upon completion of this chapter, you will be able to:

1. Describe the difference between standard enteral formulas and hydrolyzed formulas.
2. Choose the most appropriate enteral formula for a given client.
3. Discuss the advantages and disadvantages of various enteral nutrition delivery methods.
4. Give examples of barriers that prevent clients from receiving the prescribed amount of enteral formula.
5. List ways to maximize tube-feeding tolerance.
6. Identify signs of tube-feeding intolerance and recommend appropriate interventions.
7. Explain the benefits of using enteral nutrition over parenteral nutrition when enteral nutrition is not contraindicated.
8. List indications for using parenteral nutrition.
9. Discuss the components of parenteral nutrition.
10. List potential metabolic complications of parenteral nutrition.

Oral diets are the safest, easiest, and most preferred method of feeding clients. Clients who are unable to consume adequate nutrition may be fed in part or in total via enteral or parenteral nutrition (PN). This chapter describes enteral feeding routes, formulas, delivery methods, and potential complications. The indications for PN, its composition, and potential complications are presented.

ENTERAL NUTRITION

Enteral Nutrition (EN)
the delivery of nutrients by tube, catheter, or stoma into the gastrointestinal tract beyond the oral cavity; commonly known as tube feeding.

Enteral nutrition (EN) has long been considered the standard of care for providing nutrition support for clients who are unable to consume adequate calories and protein orally and have at least a partially functional gastrointestinal (GI) tract that is accessible and safe to use. EN may supplement an oral diet or may be the sole source of nutrition. Indications for EN

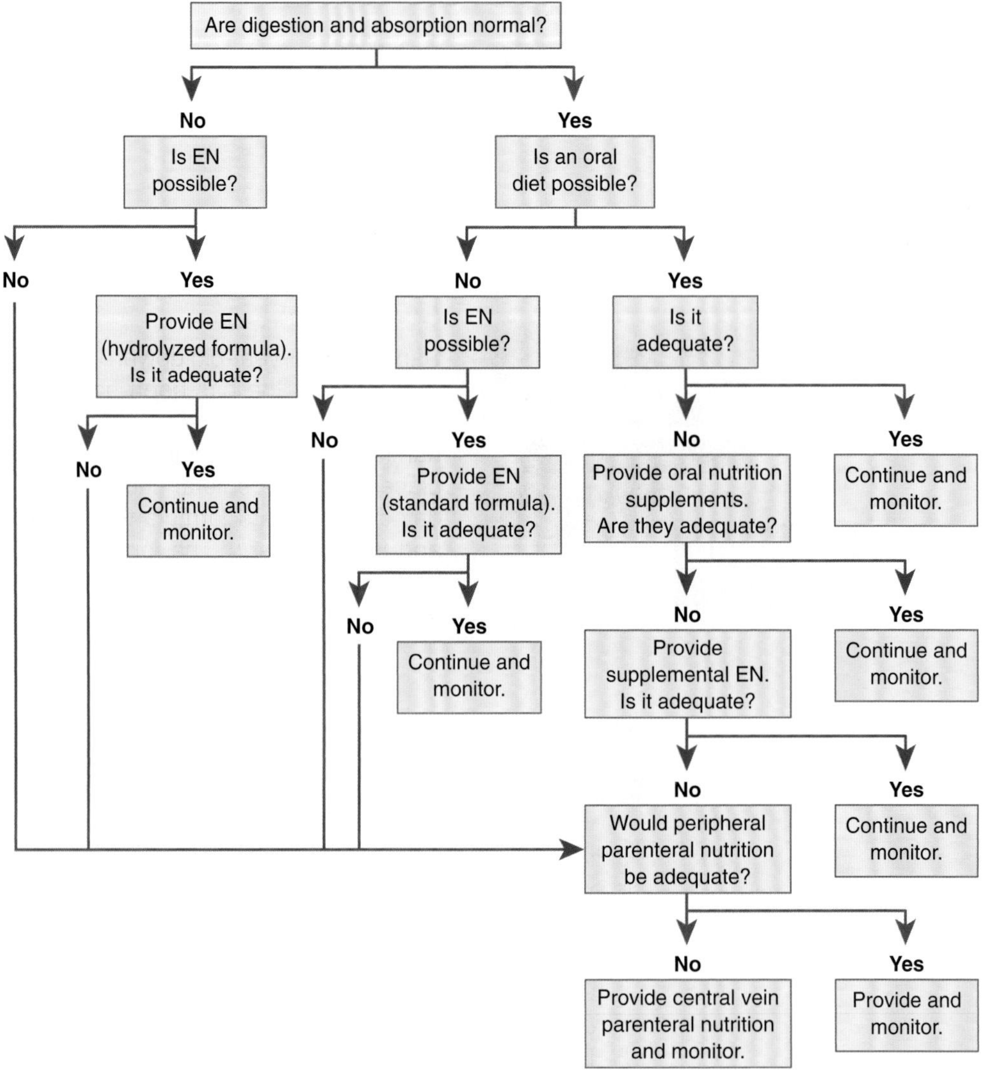

Figure 16.1 ▶ **Selecting the appropriate type and method of feeding.**

include dysphagia, mechanical ventilation, chronic history of poor oral intake, critical illness, head and neck surgeries, and malnutrition with inadequate oral intake. EN is contraindicated when the GI tract is nonfunctional or inaccessible, in severe short bowel syndrome, intractable vomiting and/or diarrhea, GI ischemia, bowel obstruction, high-output fistula, peritonitis, and paralytic ileus. Figure 16.1 illustrates the process of selecting an appropriate method of feeding based on GI function.

EN is preferred over PN because it is a cost-effective method of delivering nutrition support and is associated with less septic morbidity and fewer infectious (Academy of Nutrition and Dietetics, 2020a). Even in critically ill clients, it is practical and safe to use EN instead of PN (McClave et al., 2016).

Estimating Nutritional Needs

Calculations of the client's calorie and protein requirements are used to determine the appropriate type and volume of formula necessary to meet the client's needs. The following general guidelines may be used and revised according to the client's response to nutrition therapy:

- Calories: 25 to 30 cal/kg/day may be used as the initial estimate of need.
- Protein: Normal protein Recommended Dietary Allowance (RDA) is 0.8 g/kg body weight. Older clients and ill clients may need 1.2 to 2.0 g/kg/day. Protein needs are likely even higher for burn or multi-trauma clients (McClave et al., 2016).

BOX 16.1 Comparing Client Needs to Nutrients Provided via Enteral Nutrition Order

Example: A healthy client who weighs 165 pounds (75 kg) is ordered on standard formula that provides 1 cal/mL and 40 g protein/L. The initial rate is 50 mL/h, which will be advanced at 20 mL/h every 4 hours until the goal rate of 90 mL/h is achieved. The assumption is that the formula will infuse for 22 hours/day to allow time off to administer medications.

Calculation Guidelines

- Calories: 25 to 30 cal/kg/day
- Normal protein RDA is 0.8 g/kg body weight

Client Need Calculations

Estimated calories: 1875 to 2250 cal/day
75 kg × 25 cal/kg = 1875 cal
75 kg × 30 cal/kg = 2250 cal

Estimated protein: 60 g
75 kg × 0.8 g/kg = 60 g protein/day

Nutrients Provided via Enteral Nutrition Order

- Calories
  Initially: 50 mL/h × 22 h = 1100 mL
  1100 mL × 1 cal/mL = 1100 cal
  Goal rate: 90 mL/h × 22 h = 1980 mL
  1980 mL × 1 cal/mL = **1980 cal/day**
- Protein
  Initially: 1.1 L × 40 g/L = 44 g
  Goal rate: 1.98 L × 40 g/L = **79.2 g protein/day**

- Fluid: Common guidelines are 30 to 40 mL/water/kg/day or approximately 2.5 L/day for women and 3 L/day for men. These guidelines are not evidence based, nor do they account for conditions that impact fluid needs, such as GI fluid losses related to vomiting, diarrhea, and ostomy drains.
- Protein: Box 16.1 gives an example of calorie and protein calculations compared to nutrients provided via an EN prescription.

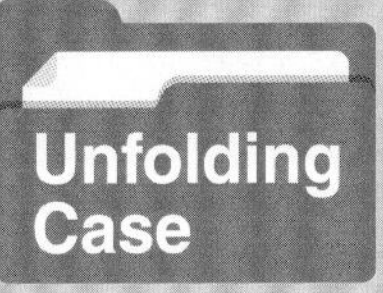

Recall Sandy. What was Sandy's body mass index (BMI) on admission? Calculate her estimated calorie, protein, and fluid needs. Will she obtain adequate calories and protein from the formula as prescribed?

Formula Selection

Formula selection is based on the client's nutritional needs and medical conditions. Standard formulas are the most commonly used formulas and are appropriate for most clients who require EN. Variations of standard formulas can meet the needs of clients who have elevated calorie and/or protein needs. Hydrolyzed formulas are intended for clients with impaired GI function. Disease-specific formulas are also available.

Standard Formulas

Standard Formulas
tube-feeding formulas that contain whole molecules of protein; known as intact or polymeric formulas.

Standard formulas, also known as polymeric or intact formulas, are made from whole proteins found in foods (e.g., milk, meat, eggs) or protein isolates.

- Because they contain complex molecules of protein, carbohydrates, and fat, standard formulas are intended for clients who have normal digestion and absorption.
- Blenderized formulas are a type of standard formula that are made from a mixture of whole foods (such as chicken, vegetables, fruits, and oil) and fortified with vitamins and minerals. They may be homemade or commercially made and appeal to people who want a more natural formula.
- Many standard formulas can be consumed as an oral supplement.
- Standard formula variations include high-protein, high-calorie, fiber-enriched as well as disease-specific formulas (Table 16.1).

Hydrolyzed Formulas

Hydrolyzed
broken down or predigested.

Hydrolyzed or elemental formulas contain very little residue and are intended for clients with impaired digestion or absorption, such as people with inflammatory bowel disease, cystic fibrosis, and pancreatic disorders.

- They contain nutrients that are partially hydrolyzed (e.g., semi-elemental formulas that contain peptides and free amino acids) or completely hydrolyzed (e.g., elemental formulas that contain 100% free amino acids).
- Carbohydrates and fat in hydrolyzed formulas are also in simple forms that require little or no digestion, such as carbohydrates in the form of maltodextrin or fructose and fat in the form of fatty acid esters or medium-chain triglyceride (MCT) oil.
- Table 16.2 features selected hydrolyzed enteral formulas.

Table 16.1 Examples and Selected Characteristics of Standard Formulas

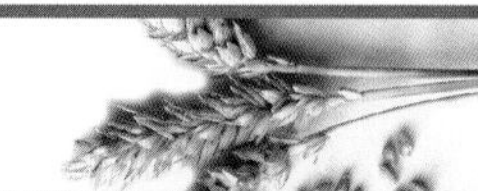

Product	Calories per Milliliter	Protein (g/L)	Water (g/L)	Volume Needed to Meet 100% RDIs for Micronutrients (mL)
Standard: Routine with varieties for high protein and high calorie needs				
Osmolite 1.0	1.0	44.3	842	1321
Nutren 1.0	1.0	40	844	1500
High protein				
Promote	1.0	63	837	1000
Isosource HN	1.2	54	808	1250
High calorie				
Osmolite 1.5 Cal	1.5	62.7	762	1000
Isosource 1.5 Cal	1.5	68	764	1000
Fiber enriched: May also contain prebiotics and probiotics				
Jevity 1.0 Cal (14.4 g fiber/L)	1.0	44.3	835	1321
Fibersource HN (15.2 g fiber/L)	1.2	54	808	1250
Blenderized: Real food ingredients				
Complete	1.06	48	828	1400

Source: Product information from https://abbottnutrition.com/therapeutic and https://www.nestlehealthscience.us/

Table 16.2 **Examples and Selected Characteristics of Hydrolyzed Enteral Nutrition Formulas**

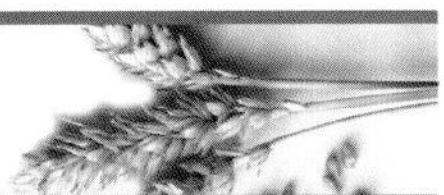

Product	Calories per Milliliter	Protein (g/L)	Water (g/L)	Volume Needed to Meet 100% RDIs for Micronutrients (mL)
Partially hydrolyzed formulas (peptides) for malabsorption				
Peptamen	1.0	40	848	1500
Vital 1.0	1.0	40	842	1422
Partially hydrolyzed formulas (peptides) with immune-modulating ingredients (e.g., arginine)				
Impact	1.0	56	852	1500
Pivot 1.5 Cal	1.5	93.8	759	1000
Completely hydrolyzed formulas (free amino acids)				
Tolerex (contains minimal fat)	1.0	20.5	842	1800
Vivonex RTF (contains 10% of total calories from fat)	1.0	50	848	1500

Source: Product information from https://abbottnutrition.com/therapeutic and https://www.nestlehealthscience.us/

Disease-specific Formulas

A variety of disease-specific formulas are available to meet the altered nutrient needs of clients with certain illnesses, such as diabetes/glucose intolerance, immunocompetence, kidney disease, and respiratory insufficiency (Table 16.3).

- Expert consensus suggests avoiding the routine use of all specialty formulas in critically ill clients in a medical intensive care unit (ICU) and disease-specific formulas in the surgical ICU (McClave et al., 2016).
- However, immune-modulating formulas containing arginine should be considered in clients with severe trauma and postop clients in the surgical ICU (McClave et al., 2016).

Table 16.3 **Examples and Selected Characteristics of Disease-Specific Enteral Nutrition Formulas**

Product	Calories per Milliliter	Protein (g/L)	Water (g/L)	Volume Needed to Meet 100% RDIs for Micronutrients (mL)
For diabetes: Composed of approximately 40% carbohydrate, 40% fat				
Glucerna 1.0 Cal	1.0	42	852	1420
Diabetisource AC	1.2	60	818	1250
Immune modulating: Contain ingredients such as arginine, glutamine, omega-3 fatty acids, and nucleotides				
Oxepa	1.5	62.7	785	946
Impact	1.0	56	852	1500
For clients on dialysis: Calorically dense for clients who require a fluid restriction; low in electrolytes				
Nepro with Carbsteady	1.8	81	727	944
Novasource Renal	2.0	90.7	717	1000
For respiratory insufficiency: Low in carbohydrate, high in fat to help reduce CO_2 production and respiratory quotient; calorically dense				
Pulmocare	1.5	62.6	785	947
Nutren Pulmonary	1.5	68	782	1000

Source: Product information from https://abbottnutrition.com/therapeutic and https://www.nestlehealthscience.us/

Formula Characteristics

As illustrated in Tables 16.1 to 16.3, enteral formulas differ in their calorie density, amount of protein/L, water content, and micronutrient density. Additional salient points are summarized in Box 16.2.

Feeding Route

The choice of enteral access or placement of the feeding tube is highly dependent on the anticipated length of time for which tube feeding will be used. Table 16.4 summarizes the advantages and disadvantages of various feeding routes.

BOX 16.2 Additional Points Regarding Enteral Formula Characteristics

Calorie Density: determines the volume of formula needed to meet the client's estimated needs.

- Most routine formulas provide 1.0 to 1.2 cal/mL, which is adequate for most clients needing EN support.
- High-calorie formulas provide 1.5 to 2.0 cal/mL and are appropriate for clients who need a fluid restriction or those who are intolerant of higher volumes of formula.

Macronutrient Content: varies with the intended use of the formula.

- Diabetes-specific formulas contain lower percentages of carbohydrate and provide fiber.
- Respiratory insufficiency formulas are high in fat to reduce respiratory quotient.
- Formulas for clients with malabsorption contain negligible to low amounts of fat in the form of MCTs. Depending on the actual fat content, some clients may not meet their essential fatty acid requirement.

Water Content: varies with the caloric concentration.

- Generally, formulas that provide 1.0 cal/mL provide approximately 850 mL of water per liter.
- The water content of high-calorie formulas is lower at 690 to 720 mL/L.
- Adults generally need at least 30 mL/kg/day, so most clients who received EN need additional free water to meet fluid requirements.
- Free water is administered when water is used to flush the tube and as a bolus administration specifically for the purpose of meeting fluid requirements.

Micronutrient Density: the amount of formula needed to meet 100% of adult Dietary Reference Intakes (DRIs) for vitamins and minerals.

- Generally, the amount of formula needed to meet nutrient DRIs ranges from 1000 to 1500 mL/day.
- When an enteral feeding is the client's sole source of nutrition, it is important to ensure nutritional adequacy within the volume of formula the client receives.

Residue Content: composed of fiber, undigested food, intestinal secretions, and other cells.

- Standard formulas come in low-residue or fiber-enriched varieties.
- Hydrolyzed formulas are essentially residue free because they are completely absorbed.

Fiber Content: Fiber stimulates peristalsis, increases stool bulk, and is degraded by GI bacteria to short-chain fatty acids that promote repair and maintenance of the intestinal lining. EN formulas containing fiber may improve digestive health and normal bowel function in noncritically ill clients (Brown et al., 2015).

- Fiber-enriched standard formulas provide 10 to 15 g fiber per liter in the form of oat, soy, pea, guar gum, or other fibers.
- Blenderized formulas are made from whole foods and thus contain natural sources of fiber, generally about 4 g fiber per liter.

Other ingredients:

- Virtually all formulas are lactose and gluten free.
- Formulas may also be kosher and halal.

Osmolality: the measure of particles in solution; determined by the concentration of sugars, amino acids, and electrolytes.

- Osmolality was once thought to contribute to diarrhea and GI intolerance in enterally fed clients, but this idea is not supported by evidence.
- Enteral formulas have lower osmolality than many common liquids (e.g., broth, soda, juices, sherbet) and medications that are routinely ordered for clients (e.g., acetaminophen elixir, sugar-free KCl elixir, liquid multivitamin).

Table 16.4 **Advantages and Disadvantages of Various Feeding Routes**

Route	Indications	Advantages	Disadvantages
Prepyloric: Feeding into the stomach			
Nasogastric (NG)	• Inability to safely and adequately consume oral intake • Short-term feeding (<4 weeks) with functional gastrointestinal tract	• Easy to place and remove tube • Can use stomach as reservoir • Can use intermittent feedings and without a pump	• Contraindicated for clients at high risk for aspiration • Potentially irritating to the nose and esophagus • May be removed by uncooperative or confused clients • Not appropriate for long-term use • Unaesthetic for client
Gastrostomy	• For long-term use in clients with a functional gastrointestinal tract • Frequently used for clients with impaired ability to swallow	• Feedings can be given intermittently and without a pump	• Moderate risk of aspiration in high-risk clients; stoma care required • Danger of peritonitis • Potential for tube dislodgment
Postpyloric: Feedings delivered beyond the pyloric sphincter			
Nasojejunal	• Short-term feeding for clients at high risk of aspiration, delayed gastric emptying, or gastroesophageal reflux disease (GERD)	• Lower risk of aspiration, especially important for clients who have impaired gag or cough reflex, decreased consciousness, ventilator dependence, or a history of aspiration pneumonia	• More difficult to insert and confirm placement • Tube may migrate into the stomach • Infusion pump required • Tube clogs easily
Jejunostomy	• For long-term use in clients at high risk for aspiration pneumonia and clients with altered gastrointestinal integrity above the jejunum • For short-term use after gastrointestinal surgery	• Low risk of aspiration • No risk of misplacing tube into the trachea • More comfortable and aesthetic for clients than transnasal tubes • Feedings can begin sooner than other feedings because motility resumes more quickly in the intestines than in the stomach after gastrointestinal surgery	• Most difficult insertion procedure • Small-diameter tubes easily become clogged • Peritonitis can occur from tube dislodgment • Cannot be used for intermittent or bolus feedings • Stoma care required • Infusion pump required

Transnasal Routes
feeding routes that extend from the nose to either the stomach or the small intestine.

Ostomy Routes
a surgically created opening (stoma) made to deliver feedings directly into the stomach or intestines.

- Short-term access (<30 days) is most commonly obtained through nasal passage of a feeding tube into the stomach via the esophagus (nasogastric [NG]). Nasoenteric feeding tubes end in the small intestine. **Transnasal routes** do not require surgery or insertions for placement, but long-term use may irritate the nasal passage, throat, and esophagus.
- For permanent or long-term enteral access (>30 days), a surgical incision or needle puncture is used to create an opening in the abdominal wall, either into the stomach (gastrostomy) or into the jejunum (jejunostomy). The advantages of **ostomy routes** are that they have a lower risk of aspiration, can be hidden under clothing, and eliminate irritation to the mucous membranes. However, enterostomy tubes must be placed by a physician or surgeon, and there is a risk of infection at the insertion site.

Delivery Methods

The type of delivery method to be used depends on the type and location of the feeding tube, the type of formula being administered, and the client's tolerance.

Intermittent Feedings
tube feedings administered in equal portions at selected intervals.

Intermittent Tube Feedings

Intermittent feedings are administered five to eight times daily in large volumes (250–500 mL) over 30 to 45 minutes or longer.

- A gravity or an enteral feeding pump may be used.
- Feedings may be spaced throughout an entire 24-hour period or may be scheduled only during waking hours to give clients time for uninterrupted sleep.
- Intermittent feedings are generally used for gastric-fed, stable clients and home tube feedings.
- They offer the advantage of resembling a more normal pattern of intake and allow the client more freedom of movement between feedings.

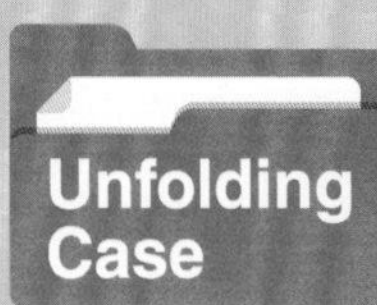

Think of Sandy. The doctor has ordered 2200 mL/day of a standard formula that provides 1.0 cal/mL to be given over 18 hours. The formula provides 842 g water/L. What will the infusion rate be? Will she meet her fluid requirement without additional free water?

Bolus Feedings

Bolus Feedings
rapid administration of a large volume of formula.

Bolus feedings are a variation of intermittent feedings.

- A relatively large volume of formula (≥250 mL) is given over 10 to 20 minutes 4 to 6 times/day by gravity via a syringe.
- They are used only for gastric feedings in stable clients and ambulatory clients.
- They are more likely to cause symptoms of GI intolerance (nausea, vomiting, abdominal pain) than the other delivery methods.

Continuous Drip Method

Continuous drip feedings are the most commonly used administration method in hospitalized clients, especially those who are critically ill, are at risk for gastroesophageal reflux, have a history of aspiration pneumonia, or require intestinal feedings. They are also used for clients who cannot tolerate intermittent or bolus feedings.

- The prescribed amount of formula volume is given at a constant rate over a specified period of time, usually 16 to 24 hours.
- An infusion pump is usually used. Feedings into the jejunum require a pump.
- This method is associated with smaller residual volumes and lower risk for aspiration when compared to other delivery methods.

Cyclic Feedings

Cyclic feedings are a variation of continuous drip feedings and deliver a constant rate of formula over 8 to 20 hours, often during sleeping hours.

- Because there is "time off," the rate of infusion tends to be higher than with continuous feedings.
- A pump is usually used.
- Cyclic feedings are usually well tolerated and often used to maintain a reliable source of nutrition while transitioning from total EN to an oral intake or in noncritical, undernourished clients unable to meet their nutritional needs orally.

Feeding Systems

EN is delivered through either open or closed feeding systems.

Open System

With an open system, formula from the original can or bottle is poured into a feeding reservoir that is either a feeding bag or a syringe (for a bolus feeding).

- Ready-to-use formulas may safely hang for 8 to 12 hours.
- Reconstituted formulas should hang for 4 hours or less.

Closed Systems

A closed or ready-to-hang system uses a sterile, prefilled container of formula (usually 1 L) that is spiked with a feeding tube and then delivered via an infusion pump.

- Closed systems may also be used to deliver bolus feedings by setting the infusion pump to deliver boluses at predetermined times.
- Although closed systems are more expensive, they may hang for 24 to 48 hours when label instructions are followed.
- Closed systems have a lower risk of microbial contamination and require less time to prepare, hang, and manage than an open-system client (Foster et al., 2015).

Initiating and Advancing the Feeding

There are no prospective randomized studies to determine the optimal rate to initiate feedings or how quickly they should be advanced (Parrish & McCray, 2019a).

- The EN order may specify starting a continuous feeding at 20 to 50 mL/h and advancing by 10 to 25 mL/h every 4 to 24 hours as tolerated until goal rate is reached.
- Intermittent or bolus feedings generally start at 120 mL every 4 hours and advance by 30 to 60 mL every 8 to 12 hours (Parrish & McCray, 2019a).
- Stable clients generally tolerate rapid rate advancement to reach goal rate and may even tolerate beginning enteral feedings at the goal rate.
- Expert consensus suggests that clients who are at high nutrition risk or severely malnourished should be advanced toward goal rate as quickly as tolerated over 24 to 48 hours with appropriate monitoring (McClave et al., 2016).
- The sooner the goal rate is achieved, the sooner the client's nutritional needs are met.
- Regardless of the access route, enteral formulas are initiated at full strength. The previous practice of diluting hypertonic feedings has not been shown to improve tolerance, prolongs the period of inadequate nutrition support, and may increase the risk of bacterial contamination.

To maximize tolerance, perform the following:

- Confirm backrest elevation is greater than 30° to 45°.
- Check **gastric residual volume** (GRV) every 8 hours or as per order.
  - Conditions where GRV checks may be useful in clients who receive EN into the stomach include head injury, abdominal surgery, obtunded or vegetative state, and critical illness following surgery or trauma (Parrish & McCray, 2019b).
  - There is no standard definition of GRV and little agreement on how frequently GRV should be checked and whether the GRV should be returned to the stomach (Parrish & McCray, 2019b).
- Consider continuous feedings if client receives bolus feedings.
- Consider post-pyloric feedings if client receives feedings into the stomach.

Gastric Residual Volume
the volume of feeding that remains in the stomach from a previous feeding.

Water Flushes

Flushing the tube periodically helps meet water requirements and ensures patency (openness). The often-cited standard for maintaining tube patency in adults is to flush with a minimum of 20 to 30 mL of warm water (Campbell, 2015):

- every 4 to 6 hours during continuous feedings (including cyclic feedings)
- before and after every bolus or intermittent feeding
- before and after checking gastric residuals
- before and after giving medication
  - If more than one medication is given at the same time, then give 5 mL of water between each

Monitoring

Monitoring ensures that the client is tolerating the EN regimen and that it is meeting the client's needs. As per facility protocol, the nurse may monitor the following:

- daily weights
- daily intake and output
- GRV
- character and frequency of bowel movements
- electrolyte levels
- tube placement
- tube site for infection
- tube-feeding tolerance

Tube-Feeding Intolerance

Although EN is an effective way to provide nutritional support to clients who are unable to consume adequate nutrition orally, many clients fail to receive the amount of EN ordered and do not receive the full benefit of nutrition support. For instance, cessation of EN occurs in >85% of ICU clients for 8% to 20% of the infusion time (McClave et al., 2016). Numerous barriers interfere with delivery of the EN prescriptions (Box 16.3) (Parrish & McCray, 2019b). Client intolerance accounts for one third of the time EN is halted, but only half of this represents true intolerance (McClave et al., 2016).

- Hospitalized clients often have significant GI issues, but they may arise from causes other than EN, such as the underlying disease process or inadequate/inappropriate medications.
- There is little evidence to support using bowel sounds or GRVs as a measurement of EN tolerance (Parrish & McCray, 2019b).
- Further assessment is needed to identify the cause of the issue and effectively intervene.
- Box 16.4 outlines signs of intolerance and suggested interventions.

BOX 16.3 Barriers to Delivering Optimal Enteral Nutrition

- "Holds"—or periods of time when the tube feeding is withheld—for surgery, bedside procedures, respiratory procedures, diagnostic procedures, extubation
- Issues with enteral access, such as clogged tubes, dislodged tubes, staffing unavailable to place tubes
- Inaccurate calculation of client nutrient needs
- Certain medical issues, such as hypotensive episodes or GI bleeding
- Perceived or actual tube-feeding intolerance
- Client psychosocial barriers such as fear of advancing formula, anxiety, depression

BOX 16.4 Signs of Tube-Feeding Intolerance and Suggested Interventions

Abdominal distress: distention, pain, abdomen is firm or tense.

- Hold feeding.
- Check for constipation.

Nausea

- Give antiemetics.
- Minimize narcotics.
- Check for constipation.

Emesis

- Hold feeding.
- Check for constipation.

Constipation

- EN does not cause constipation: underlying risk factors include the use of certain medications, immobility, and poor bowel habits or secondary to an underlying condition such as irritable bowel syndrome, neurologic disorders, or endocrine disorders.
- Minimize the use of narcotics or consider a narcotic antagonist to promote intestinal contractility.

Diarrhea

- EN is rarely the cause and does not indicate the need to hold EN (Parrish & McCray, 2019a).
- Assess normal stooling pattern prior to illness.
- Assess for causes:
  - Medications are a common, but often unrecognized, cause of diarrhea in tube-fed clients (Parrish & McCray, 2019a). Liquid medications that contain sorbitol or other sugar alcohols can cause osmotic diarrhea when consumed in excess of the individual's tolerance threshold. Examples of liquid medications with sugar alcohols include Tylenol Elixir, multivitamin/mineral liquid, potassium chloride elixir, and proton pump inhibitor suspensions.
  - Other medications known to cause diarrhea include antibiotics, lactulose, magnesium supplements, and phosphate.
  - Other causes include infections (particularly *Clostridium difficile*) and underlying diseases such as inflammatory bowel disease, pancreatic insufficiency, and diabetes enteropathy.
- Monitor stool frequency, volume, and consistency.

Source: Parrish, C., & McCray, S. (2019a). Part II enteral feeding: Eradicate barriers with root cause analysis and focused intervention. *Practical Gastroenterology*. https://med.virginia.edu/ginutrition/wp-content/uploads/sites/199/2019/02/Parrish-Barriers-in-EN-February-2019.pdf; Parrish, C., & McCray, S. (2019b). Part I enteral feeding barriers: Pesky bowel sounds & gastric residual volumes. *Practical Gastroenterology*. https://med.virginia.edu/ginutrition/wp-content/uploads/sites/199/2019/02/Parrish-Bowel-Sounds-and-GRVs-January-2019.pdf

Aspiration

EN is generally considered safe, but there can be various complications. Potential metabolic complications include fluid imbalance, electrolyte imbalances, and altered glucose levels. The tube may become clogged, become dislodged, or cause irritation at the insertion site. Aspiration is the most serious potential complication with gastric feedings.

- Factors contributing to aspiration risk include inability to protect the airway, presence of an NG tube, mechanical ventilation, client age of 70 years or older, reduced level of consciousness, poor oral care, inadequate amount of nurses for the number of clients, supine positioning, neurologic deficits, gastroesophageal reflux, and use of bolus EN (McClave et al., 2016).
- Aspiration risk is reduced by switching from bolus gastric feedings to continuous infusion and delivering EN into the small bowel instead of the stomach.
- Elevate the head of the bed to 30° to 45°. Position the client upright in a chair if doing so is not contraindicated.
- Confirm the tip of the feeding tube is properly placed before the feeding starts. Verify that feeding tube is correctly placed at least every 4 hours during continuous feedings or in the time frame according to institutional protocol.

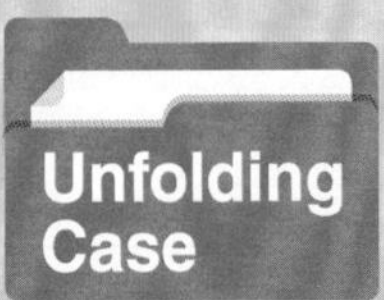

Recall Sandy. She developed diarrhea after 2 days on a tube feeding. What are the possible causes? What would you recommend to resolve her diarrhea?

Giving Medications by Tube

Although many medications are frequently given through feeding tubes to clients who are unable to swallow, they should never be given while a feeding is being infused. Some drugs become ineffective if added directly to the enteral formula. Adding acidic drugs to the formula may cause the protein to coagulate and clog the tube. It is important to stop the feeding before administering drugs and to make sure the tube is flushed with 10 to 30 mL of water before and after the drug is given. If more than one drug is given, then flush the tube between doses with 5 mL of water. Drugs absorbed from the stomach should never be given through an NI tube.

Transition to an Oral Diet

The goal of diet intervention during the transition period between EN and oral diet is to ensure adequate nutritional intake while promoting an oral diet. The tube feeding should be stopped for 1 hour before each meal to begin the transition process. Gradually increase meal frequency until six small oral feedings are accepted. Actual intake should be recorded and evaluated daily. Tube feedings may be limited to only during night when oral calorie intake consistently reaches 500 to 700 cal/day. The tube feeding may be totally discontinued when the client consistently consumes two thirds of protein and calorie needs and 1000 mL fluid orally for 3 consecutive days.

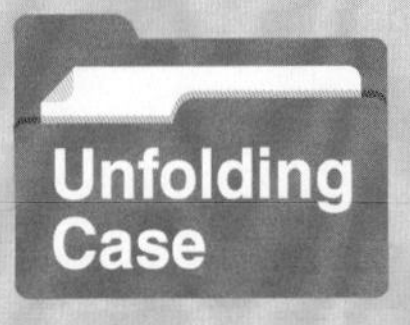

Consider Sandy. Her condition improves, and she desperately wants to have the feeding tube removed. She knows she must demonstrate that she can orally consume a "fair" intake. What measures can you take to encourage and maximize her oral intake?

NURSING PROCESS Enteral Nutrition Support

Vince is 48 years old, is 6 ft tall, and has weighed 170 to 175 pounds throughout his adult life. Two weeks ago, he was admitted to the ICU after an industrial accident caused first- and second-degree burns over 20% of his body. He was initially fed via an NG tube and then started on an oral diet. Vince was able to achieve only 40% of the calorie goal set by the dietitian, so he has reluctantly agreed to be fed by tube for 8 hours during the night to supplement his daytime oral intake.

Assessment

Medical–Psychosocial History	• Medical history that may have nutrition implications, such as diabetes or GI disorder. • Medications that may affect nutrition. • Current treatment plan. • Level of tube-feeding acceptance, including fears or apprehension about being tube fed during the night. • If Vince may need a tube feeding after discharge, assess living situation: availability of running water, electricity, refrigeration, cooking and storage facilities, employment, social support system, and financial status.

NURSING PROCESS — Enteral Nutrition Support (continued)

Anthropometric Assessment
- Height, current weight, BMI
- Percentage of weight loss

Biochemical and Physical Assessment
- Check laboratory values: hemoglobin, hematocrit, glucose, electrolytes, and other abnormal values for their nutritional significance.
- Check tube for proper positioning: Check external length of tube every 4 hours to monitor tube placement.
- Monitor hydration status.
- Ask if the client has any physical complaints associated with oral food intake or tube feeding, such as nausea or bloating.
- Observe abdomen for distention.
- Measure GRVs if indicated.
- Monitor stool frequency, volume, and consistency.

Dietary Assessment
- How many calories and how much protein are being provided via the tube feeding?
- Do the nocturnal tube feedings affect the amount of food consumed orally during the day?
- Is protocol being followed for administering the tube feeding and documenting administration and tolerance?
- Is Vince able and willing to learn how to use tube feeding at home if necessary?

Analysis

Possible Nursing Analyses

Malnutrition risk related to hypermetabolism secondary to thermal injuries as evidenced by oral calorie intake of 40% of goal.

Planning

Client Outcomes

The client will
- meet calorie and protein goals via combination of oral and tube feeding,
- be free of any signs or symptoms of aspiration and other complications, and
- discontinue tube feedings when oral intake is consistently two thirds of calorie and protein goal

Nursing Interventions

Nutrition Therapy
- Administer tube feeding as ordered.
- Encourage oral intake.

Client Teaching

Instruct the client
- on the importance of tube feedings for supplemental nutrition until oral intake meets at least two thirds of goal,
- on the signs and symptoms of intolerance of tube feeding and to alert the nurse if any problems arise,
- not to adjust the flow rate unless otherwise instructed, and
- on formula preparation, administration, and monitoring as well as the rationales and interventions for tube-feeding complications, if home EN is indicated.

Evaluation

Evaluate and Monitor
- Monitor weight.
- Monitor calorie and protein intake.
- Monitor flow rate and administration.
- Monitor for signs and symptoms of intolerance: complaints of abdominal distress, nausea, emesis, constipation, and diarrhea.

PARENTERAL NUTRITION

Parenteral Nutrition (PN) the delivery of nutrients by vein; *parenteral* literally means "outside the intestinal tract."

Parenteral Nutrition (PN) was developed in the 1960s when researchers from the University of Pennsylvania discovered how to deliver nutrients into the bloodstream via central venous access, thereby bypassing the GI tract (Koretz, 2007). PN may be provided via a central or a peripheral vein and may be the sole or supplemental source of nutrition. The term *PN* implies central PN unless otherwise specified.

Indications for Parenteral Nutrition

PN is used in adult clients who are malnourished or at risk for malnutrition when a contraindication to EN exists. It is also used when the client does not tolerate adequate EN or lacks sufficient bowel function to maintain or restore nutritional status (Worthington et al., 2017). Conditions that are likely to require PN include impaired absorption or loss of nutrients (e.g., short bowel syndrome, radiation enteritis), mechanical bowel obstruction (e.g., stenosis or strictures), the need for bowel rest (e.g., ischemic bowel, severe pancreatitis), motility disorders (e.g., prolonged ileus), and the inability to achieve or maintain enteral access (e.g., active GI bleeding). It is recommended that PN not be used solely on the basis of medical diagnosis or disease state (Worthington et al., 2017).

Disadvantages and Contraindications of Parenteral Nutrition

Although PN is a life-sustaining treatment, clinical practice guidelines uniformly support the use of EN as the preferred route for nutrition support when possible (Worthington et al., 2017). PN is invasive, costly, and associated with numerous mechanical and infectious complications. Potential metabolic complications that impact nutrition are listed in Box 16.5.

- PN is never an emergency procedure, and it should be discontinued as soon as possible.
- It should not be used to solely treat poor oral intake and/or cachexia associated with advanced malignancy (Worthington et al., 2017).
- PN is not indicated when the prognosis does not warrant aggressive nutrition support (Academy of Nutrition and Dietetics, 2020b).

Access Sites

PN may be infused via peripheral or central veins.

Peripheral Parenteral Nutrition

Peripheral parenteral nutrition (PPN) is not widely used because solutions infused into peripheral veins must have lower osmolarity (i.e., they must have low concentrations of

BOX 16.5 Potential Metabolic Complications of Parenteral Nutrition

Hyperglycemia, hypoglycemia
Electrolyte imbalances
Liver dysfunction
    Elevated liver enzymes
    Hypertriglyceridemia
Steatosis, cholestasis, gallstones
Refeeding syndrome
Metabolic bone disease (from long-term use)

dextrose and amino acids) to prevent phlebitis and increased risk of thrombus formation (Worthington et al., 2017).

- Because the caloric and nutritional value of PPN is limited, it is best suited for clients who need short-term nutrition support (≤7–10 days).
- It is intended to prevent, rather than correct, nutritional deficits.
- PPN is contraindicated in clients who need a fluid restriction, such as in clients with renal failure, liver failure, or congestive heart failure.

Central Parenteral Nutrition

Central PN
the infusion of nutrients into the bloodstream by way of a central vein. Central PN solutions are nutritionally complete.

- **Central PN** is administered via central venous catheters (CVCs). Their distal tip lies in the distal vena cava or right atrium. Using a large-diameter central vein allows for the infusion of a hypertonic formula because it is quickly diluted. Smaller veins are not able to handle such concentrated solutions.
- CVC catheter types include non-tunneled, peripherally inserted central catheter, tunneled, or implanted ports.

Parenteral Nutrition Solutions

PN solutions are a complex mixture of protein, carbohydrate, fat, electrolytes, vitamins, and trace elements in sterile water. Established clinical guidelines define the ratio of carbohydrates, amino acids, and lipids.

- PN regimens can be individualized to meet specific requirements or standardized to cover nutrition needs of a larger client population (Yu et al., 2017).
- PN admixture formulations come with and without lipids.
  - Total nutrient admixture (TNA) or "3 in 1" solution contains all the macronutrients (dextrose, amino acids, and intravenous fat emulsions [IVFE]) in one intravenous solution. Commercial preparations of electrolytes, vitamins, and trace elements are added to provide total nutrition.
  - A "2 in 1" solution contains everything in the "3 in 1" solution except the IVFE. IVFE is infused separately for calories and to prevent fatty acid deficiency on a daily or intermittent basis.

Calories

The client's total calorie needs are determined according to recommended guidelines (ASPEN, 2019b).

- **Stable clients:** 20 to 30 cal/kg/day
- **Critically ill, trauma, and septic clients:** 20 to 30 cal/kg/day
- **Obese clients:** 22 to 25 cal/kg of ideal body weight/day

Protein

Protein is provided as a solution of crystalline essential and nonessential amino acids with the amounts of specific amino acids varying insignificantly among manufacturers.

- Protein usually provides 15% to 20% of total calories in PN formulas.
- Recommended protein amounts are 0.8 to 1.5 g/kg/day for stable clients and 1.2 to 2.5 g/kg/day for critically ill clients or those with trauma or sepsis (ASPEN, 2019b).
- Because protein has minimal metabolic consequences, amino acids can be initiated at the goal rate.

Carbohydrate

Dextrose Monohydrate a molecule of glucose combined with a molecule of water.

Glucose in the form of **dextrose monohydrate** is the main source of calories in PN.

- Dextrose provides 3.4 cal/g.
- Dextrose concentrations for central PN range from 25% to 70%. Only concentrations at 10% or less are used for PPN to avoid damage to the peripheral vein. The amount and concentration provided varies with the client's nutritional needs, the amount of intravenous lipid emulsion (IVLE) given, and tolerance.
- Dextrose infusion rate starts at a moderate dose and progresses gradually.
- The goal recommendation for dextrose is 4 to 5 mg/kg/min in stable clients and <4 mg/kg/min in critically ill clients (ASPEN, 2019b).
- Carbohydrate is an important energy source but giving a client too much can have negative consequences.
  - Hyperglycemia contributes to severe infection, organ dysfunction, and death in critically ill clients (Cotogni, 2017).
  - To achieve glycemic control in clients with hyperglycemia, short-acting insulin is given either by intravenous (IV) pump infusion or by adding it to the infusion bag.
  - A high carbohydrate load may also lead to excessive carbon dioxide production, which may complicate weaning from mechanical ventilation. The trend toward less aggressive feeding has decreased the incidence of this complication.

Fat

IVLEs provide essential fatty acids and calorie-dense nonprotein calories in an isotonic solution.

- In the United States, soybean oil has been the mainstay of PN lipid formulations since the 1970s. Within the last decade, newer-generation lipid products have been developed using various combinations of fats, namely, MCT oil, olive oil, and fish oil, to alter the content of fatty acids that may play a role in immunity and inflammation (Raman et al., 2017).
- IVLEs are available in 10%, 20%, and 30% concentrations and supply 1.1, 2.0, and 3.0 cal/mL, respectively.
- The recommendations for IVLEs are to dose at <1 g/kg/day in critically ill and septic clients and not greater than 1 g/kg/day in stable clients (ASPEN, 2019b).
- Lipids are a significant source of calories and so are useful when volume must be restricted or when dextrose must be lowered because of persistent hyperglycemia.
- Allergy contraindications with standard soybean IVLEs include hypersensitivities to egg, soy, or peanut proteins (Raman et al., 2017).
- IVLEs should be avoided or used with caution in clients with severe hyperlipidemia, severe liver insufficiency, or recent myocardial infarction, stroke, or embolism.

Micronutrients

The American Society for Parenteral and Enteral Nutrition (ASPEN) has put forth recommendations for PN micronutrient dosing for adults, neonatal, and pediatric clients (ASPEN, 2019b).

- Standard electrolyte packages include sodium, potassium, chloride, calcium, magnesium, acetate, and phosphorus.
- Most PN multivitamin products in the United States contain 13 vitamins that provide the daily requirements for parenteral vitamins when administered at full daily dose. Both fat and water soluble vitamins are provided.
- The trace elements typically added to PN solutions include chromium, copper, manganese, selenium, and zinc. Iron destabilizes other ingredients in PN solutions, so a special form of it is injected separately as needed.
- Shortages of vitamins, electrolytes, and other PN nutrition components have critically impacted hospitals and home infusion companies throughout the United States over the last several years (ASPEN, 2019a).

BOX 16.6 Nursing Management Considerations for Parenteral Nutrition

- Once PN solutions are prepared, they must be used immediately or refrigerated.
- Remove PN bag from refrigerator at least 1 to 2 hours before hanging to allow solution to warm to room temperature. Do not place in hot water or microwave.
- Verify PN orders with the label on the bag.
- Once hung, the solution is infused or discarded within 24 hours.
- Inspect the solution for "creaming," which occurs as larger fat droplets aggregate and rise to the surface. This reaction is reversible with mixing. If the fat in the formula has coalesced or is "oiling out," the mixture is unusable. The PN order may need to be adjusted to prevent reoccurrence.
- Monitor the flow rate to avoid complications and ensure adequate intake.
- Perform physical assessment per protocol.
- Monitor laboratory data and clinical signs to prevent the development of nutrient deficiencies or toxicities.
- Measure and record fluid intake and output.
- Monitor weight. Weight gain >1 kg/day indicates fluid overload.
- Some clients may feel hungry while receiving PN and should be allowed to eat, if possible. If oral intake is contraindicated, give mouth care.
- Begin weaning the client from PN to EN or oral intake as soon as possible. Gradual weaning is necessary to prevent rebound hypoglycemia.
- Clients who have permanently nonfunctional GI tracts require PN indefinitely. For home PN to be successful, clients and their families must be physically and emotionally prepared. Intensive counseling focuses on preparation and administration of the solution, catheter and equipment care, and assessment skills as well as the psychological impact of permanent PN.

Note. EN = enteral nutrition; PN = parenteral nutrition.

Initiation and Administration

PN is initiated and administered according to client characteristics and facility protocol. Nutrition-related nursing management considerations appear in Box 16.6. Recommendations for initiating PN are based on the client's status (Worthington et al., 2017):

- after 7 days for well-nourished, stable adult clients who have been unable to receive 50% or more of their estimated requirements via oral and/or EN
- within 3 to 5 days in clients who are nutritionally at risk and unlikely to achieve desired intake orally or via EN
- as soon as feasible for clients with existing moderate or severe malnutrition in whom oral intake or EN is not possible or adequate
- delayed initiation in a client with severe metabolic instability until the client's condition has improved

Infusions may be continuous or cyclical.

- PN is typically infused continuously over 24 hours. Continuous infusions are given to clients who are malnourished or critically ill.
- **Cyclical PN infusions** given over a period of 8 to 16 hours or more are widely used in clients who require long-term PN and/or PN on an outpatient basis.
  - Compared to continuous infusions, cyclic infusions cause metabolic changes that must be considered: the body must adapt to changes in blood levels of nutrients (e.g., glucose) that occur when the infusion stops and higher infusion rates are required to compensate for the off periods.
  - Cyclical PN is often used as a transition between PN and EN or an oral intake. During the switch from continuous to cyclic PN, the infusion time may be gradually decreased by several hours each day, as ordered, and assessment is ongoing for signs of glucose intolerance.

Cyclical PN Infusions infusing PN at a constant rate for 8 to 16 hours/day.

Refeeding Syndrome

When PN was first introduced, it was widely and enthusiastically embraced as state-of-the-art therapy. The prevailing school of thought was that "if some is good, more is better" and overfeeding was common practice (Koretz, 2007). At that time, PN was called "hyperalimentation"—literally excessive nourishment. The practice of overfeeding has been replaced with a more conservative, lower-in-calories approach because it is now known that overfeeding, particularly overfeeding carbohydrates in nutritionally debilitated clients, can lead to a life-threatening complication known as the **refeeding syndrome**.

Refeeding Syndrome
a potentially fatal complication that occurs from an abrupt change from a catabolic state to an anabolic state and an increase in insulin caused by a dramatic increase in carbohydrate intake.

- Refeeding syndrome is characterized by metabolic and physiological shifts of fluid, electrolytes, and minerals from the extracellular fluid to intracellular fluid from the infusion of dextrose. The spike in insulin following the infusion of dextrose promotes anabolism; cells quickly draw potassium, phosphate, and magnesium out of the bloodstream.
- The resulting decrease in serum electrolyte levels can lead to fluid retention, heart failure, and respiratory failure.
- Symptoms include edema, cardiac arrhythmias, muscle weakness, and confusion.
- Thiamin deficiency occurs from the increased metabolism of carbohydrates and may cause acidosis, hyperventilation, and neurological impairments.
- The risk of refeeding syndrome can be minimized by ensuring normal electrolyte levels prior to initiating PN and beginning PN at a 25% of estimated daily needs and advancing the infusion slowly. A higher-protein, low-carbohydrate regimen is recommended. Supplemental thiamin is provided.
- Monitoring of glucose and electrolyte levels is essential.

Transitioning from Parenteral Nutrition

The transition from PN to EN and/or an oral intake begins only after GI function is adequate. PN is usually tapered as EN feedings or oral intake resumes; the transition rate is influenced by how long the client has been dependent on PN and their overall health. When the client is able to consume 50% to 75% of calorie, protein, and micronutrient requirements through EN and/or an oral intake, PN may be discontinued (Worthington et al., 2017).

How Do You Respond

My client claims they can taste their tube feeding. Can they? Except for clients who experience gastric reflux, clients cannot truly taste a tube feeding. However, the appearance and aroma of the formula may influence the client's acceptance and perception of palatability. If the formula's appearance is offensive, cover the feeding reservoir or remove it from the client's field of vision, if possible.

What are modular enteral nutrition formulas? Modular formulas are an infrequently used option to improve a client's intake. They are powdered or liquid products usually composed of a single nutrient, such as carbohydrate (e.g., hydrolyzed cornstarch), protein (e.g., whey protein), or fat (e.g., MCT oil). These products can be added to enteral formulas, food, or beverages to boost calorie or nutrient density. For instance, a client with chronic kidney failure may receive carbohydrate-fortified mashed potatoes to increase calorie intake without adding protein or altering taste. The disadvantages of adding a modular product EN is ineffective quality control (calculation errors), risk of bacterial contamination, and higher costs than standard formulas. They also increase the risk of clogged tubes and nutrient imbalances.

REVIEW CASE STUDY

Eugene is a 73-year-old man who weighs 168 pounds and is 5 ft 10 in. tall. He has had progressive difficulty swallowing related to supranuclear palsy. He has no other medical history other than hypertension, which is controlled by medication. He denies that the disease interferes with his ability to eat, even though he coughs frequently while eating and has lost 20 pounds over the last 6 months. He is currently hospitalized with pneumonia, and a swallowing evaluation concluded that he should have NPO. He has agreed to an NG tube because he believes the "problem" will be short term and he will be able to resume a normal oral diet after he is discharged from the hospital. Based on his age and activity, and considering his weight and health status, the dietitian has determined he needs 2000 cal/day and approximately 90 g protein per day to help maintain muscle mass.

- What type of formula would be most appropriate for him? How much formula would he need to meet his calorie requirements? How much formula would he need to meet his vitamin and mineral requirements?
- What type of delivery would you recommend? What would the goal rate be?
- If the doctor convinces him to agree to having a percutaneous endoscopic gastrostomy (PEG) tube placed, what formula and feeding schedule would you recommend for use at home? What does his family need to be taught about tube feedings?

STUDY QUESTIONS

1 Which tube is appropriate for a short-term enteral feeding?
   a. gastrostomy
   b. PEG
   c. NG
   d. jejunostomy

2 What is the underlying difference between standard and hydrolyzed formulas?
   a. Standard formulas cannot meet the needs of clients who have high protein needs.
   b. Standard formulas contain intact nutrients. Hydrolyzed formulas contain nutrients in more readily absorbable form.
   c. Standard formulas can be infused in the stomach or intestine. Hydrolyzed formulas can be infused only into the stomach.
   d. Standard formulas are nutritionally complete. All hydrolyzed formulas intentionally lack one or more nutrients.

3 Which type of enteral formula would be most appropriate for a client experiencing malabsorption related to inflammatory bowel disease?
   a. a standard intact formula
   b. a fiber-enriched intact formula
   c. a hydrolyzed formula for malabsorption
   d. a client with malabsorption cannot receive EN

4 Which of the following conditions indicate that IVLEs should be used with caution or avoided? Select all that apply.
   a. recent myocardial infarction
   b. hyperglycemia
   c. severe hyperlipidemia
   d. allergy to eggs

5 Which tube-feeding delivery method is most likely to cause symptoms of GI intolerance?
   a. intermittent feedings
   b. bolus feedings
   c. cyclic feedings
   d. continuous drip feedings

6 Which of the following statements is true?
   a. Medications may be the primary cause of diarrhea in tube-fed clients.
   b. Diarrhea is most commonly caused by infusing EN at too high a rate.
   c. Diarrhea indicates the tube feeding should be held.
   d. Diluting the formula and gradually increasing the concentration helps avoid diarrhea.

7 Which of the following conditions are likely to require PN? Select all that apply.
   a. paralytic ileus
   b. severe short bowel syndrome
   c. dysphagia
   d. coma

8 When oral or EN is not possible or adequate, when should PN be initiated in clients who are moderately to severely malnourished?
   a. as soon as feasible
   b. within 2 to 3 days
   c. within 3 to 5 days
   d. within 7 days

CHAPTER SUMMARY ENTERAL AND PARENTERAL NUTRITION

Enteral Nutrition

Enteral nutrition (EN) is commonly referred to as tube feeding. EN is preferred whenever the GI tract is at least partially functional, accessible, and safe to use. The client's nutritional needs are estimated before selection decisions are made.

Formula Selection

- **Standard formulas** contain intact nutrients and are suitable for most clients who need EN.
- **Hydrolyzed formulas** are composed of nutrients in simple form for clients with altered digestion and/or absorption.
- **Disease-specific formulas** are specially designed for clients with certain disorders, such as diabetes, pulmonary disorders, and immune disorders.

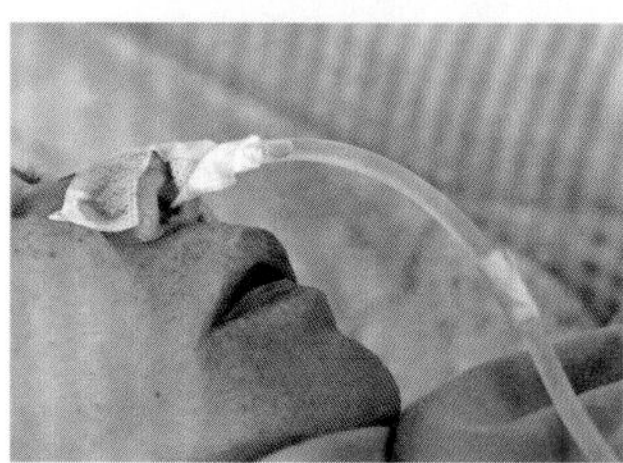

- **Formula characteristics** differ in caloric density, amount of protein/L, water content, micronutrient density, and other features.
- **Feeding routes** are NG, NI, gastrostomy, and jejunostomy.

Delivery Methods

- **Intermittent:** 250 to 500 mL given 4–8 times/day
- **Bolus:** variation of intermittent; >250 mL given 4–6 times/day via gravity using a syringe
- **Continuous drip:** consistent rate over 16 to 24 hours
- **Cyclic:** variation of continuous drip given over 8 to 20 hours

Feeding Systems

- **Open system:** Formula is poured from original container into feeding reservoir.
- **Closed system:** Formula is in ready-to-hang form

Initiating and Advancing the Feeding

- The optimal rate to initiate feedings and how quickly they should be advanced are not known.
- Formulas are infused at full strength.
- Stable clients may be able to tolerate starting feeding at goal rate.

Water flushes keep the tube clear, meet fluid requirements, and are completed before and after medication and feedings.

Monitoring is necessary to ensure tolerance and nutritional adequacy. Real or perceived tube-feeding intolerance is a common reason for holding EN.

- Tube-feeding complications include altered fluid balance, electrolyte imbalances, altered glucose levels, mechanical problems with the tube, and aspiration of gastric feedings.

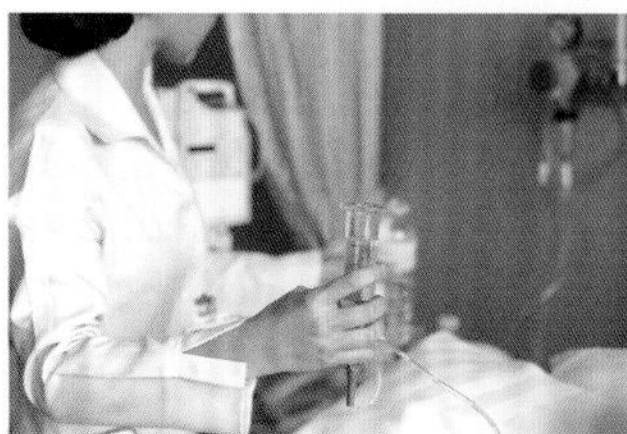

Medications by tube must be given separately and after flushing the tube with water. Many medications contain sorbitol, which may cause diarrhea.

Transition to oral diet: EN may be discontinued when oral intake provides two thirds of protein and calorie needs.

Parenteral Nutrition

Parenteral nutrition (PN) is the delivery of a nutritionally complete sterile solution into a major vein.

- **Indications:** clients who are unable to absorb adequate nutritional enterally.
- **Disadvantages** are that it is invasive, costly, associated with numerous metabolic, mechanical, and infections complications.

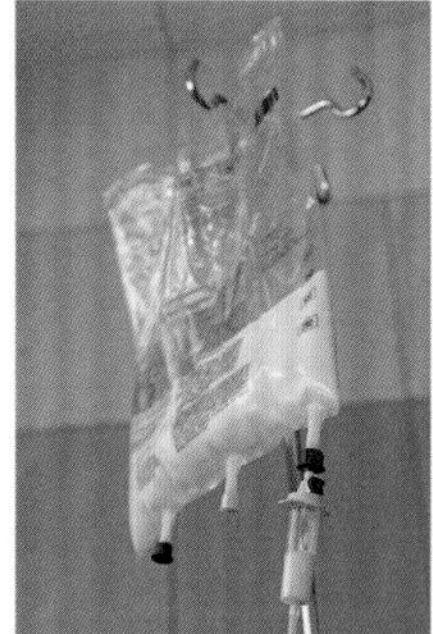

- **Access sites:** may be delivered peripherally (PPN) or via central vein (PN). PPN solutions must be isotonic and therefore are limited in calories.
- **PN solutions:** TNAs ("3 in 1") contain all 3 macronutrients in one IV solution. "2 in 1" solutions contain everything except IVFE, which can be administered separately, often by piggyback infusion. Electrolytes, vitamins, and trace minerals are added to parenteral solutions.

Composition

- **Protein:** crystalline essential and nonessential amino acids that can be initiated at goal rate.
- **Carbohydrate:** dextrose monohydrate that is initiated at low rate and progressed slowly.
- **Fat:** IVLEs prevent essential fatty acid deficiency and are a concentrated source of calories.
- **Micronutrients:** Electrolytes, multivitamins, and trace minerals are added.

CHAPTER SUMMARY ENTERAL AND PARENTERAL NUTRITION (continued)

Initiation and Administration

- as per facility protocol
- infused continuously to begin PN and appropriate for malnourished and critically ill clients
- cyclic PN is widely used by clients who need PN permanently

Refeeding Syndrome: a life-threatening complication from the abrupt change from a catabolic to an anabolic state from the increase in carbohydrate in debilitated clients.

- prevention strategies: correct electrolyte levels before beginning PN, initiate at a low rate, advance PN slowly.

Transitioning from PN: PN may be discontinued when oral/enteral intake provides 50% to 75% of client needs.

Figure sources: *shutterstock.com/nampix, shutterstock.com/Bignai, and shutterstock.com/Martin Carlsson*

Student Resources on thePoint®
For additional learning materials, activate the code in the front of this book at https://thePoint.lww.com/activate

Websites

American Society for Parenteral and Enteral Nutrition at www.nutritioncare.org

Enteral product information at www.abbottnutrition.com; https://www.nestlehealthscience.us/

European Society for Parenteral and Enteral Nutrition at www.ESPEN.org

The Oley Foundation, a nonprofit organization to help clients, families, and clinicians involved with home parenteral or enteral nutrition at www.oley.org

References

Academy of Nutrition and Dietetics. (2020a). *Nutrition care manual: Enteral nutrition.* https://www.nutritioncaremanual.org/topic.cfm?ncm_category_id=1&lv1=255693&lv2=255696&lv3=273259&ncm_toc_id=273259&ncm_heading=Nutrition%20Care

Academy of Nutrition and Dietetics. (2020b). *Nutrition care manual: Parenteral nutrition.* https://www.nutritioncaremanual.org/topic.cfm?ncm_category_id=1&lv1=255693&lv2=255697&lv3=273260&ncm_toc_id=273260&ncm_heading=Nutrition%20Care

ASPEN. (2019a). *Product shortages.* https://www.nutritioncare.org/ProductShortages/

ASPEN. (2019b). *Appropriate dosing for parenteral nutrition: ASPEN recommendations.* http://www.nutritioncare.org/PNDosing

Brown, B., Roehl, K., & Betz, M. (2015). Enteral nutrition formula selection: Current evidence and implications for practice. *Nutrition in Clinical Practice, 30*(1), 72–85. https://doi.org/10.1177/0884533614561791

Campbell, S. (2015). Best practices for managing tube feeding. A nurse's pocket manual. Abott Laboratories. https://static.abbottnutrition.com/cms-prod/abbottnutrition-2016.com/img/M4619.005%20Tube%20Feeding%20manual_tcm1411-57873.pdf

Cotogni, P. (2017). Management of parenteral nutrition in critically ill patients. *World Journal of Critical Care Medicine, 6*(1), 13–20. https://doi.org/10.5492/wjccm.v6.i1.13

Foster, M., Phillips, W., & Parrish, C. (2015). Transition to ready to hang enteral feeding system: One institution's experience. *Practical Gastroenterology.* https://med.virginia.edu/ginutrition/wp-content/uploads/sites/199/2014/06/Parrish-Dec-15-Updated.pdf

Koretz, R. (2007). Do data support nutrition support? Part I: Intravenous nutrition. *Journal of the American Dietetic Association, 107*(6), 988–996. https://doi.org/10.1016/j.jada.2007.03.015

McClave, S., Taylor, B., Martindale, R., Warren, M., Johnson, D. R., Braunschweig, C., McCarthy, M., Davanos, E., Rice, T., Cresci, G., Gervasio, J., Sacks, G., Roberts, P., Compher, C., & the Society of Critical Care Medicine and American Society for Parenteral and Enteral Nutrition. (2016). Guidelines for the provision and assessment of nutrition support therapy in the adult critically ill client: Society of Critical Care Medicine (SCCM) and American Society for Parenteral and Enteral Nutrition (A.S.P.E.N.). *Journal of Parenteral and Enteral Nutrition, 40*(2), 159–211. https://doi.org/10.1177/0148607115621863

Parrish, C., & McCray, S. (2019a). Part II enteral feeding: Eradicate barriers with root cause analysis and focused intervention. *Practical Gastroenterology.* https://med.virginia.edu/ginutrition/wp-content/uploads/sites/199/2019/02/Parrish-Barriers-in-EN-February-2019.pdf

Parrish, C., & McCray, S. (2019b). Part I enteral feeding barriers: Pesky bowel sounds & gastric residual volumes. *Practical Gastroenterology.* https://med.virginia.edu/ginutrition/wp-content/uploads/sites/199/2019/02/Parrish-Bowel-Sounds-and-GRVs-January-2019.pdf

Raman, M., Almutairdi, A., Mulesa, L., Alberda, C., Beattie, C., & Gramlich, L. (2017). Parenteral nutrition and lipids. *Nutrients, 9*(4), 388. https://doi.org/10.3390/nu9040388

Worthington, P., Balint, J., Bechtold, M., Bingham, A., Chan, L.-N., Durfee, S., Jevenn, A., Malone, A., Mascarenhas, M., Robinson, D., & Holcombe, B. (2017). When is parenteral nutrition appropriate? *Journal of Parenteral and Enteral Nutrition, 41*(3), 324–377. https://doi.org/10.1177/0148607117695251

Yu, J., Wu, G., Tang, Y., Ye, Y., & Zhang, Z. (2017). Efficacy, safety, and preparation of standardized parenteral nutrition regimens: Three-chamber bags vs compounded monobags-a prospective, multicenter, randomized single-blind clinical trial. *Nutrition in Clinical Practice, 32*(4), 545–551. https://doi.org/10.1177/0884533617701883

Chapter 17

Nutrition for Obesity and Eating Disorders

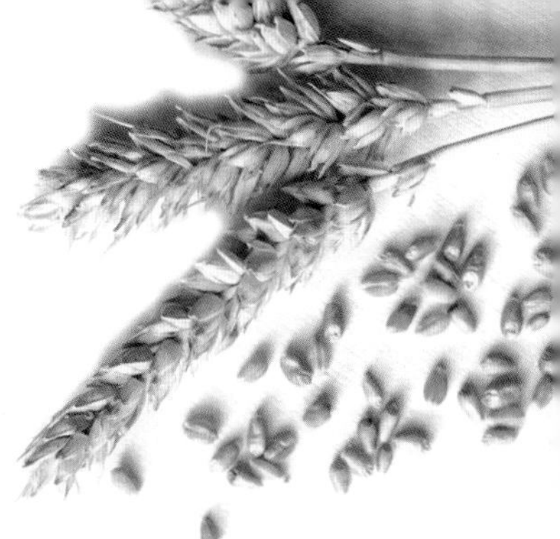

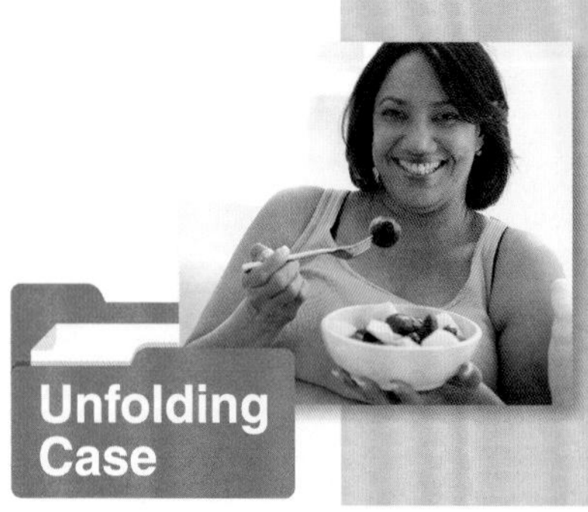

Emma Guido

Emma is 33 years old, stands 5 ft 1 in. tall, and weighs 160 pounds. Since the age of 21 years, her weight has ranged from 100 to 160 pounds. Her goal is to weigh 110 pounds. She is a certified personal trainer but changed professions because it was "fueling bad behaviors." She does not have a medical history, although she admits to being hospitalized at one point because of very low potassium levels. She wants to achieve "more normal" eating behaviors.

Learning Objectives

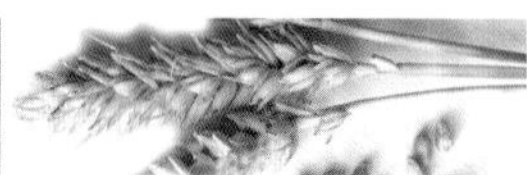

Upon completion of this chapter, you will be able to:

1 Discuss the value and shortcomings of using body mass index (BMI) and abdominal waist circumference to quantify and classify obesity.
2 Assess a person's level of disease risk based on BMI and waist circumference.
3 Discuss the three components of lifestyle therapy for weight management.
4 Identify general calorie targets for weight-loss diets for men and women.
5 Discuss the potential health benefits that may be realized when a Mediterranean diet or Dietary Approaches to Stop Hypertension diet is used for weight loss.
6 Give examples of evidence-based diets that are associated with weight loss if calorie intake is appropriately lowered.
7 Give examples of lifestyle behaviors of people who are successfully able to maintain weight loss.
8 Explain when weight-loss medications are appropriate in weight-loss treatment.
9 Describe a general diet progression after bariatric surgery.
10 Suggest possible nutritional interventions for nutritional complications that may occur after bariatric surgery.
11 Contrast nutrition therapies for anorexia nervosa, bulimia nervosa, and binge-eating disorder.

Obesity is a complex chronic condition that typically develops over an individual's lifetime. At its most basic level, obesity is a problem of excessive calorie intake. A far less common weight issue is disordered eating manifested as anorexia nervosa (AN) or bulimia nervosa. Historically, the studies of obesity and eating disorders have been separate, with the former rooted in medicine and the latter the focus of psychiatry and psychology. Yet there are commonalities between them, such as questions of appetite regulation, concerns with body image, and similar etiologic risk factors.

This chapter focuses on obesity—its causes, complications, and treatment approaches, including nutrition therapy, behavioral intervention, physical activity, pharmacology, and surgery. Eating disorders and their nutrition therapy are described.

OBESITY

Obesity can be defined as abnormal or excessive body fat accumulation that leads to adverse health consequences. The cause of obesity seems obvious: excessive calorie intake compared to calorie expenditure over a period of time (i.e., people eat more calories than they use). Although we know *how* obesity occurs, *why* it occurs is not fully understood despite intensive study. Certainly, dietary patterns and inactivity are among the primary contributing factors. However, the causes are multifactorial and complex. It is likely that obesity results from a dynamic interaction of genetic, physiological, behavioral, sociocultural, and environmental factors (Bray et al., 2016). Examples of these factors are outlined in Table 17.1.

Measures of Obesity

Body mass index (BMI) and waist circumference are ways to quantitatively define and classify obesity and assess the risk of disease (Table 17.2).

Table 17.1 Factors That May Contribute to Obesity

Causative Factors	Examples
Genetic	• More than 50 genes are strongly associated with obesity (Sicat, 2018). • Rarely, single gene defects (e.g., leptin deficiency) cause severe obesity in early childhood related to very high levels of hunger. • More commonly, predisposition occurs from multiple genes (e.g., fat mass and obesity-associated gene [FTO]) that may promote hunger, lower satiety, or lower control overeating.
Physiological	
Diseases	• Hypothyroidism • Cushing syndrome
Metabolic/hormonal	• Leptin helps regulate energy balance and suppresses appetite; leptin resistance may promote higher intake of calories and prevent sustained weight loss • During dieting and weight loss, ghrelin levels increase (ghrelin stimulates appetite, particularly for high-fat, high-sugar foods)
Side effect of medications	• Antidepressants • Antipsychotics • Corticosteroids • Insulin
Mental disorders	• Depression • Binge-eating disorder • Bulimia nervosa
Sociocultural/behavioral	• Preference for foods high in fat and/or carbohydrates • "Value meals," increased intake of food away from home • Increase in sedentary occupations • Increase in sedentary leisure time • Labor-saving devices (e.g., motorized walkways) • Lack of adequate sleep
Environmental	• Communities not conducive to physical activity • Distances between homes and work/shopping too far for walking • Living near high concentration of fast-food restaurants

Source: Sicat, J. (2018, July 23). *Obesity and genetics: Nature and nurture*. Obesity Medicine Association. https://obesitymedicine.org/obesity-and-genetics; AACE Obesity Resource Center. (n.d.). What is the disease of obesity? Obesity pathophysiology. https://www.aace.com/sites/default/files/pdfs/disease_state_resources/nutrition_and_obesity/slide_library/1.2.obesity-pathophysiology.pdf; van der Valk, E., van den Akker, E., Savas, M., Kleinendorst, L., Visser, J. A., Van Haelst, M. M., Sharma, A. M., & van Rossum, E. F. C. (2019). A comprehensive diagnostic approach to detect underlying causes of obesity in adults. *Obesity Reviews*, *20*, 795–804. https://doi.org/10.1111/obr.12836

Table 17.2 **Classification of Overweight and Obesity by Body Mass Index, Waist Circumference, and Associated Disease Risks**

	BMI[b] (kg/m²)	Obesity Class	Disease Risk[a] Relative to Normal Weight and Waist Circumference: Men 102 cm (<40″) Women 88 cm (<35″)	Disease Risk[a] Relative to Normal Weight and Waist Circumference: Men > 102 cm (≥40″) Women > 88 cm (≥35″)
Underweight	<18.5		—	—
Normal	18.5–24.9		—	—
Overweight	25.0–29.9		Increased	High
Obesity	30.0–34.9	I	High	Very high
	35.0–39.9	II	Very high	Very high
Extreme obesity	40.0 +	III	Extremely high	Extremely high

[a] Disease risk for type 2 diabetes, hypertension, and CVD.
[b] BMI ranges that define underweight, normal weight, overweight, and obesity begin at lower levels for Asians.
+ Increased waist circumference also can be a marker for increased risk, even in persons of normal weight.
Source: U.S. Department of Health and Human Services. (n.d.). *Classification of overweight and obesity by BMI, waist circumference, and associated disease risks*. National Heart, Lung, and Blood Institute. https://www.nhlbi.nih.gov/health/educational/lose_wt/BMI/bmi_dis.htm

Body Mass Index

BMI is calculated by dividing weight in kilograms by height in meters squared.

- It often correlates with the degree of body "fatness," but it does not differentiate for gender, ethnicity, muscle mass, and frame size (Welcome, 2017).
- BMI should be considered a screening tool to identify obesity, not a diagnostic method (Bray et al., 2016).
- The classification of underweight, normal weight, overweight, and obesity begins at lower levels for Asians than at the ranges given in Table 17.2.

Waist Circumference

Waist circumference is a measure of central obesity.

Overweight
a BMI of 25 or greater.

Obesity
a BMI of 30 or greater.

- Although it is not used routinely to diagnose **overweight** and **obesity**, waist circumference is a strong predictor of obesity-related, long-term health problems and correlates well with metabolic disease risk (Welcome, 2017).
- Like BMI, suggested cutoff points for health risk based on waist circumferences are lower for Asians (≥35 in. for men and ≥31 in. for women) than for Caucasians (International Diabetes Federation, 2006).

Obesity Prevalence

Obesity is a worldwide epidemic and a global public health challenge. According to the World Health Organization, more people are obese than underweight in every region of the world except parts of sub-Saharan Africa and Asia (World Health Organization [WHO], 2018). Worldwide, obesity has almost tripled from 1975 to 2016. In 2016, more than 1.9 billion adults aged 18 and older were overweight, 650 million of whom were obese.

From 1960–1962 to 2015–2016, obesity and severe obesity increased dramatically in both men and women (Fig. 17.1) (Fryar et al., 2018). In 2015–2016, the prevalence of obesity among American adults was 39.8%, or approximately 93.3 million adults (Hales et al., 2017). Obesity

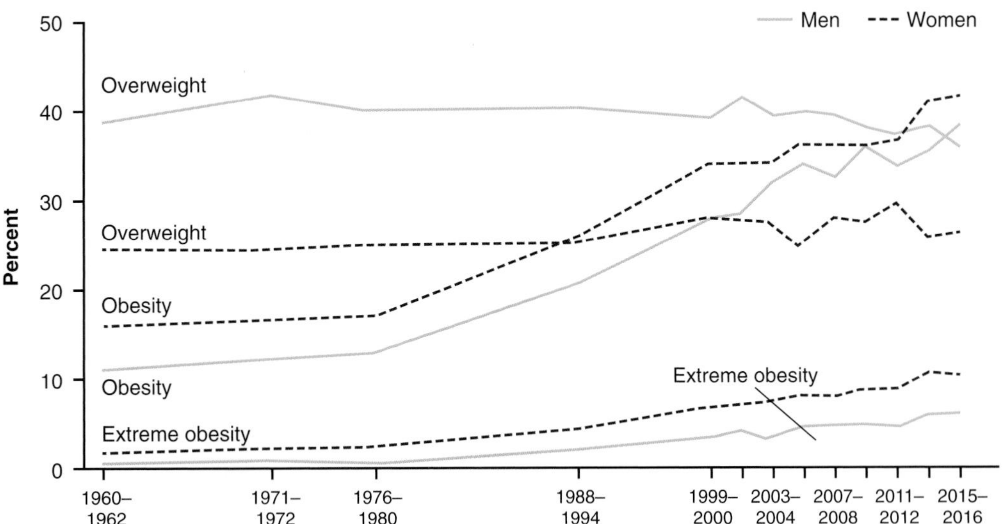

Figure 17.1 ▲ Trends in adult overweight, obesity, and extreme obesity among men and women aged 20 to 74 years, 1960–1962 to 2015–2016. (*Source:* Carroll, M., Fryar, C., & Ogden, C. [2018, September]. *NCHS Health E-Stats.* Centers for Disease Control and Prevention. https://www.cdc.gov/nchs/data/hestat/obesity_adult_15_16/obesity_adult_15_16.pdf)

Note. Data are age adjusted by the direct method to U.S. Census 2000 estimates using age groups 20–39, 40–59, and 60–74. Overweight is a body mass index (BMI) of 25.0–29.9 kg/m^2; obesity is a BMI at or above 30.0 kg/m^2; and severe obesity is a BMI at or above 40.0 kg/m^2. Pregnant women are excluded from the analysis.

prevalence has increased in all age groups and in all racial and ethnic groups. Overall, obesity prevalence is higher among the following:

- adults ages 40 to 59 than among adults aged 20 to 39
- women than men (Fig. 17.2)
- Hispanic adults compared to other races (Fig. 17.2)

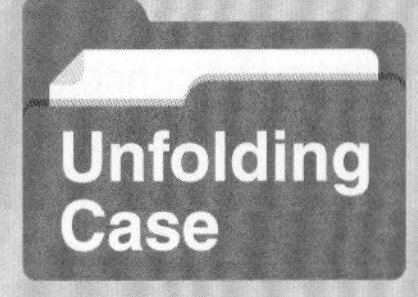

Consider Emma. What is her current BMI? Does it present a health risk? What was her BMI when she weighed 100 pounds? Was that a healthier weight?

Obesity Complications

Overweight and obesity are associated with increased risk of all-cause mortality (Aune et al., 2016). High BMI is a major risk factor for cardiovascular disease, diabetes, musculoskeletal disorders, and some cancers (Box 17.1) (WHO, 2018). Most of the world's population live in countries where overweight and obesity kill more people than underweight (WHO, 2018). Obesity also increases the risk of the following:

- morbidity from hypertension, dyslipidemia, type 2 diabetes, coronary heart disease, stroke, gallbladder disease, osteoarthritis, sleep apnea, respiratory problems, and some cancers (Jensen et al., 2014)
- complications during and after surgery
- complications during pregnancy, labor, and delivery

Where excess body fat is stored also influences the risk of comorbidities.

- Central obesity, as part of the **metabolic syndrome**, increases the risk of coronary heart disease and type 2 diabetes (see Chapters 21 and 22).

Metabolic Syndrome
a cluster of interrelated symptoms, including obesity, insulin resistance, hypertension, and dyslipidemia, which together increase the risk of cardiovascular disease and diabetes.

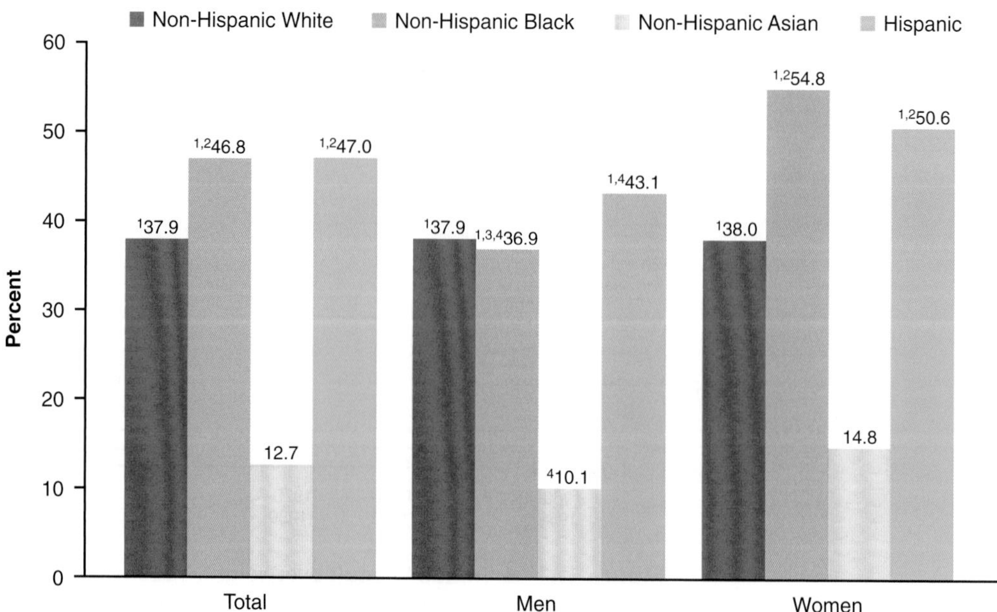

Figure 17.2 ▲ **Age-adjusted prevalence of obesity among adults aged 20 and over, by sex and race and Hispanic origin: United States, 2015–2016.** (*Source:* Hales, C., Carroll, M., Fryar, C., & Ogden, C. [2017, October]. *NCHS data brief.* Centers for Disease Control and Prevention. https://www.cdc.gov/nchs/data/databriefs/db288.pdf)

Note. All estimates are age adjusted by the direct method to the 2000 U.S. census population using the age groups 20–39, 40–59, and 60 and over. Access data table for figure at https://www.cdc.gov/nchs/data/databriefs/db288_table.pdf#2.

[1] Significantly different from non-Hispanic Asian persons.
[2] Significantly different from non-Hispanic White persons.
[3] Significantly different from Hispanic persons.
[4] Significantly different from women of the same race and Hispanic origin.

BOX 17.1 Potential Complications of Overweight/Obesity

Metabolic complications:

- Prediabetes
- Metabolic syndrome
- Type 2 diabetes mellitus
- Nonalcoholic fatty liver disease and nonalcoholic steatohepatitis

Cardiovascular complications:

- Dyslipidemia
- Hypertension
- Cardiovascular disease

Certain cancers:

- Postmenopausal breast
- Colorectal
- Endometrial
- Esophagus
- Kidney
- Pancreas
- Possibly linked to cancers of: gallbladder, liver, cervix, ovary, and aggressive prostate cancer
- Possibly linked to non-Hodgkin's lymphoma and multiple myeloma

Organ-specific, hormonal, and mechanical complications:

- Polycystic ovary syndrome and infertility in women
- Hypogonadism in men
- Obstructive sleep apnea
- Asthma/respiratory disease
- Osteoarthritis
- Urinary stress incontinence
- Gastroesophageal reflux disease

Psychological complications:

- Depression
- Anxiety
- Binge-eating disorder
- Stigmatization

Source: Garvey, W. T., Mechanick, J., Brett, E., Garber, A., Hurley, D., Jastreboff, A., Nadolsky, K., Pessah-Pollack, R., Plodkowski, R., & Reviewers of the AACE/ACE Obesity Clinical Practice Guidelines. (2016). American association of clinical endocrinologists and American college of endocrinology comprehensive clinical practice guidelines for medical care of patients with obesity. *Endocrine Practice*, *22*(supplement 3), 1–203. https://doi.org/10.4158/EP161365.GL; Simon, S. (2019). *The link between weight and cancer risk.* https://www.cancer.org/latest-news/the-link-between-weight-and-cancer-risk.html; Sarwer, D., & Polonsky, H. (2016). The psychosocial burden of obesity. *Endocrinology and Metabolism Clinics of North America*, *45*(3), 677–688. https://doi.org/10.1016/j.ecl.2016.04.016

Central Obesity
waist circumference exceeding 35 in. in women or 40 in. in men.

- **Central obesity** also increases the risk of stroke, sleep apnea, hypertension, dyslipidemia, insulin resistance, inflammation, and some types of cancer (Tchernof & Després, 2013). This risk is usually confirmed at any degree of total body fatness.
- Evidence shows that as waist circumference increases, so does risk of obesity comorbidities (Jensen et al., 2014).

MANAGEMENT OF OVERWEIGHT AND OBESITY

While prevention may be key to reversing the obesity epidemic, prevention strategies tested in schools, work places, and communities have shown little effect, emphasizing the need for effective treatment (Bray et al., 2016). Treatment guidelines have been issued by leading health organizations such as the American Heart Association/American College of Cardiology/The Obesity Society (Jensen et al., 2014) and the American Association of Clinical Endocrinologists and American College of Endocrinology (Garvey et al., 2016). Assessment begins with identifying clients who need to lose weight. Table 17.3 identifies who should lose weight based on BMI and the presence/severity of weight-related complications.

Evaluating Readiness to Lose Weight

Objectively identifying who may benefit from weight loss is not the only criterion to be considered before beginning treatment; assessing the client's level of readiness to make changes is crucial. Because clients at the two earliest stages of the transtheoretical stages of behavior change model are ambivalent about behavior change, clients in those stages are not likely to benefit from weight-loss counseling (Fig. 17.3) (Wee et al., 2005). Even worse, counseling before readiness may preclude subsequent attempts at weight loss, when the client may be more likely to succeed. The question that needs to be answered is, Is the client committed to making permanent changes for long-lasting success?

Table 17.3 Obesity Treatment Based on Body Mass Index and Complications

BMI	Weight Status	Weight-Related Complications	Goals of Treatment	Treatment
<25	Normal		Prevent overweight/obesity	Healthy eating pattern Increased physical activity Health education
≥25	Overweight or obese	None	Weight loss or prevent additional weight gain to prevent complications	**Lifestyle/behavioral therapy**[a] Possible weight-loss medication if lifestyle therapy is not effective and BMI ≥ 27
		1 or more mild to moderate complications or may be treated effectively with moderate weight loss	Achieve sufficient weight loss to ameliorate complications and prevent further problems	**Lifestyle/behavioral therapy**[a] Consider weight-loss medication if BMI ≥ 27
		At least 1 severe complication or requires more aggressive weight loss for effective treatment	Achieve sufficient weight loss to ameliorate complications and prevent further problems	**Lifestyle/behavioral therapy**[a] Weight-loss medication if BMI ≥ 27 Consider bariatric surgery if BMI ≥ 35

[a]Lifestyle/behavioral therapy: A three-pronged approach that includes a healthy, calorie-reduced eating plan, an increase in physical activity, and behavioral interventions to facilitate adherence to eating and activity changes.

Source: Garvey, W. T., Mechanick, J., Brett, E., Garber, A., Hurley, D., Jastreboff, A., Nadolsky, K., Pessah-Pollack, R., Plodkowski, R., & Reviewers of the AACE/ACE Obesity Clinical Practice Guidelines. (2016). American association of clinical endocrinologists and American college of endocrinology comprehensive clinical practice guidelines for medical care of patients with obesity. *Endocrine Practice*, *22*(supplement 3), 1–203. https://doi.org/10.4158/EP161365.GL

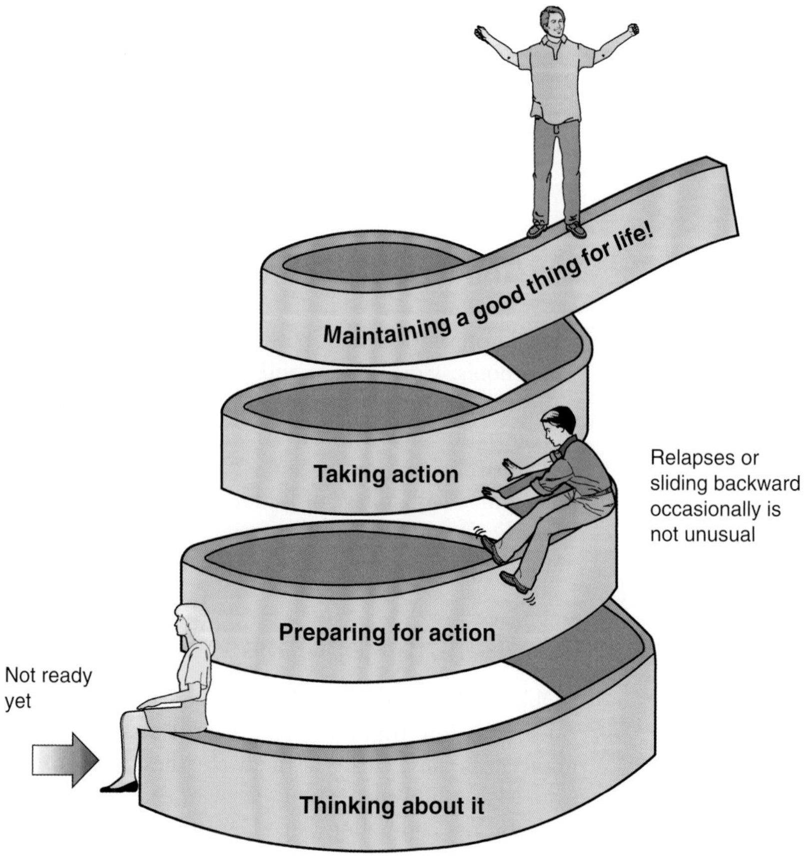

Figure 17.3 ▶ Stages of change.

Treatment Goals

As indicated in Table 17.3, treatment goals for weight management focus on preventing or ameliorating weight-related complications through weight loss, not "curing" overweight and obesity. In reality, achieving a permanent decrease in BMI to 25 or less is seldom achieved. The goal of losing large amounts of weight may be unrealistic, overwhelming, and, from a health perspective, not necessary to achieve medically significant health benefits.

- A sustained weight loss of as little as 3% to 5% of body weight can cause clinically significant reductions in triglycerides, blood glucose, and hemoglobin A1c and lowered risk of type 2 diabetes (Jensen et al., 2014).
- Greater weight loss leads to greater benefits, such as lowering blood pressure, improving low-density lipoprotein (LDL) cholesterol and high-density lipoprotein (HDL), and reducing the need for medications to control blood pressure, blood glucose, and lipids (Jensen et al., 2014).
- A 5% to 10% weight loss within 6 months is recommended.
- For some people, even modest weight loss may be unattainable, so a more appropriate goal may be to prevent additional weight gain. Although this may sound like a passive approach, it requires active intervention, not simply maintenance of the status quo.

Think of Emma. Would you identify her as a candidate for weight loss? If so, what would a reasonable weight goal be?

WEIGHT-LOSS THERAPIES

Weight-loss therapies include lifestyle/behavioral therapy (healthy calorie-reduced eating plan, physical activity, and behavioral interventions), weight-loss medications, and bariatric surgery.

Lifestyle/Behavioral Therapy

Lifestyle/behavioral therapy serves as the foundation of weight management for all people who are overweight or obese regardless of complications (see Table 17.3). It is a three-pronged approach that includes a healthy, calorie-reduced eating plan, an increase in physical activity, and behavioral interventions to facilitate adherence to eating and activity changes (Box 17.2). Lifestyle/behavioral therapy alone will cause a substantial proportion of clients to lose enough weight to improve health (Jensen et al., 2014).

Interestingly, it is recommended that people with a healthy BMI use similar approaches to prevent overweight and obesity: Eat a healthy eating pattern, increase physical activity, and participate in health education.

Healthy Calorie-Reduced Eating Plan

Reducing calorie intake is the main component of any weight-loss intervention (Garvey et al., 2016). A hypocaloric eating plan may be achieved by any of the following methods (Jensen et al., 2014):

- choosing a general target to create a calorie deficit, such as 1200 to 1500 cal/day for women and 1500 to 1800 cal/day for men
- prescribing a calorie level that is 500 to 750 cal/day less than estimated need; a 500-cal/day deficit theoretically causes a 1-pound weight loss/week (see Box 17.3)

BOX 17.2 Components of Evidence-Based Lifestyle/Behavior Therapy for Obesity Treatment

Eating Plan

- Reduce total calorie intake by 500 to 750.
- Individualize plan according to personal and cultural preferences.
- Use a healthy meal pattern: Mediterranean, DASH, low-carb, low-fat, volumetric, high-protein, vegetarian.
- Meal replacements may aid weight loss.
- VLCD for limited circumstances and with medical supervision.

Physical Activity

- Increase aerobic activity.
- Engage in resistance training exercises.
- Decrease sedentary time.

Behavioral Interventions

Any number of the following:

- Self-monitoring, such as with food intake, exercise, and weight.
- Goal setting, such as regarding food intake, physical activity, or behavioral changes.
- Problem-solving strategies, such as planning appropriate behaviors for high-risk situations.
- Stimulus control, such as restructuring the environment to avoid triggers for overeating.
- Behavioral contracting to promote behavior change.
- Stress reduction to decrease the risk that food will be used to reduce stress.
- Cognitive restructuring such as changing inaccurate beliefs.
- Motivational interviewing to resolve ambivalent feelings and find internal motivation.
- Mobilization of social support structures, which is important for long-term weight-loss success.
- Education via face-to-face meetings, group sessions, or remote technologies.

Source: American Association of Clinical Endocrinologists, American College of Endocrinology. *AACE/ACE Algorithm for medical care of patients with obesity.* https://pro.aace.com/disease-state-resources/nutrition-and-obesity/treatment-algorithms/obesity-algorithm#/start

BOX 17.3 One Pound of Body Fat Equals Approximately 3500 Calories

- **To lose 1 pound per week:** reduce intake by 3500 cal/week or 500 cal/day (3500 calories ÷ 7 days/week).
- **To lose 2 pounds per week:** reduce intake by 7000 cal/week or 1000 cal/day (7000 cal ÷ 7 days/week.).

- adopting an *ad lib* approach that does not necessarily prescribe a specific calorie level but achieves a calorie deficit by restricting or eliminating particular food groups, as seen in a low-carbohydrate or low-fat eating plan

The "Best" Weight Loss Diet

The question of which diet is the "best" diet for weight loss has been debated for decades. Attention has focused on the relevance of the macronutrient composition of the diet—the proportion of carbohydrates, protein, and fat—in achieving and maintaining weight loss.

- Data are insufficient to support any particular macronutrient distribution for the specific purpose of promoting weight loss (Garvey et al., 2016). In other words, when designed to provide fewer calories for weight loss, numerous evidence-based dietary approaches can be effective (Table 17.4). From a weight-loss standpoint, calories matter more than the percent contribution of carbohydrates, protein, and fat. Table 17.5 illustrates the amount from each food group in a low-fat, balanced, and low-carbohydrate 1500-calorie eating plan.
- Because most low-calorie diets lead to clinically important weight loss *if the diet is followed*, the "best" diet is the one the client will adhere to (Johnston et al., 2014).
- However, in terms of overall health, certain meal patterns or approaches may be beneficial for certain populations, as described in the following section.

The Dietary Approaches to Stop Hypertension Diet

The Dietary Approaches to Stop Hypertension (DASH) diet may be preferable for clients with hypertension.

- It lowers blood pressure even when weight loss is not the goal (Svetkey et al., 1999).
- It has also been shown to be an effective weight-loss meal pattern when modified to provide a calorie deficit of 500 cal/day (Appel et al., 2003).
- The DASH diet is rich in fruit, vegetables, low-fat dairy products, and whole grains; moderate in poultry, fish, and nuts; and low in fat, red meat, and added sugar.
- For more on the DASH diet, see Chapters 7 and 22.

The Mediterranean Diet

The Mediterranean diet may be beneficial for clients with cardiometabolic risk (e.g., high glucose, high triglycerides, low HDL cholesterol, central obesity, and hypertension) (Garvey et al., 2016).

- A Mediterranean-Style Eating Pattern is associated with a decrease in BMI, hemoglobin A1c, fasting glucose, and fasting insulin (Huo et al., 2014).
- The PREvención con Dieta MEDiterránea study showed that better conformity with the traditional Mediterranean-Style Eating Pattern is associated with better cardiovascular disease (CVD) outcomes, including reductions in the rates of coronary heart disease, ischemic stroke, and total CVD (Martinez-Gonzalez et al., 2019).
- The Mediterranean-Style Eating Pattern is rich in fruit, vegetables, nuts, legumes, unprocessed cereals, and olive oil; moderate in fish and wine with meals; and low in meat, meat products, and dairy products. It is a relatively high-fat diet (e.g., 40% of total calories), particularly monounsaturated fat, largely due to the liberal use of olive oil.
- For more on the Mediterranean diet, see Chapters 2 and 14.

Table 17.4 Evidence-Based Dietary Approaches Associated with Weight Loss if Low-Calorie Intake Is Achieved

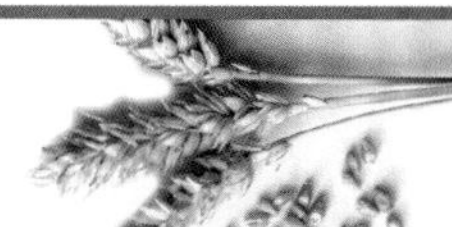

Dietary Approach	Description[a]
Diet from the European Association for the Study of Diabetes Guidelines	Food group approach without formal prescribed calorie restriction
Higher-protein diet	Prescribed calorie restriction of 25% protein, 30% fat, and 45% carbohydrate
Higher-protein zone-type diet	Five meals a day, each composed of 30% protein, 30% fat, and 40% carbohydrate without prescribed calorie restriction
Lacto-ovo vegetarian-style diet	Prescribed calorie restriction
Low-calorie diet	Prescribed calorie restriction
Low-carbohydrate diet	Initial carbohydrate intake of <20 g/day without prescribed calorie restriction
Low-fat vegan-style diet	10%–25% of calories from fat without prescribed calorie restriction
Low-fat diet	20% of calories from fat without prescribed calorie restriction
Low–glycemic load diet	With or without prescribed calorie restriction
Lower-fat, high-dairy diet	Less than 30% fat, four servings of dairy per day, with or without increased fiber and/or low-glycemic index foods with prescribed calorie restriction
Macronutrient-targeted diets	Prescribed calorie restriction with 15%–25% protein, 20%–40% fat, and 35%, 45%, 55%, or 65% carbohydrates
Mediterranean-style diet	Prescribed calorie restriction
Moderate-protein diet	12% protein, 30% fat, 58% carbohydrates without prescribed calorie restriction
The American Heart Association–style step 1 diet	Prescribed calorie restriction of 1500–1800 cal/day with <30% fat, <10% saturated fat

[a]In diets without a prescribed calorie restriction, calorie deficits result from restricting or eliminating specific foods or food groups.

Source: Jensen, M., Ryan, D., Apovian, C., Ard, J. D., Comuzzie, A. G., Donato, K. A., Hu, F., Hubbard, V., Jakicic, J., Kushner, R., Loria, C., Millen, B., Nonas, C., Pi-Sunyer, X., Stevens, J., Stevens, V., Wadden, T., Wolfe, B., & Yanovski, S. Z. (2014). 2013 AHA/ACC/TOS guideline for the management of overweight and obesity in adults. A report of the American College of Cardiology/American Heart Association Task Force on Practice Guidelines and the Obesity Society. *Journal of the American College of Cardiology*, *63*(25), 2985–3023. https://doi.org/10.1016/j.jacc.2013.11.004.

Table 17.5 Sample 1500-Calorie Eating Plans for Low-Fat, Balanced, and Low-Carb Diets

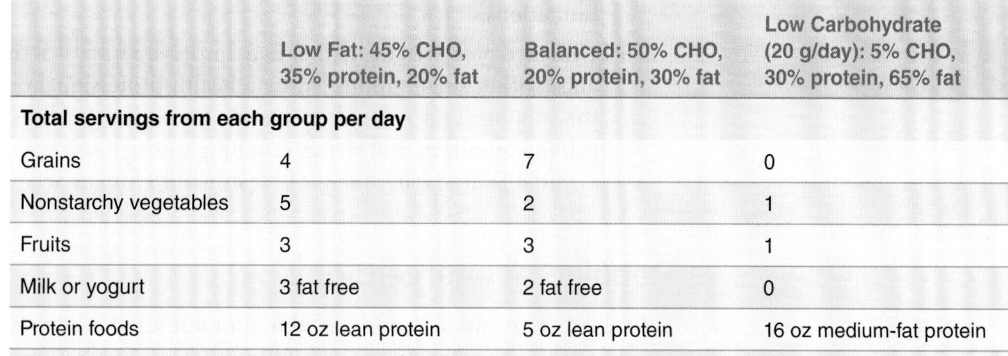

	Low Fat: 45% CHO, 35% protein, 20% fat	Balanced: 50% CHO, 20% protein, 30% fat	Low Carbohydrate (20 g/day): 5% CHO, 30% protein, 65% fat
Total servings from each group per day			
Grains	4	7	0
Nonstarchy vegetables	5	2	1
Fruits	3	3	1
Milk or yogurt	3 fat free	2 fat free	0
Protein foods	12 oz lean protein	5 oz lean protein	16 oz medium-fat protein
Fats	2	5	5

Meal Replacement Approach

Consuming liquid meal replacements or prepackaged foods is one approach that may promote more weight loss than standard low-calorie diets and behavior counseling (Rock et al., 2016).

- Prepacked foods overcome several barriers to dietary adherence, including portion control, convenience, and reduced decision-making.
- Commercial diet programs, such as Jenny Craig and Nutrisystem, feature one to two meals per day of vitamin- and mineral-fortified, low-calorie meals, which may be in the form of a shake, frozen entrée, or meal bar.
- In overweight and obese women, the use of liquid and bar meal replacements is associated with greater weight loss at up to 6 months compared to a balanced low-calorie diet of conventional food (Jensen et al., 2014).
- Long-term studies are needed to determine how meal replacements impact weight-loss maintenance.

Very-Low-Calorie Diet

Very-low-calorie diets (VLCDs) provide <800 cal/day, usually in the form of a liquid shake that is enriched with high biologic value protein and 100% of the daily value for micronutrients.

- Initial weight loss is quick and substantial, but VLCDs are associated with gallstones and sudden death and greater weight regain compared with weight loss achieved through a more moderate calorie restriction (Hemmingsson et al., 2012).
- VLCDs should be used only in limited circumstances in a medical care setting, with the provision of medical supervision and high-intensity lifestyle intervention (Jensen et al., 2014).
- VLCDs are a common method to reduce weight prior to bariatric surgery to reduce overall surgical risk in people with severe obesity (Yolsuriyanwong et al., 2019).

Physical Activity

Evidence-based lifestyle therapy for the treatment of obesity includes the following physical activity recommendations (Garvey et al., 2016):

- Aerobic physical activity progressing to 150 minutes/week or more performed on 3 to 5 separate days/week. Greater amounts of exercise are associated with better long-term weight-loss maintenance (Vanderwood et al., 2011; Wadden et al., 2011).
- Resistance training of single-set exercises involving the major muscle groups performed 2–3 times/week. Resistance training exercises help promote fat loss while preserving muscle mass during weight-loss therapy.
- Reduce sedentary behavior, which in general means any waking behavior with low energy output done while sitting, reclining, or lying down.
- Physical activity should be individualized according to the client's preferences and physical limitations.
- Evidence-based strategies that may improve physical activity levels include receiving guidance within small groups led by a health professional or trainer; using a "buddy system" for support; and technology-based approaches, such as pedometers and other wearable activity monitors, and virtual coaching through text messaging, telephone, or the Internet (United States Department of Health and Human Services, 2018).

Behavioral Interventions

Behavioral interventions are intended to promote adherence to nutrition and physical activity prescriptions through activities such as self-monitoring, goal setting, and stimulus control (Box 17.2). Box 17.4 lists specific strategies to promote adherence to a reduced-calorie eating plan.

BOX 17.4 Behavior Change Ideas

Change the Environment

- Keep food only in the kitchen, not scattered around the house.
- Stay out of the kitchen except when preparing and cleaning up after meals.
- Avoid tasting food while cooking; don't take extra portions to get rid of a food.
- Place the low-calorie foods in the front of the refrigerator; keep the high-calorie foods hidden.
- Remove temptation to better resist it: "Out of sight, out of mind."
- Plan meals and snacks to help eliminate hasty decisions and impulses that may sabotage healthy eating.

Eat Wisely

- Wait 10 minutes before eating when you feel the urge; hunger pangs may go away if you delay eating.
- Never skip meals.
- Eat before you're starving and stop when satisfied, not stuffed.
- Eat only in one designated place and devote all your attention to eating. Activities such as reading and watching television can be so distracting that you may not even realize you ate.
- Serve food directly from the stove to the plate instead of family style, which can lead to second helpings.
- "Right size" portions by estimating portion sizes according to common household items, such as using the size of a woman's palm to estimate a 3 oz serving of meat.
- Eat the low-calorie foods first.
- Drink water with meals.
- Use a small plate to give the appearance of eating a full plate of food.
- Chew food thoroughly and eat slowly.
- Put utensils down between mouthfuls.
- Leave some food on your plate to help you feel in control of food rather than feeling that food controls you.
- Eat before attending a social function that features food; while there, select low-calorie foods to nibble on.
- Give yourself permission to enjoy an occasional planned indulgence and do so without guilt; don't let disappointment lead to an eating binge.
- Eat satisfying foods and do not restrict particular foods.
- Replace sugar-sweetened beverages with water.

Shop Smart

- Never shop while hungry.
- Shop only from a list; resist impulse buying.
- Buy food only in the quantity you need.
- Don't buy foods you find tempting.
- Stock on fruits and vegetables for low-calorie snacking.

Practice Healthy Habits

- Keep busy with hobbies or projects that are incompatible with eating to take your mind off eating.
- Brush your teeth immediately after eating.
- Keep food and activity records.
- Keep hunger records.
- Get more sleep if fatigue triggers eating.
- Weigh yourself regularly.

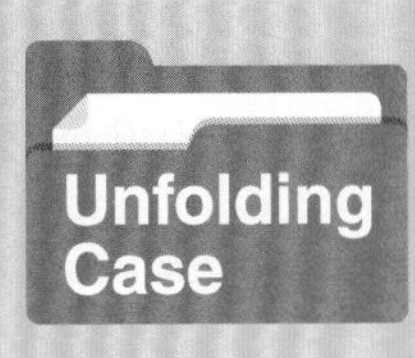

Recall Emma. In an effort to lose weight, she has been weighing and measuring her food and tracking her total daily intake, which averages between 900 and 1100 cal/day. Her food records show that she eats grains and protein foods but no vegetables, fruits, or dairy. What would you tell Emma about appropriate calories and weight-loss diets? What would you tell her about healthy eating?

Comprehensive Lifestyle Programs

Comprehensive lifestyle programs are structured multidisciplinary programs that include all three lifestyle therapies: hypocaloric eating plan, physical activity prescriptions, and behavioral interventions. Multiple studies show that structured comprehensive programs produce substantially greater weight loss than standard or usual care (Garvey et al., 2016). Frequent contact between health care professionals and accommodations for personal and cultural client preferences may contribute to improved success.

- Overweight and obese adults who want to lose weight should be advised to participate in a comprehensive lifestyle program for at least 6 months. Such programs help participants adhere to a lower-calorie diet and increase physical activity through the use of behavioral strategies (Jensen et al., 2014).

- Longer-duration programs (longer than 1 year) result in greater weight loss and are more effective in preventing weight regain (Millen et al., 2014).
- Electronically delivered weight-loss programs are useful but may result in smaller weight loss than in-person interventions (Raynor & Champagne, 2016).
- Commercial weight-loss diets that include comprehensive lifestyle intervention, such as Weight Watchers, can be used provided there is peer-reviewed published evidence of their safety and efficacy (Raynor & Champagne, 2016).

Weight Maintenance after Loss

Although losing weight may be difficult, keeping it off is even harder. Calorie expenditure is lower after weight loss because a lighter/smaller body requires fewer calories than a heavier/larger body when performing the same activity. Metabolic changes that occur during weight loss may also contribute to the risk of regain. Evidence shows that weight loss causes an adaptive thermogenesis which is a lowering of calorie expenditure beyond what can be predicted by changes in body weight and composition (Camps et al., 2013). This metabolic adaptation is a survival mechanism to conserve energy during periods of famine. After weight loss, adaptive thermogenesis may be responsible for a decrease in calorie expenditure of 20 to 200 cal/day—meaning someone who has lost significant weight may burn up to 200 fewer calories per day compared to someone of the same weight who has not experienced weight loss. Camps et al. (2013) found that people with a larger weight loss show a greater decrease in resting metabolic rate and that adaptive thermogenesis may persist for up to 44 weeks after weight loss. Adaptive thermogenesis was no longer observed when weight was regained to preloss or higher weight. The disproportionate decrease in calorie expenditure after weight loss could be one of the factors contributing to the high rate of regain (Camps et al., 2013).

Typically, clients who participate in a lifestyle intervention program reach maximum weight loss at 6 months, followed by a plateau and gradual regain over time (Jensen et al., 2014). Weight regain is most likely to occur in people who ease up on physical activity, increase their fat intake, use less dietary restraint, and weigh themselves less often. Better long-term weight maintenance is associated with larger initial weight loss and longer duration of maintenance (Thomas et al., 2014). Long-term weight-loss maintenance is possible but requires sustained behavior change (Thomas et al., 2014), namely, high levels of physical activity (>200 minutes/week), continuation of a low-calorie eating plan, and weekly self-monitoring of weight (Jensen, 2014).

The National Weight Control Registry (NWCR), founded in 1994 to identify and investigate behavioral and psychological characteristics of people who are successful in maintaining significant weight loss, is currently tracking more than 10,000 people in the registry. The average participant has lost an average of 66 pounds and kept it off for 5½ years. Participants are surveyed annually to examine the behavioral and psychological characteristics of weight maintainers and to identify the strategies they use to maintain their weight loss. Characteristics of successful weight maintainers appear in Box 17.5.

BOX 17.5 Successful Weight Maintenance

The main strategies used by participants in the National Weight Control Registry (NWCR) to successfully maintain long-term weight loss are the following:

- High levels of physical activity (about 1 hour/day), walking being the exercise of choice for most people
- Eating a low-calorie, low-fat diet
- Eating breakfast every day
- Weighing themselves at least once a week
- Limiting TV viewing to <10 hours/week
- Maintaining a consistent pattern across weekdays and weekends

Source: National Weight Control Registry. (n.d.). *NWCR facts*. http://nwcr.ws/Research/default.htm

Weight-Loss Medications

While lifestyle modification alone is effective in achieving some weight loss, virtually all obesity medication studies show that adding weight-loss medication to lifestyle therapy consistently produces greater weight loss and weight-loss maintenance than lifestyle therapy alone (Garvey et al., 2016). Similarly, data show that weight-loss medication alone does not result in as much weight loss as when medications are combined with lifestyle therapy (Garvey et al., 2016).

- Weight-loss medications are approved by the Food and Drug Administration (FDA) for clients with a BMI ≥ 30 without weight-related complications or ≥27 in clients with at least one weight-related complication (Mechanick et al., 2019).
- Weight-loss medications are used long term for chronic management of obesity. Short-term use (3–6 months) has not been shown to produce long-term health benefits (Garvey et al., 2016).
- In clients with weight-related complications that can be ameliorated by weight loss, it is recommended that lifestyle therapy and weight-loss medications be combined at the initiation of treatment.
- Weight-loss medications are increasingly used in clients who have had bariatric surgery but have failed to lose adequate weight or have had weight regain (Mechanick et al., 2019).
- Table 17.6 features the drugs approved by the U.S. FDA for the treatment of obesity.
- Evidence is generally lacking on the usefulness of dietary supplements in promoting weight loss (Box 17.6).

Table 17.6 U.S. Food and Drug Administration–Approved Drugs for Long-Term Obesity Treatments

Generic Name/Trade Name	Drug Type	Effects	Common Side Effects
Orlistat/Xenical (Alli is the over-the-counter lower-dose version of orlistat)	Pancreatic lipase inhibitor	Reduces absorption of dietary fat; fat-soluble vitamin supplement recommended at bedtime or 2 hours after orlistat dose; fewer side effects when low-fat diet consumed	Gastrointestinal (GI) issues (cramping, diarrhea, oily spotting, fecal incontinence), headache, rare cases of severe liver injury reported; GI side effects limit its popularity in clients
Phentermine-topiramate/ Qsymia	Phentermine is an appetite suppressant; topiramate is an antiepileptic	Decreases hunger and promotes satiety; associated with greater mean weight loss than the other medications	Paresthesia, dizziness, altered taste sensation, insomnia, constipation, dry mouth
Liraglutide 3.0 mg/Saxenda (available by injection only)	Glucagon-like 1 receptor agonist	Impairs appetite and increases satiety	Nausea, diarrhea, constipation, abdominal pain, dyspepsia, vomiting, headache, increased heart rate, pancreatitis; found to cause a rare type of thyroid tumor in animals
Naltrexone-bupropion ER/ Contrave	Naltrexone is an opioid receptor blocker; bupropion is a dopamine and norepinephrine reuptake inhibitor	Subjectively, clients report decreased appetite and fewer cravings	Nausea, constipation, diarrhea, headache, vomiting, dizziness, insomnia, dry mouth, anxiety

Source: National Institute of Diabetes and Digestive and Kidney Diseases. (2016). *Prescription medications to treat overweight and obesity*. https://www.niddk.nih.gov/health-information/weight-management/prescription-medications-treat-overweight-obesity; Garvey, W. T., Mechanick, J., Brett, E., Garber, A., Hurley, D., Jastreboff, A., Nadolsky, K., Pessah-Pollack, R., Plodkowski, R., & Reviewers of the AACE/ACE Obesity Clinical Practice Guidelines. (2016). American association of clinical endocrinologists and American college of endocrinology comprehensive clinical practice guidelines for medical care of clients with obesity. *Endocrine Practice*, *22*(supplement 3), 1–203. https://doi.org/10.4158/EP161365.GL; Bray, G., Fruhbeck, G., Ryan, D., & Wilding, J. (2016). Management of obesity. *Lancet*, *387*, 1947–1956. http://media.mycme.com/documents/294/bray_2016_73259.pdf

BOX 17.6 Selected Weight-Loss Supplements

- *Acai*: No definitive evidence exists that it promotes weight loss; little information exists regarding its safety when consumed in supplement form.
- *Bitter orange*: Evidence is insufficient to support its use for any health purpose. Safety concerns have been raised, especially in people with cardiac issues or hypertension.
- *Ephedra (ma huang)*: There is little evidence of its effectiveness except for short-term weight loss. It is associated with serious adverse events, such as cardiovascular complications and death. Sale has been banned in the United States since 2004.
- *Green tea*: There is not enough reliable data to assess its effect on weight loss. A few, small studies found that the loss of weight in overweight or obese adults who had taken a green tea preparation was very small, not statistically significant, and not likely to be clinically important.
- *Hoodia*: No reliable evidence supports its use for any health condition. Safety has not been studied.

Source: National Institutes of Health, National Center for Complementary and Integrative Health. (2015). *Weight-control and complementary and integrative approaches: What the science says*. https://nccih.nih.gov/health/providers/digest/weightloss-science#acai

Weight-Loss Devices

A relatively new approach in treating obesity is the use of FDA-approved nonsurgical procedures using certain devices. For instance, various endoscopic bariatric therapies work by reducing stomach capacity, such as the insertion of an intragastric balloon to occupy space in the stomach. Three gastric balloons have been approved by the FDA for clients with a BMI of 30 to 40. Although the devices are associated with short-term weight loss, their effectiveness and safety in long-term obesity management remain uncertain (Mechanick et al., 2019).

Recently, the popular press has touted FDA approval for a new weight-loss pill called Plenity™ that expands in the stomach to provide a feeling of fullness. However, the FDA approved Plenity™ as an adjunct to diet and exercise and as "a transient, space-occupying devise for weight management and/or weight loss for people with BMI of 25–40" (U.S. Food and Drug Administration, 2019). It is composed of hydrogel that acts like a fiber supplement to absorb water thereby causing the stomach to lose about 25% of its available volume. The "device" then passes from the body via the GI tract. Preliminary studies show promise, but long-term safety and usefulness are yet to be determined.

Bariatric Surgery

Bariatric surgery is the most effective treatment for obesity. Weight-loss surgeries are considered both bariatric and metabolic surgeries. In addition to leading to significant weight loss, these surgeries cause significant improvements in glycemic-control metrics in clients with type 2 diabetes and in cardiovascular outcomes, such as hypertension, dyslipidemia, myocardial infarction, and stroke (Mechanick et al., 2019). The underlying mechanisms of the beneficial effects are complex and include changes in GI anatomy and motility, diet and behavior, gut hormones (e.g., ghrelin), bile acid flow, and gut bacteria (Dagan et al., 2017). Candidates for bariatric surgery are listed in Box 17.7.

Surgical procedures for obesity restrict the stomach's capacity or combine a reduced stomach capacity with malabsorption by bypassing part of the small intestine. The type of procedure used is based on individualized goals, local expertise, client preferences, and other variables. Laparoscopic procedures are preferred over open procedures because they are associated with lower early postoperative morbidity and mortality (Mechanick et al., 2019). Vitamin and mineral deficiencies are one of the disadvantages of bariatric surgery. They are most likely to develop after the first year of surgery. Clients take vitamin and mineral supplements for the rest of their lives.

Seventy percent of total bariatric surgeries in the United States are laparoscopic sleeve gastrectomy (SG), 5% are laparoscopic gastric bypass, and 3% are adjustable gastric banding (Mechanick et al., 2019).

BOX 17.7 Candidates[a] for Bariatric Surgery

Candidates for bariatric surgery are clients with

- BMI ≥40 without medical complications in whom bariatric procedures would not be associated with excessive risk,
- BMI ≥35 and ≥1 severe obesity-related complications remediable by weight loss such as type 2 diabetes, high risk for type 2 diabetes, poorly controlled hypertension, nonalcoholic fatty liver disease, obstructive sleep apnea, osteoarthritis of the knee or hip, and urinary stress incontinence, and
- BMI 30–34.9 and type 2 diabetes with inadequate glucose control despite optimal lifestyle and medical therapy.
- Bariatric surgery should also be considered to achieve optimal health and quality-of-life outcomes when the amount of weight loss needed to prevent or treat clinically significant obesity-related complications cannot be obtained using only structured lifestyle change with medical therapy.

[a]BMI criterion may be adjusted for ethnicity (e.g., lowered for Americans of Asian descent).

Source: Mechanick, J., Apovian, C., Brethauer, S., Garvey, T., Joffe, A., Kim, J., Kushner, R., Lindquist, R., Pessah-Pollack, R., Seger, J., Urman, R., Adams, S., Cleek, J., Correa, R., Figaro, M., Flanders, K., Grams, J., Hurley, D., Kothari, S., ... Still, S. (2019). Clinical practice guidelines for the perioperative nutrition, metabolic, and nonsurgical support of patients undergoing bariatric procedures-2019 update: Cosponsored by American Association of Clinical Endocrinologists/American College of Endocrinology, The Obesity Society, American Society for Metabolic & Bariatric Surgery, Obesity Medicine Association, and American Society of Anesthesiologists. *Endocrine Practice*, *25*(supplement 2), 1–75. https://journals.aace.com/doi/pdf/10.4158/GL-2019-0406

Sleeve Gastrectomy

Sleeve Gastrectomy (SG) removes approximately 80% of the stomach longitudinally, resulting in a small pouch resembling a sleeve (hence the name) or long thin banana (Fig. 17.4).

- The pyloric sphincter and intestines remain intact so the food pathway is not altered.
- Removal of most of the stomach results in increases in gut hormone levels that induce satiety, inhibit food intake, increase insulin sensitivity, and slow gastric emptying (Weight Management Dietetic Practice Group et al., 2015).
- Weight loss is somewhat less than that produced by Roux-en-Y Gastric Bypass (RYGB), but it is achieved at lower cost, lower morality, lower rates of complications, and fewer metabolic complications (Raynor & Champagne, 2016).
- Common micronutrient deficiencies after SG include calcium, iron, vitamin B_{12}, thiamin, and vitamin D (Weight Management Dietetic Practice Group et al., 2015).

Roux-en-Y Gastric Bypass

Roux-en Y Gastric Bypass (RYGB) has long been considered the gold standard procedure for obesity (Raynor & Champagne, 2016). The GI tract is permanently altered as a small pouch is created at the top of the stomach and the jejunum is attached via a small hole in the pouch. Food bypasses most of the stomach, the entire duodenum, and a small portion of the proximal jejunum (Fig. 17.5). Removal of the pyloric sphincter increases the risk of **dumping syndrome**.

Dumping Syndrome
symptoms (e.g., nausea, abdominal cramping, diarrhea, hypoglycemia) that occur from rapid emptying of an osmotic load from the stomach into the small intestine.

- Weight loss and/or improvement in obesity-related comorbidities such as diabetes and hyperlipidemia are greater for RYGB than the currently more popular procedure SG (Lager et al., 2017).
- Mortality rate and rate of complications are higher in RYGB than the other two surgeries (Raynor & Champagne, 2016).
- The most common micronutrient deficiencies after RYGB include calcium, iron, folate, vitamin B_{12}, thiamin, and vitamin D (Weight Management Dietetic Practice Group et al., 2015).

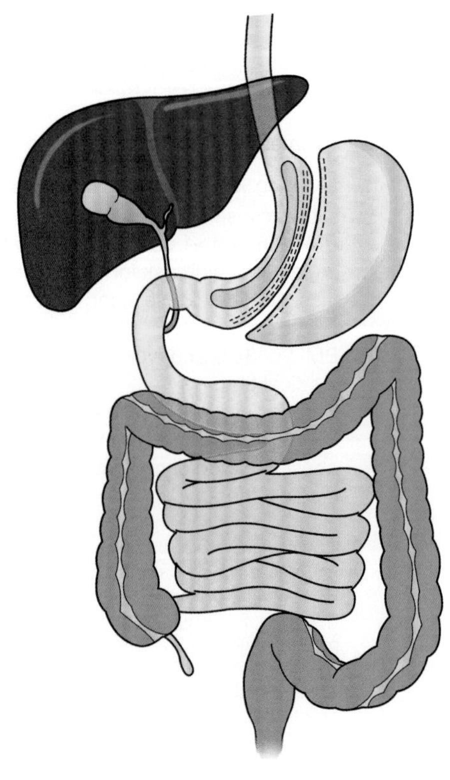

Figure 17.4 ▶
Sleeve gastrectomy.

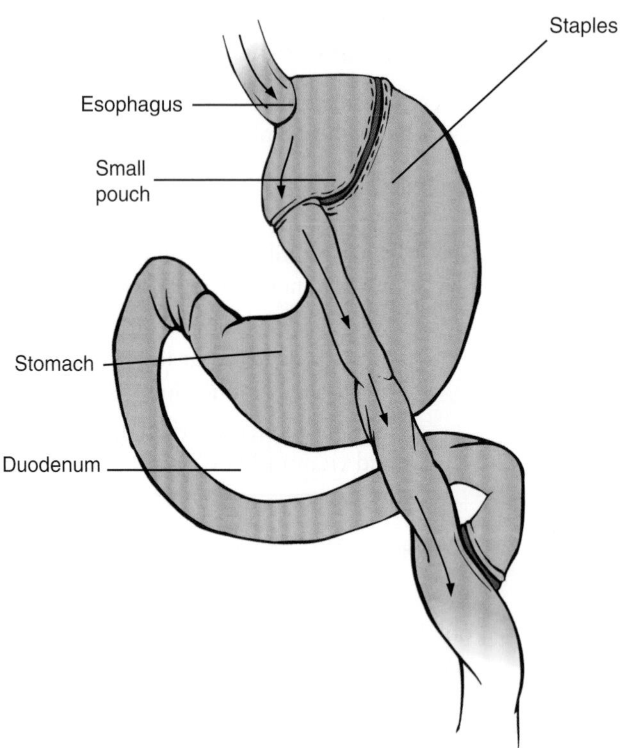

Figure 17.5 ▶
Roux-en-Y gastric bypass.

Laparoscopic Adjustable Gastric Banding

Laparoscopic adjustable gastric banding (LAGB) works purely by restricting the capacity of the stomach.

- An inflatable band encircles the uppermost stomach to create a 15- to 30-mL capacity gastric pouch with a limited outlet between the pouch and the main section of the stomach (Fig. 17.6).

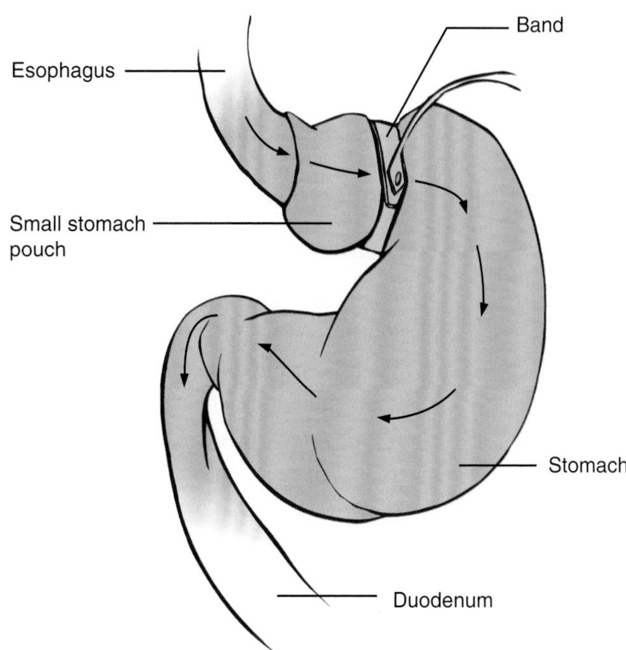

Figure 17.6 ▶ Laparoscopic adjustable gastric banding.

- The outlet diameter can be adjusted by inflating or deflating a small bladder inside the "belt" through a small subcutaneous reservoir. The size of the outlet can be repeatedly changed as needed.
- Clients must understand the importance of eating small meals, eating slowly, chewing food thoroughly, and progressing the diet gradually from liquids, to pureed foods, to soft foods.
- The popularity of LAGB has decreased in the United States, primarily due to inferior weight loss, complex follow-up, a lower remission rate of diabetes, and a high rate of reoperation due to complications (Raynor & Champagne, 2016).
- Common micronutrient deficiencies after LAGB include calcium, iron, thiamin, and vitamin D.

Nutrition Therapy for Bariatric Surgery

Bariatric surgery is not a magical cure for weight loss but rather an adjunct to comprehensive lifestyle treatment that includes diet, physical activity, and behavioral intervention. Bariatric surgery requires dramatic and dynamic changes in intake. Nutrition therapy is important presurgically, postsurgically, and long term for weight management and overall health.

Presurgical Phase

Preoperative nutrition counseling addresses presurgical weight loss and behavior change. Modest presurgical weight loss has been associated with surgical advantages, such as shortened surgery time and improved glycemic state (Dagan et al., 2017).

- There is no consensus regarding how long a diet should be followed. Recommendations for the duration of the diet range from 2 to 6 weeks (Dagan et al., 2017).
- Likewise, the ideal macronutrient distribution of the presurgical diet is not known, although a low-carbohydrate diet may be more effective in promoting short-term weight loss and improved insulin sensitivity (Dagan et al., 2017).
- Despite short-term benefits of preoperative weight loss, evidence is inconclusive regarding the long-term benefits.
- Vitamin and mineral deficiencies should be identified and corrected before surgery. Studies show vitamin B_{12}, iron, folic acid, vitamin D, and thiamin are the most common presurgical nutrient deficiencies (Dagan et al., 2017).

- Clients are screened for problematic eating behaviors that are barriers to postsurgical success, such as binge eating, emotional eating, and boredom eating (Tempest, 2012).
- Preoperative counseling also gives clients a realistic expectation of the postoperative phase, dispelling any notions that the surgery guarantees success.

Initial Postsurgical Phase: The First 2 Months after Surgery

General nutrition and eating behavior guidelines after bariatric surgery are listed in Box 17.8.

- The initial postsurgical diet begins with small portions of room-temperature clear liquids and progresses in texture and consistency over the first 2 months.
- There is no evidence to support a specific protocol of postsurgical diet stages, though many guidelines are available.
- A sample diet progression is outlined in Box 17.9.
- Although nutrition complications can occur any time after bariatric surgery, they are most likely in the initial 2 months (Table 17.7).

Later Postsurgical Phase: 2 Months to 1 Year after Surgery

About 2 months after surgery, clients are ready to follow a regular healthy eating pattern.

- Eating nutrient-dense foods helps clients distinguish between physical and emotional hunger.
- Three meals with one to two snacks daily comprise the structured pattern.
- Food portions and speed of eating are monitored to promote weight loss and maintenance (Weight Management Dietetic Practice Group et al., 2015).

BOX 17.8 General Postsurgical Nutrition Guidelines and Eating Behavior Recommendations

Nutrition Guidelines

- Fluids: Throughout all diet stages, consume adequate fluid to prevent dehydration (at least 1.5 L/day).
- Protein: Recommendations vary. Client may need 60–80 g/protein/day or 1.1 to 1.5 g/kg ideal body weight (using an "ideal" body weight as what the patient's weight would be at a BMI of 25).
- Limit carbohydrates during early postop period (50 g/day) and gradually increase to 130 g/day.
- Avoid concentrated sugars (e.g., sugar-sweetened beverages, sugar, honey, and sweet foods) to decrease the risk of dumping syndrome (for post RYGB) and because they are empty calories.
- Eating fiber (after 1 month postsurgery) promotes weight loss and enhances healthy eating.
- Fat recommendations do not differ from those of the general population.
- Avoid carbonated beverages (e.g., seltzer water).
- Progression to solid foods is important because solids provide greater satiety than liquids.

Eating Behavior Recommendations

- Consume 4 to 6 meals/day. Avoid eating small amounts throughout the day (known as "grazing") because it reduces long-term success.
- Eat protein foods before eating other foods in the meal.
- Eat slowly.
- Take small bites.
- Chew food thoroughly so that it becomes the consistency of applesauce.
- Stop eating when satiated instead of stopping only when feeling satiated (or "full").
- Avoid fluids 15 minutes before and for at least 30 minutes after eating solids.

Source: Dagan, S., Goldenshluger, A., Globus, I., Schweiger, C., Kessler, Y., Sandbank, G., Ben-Porat, T., & Sinai, T. (2017). Nutritional recommendations for adult bariatric surgery patients: Clinical practice. *Advances in Nutrition*, *8*, 382–394. https://doi.org/10.3945/an.116.014258

BOX 17.9 Sample Postsurgical Diet Progression

For 24 to 48 hours after surgery

- Consume room-temperature clear liquids, such as water, decaffeinated herbal tea, and broth at a rate of about 2 to 4 oz/hour during waking hours.
  - Gradually increase volume to at least 8 cups/day.
  - Consume in small portions (one-half cup/serving).

At 3 to 7 days postsurgery,

- add full liquids, such as milk, soy drinks, and plain yogurt.
  - Bariatric protein powder supplements mixed with water or milks may be used as "meal replacements."

At 1 to 2 week postsurgery,

- progress to mashed/pureed diet using smooth foods,
- slowly progress texture as tolerated, and
- avoid liquids with solids and for 30 minutes after eating.

At 2 weeks postsurgery,

- add soft foods, such as scrambled eggs, soft-cooked vegetables, and soft-peeled fruit;
- add crackers.

One month postsurgery,

- add solid foods, including legumes, fresh vegetables, fresh fruit, and bread;
- protein should be emphasized; and
- consume fiber-rich foods to promote weight loss.

At 2 months postsurgery,

- consume a regular, well-balanced eating pattern, such as the DASH diet.

Long-term nutritional and lifestyle recommendations:

- Continue with a healthy eating pattern, such as the DASH diet or Mediterranean diet.
- Engage in 150 minutes/week of aerobic exercise and gradually increase to 300 minutes/week.
- Do resistance training exercises 2 to 3 times/week.
- Avoid smoking and tobacco products as a general health practice, not one specific to bariatric surgery.
- Avoid or reduce alcohol intake after RYGB due to increased alcohol absorption and longer time to eliminate alcohol.
- Other postsurgical clients who want to drink alcohol should eat 15 to 30 minutes before consuming.
- Avoid complete fasting (e.g., for religious reasons) for 12 to 18 months after bariatric surgery (until vomiting risk decreases). Clients who participate in fasting after that period should be sure to fully hydrate before fasting.
- Take lifelong vitamin and mineral supplements as prescribed.

Source: Dagan, S., Goldenshluger, A., Globus, I., Schweiger, C., Kessler, Y., Sandbank, G., Ben-Porat, T., & Sinai, T. (2017). Nutritional recommendations for adult bariatric surgery patients: Clinical practice. *Advances in Nutrition*, *8*, 382–394. https://doi.org/10.3945/an.116.014258

Success of Bariatric Surgery

Evidence shows that bariatric surgery results in greater weight loss and is more effective in inducing remission of type 2 diabetes than nonsurgical treatments (Courcoulas et al., 2015). The Longitudinal Assessment of Bariatric Surgery Study looked at RYGB and LAGB and found (Courcoulas et al., 2018) the following:

- Long-term health improvements vary with the procedure.
  - RYGB produces high rates of comorbid disease remission, most of which are evident by the first 2 years after surgery. Some decline in disease remission occurs from years 3 to 7, especially for diabetes and hypertension.

Table 17.7 Potential Nutrition Complications after Bariatric Surgery

Complication	Possible Causes	Possible Interventions
Dehydration	• Inadequate fluid intake related to separating solids from liquids and avoidance of sugar-sweetened beverages and carbonated beverages • Excessive losses through vomiting or severe diarrhea	• Encourage client to consume at least 1.5 L fluid/day • Encourage client to consume fluid even if the sensation of thirst is absent • Intravenous hydration if necessary • Antiemetics
Diarrhea	• Lactose intolerance • Drinking fluids with meals • Infection • Dumping syndrome • Intake of sugar alcohols • LAGB, RYGB, and SG do not cause diarrhea	• Increase fluid intake • Reduce intake of lactose, fat, sugar alcohols, and fiber
Dumping syndrome	• Rapid emptying of hyperosmolar load (high-sugar and high-carbohydrate foods) into the small bowel followed by a shift of intravascular fluid into the intestinal lumen • Most often occurs with RYGB	• Avoid refined carbohydrates, such as juice, soda, concentrated sweets, foods with added sugars (sugar, honey, and high-fructose corn syrup) • Increase intake of protein, fiber, and complex carbohydrates • Separate liquids and solids by at least 30 minutes
Protein malnutrition (associated with malabsorptive procedures)	• Poor oral intake • Prolonged vomiting or diarrhea • Acquired food intolerance for protein-rich foods	• Exact protein requirements after bariatric surgery are unknown • Suggested goals may be 60–80 g protein/day or 1–1.5 g protein/kg ideal body weight/day
Constipation	• Use of narcotics • Inadequate fluid intake • Low-fiber intake • Calcium or iron supplementation	• Assess fluid and fiber intake for adequacy • Reduce iron dosage to the lowest possible dose • Stool softener or laxative may be needed
Eating issues, such as food intolerances, regurgitation without nausea or true vomiting, food gets "stuck"	• Altered taste • Eat or drink too much or too rapidly • Failure to chew food thoroughly • Improperly moistened food	• Avoid foods not tolerated • Remind client to eat and drink mindfully and slowly • Avoid problem foods until tolerance improves

Source: Weight Management Dietetic Practice Group, Cummings, S., & Isom, K. (Eds.). (2015). *Academy of nutrition and dietetics pocket guide to Bariatric surgery* (2nd ed.). American Academy of Nutrition and Dietetics; Dagan, S., Goldenshluger, A., Globus, I., Schweiger, C., Kessler, Y., Sandbank, G., Ben-Porat, T., & Sinai, T. (2017). Nutritional recommendations for adult bariatric surgery patients: Clinical practice. *Advances in Nutrition*, *8*, 382–394. https://doi.org/10.3945/an.116.014258

  - The only comorbid conditions with lower prevalence 7 years after LAGB are low HDL cholesterol and high triglyceride.
- The greater the amount and speed of the initial weight loss the better the long-term weight outcomes.
  - Seventy-five percent of RYGB participants maintained at least 20% of weight loss through 7 years.
  - Fifty percent of LAGB participants maintained at least 16% of weight loss through 7 years.
- Weight regain may be more common after SG than RYGB; however, poor reporting and a lack of a consensus definition of weight regain hamper comparisons (Lauti et al., 2017).
- Postoperative behavioral intervention appears to result in greater weight loss than surgery alone (Stewart & Avenell, 2016). Even cognitive behavior therapy via telephone for clients 6 months postsurgery has been shown to result in significant improvements in binge eating, emotional eating, depressive symptoms, and anxiety symptoms (Sockalingam et al., 2017).

Nutrition for Weight Maintenance

A healthy lifestyle is vital to optimize and sustain long-term weight loss after bariatric surgery. Weight maintenance requires that clients eat mindfully with attention to hunger and satiety cues. Factors associated with successful weight maintenance after bariatric surgery include the following:

- compliance to nutrition recommendations
- eating regularly scheduled meals instead of "grazing"
- heeding satiety cues
- realistic expectations
- regular moderate aerobic physical activity
- tracking food intake
- monitoring weight
- adequate sleep
- meal planning
- limiting fluids with and immediately after meals
- avoiding alcohol
- periodic assessment to identify and treat eating or other psychiatric disorders

NURSING PROCESS Obesity

Rosa is 37 years old, 5 ft 4 in. tall, and the mother of two children. Before her first child was born 10 years ago, her normal weight was 140 pounds. She gained 35 pounds during pregnancy and didn't regain her normal weight before her second pregnancy a year later. She is now at her heaviest weight of 180 pounds. She complains of fatigue and thinks her weight contributes to her asthma. She admits to "out of control eating" and has tried several diets but has been unable to take weight off and keep it off. Her doctor told her she has prehypertension and encouraged her to lose weight to lower both her blood pressure and serum glucose levels. The fear of needing medication for hypertension or diabetes has motivated her to lose weight.

Assessment

Medical–Psychosocial Data

- Medical history and comorbidities, such as hypertension, dyslipidemia, cardiovascular disease, diabetes, sleep apnea, osteoarthritis, and esophageal reflux
- Medications that may promote weight gain or interfere with weight loss, such as steroid hormones, psychotropic drugs, mood stabilizers, antidepressants, and antiepileptic drugs
- Level of motivation to lose weight including previous history of successful and unsuccessful attempts to lose weight, social support, and perceived barriers to success

Anthropometric Assessment

- Height, current weight, BMI
- Weight history
- Waist circumference

Biochemical and Physical Assessment

- Lab values related to possible comorbidities, such as total cholesterol, LDL cholesterol, HDL cholesterol, triglycerides, glucose, hemoglobin A1c
- Triiodothyronine (T_3) and thyroxine (T_4) for thyroid function
- Blood pressure

Dietary Assessment

- How many daily meals and snacks do you usually eat?
- Do you skip meals?
- What is a typical day's intake?
- How do you think your usual intake needs to change to be healthier or to help you lose weight?
- What will be hardest for you to change? What will be easiest?
- What triggers cause you to overeat?

NURSING PROCESS

Obesity (continued)

- How many servings of fruits and vegetables do you eat daily?
- How much sweetened soda do you drink daily?
- Do you limit any particular foods?
- How many meals per week do you eat out?
- What triggers your "out of control" eating?
- Do you take vitamins, minerals, or supplements to help with weight loss? If so, what?
- What is your goal weight?
- How much aerobic physical activity do you do on a daily basis?
- Do you do resistance training exercises?
- How much of your day is spent on sedentary activities?
- How much alcohol do you consume?
- Do you have any cultural, religious, or ethnic food preferences?
- Do you have any food allergies or intolerances?

Analysis

Possible Nursing Analyses

Obesity related to excess calorie intake as evidenced by a BMI of 31.

Planning

Client Outcomes

The client will
- gradually increase physical activity (aerobic and resistance training) while reducing sedentary activity,
- consume a nutritionally adequate, hypocaloric diet consisting of healthy carbohydrates, healthy fats, and lean protein,
- eat three meals per day,
- practice behavior change to modify undesirable eating habits,
- self-monitor food intake, physical activity, and weight loss,
- lose 1–2 pounds/week on average until 10% of initial weight is lost,
- verbalize the components of a hypocaloric healthy eating pattern.

Nursing Interventions

Nutrition Therapy

- Decrease calorie intake to 1500 a day in three meals using an evidence-based dietary approach selected by the client.
- Encourage ample fluid intake, preferably water and other noncalorie drinks, to promote excretion of metabolic wastes.

Client Teaching

Instruct the client on the following:
- The interrelationship between a hypocaloric diet, increased physical activity, and behavior change in managing weight
- The eating plan essentials with emphasis on high-satiety foods, such as whole grains, fruit and vegetables, low-fat or nonfat dairy, and lean protein
- Behavioral matters, including
  - eating only in one place while sitting down
  - putting utensils down between mouthfuls
- Monitoring hunger on a scale of 1 to 10, with 1 corresponding to "famished" and 10 corresponding to "stuffed": Encourage clients to eat when the hunger scale is at about 3 and to stop when satisfied (not full) at about 6 or 7
- Weighing oneself at least once a week
- Periodically keeping a record of food intake and activity
- Planning splurges instead of eating on impulse: Planned splurges involve making a conscious decision to eat something, enjoying every mouthful of the food, and then moving on from the experience without feelings of guilt or failure

NURSING PROCESS

Obesity (continued)

- Changing eating attitudes by
  - replacing negative self-talk with positive talk,
  - replacing the attitude of "always being on a diet" with an acceptance of eating healthier and less as a way of life
- Consulting a physician or dietitian if questions concerning the eating plan or weight loss arise

Evaluation

Evaluate and Monitor

- Monitor weight.
- Evaluate food and activity records to assess adherence; suggest changes in the meal plan as needed.
- Provide periodic feedback and reinforcement.
- Monitor biochemical data for improvements attributable to weight loss.

EATING DISORDERS: ANOREXIA NERVOSA, BULIMIA NERVOSA, BINGE-EATING DISORDER, AND EATING DISORDERS NOT OTHERWISE SPECIFIED

Body Dysmorphic Disorder excessive preoccupation with a real or imagined defect in physical appearance.

Anorexia Nervosa (AN) a condition of self-imposed fasting or severe self-imposed dieting.

Bulimia Nervosa (BN) an eating disorder characterized by recurrent episodes of bingeing and purging.

Eating disorders are serious psychological disorders. They are characterized by severe disturbances in eating behaviors (Box 17.10) that can have a profound effect on health and/or psychosocial functioning. Other characteristics include obsessive ideation about body size and weight and **body dysmorphic disorder** or distorted body image. Table 17.8 compares **anorexia nervosa (AN)** and **bulimia nervosa (BN)**. Binge-eating disorder (BED) is the other eating disorder defined in the *Diagnostic and Statistical Manual of Mental Disorders, Fifth Edition* (*DSM-5*) (American Psychiatric Association [APA], 2013).

Eating disorders result from complex interaction of genetic, developmental, family influences, and sociocultural factors; however, the etiology of eating disorders in not known. Studies indicate

BOX 17.10 Examples of Disordered Eating Behaviors

- Calorie restriction for weight loss
- Avoidance of specific foods, especially high-calorie foods that are perceived to be fattening
- Eating a limited variety of foods
- Restricting dietary fat intake
- Inflexibility with food
- Filling up on low-calorie foods, such as fruits and vegetables
- Excessive use of artificial sweeteners
- Use of nonnutritive beverages such as water and diet soft drinks to suppress appetite
- Excessive caffeine intake
- Abnormal timing of meals and snacks
- Over-involvement in food preparation
- Collecting recipes and menus
- Excessive use of condiments
- Overestimating portion sizes
- Confusion about how much to eat

Source: Hart, S., Marnane, C., McMaster, C., & Thomas, A. (2018). Development of the "Recovery from Eating Disorders for Life" Food Guide (REAL Food Guide)-a food pyramid for adults with an eating disorder. *Journal of Eating Disorders*, *6*, 6. https://doi.org/10.1186/s40337-018-0192-4

Table 17.8 A Comparison of Anorexia Nervosa and Bulimia Nervosa

	Anorexia Nervosa	Bulimia Nervosa
Major characteristics	• Preoccupation with food • Irrational fear of normal body weight • Body image distortion • Self-worth based on size and shape • Compulsive pursuit of thinness • Terrified of gaining weight or becoming fat	• Preoccupation with food • Irrational fear of normal body weight • Body image distortion • Self-worth based on size and shape • Binge eating accompanied by a lack of sense of control
Onset	• Usually develops during adolescence or young adulthood	• Usually develops during adolescence or young adulthood
Overall adult prevalence	• 0.6% • Lifetime prevalence 3 times higher in women than men	• 0.3% • 5 times higher among women than men

Typical eating and exercise behaviors	• Semi-starvation with compulsive exercise
	• Onset of disorder is usually preceded by dieting behavior
		• Gorging (e.g., 1200–11,500 calories in a short amount of time) followed by purging:
		  ◦ Self-induced vomiting
		  ◦ Excessive exercise
		  ◦ Abuse of laxatives
		  ◦ Diuretics
		  ◦ Enemas
		  ◦ Fasting
		• "Dieting" is a way of life but bingeing may occur several times per day and may be planned

Weight	Significantly low body weight (e.g., <85% ideal body weight) compared to what is minimally expected for age, sex, developmental trajectory, and physical health	• Fluctuations are normal • Weight may be normal or slightly above normal
Emotional symptoms	• Denial of the condition can be extreme • Body image disturbance • Pronounced emotional changes • Low self-esteem • 56% of survey respondents met criteria for at least one of the core *DSM-5* disorders with any anxiety disorder, the most common cormorbidity (National Institute of Mental Health, 2017)	• Displays mood swings • Full recognition of the behavior as abnormal • Ongoing feelings of isolation, guilt, depression, and low self-esteem • 94% of survey respondents met criteria for at least one of the core *DSM-5* disorders with any anxiety disorder, the most common cormorbidity (National Institute of Mental Health, 2017)
Physical consequences	• Hypotension • Bradycardia • Electrolytes imbalances, which can be life threatening • Hypothermia • Loss of GI functions: decreased peristalsis, delayed gastric emptying, atrophy of GI lining, diarrhea • Lanugo (fine, downy hair on extremities) • Hormonal imbalances: amenorrhea or delayed onset of menstruation, osteoporosis	• Hypotension • Bradycardia • Electrolytes imbalances, which can be life threatening • Erosion of teeth enamel • Swollen salivary glands in cheeks • Sores, scars, or calluses on knuckles or hands
Nutrient deficiencies	• Protein–calorie malnutrition • Various micronutrient deficiencies	• Varies

Source: Eating disorders. (2020). Available at www.nutritioncaremanual.org. and learn at Nationaleatingdisorders.org/learn (n.d.); National Institute of Mental Health. (2017, November). *Eating disorders*. https://www.nimh.nih.gov/health/statistics/eating-disorders.shtml

that genetic heritability may account for 50% to 80% of the risk of developing anorexia and BN (Trace et al., 2013). Dieting may be the initial impetus in the development of eating disorders. Other risk factors include early childhood eating and GI problems, increased concern about weight and size, negative self-evaluation, sexual abuse, and other traumas (Ozier & Henry, 2011). Major stressors, such as the onset of puberty, parental divorce, death of a family member, and ridicule of being or becoming fat, may be precipitating factors. Athletes may develop eating disorders to improve their performance. People with eating disorders often have anxiety and depression. Each person's recovery process is unique; therefore, treatment plans are highly individualized.

A multidisciplinary approach that includes nutrition counseling, behavioral interventions, psychotherapy, family counseling, and group therapy is most effective. Antidepressant drugs effectively reduce the frequency of problematic eating behaviors but do not eliminate them. Most eating disorders are treated on an outpatient basis; however, life-threatening consequences of malnutrition in severe cases of AN may necessitate inpatient treatment (Rocks et al., 2014). Treatment can be complex and protracted.

Anorexia Nervosa

AN is characterized by restriction of food intake, intense fear of gaining weight, and a distorted body image (Fig. 17.7) (APA, 2013). Eating issues may include self-imposed starvation, avoidance of social eating, disassociation from internal hunger cues, and food rituals that delay or extend a meal, such as repeated cutting or reheating of food. Denial of the condition can be extreme.

Malnutrition and low body weight may result in major impairment in health (Resmark et al., 2019). There is no proven treatment for AN, and rates of relapse and chronicity are high. For instance, it may take years for clients with AN to achieve a first remission or to recover permanently. It is estimated that 25% of adult clients develop a chronic form of the disorder and 33% of clients suffer long-term residual symptoms (Resmark et al., 2019).

Nutrition Therapy for Anorexia Nervosa

Although nutritional and weight restoration is a core focus of most AN programs, there has been very little research on this area of AN (Marzola et al., 2013). The American Psychiatric Association (APA) guidelines for AN state that the goals of nutritional rehabilitation for seriously underweight clients are to (Marzola et al., 2013)

- restore weight,
- normalize eating pattern,

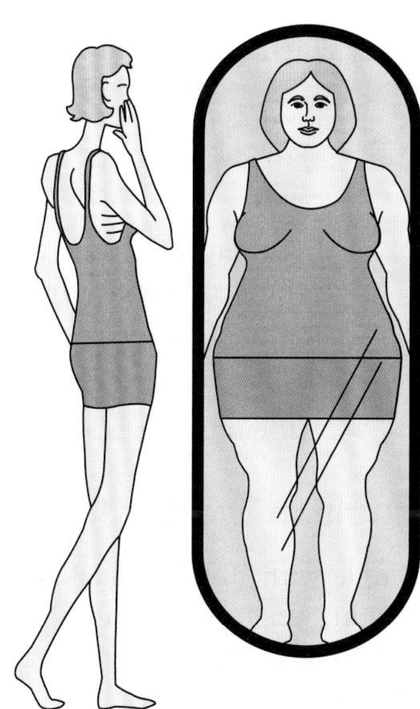

Figure 17.7 ▶ A woman suffering from anorexia sees herself as overweight.

- achieve normal perceptions of hunger and satiety, and
- correct biological and psychological sequelae of malnutrition.

APA guidelines for anorexia nervosa are as follows:

- Provide initial calorie intake of 1000 to 1600 cal/day or 30 to 40 cal/kg with gradual progression to 70–100 cal/kg/day is used (Marzola et al., 2013). The "low and slow" calorie initiation is for the purpose of reducing the risk of refeeding syndrome. Monitoring of vitals, electrolytes, and cardiac function is required to prevent **refeeding syndrome**.
- The necessity of this conservative approach has been challenged; newer guidelines state that an initial low-calorie intake with gradual increase is not required for safe weight gain in clients with mild to moderate AN (Resmark et al., 2019). However, recommended initial calorie amounts were not specified.
- Weight gain targets suggested 2 to 3 pounds/week for hospitalized clients and 0.5 to 1 pound/week for people in outpatient programs (Marzola et al., 2013).
- Clients who refuse to eat may need nasogastric feeding.

Refeeding Syndrome
a potentially life-threatening condition characterized by severe shifts in fluid and electrolytes, especially phosphorus, from the extracellular to intracellular fluid when refeeding begins in a person who is severely malnourished and depleted in total body phosphorus. Thiamin deficiency may also occur secondary to increased metabolism of carbohydrates.

Additional considerations (Marzola et al., 2013) are as follows:

- For weight maintenance, clients with AN may need 50 to 60 cal/kg, amounts higher than those required by the general population. The high need may be due to exercise and changes in metabolism.
- During refeeding, treatment should focus on correcting disordered eating patterns, such as irregular eating, vegetarianism, and restricted variety of foods.

Strategies to promote compliance and feelings of trust include

- involving the client in formulating individualized goals and meal plans;
- offering rewards linked to the quantity of calories consumed, not to weight gain;
- having the client record food intake and exercise activity; diet diversity may be predictive of weight maintenance in clients with AN (Schebendach et al., 2008);
- meal planning tips and eating behavior strategies for AN (see Box 17.11).

Bulimia Nervosa

BN is characterized by binge-eating episodes followed by behaviors to prevent weight gain, such as self-induced vomiting, fasting, or excessive exercise. Although the mortality rate associated with BN is less than that of AN, it is still increased due to severe electrolyte and acid–base imbalances related to recurrent vomiting or stimulant laxative abuse (Westmoreland et al., 2016). The diagnostic criteria are as follows (APA, 2013):

- Recurrent episodes of binge eating occur, which are characterized by eating a large amount of food within any 2-hour period that is accompanied by a feeling of lack of control overeating.
- Recurrent behaviors to prevent weight gain from bingeing occur, such as self-induced vomiting; laxative, diuretic, or diet pill abuse; or excessive exercise.
- Binge and purge episodes occur on average at least once a week for 3 months but may occur several times a day
- Self-evaluation is strongly based on body shape and weight.

Nutrition Therapy for Bulimia Nervosa

People with BN are usually within their normal weight range, although some may be overweight; weight fluctuations are common. The major goals of nutrition therapy are to stabilize weight by decreasing bingeing and purging and achieve normal perceptions of hunger, fullness, and satiety.

BOX 17.11 Meal Planning Tips and Eating Behavior Strategies for Anorexia Nervosa

Meal Planning Tips

- Eat a meal or snack every 3 to 4 hours even if not hungry during initial phase of treatment.
- Eat sources of protein, fat, and complex carbohydrates, preferably whole grains, at every meal and snack.
- If a small amount of food causes a feeling of fullness, recognize that it does not mean you have overeaten. Fullness is a temporary feeling.
    - Consume the planned amounts of all foods. Do not overconsume fruits and vegetables, which may then displace the intake of other more calorically dense foods. Gradually increase portion sizes of "safe" foods.
    - Gradually increase variety of foods and food groups consumed.
    - Drink water and other beverages to meet fluid needs but avoid all diet drinks.
    - Supplements may be prescribed to meet nutrient needs until intake is adequate.

Eating Behaviors

- Avoid ritualistic eating behaviors that may impair the ability to recognize hunger or satiety.
- Learn to trust that there are no "good foods" or "bad foods" but that all foods can fit into a healthy meal plan.
- Reduce obsessive thoughts about food, eating, weight, and body image. Instead, develop alternative activities and rewards to replace these thoughts.
- Be patient with learning to self-nourish.
- Use a hunger scale to identify internal cues for hunger, satiety, and fullness.
- Understand that weight restoration is necessary for recovery, which will allow the body and mind to function more effectively.

Source: Academy of Nutrition and Dietetics. (2020). Nutrition care manual. Anorexia nervosa meal planning tips. https://www.nutritioncaremanual.org/client_ed.cfm?ncm_client_ed_id=64

- Nutritional counseling focuses on identifying and correcting food misinformation and fears and includes discussing normal weight fluctuations, hunger and satiety cues, meal planning, establishing a normal pattern of eating, and identifying the dangers of dieting.
- People with BN must understand that gorging is only one aspect of a complex pattern of altered behavior; in fact, excessive dietary restriction is a major contributor to the disorder.
- Although most clients with BN want to lose weight, dieting and recovery from an eating disorder are incompatible. Normalization of eating behaviors is a primary goal.
- Nutrition strategies for BN are listed in Box 17.12.

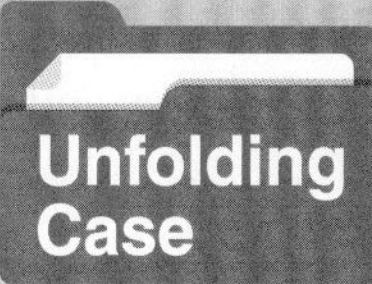

Recall Emma. She admits that she has seen a counselor for an eating disorder and that she binges and purges when she's "bad." She recognizes that bingeing and purging are not normal behaviors and admits to feeling out of control when a binge begins. Restrictive dieting always precedes her periods of bingeing. She purges with vomiting and laxatives, which caused her to be hospitalized for hypokalemia. Is counting calories a good strategy for Emma? What strategies would you recommend to help Emma normalize her eating behaviors?

Binge-Eating Disorder

BED, previously referred to as compulsive overeating, was included as its own category of eating disorder in the *DSM-5*. Before then, it was not recognized as a separate disorder and was diagnosable only under the catch-all category of Eating Disorder Not Otherwise Specified. The diagnostic criteria for BN include recurrent episodes of binge eating with an episode

BOX 17.12 Meal Planning Tips and Eating Goals for Bulimia Nervosa

Daily Meal Planning Tips

- Eat three meals and 2 to 3 snacks daily to regain structure.
- Eat every 4 to 5 hours while learning to recognize hunger cues.
- Use a hunger scale to identify internal cues for hunger, satiety, and fullness.
- Eat slowly.
- All foods are acceptable. Restricting foods can lead to binge eating.
- Strive for variety, balance, and moderation in food choices.
- Eat protein, fat, and high-fiber foods at each meal and snack for satiety and bulk.
- Eat fruit and vegetables when able to do so without feeling an uncomfortable fullness.
- Consume adequate but not excessive water and fluid to meet needs.

Recognize and identify eating habits, feelings, or situations that may trigger binges or out-of-control eating, such as

- certain food triggers,
- body image concerns,
- social settings or being alone,
- frustration, stress, or particular emotions, and
- feeling full.

Identify alternative activities to manage feelings that may lead to bingeing, such as

- moderate physical activity,
- journaling or talking to a friend,
- listening to music,
- diversionary activities such as homework or gardening, and
- creating art.

Source: Academy of Nutrition and Dietetics. (2020). Nutrition care manual. Anorexia nervosa meal planning tips. https://www.nutritioncaremanual.org/client_ed.cfm?ncm_client_ed_id=65

characterized by eating significantly more food in a short period of time than most people would eat under similar circumstances, with episodes marked by of lack of control (APA, 2013). Unlike BN, people with BED do not purge. Binge eating occurs on average, at least once a week for 3 months. Episodes produce significant distress regarding binge eating and are associated with three or more of the following:

- eating more quickly than normal
- eating until comfortably full
- eating large amounts of foods when not physically hungry
- eating alone because of embarrassment of how much is eaten
- feeling disgusted with oneself, depressed, or very guilty after overeating

BED differs from common overeating in that it is more severe, is associated with more subjective distress regarding the eating behavior, and is accompanied with physical and psychological problems. People with BED may be of normal weight, but it is often associated with obesity and its comorbid nutritional and medical complications. Risk factors include childhood obesity, parental obesity, high degree of body dissatisfaction, dysfunctional attitudes regarding weight and shape, poor self-esteem, and impaired social functioning (Academy of Nutrition and Dietetics, 2020). Comorbidities include major depressive disorder, anxiety disorders, and alcoholism. BED is more prevalent than AN and BN combined (National Institute of Mental Health, 2017).

Psychotherapy, particularly cognitive behavior therapy, and medication are the main treatment modalities for BED (Westerberg & Waitz, 2013). The focus of nutrition therapy is to normalize eating behaviors with emphasis on recognizing internal hunger and satiety cues (Box 17.13). Reducing binge eating may be followed by participation in a weight-control program.

BOX 17.13 **Binge-Eating Disorder Meal Planning Tips**

- Use a hunger rating scale to identify hunger, satiety, and fullness. For instance, on a scale of 1 to 10, 1 represents "starving," 10 represents "stuffed," and satiety may be 6 or 7. A workable range may be to eat at a 3 or 4 and stop at 6 or 7.
- Identify signs of hunger, such as empty stomach, stomach noise, feeling irritable, headache, and feeling weak or light-headed.
- Eat slowly and allow 20 to 30 minutes for each meal to let the brain to signal that the body has eaten enough.
- Make eating its own activity; avoid TV and other electronics, reading, cooking, and driving while eating.
- Eat seated and avoid eating alone.
- Enjoy the food.
- Know that you can have more when hunger returns.
- Do not label any foods "forbidden."
- Identify triggers and alter your environment accordingly.

Source: Academy of Nutrition and Dietetics. (2020). Nutrition care manual. Binge-eating disorder meal planning tips. https://www.nutritioncaremanual.org/client_ed.cfm?ncm_client_ed_id=63

Eating Disorders Not Otherwise Specified

The prevalence of eating disorders not otherwise specified (EDNOS) is unknown because there is no simple definition of EDNOS. This group represents people who diet frequently, who use unhealthful methods to lose weight such as restricting food, and people who meet some, but not all, of the criteria for the diagnosable eating disorders (Academy of Nutrition and Dietetics, 2020).

How Do You Respond

If 1200 calories can promote a 1- to 2-pound loss per week, will a more drastic calorie reduction speed the weight-loss process?
People often think that the greater the calorie deficit, the quicker the weight loss. In reality, cutting calories too much may result in higher proportions of lean tissue loss. This leads to a lowering of basal energy expenditure and reduced exercise tolerance, making weight loss and maintenance more difficult (Blackburn et al., 2010).

REVIEW CASE STUDY

"I hate being fat."

Client history: C.C. is a 43-year-old mother of three who has experienced gradual weight gain after the birth of each of her children. She is 5 ft 7 in. tall, weighs 189 pounds, works full time, and does not engage in regular exercise. She has prediabetes and prehypertension and appears eager to make lifestyle changes to improve her health and be a better nutritional role model for her children. She has successfully lost weight in the past through Weight Watchers but eventually got bored and regained all of the weight she lost. Her usual intake is no breakfast, snacks at a vending machine twice a day, fast food for lunch, and dinner with the family. Her dinner usually consists of about 6 oz of meat, potatoes, sometimes a vegetable, bread with butter, and dessert. C.C. admits to a weakness for sweets but wants to try a low-carbohydrate diet because she heard it is the best and easiest way to lose weight.

- What is C.C.'s weight status based on her BMI?
- What would be an appropriate calorie diet for her to lose weight?
- What would you tell her about the "best and easiest" way to lose weight?
- What foods does she eat that provide carbohydrates? Compared to the low-carbohydrate eating plan outlined in Table 17.4, what food groups would she need to increase? Decrease?
- What other lifestyle changes would you recommend for her?
- Create a nursing care plan complete with nursing diagnosis, client goal, interventions, and monitoring recommendations.

STUDY QUESTIONS

1 The client asks if it is okay to follow a low-carbohydrate, ketogenic-type diet in the short term to get started on weight-loss efforts. Which of the following would be the nurse's best response?
   a. "No, low-carbohydrate diets are not healthy and would only sabotage your weight-loss efforts."
   b. "A ketogenic-type diet can help you lose weight as can many other types of diets. The important factor that determines whether you lose weight is the number of calories you eat, not the proportion of carbohydrates, protein, and fat you eat."
   c. "A low-carbohydrate diet is better than any other type of diet and is a good choice for you to use."
   d. "A low-fat diet is easier. Try that instead."

2 What behavioral factors are associated with successful long-term weight maintenance after weight loss? Select all that apply.
   a. high levels of daily physical activity
   b. weighing oneself at least weekly
   c. consuming a low-calorie, low-fat diet
   d. eating only two meals/day

3 The client asks if meal replacements, such as Jenny Craig products, are a good idea to help with weight loss. Which of the following would be the nurse's best response?
   a. "They are a great way to control portions and can help you adhere to your hypocaloric meal plan when used as suggested."
   b. "They are gimmicks that fail to teach you how to control your own intake. They are not recommended."
   c. "Most people gain weight while using them. You should stay away from them."
   d. "They are not nutritionally balanced so you actually have to overeat in order to meet your nutritional requirements if you use them."

4 A 32-year-old client has learned that their BMI has increased to 28 since their last annual physical. They are determined to lose weight and asks if they can use weight-loss medication instead of going on a diet because they have had trouble following diets. Which is the best response?
   a. "You are not a candidate for weight-loss medications because they can only be prescribed for people with complications related to weight, such as diabetes."
   b. "You are an ideal candidate for weight-loss medications. Tell the doctor you are interested in them when they arrive."
   c. "For people with a BMI of 28 and no weight-related complications, weight-loss medications are considered only if you are unsuccessful at losing weight with lifestyle therapy. See how successful you can be with lifestyle therapy."
   d. "Weight-loss medications are associated with serious risks so they are reserved for people with BMI > 35."

5 Which of the following calorie level ranges is considered appropriate for weight-loss diets for most women?
   a. 1800 to 2000 cal/day
   b. 1200 to 1500 cal/day
   c. 1000 to 1200 cal/day
   d. 800 to 1000 cal/day

6 The nurse knows the instructions on how to reduce the risk of dumping syndrome after RYGB surgery are effective when the client verbalized they will
   a. avoid high-sugar foods and fluids with meals and for 30 minutes afterward.
   b. eat less fat.
   c. limit complex carbohydrates.
   d. eat larger, less frequent meals.

7 What is the priority when instituting nutrition therapy to a client diagnosed with BN?
   a. Teach the client about nutrient and calorie requirements.
   b. Halt weight loss.
   c. Reduce bingeing and purging.
   d. Provide sufficient calories for weight gain.

8 What is the priority when instituting nutrition therapy for a client diagnosed with AN?
   a. Teach the client about nutrient and calorie requirements.
   b. Restore weight.
   c. Motivate the client by offering rewards linked to weight gain.
   d. Halt purging behaviors.

CHAPTER SUMMARY NUTRITION FOR OBESITY AND EATING DISORDERS

Obesity can be defined as abnormal or excessive body fat accumulation that leads to adverse health consequences. It is a chronic, complex condition with potentially many contributing factors.

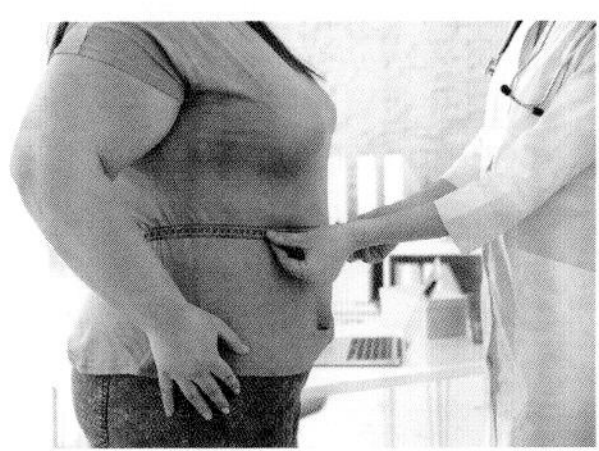

Measures of obesity: BMI and waist circumference are screening tools, not diagnostic measures, to quantify and classify obesity.

Obesity prevalence: Obesity is a worldwide epidemic. In the United States, approximately 40% of adults are obese. The prevalence has increased in both genders, in all age groups, and among all races and ethnicities.

Obesity complications: Overweight and obesity increase the risk of all-cause mortality. High BMI is a major risk factor for cardiovascular disease, diabetes, musculoskeletal disorders, and some cancers. Central obesity is linked to increased risk of obesity comorbidities.

Management of Overweight and Obesity

The treatment of obesity is based on BMI and the presence/severity of complications. Clients' readiness to lose weight should be evaluated before initiating a weight-loss attempt. Although restoration of healthy or normal BMI is ideal, as little as 3% to 5% of body weight loss results in clinical improvements, especially in glycemic metrics. Over 6 months, 5% to 10% weight loss is recommended.

Weight-Loss Therapy: Lifestyle/Behavioral Therapy

Lifestyle therapy serves as the foundation of weight management for all people, regardless if other therapies are also used.

Healthy, calorie-reduced eating plan: Generally, low-calorie diets provide 1200 to 1500 cal/day for women and 1500 to 1800 cal/day for men. A variety of eating patterns can produce weight loss as long as the appropriate amount of calories is consumed. The best diet is the one the client will stick to. Certain populations may benefit from certain low-calorie eating patterns.

- The DASH diet lowers blood pressure and may be preferable for people with hypertension.
- The Mediterranean diet improves glycemic metrics and decreases the risk of cardiovascular disease.

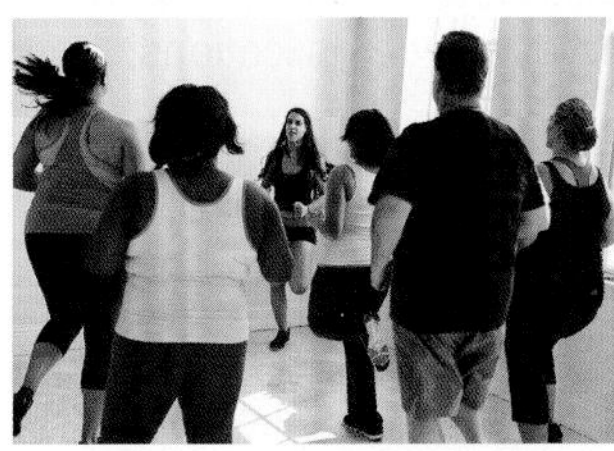

Physical activity: Recommendations include increasing aerobic activity, resistance training, and reducing sedentary time.

Behavioral therapy: Behavioral therapy is used to improve adherence to diet and exercise changes. Strategies include self-monitoring, goal setting, stimulus control, and cognitive structuring.

Comprehensive lifestyle programs: Comprehensive lifestyle programs run by a multidisciplinary team help participants adhere to diet, exercise, and behavioral changes. At least 6 months of participation is recommended, with longer durations producing better results.

Weight maintenance after loss: Long-term weight-loss maintainers tend to continue to eat a low-calorie and low-fat diet, exercise about 1 hour/day, weigh themselves weekly, and limit TV viewing.

Weight-Loss Medications

Medications are approved for obesity treatment in people who have a BMI ≥30 or ≥27 with at least one weight-related complication. They work best when combined with lifestyle modification; lifestyle modification produces greater loss when medications are used. Medications are a long-term intervention. Weight-loss devices, such as endoscopically place intragastric balloons, are additional options.

Bariatric Surgery

Bariatric surgeries are the more effective and long-lasting treatment for obesity. They can result in significant weight loss, treat type 2 diabetes, and improve cardiometabolic risk factors. Nutrient deficiencies are common and lifelong supplementation with micronutrients is necessary.

Sleeve gastrectomy is performed more often than other bariatric surgeries. It significantly reduces gastric capacity. It produces less weight loss than gastric bypass but has lower rates of complications.

Roux-en-Y gastric bypass promotes weight loss by restricting gastric capacity and bypassing part of the small intestine where nutrient absorption takes place. Weight loss and complications are greater than with other procedures.

Adjustable gastric banding restricts the capacity of the stomach. The outlet diameter can be adjusted repeatedly as needed. It produces inferior weight loss, requires

(continued)

CHAPTER SUMMARY NUTRITION FOR OBESITY AND EATING DISORDERS (continued)

follow-up, has a lower remission rate of diabetes, and has a high rate of reoperation due to complications.

Nutrition for bariatric surgery: Surgery is not a magic cure for weight loss but rather an adjunct to lifestyle therapy.

Presurgery: Weight loss may help improve surgical outcomes, although the long-term benefits are not known. Preoperative nutrition counseling prepares clients for dietary changes needed and helps them set realistic expectations for weight loss.

Postsurgery: Oral intake progresses from room-temperature clear liquids to a regular healthy eating plan by around 2 months. Protein needs are elevated; fluid is not consumed with meals or for 30 minutes afterward to reduce the risk of dumping syndrome. Clients are urged to chew food thoroughly, avoid sugars, eat slowly and mindfully, and stop eating when satisfied.

Long-term maintenance: A healthy diet, such as the DASH or Mediterranean diet, along with exercise and micronutrient supplements is needed.

Eating Disorders

Eating disorders are psychological disorders characterized by severe disturbances in eating behaviors that can profoundly affect health and psychological functioning.

Anorexia nervosa: AN is virtually self-imposed starvation as part of a compulsive pursuit of thinness. Restoration of weight is the primary goal; little is known about the optimal approach. Oral feedings are preferred; nasogastric feedings may be necessary in hospitalized clients who refuse to eat.

Bulimia nervosa: BN is binge eating characterized by a lack of sense of control and accompanied by purging via self-induced vomiting, laxative abuse, diuretics, or fasting. Body weight may be normal or slightly above normal. Weight stabilization and normalization of eating behaviors are the primary goals.

Binge-eating disorder refers to binge eating without purging accompanied by physical and psychological problems. Clients may be normal weight but most are obese. The focus of nutrition therapy is normalization of eating behaviors with an emphasis on recognizing hunger and satiety cues.

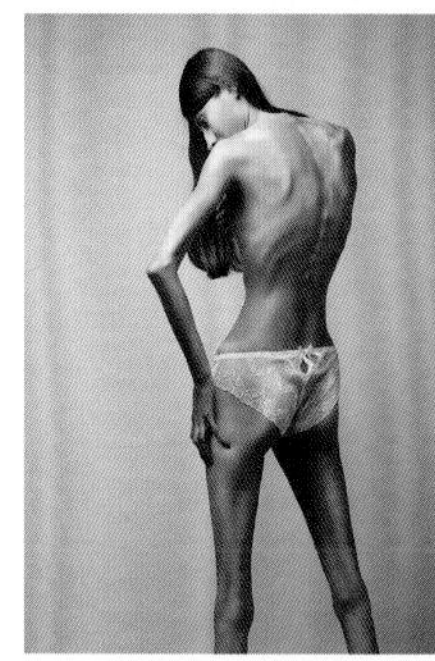

Eating Disorders Not Otherwise Specified refers to disordered eating behaviors that meet some—but not all—of the criteria for the diagnosable eating disorders

Figure sources: *shutterstock.com/New Africa, shutterstock.com/Monkey Business Images, shutterstock.com/Den Rise*

Student Resources on thePoint®
For additional learning materials, activate the code in the front of this book at https://thePoint.lww.com/activate

Websites

For reliable information on weight, dieting, physical fitness, and obesity

Calorie Control Council at www.caloriecontrol.org
Division of Nutrition, Physical Activity, and Obesity, National Center for Chronic Disease Prevention and Health Promotion at www.cdc.gov/nccdphp/dnpa
National Heart, Lung, and Blood Institute Obesity Education Initiative at www.nhlbi.nih.gov/about/oei/index.htm
Obesity Society at www.obesity.org
Weight-Control Information Network at http://www.niddk.nih.gov/health-information/health-communication-programs/win/Pages/default.aspx

For free intake/diet analysis

FitDay at www.fitday.com

For eating disorders

Anorexia Nervosa & Related Eating Disorders (ANRED) at www.anred.com
National Eating Disorders Association at www.nationaleatingdisorders.org
Overeaters Anonymous, Inc. at www.oa.org

References

Academy of Nutrition and Dietetics. (2020). Nutrition care manual. www.nutritioncaremanual.org

American Psychiatric Association. (2013). *Diagnostic and statistical manual of mental disorders* (5th ed.). American Psychiatric Association.

Appel, L. J., Champagne, C. M., Harsha, D. W., Cooper, L. S., Obarzanek, E., Elmer, P. J., Stevens, V. J., Vollmer, W. M., Lin, P.-H., Svetkey, L. P., Young, D. R., & Writing Group of the PREMIER Collaborative Research Group. (2003). Effects of comprehensive lifestyle modification on blood pressure control: Main results of the

PREMIER clinical trial. *Journal of the American Medical Association, 289*(16), 2083–2093. https://doi.org/10.1001/jama.289.16.2083

Aune, D., Sen, A., Prasad, M., Norat, T., Janszky, I., Tonstad, S., Romundstad, P., & Vatten, L. J. (2016). BMI and all cause mortality: Systematic review and non-linear dose-response meta-analysis of 230 cohort studies with 3.74 million deaths among 30.3 participants. *British Medical Journal, 353*, i2156. https://doi.org/10.1136/bmj.i2156

Blackburn, G., Wollner, S., & Heymsfield, S. (2010). Lifestyle interventions for the treatment of class III obesity: A primary target for nutrition medicine in the obesity epidemic. *The American Journal of Clinical Nutrition, 91*(1), 289S–292S. https://doi.org/10.3945/ajcn.2009.28473D

Bray, G., Fruhbeck, G., Ryan, D., & Wilding, J. (2016). Management of obesity. *Lancet, 387*(10031), 1947–1956. https://doi.org/10.1016/S0140-6736(16)00271-3

Camps, S., Verhoef, S., & Westerterp, K. (2013). Weight loss, weight maintenance, and adaptive thermogenesis. *The American Journal of Clinical Nutrition, 97*(5), 990–994. https://doi.org/10.3945/ajcn.112.050310

Courcoulas, A., Belle, S., Neilberg, R., Pierson, S., Eagleton, J., Kalarchian, M., DeLany, J., Lang, W., & Jakicic, J. (2015). Three-year outcomes of bariatric surgery vs lifestyle intervention for type 2 diabetes mellitus treatment: A randomized clinical trial. *JAMA Surgery, 150*(10), 931–940. https://doi.org/10.1001/jamasurg.2015.1534

Courcoulas, A., King, W., Belle, S., Berk, P., Flum, D., Garcia, L., Gourash, W., Horlick, M., Mitchell, J., Pomp, A., Pories, W., Purnell, J., Singh, A., Spaniolas, K., Thirlby, R., Wolfe, B., & Yanovski, S. (2018). Seven-Year weight trajectories and health outcomes in the Longitudinal Assessment of Bariatric Surgery (LABS) Study. *JAMA Surgery, 153*(5), 427–434. https://doi.org/10.1001/jamasurg.2017.5025

Dagan, S., Goldenshluger, A., Globus, I., Schweiger, C., Kessler, Y., Sandbank, G., Ben-Porat, T., & Sinai, T. (2017). Nutritional recommendations for adult bariatric surgery clients: Clinical practice. *Advances in Nutrition, 8*(2), 382–394. https://doi.org/10.3945/an.116.014258

Fryar, C., Carroll, M., & Ogden, C. (2018). Prevalence of overweight, obesity, and extreme obesity among adults: United States, 1960–1962 through 2015–2016. https://www.cdc.gov/nchs/data/hestat/obesity_adult_15_16/obesity_adult_15_16.pdf.

Garvey, W. T., Mechanick, J., Brett, E., Garber, A., Hurley, D., Jastreboff, A., Nadolsky, K., Pessah-Pollack, R., Plodkowski, R., & Reviewers of the AACE/ACE Obesity Clinical Practice Guidelines. (2016). American association of clinical endocrinologists and American college of endocrinology comprehensive clinical practice guidelines for medical care of patients with obesity. *Endocrine Practice, 22*(supplement 3), 1–203. https://doi.org/10.4158/EP161365.GL

Hales, C., Carroll, M., Fryar, C., & Ogden, C. (2017). Prevalence of obesity among adults and youth: United States, 2015–2016. *NCHS Data Brief, 288*, 1–8. National Center for Health Statistics.

Hemmingsson, E., Johansson, K., Eriksson, J., Sundström, J., Neovius, M., & Marcus, C. (2012). Weight loss and dropout during a commercial weight-loss program including a very-low-calorie diet, a low-calorie diet, or restricted normal food: Observational cohort study. *The American Journal of Clinical Nutrition, 96*(5), 953–961. https://doi.org/10.3945/ajcn.112.038265

Huo, T., Du, T., Xu, Y., Xu, W., Chen, S., Sun, K., & Yu, X. (2014). Effects of Mediterranean-style diet on glycemic control, weight loss and cardiovascular risk factors among type 2 diabetes individuals: A meta-analysis. *European Journal of Clinical Nutrition, 69*, 1200–1208. https://doi.org/10.1038/ejcn.2014.243

International Diabetes Federation. (2006). *The IDF consensus worldwide definition of the metabolic syndrome*. https://www.idf.org/e-library/consensus-statements/60-idfconsensus-worldwide-definitionof-the-metabolic-syndrome.html

Jensen, M., Ryan, D., Apovian, C., Ard, J. D., Comuzzie, A. G., Donato, K. A., Hu, F., Hubbard, V., Jakicic, J., Kushner, R., Loria, C., Millen, B., Nonas, C., Pi-Sunyer, X., Stevens, J., Stevens, V., Wadden, T., Wolfe, B., & Yanovski, S. Z. (2014). 2013 AHA/ACC/TOS guideline for the management of overweight and obesity in adults. A report of the American College of Cardiology/American Heart Association Task Force on Practice Guidelines and the Obesity Society. *Journal of the American College of Cardiology, 63*(25), 2985–3023. https://doi.org/10.1016/j.jacc.2013.11.004

Johnston, B., Kanters, S., Bandayrel, K., Wu, P., Naji, F., Siemieniuk, R. A., Ball, G., Busse, J., Thorlund, K., Guyatt, G., Jansen, J., & Mills, E. J. (2014). Comparison of weight loss among named diet programs in overweight and obese adults: A meta-analysis. *The Journal of the American Medical Association, 312*(9), 923–933. https://doi.org/10.1001/jama.2014.10397

Lager, C., Esfandiari, N., Subauste, A., Kraftson, A., Brown, M., Cassidy, R., Nay, C., Lockwood, A., Varban, O., & Oral, E. (2017). Roux-En-Y gastric bypass vs. sleeve gastrectomy: Balancing the risks of surgery with the benefits of weight loss. *Obesity Surgery, 27*, 154–161. https://doi.org/10.1007/s11695-016-2265-2

Lauti, M., Lemanu, D., Zeng, I., Su'a, B., Hill, A., & MacCormick, A. (2017). Definition determines weight regain outcomes after sleeve gastrectomy. *Surgery for Obesity and Related Diseases, 13*(7), 1123–1129. https://doi.org/10.1016/j.soard.2017.02.029

Martinez-Gonzalez, M., Gea, A., & Ruiz-Canela, M. (2019). The Mediterranean diet and cardiovascular health: A critical review. *Circulation Research, 124*(5), 779–798. https://doi.org/10.1161/CIRCRESAHA.118.313348

Marzola, E., Nasser, J., Hashim, S., Shih, P.-a., & Kaye, W. (2013). Nutrition rehabilitation in anorexia nervosa: Review of the literature and implications for treatment. *BMC Psychiatry, 13*, 290. https://doi.org/10.1186/1471-244X-13-290

Mechanick, J., Apovian, C., Brethauer, S., Garvey, T., Joffe, A., Kim, J., Kushner, R., Lindquist, R., Pessah-Pollack, R., Seger, J., Urman, R., Adams, S., Cleek, J., Correa, R., Figaro, M., Flanders, K., Grams, J., Hurley, D., Kothari, S., … Still, S. (2019). Clinical practice guidelines for the perioperative nutrition, metabolic, and nonsurgical support of patients undergoing bariatric procedures-2019 update: Cosponsored by American Association of Clinical Endocrinologists/American College of Endocrinology, The Obesity Society, American Society for Metabolic & Bariatric Surgery, Obesity Medicine Association, and American Society of Anesthesiologists. *Endocrine Practice, 25*(supplement 2), 1–75. https://journals.aace.com/doi/pdf/10.4158/GL-2019-0406

Millen, B., Wolongevicz, D., Nonas, C., & Lichtenstein, A. (2014). 2013 American Heart Association/American College of Cardiology/The Obesity Society Guideline for the management of overweight and obesity in adults: Implications and new opportunities for registered dietitian nutritionists. *Journal of the Academy of Nutrition and Dietetics, 114*(11), 1730–1735. https://doi.org/10.1016/j.jand.2014.07.033

National Institute of Mental Health. (2017, November). *Eating disorders*. https://www.nimh.nih.gov/health/statistics/eating-disorders.shtml

National Weight Control Registry. (n.d.). The National Weight Control Registry. http://www.nwcr.ws/

Ozier, A., & Henry, B. (2011). Position of the American Dietetic Association: Nutrition intervention in the treatment of eating disorders.

Journal of the American Dietetic Association, 1111(8), 1236–1241. https://doi.org/10.1016/j.jada.2011.06.016

Raynor, H., & Champagne, C. (2016). Position of the Academy of Nutrition and Dietetics: Interventions for the treatment of overweight and obesity in adults. *Journal of the Academy of Nutrition and Dietetics, 116*(1), 129–147. https://doi.org/10.1016/j.jand.2015.10.031

Resmark, G., Herpertz, S., Herpertz-Dahlmann, B., & Zeeck, A. (2019). Treatment of anorexia nervosa-new evidence-based guidelines. *Journal of Clinical Medicine, 8*, 153. https://doi.org/10.3390/jcm8020153

Rock, C., Flatt, S., Pakiz, B., Barkai, H. S., Heath, D. D., & Krumhar, K. C. (2016). Randomized clinical trial of portion-controlled prepackaged foods to promote weight loss. *Obesity, 24*(6), 1230–1237. https://doi.org/10.1002/oby.21481

Rocks, T., Pelly, F., & Wilkinson, P. (2014). Nutrition therapy during initiation of refeeding in underweight children and adolescent in patients with anorexia nervosa: A systematic review of the evidence. *Journal of the Academy of Nutrition and Dietetics, 114*(6), 897–907. https://doi.org/10.1016/j.jand.2013.11.022

Schebendach, J., Mayer, L., Devlin, M., Attia, E., Contento, I. R., Wolf, R. L., & Walsh, B. T. (2008). Dietary energy density and diet variety as predictors of outcome in anorexia nervosa. *The American Journal of Clinical Nutrition, 87*(4), 810–816. https://doi.org/10.1093/ajcn/87.4.810

Sicat, J. (2018, July 23). *Obesity and genetics: Nature and nurture.* Obesity Medicine Association. https://obesitymedicine.org/obesity-and-genetics

Sockalingam, S., Cassin, S., Wnuk, S., Du, C., Jackson, T., Hawa, R., & Parikh, S. (2017). A pilot study on telephone cognitive behavioral therapy for patients six-months post-bariatric surgery. *Obesity Surgery, 27*, 670–675. https://doi.org/10.1007/s11695-016-2322-x

Stewart, F., & Avenell, A. (2016). Behavioural interventions for severe obesity before and/or after bariatric surgery: A systematic review and meta-analysis. *Obesity Surgery, 26*, 1203–1214. https://doi.org/10.1007/s11695-015-1873-6

Svetkey, L., Simons-Morton, D., Vollmer, W., Appel, L., Conlin, P., Ryan, D., Ard, J., Kennedy, B.; for the DASH Research Group. (1999). Effects of dietary patterns on blood pressure: Subgroup analysis of the Dietary Approaches to Stop Hypertension (DASH) randomized clinical trial. *Archives of Internal Medicine, 159*(3), 285–293. https://doi.org/10.1001/archinte.159.3.285

Tchernof, A., & Després, J. P. (2013). Pathophysiology of human visceral obesity: An update. *Physiological Reviews, 93*(1), 359–404. https://doi.org/10.1152/physrev.00033.2011

Tempest, M. (2012). Counseling the outpatient bariatric client. *Today's Dietitian, 14*(1), 38–41.

Thomas, J., Bond, D., Phelan, S., Hill, J. O., & Wing, R. R. (2014). Weight-loss maintenance for 10 years in the National Weight Control Registry. *American Journal of Preventive Medicine, 46*(1), 17–23. https://doi.org/10.1016/j.amepre.2013.08.019

Trace, S., Baker, J., Penas-Lledo, E., & Bulick, C. (2013). The genetics of eating disorders. *Annual Review of Clinical Psychology, 9*, 589–620. https://doi.org/10.1146/annurev-clinpsy-050212-185546

United States Department of Health and Human Services. (2018). *Physical activity guidelines for Americans* (2nd ed.). U.S. Department of Health and Human Services.

U.S. Food and Drug Administration. (2019, April 12). https://www.accessdata.fda.gov/cdrh_docs/pdf18/DEN180060.pdf

Vanderwood, K., Hall, T., Harwell, T., Arave, D., Butcher, M., Helgerson, S., Montana Cardiovascular Disease and Diabetes Prevention Workgroup. (2011). Factors associated with the maintenance or achievement of the weight loss goal at follow-up among participants completing an adapted diabetes prevention program. *Diabetes Research and Clinical Practice, 91*(2), 141–147. https://doi.org/10.1016/j.diabres.2010.12.001

Wadden, T., Neiberg, R., Wing, R., Clark, J., Delahanty, L., Hill, J., Krakoff, J., Otto, A., Ryan, D., Vitolins, M.; the Look AHEAD Research Group. (2011). Four-year weight losses in the Look AHEAD study: Factors associated with long-term success. *Obesity, 19*(10), 1987–1998. https://doi.org/10.1038/oby.2011.230

Wee, C., Davis, R., & Phillips, R. (2005). Stage of readiness to control weight and adopt weight control behaviors in primary care. *Journal of General Internal Medicine, 20*(5), 410–415. https://doi.org/10.1111/j.1525-1497.2005.0074.x

Weight Management Dietetic Practice Group, Cummings, S., & Isom, K. (Eds.). (2015). *Academy of nutrition and dietetics pocket guide to bariatric surgery* (2nd ed.). American Academy of Nutrition and Dietetics.

Welcome, A. (2017). *Definition of obesity.* Obesity Medicine Association website. https://obesitymedicine.org/definition-of-obesity

Westerberg, D., & Waitz, M. (2013). Binge-eating disorder. *Osteopathic Family Physician, 5*(6), 230–233. https://doi.org/10.1016/j.osfp.2013.06.003

Westmoreland, P., Krantz, M. J., & Mehler, P. S. (2016). Medical complications of anorexia nervosa and bulimia. *The American Journal of Medicine, 129*(1), 30–37. https://doi.org/10.1016/j.amjmed.2015.06.031

World Health Organization. (2018). *Obesity and overweight.* https://www.who.int/en/news-room/fact-sheets/detail/obesity-and-overweight

Yolsuriyanwong, K., Thanavachirasin, K., Sasso, K., Zuro, L., Bartfield, J., Marcotte, E., & Chand, B. (2019). Effectiveness, compliance, and acceptability of preoperative weight loss with a liquid very low-calorie diet before bariatric surgery in real practice. *Obesity Surgery, 29*, 54–60. https://doi.org/10.1007/s11695-018-3444-0

Chapter 18

Nutrition for Clients with Critical Illness

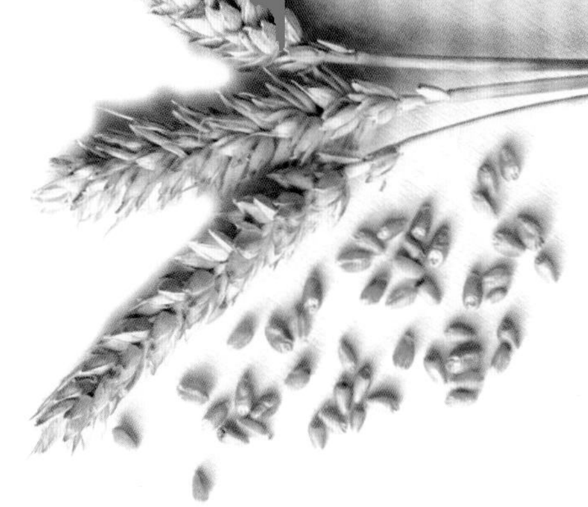

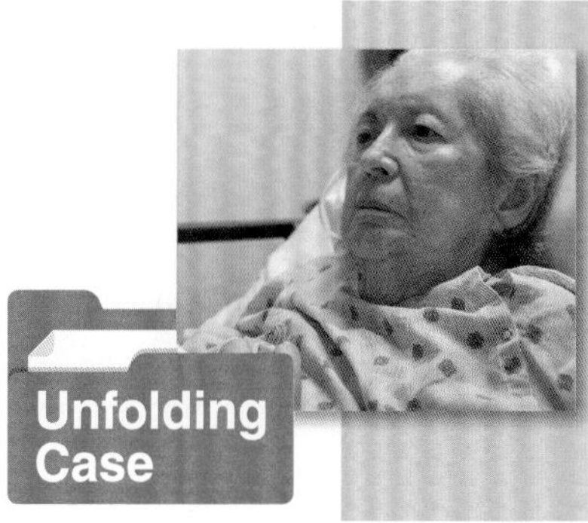

Unfolding Case

Franny Werts

Franny is a 70-year-old woman recently admitted to the hospital after sustaining five thoracic spine compression fractures from falling backward down a flight of stairs. She is confused and a neurologic consult is ordered. Shortly after admission, she developed a fever and tachycardia. Pneumonia was suspected, and she was diagnosed with sepsis and transferred to the intensive care unit (ICU). She is 5 ft tall and weighs 112 pounds, with a body mass index (BMI) of 22.

Learning Objectives

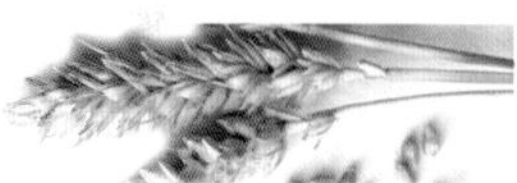

Upon completion of this chapter, you will be able to:

1 Explain how the stress response affects metabolism.
2 Explain why enteral nutrition, when feasible, is superior to parenteral nutrition in clients who are critically ill.
3 Calculate the calorie and protein requirements of a client with critical illness.
4 Explain why underfeeding calories may be preferable in the early phase of critical illness.
5 Discuss the cause and signs of refeeding syndrome.
6 Teach a client how to increase protein and calorie intake.
7 Devise a high-calorie, high-protein menu with small frequent meals.

Critical illness generally refers to any acute, life-threatening illness or injury that requires treatment in the ICU, such as trauma (e.g., gunshot wounds, motor vehicle accidents, severe burns), certain diseases (e.g., pancreatitis, acute renal failure), extensive surgery, or infection. It is typically associated with a state of catabolic stress characterized by a systemic inflammatory response and carries the risk of increased infectious morbidity, multiple-organ dysfunction, prolonged hospitalization, and disproportionate mortality (McClave et al., 2016).

Once considered adjunct therapy, nutrition support is now thought to help mitigate the metabolic response to stress, prevent oxidative cellular injury, and favorably dampen exaggerated immune responses. Early enteral nutrition (EN), appropriate macro- and micronutrient delivery, and tight glycemic control may reduce the severity of the illness, reduce complications, decrease length of stay in the ICU, and improve outcomes (McClave et al., 2016).

This chapter discusses the stress response and nutrition therapy for critical illness. Nutrition therapy for burns and acute respiratory distress syndrome (ARDS) is presented.

STRESS RESPONSE

Stress Response
a complex series of hormonal and metabolic changes that occur to enable the body to adapt to stressors.

Disruptions to homeostasis elicit a body-wide **stress response** characterized by hormonal and inflammatory changes to promote healing and resolve inflammation. The ebb and flow phases generally describe the course of the stress response (Box 18.1). The intensity of the stress response

BOX 18.1 Overview of the Stress Response Phases

Initial shock or ebb phase is marked by hemodynamic instability:

- **Typical duration:** 24 to 48 hours postinjury until the client is hemodynamically stable
- **Characteristics:**
  - shock with hypovolemia and diminished tissue oxygenation
  - decreased cardiac output, oxygen consumption, and body temperature
  - increase in heart rate
  - increased blood glucose level
  - increase in acute phase proteins
  - immune system activated
- **Treatment goals:** Restore blood flow to organs, maintain adequate oxygenation to all tissues, stop bleeding, and replace fluids.

The catabolic flow phase is marked by metabolic instability and catabolism. It lasts 3 to 10 days.

- Spike in circulating levels of hormones that direct the "fight-or-flight response" (e.g., glucagon, catecholamines, cortisol) promotes the breakdown of stored nutrients to meet energy needs:
  - glucose from glycogen
  - amino acids from skeletal muscle tissue
  - fatty acids from adipose
- Characteristics:
  - insulin resistance
  - increased cardiac output, oxygen consumption, body temperature, basal metabolic rate (BMR), and total body protein catabolism (negative nitrogen balance)
  - length of this phase is dependent on the severity of injury or infection and whether complications develop
- Nutrition goals: achieve and maintain fluid and electrolyte balance; minimize body protein catabolism; and meet calorie, protein, and micronutrient needs.

The anabolic flow phase is characterized by a positive nitrogen balance as protein synthesis begins. Adequate calories, protein, and nutrients are needed for anabolism.

depends to some extent on the cause and/or severity of the initial injury; for instance, the larger the body surface area burned, the greater the intensity of the stress response that follows.

Hormonal Response

Hormones released in response to stress include the following:

- catecholamines, glucagon, and cortisol
  - The metabolic effects from these hormones is to release stored macronutrients to meet the increased demands for energy. Their combined effects contribute to hyperglycemia.
  - Excess cortisol is damaging when stress is prolonged. It inhibits protein synthesis even when protein intake is high, promotes insulin resistance, contributes to hyperglycemia, and suppresses immune responses.
- aldosterone and antidiuretic hormone, which conserve water and sodium to help maintain blood volume

Inflammatory Response

In reaction to infection or tissue injury, the immune system mounts a quick, **acute-phase response** to destroy infection agents, prevent further tissue damage, and promote healing. Inflammation causes positive acute-phase proteins, such as C-reactive protein, to increase in concentration. Negative acute-phase proteins, such as albumin, prealbumin, and transferrin, decrease in response to inflammation. **Cytokines** and other immune system molecules are responsible for regulating acute-phase proteins; they also produce changes in other cells that cause systemic symptoms of inflammation, such as anorexia, fever, lethargy, and weight loss.

Acute-Phase Response
trauma- or inflammation-induced release of inflammatory mediators that cause changes in the levels of plasma proteins and clinical symptoms of inflammation.

Cytokines
a group name for more than 100 different proteins involved in immune responses. Prolonged production of proinflammatory cytokines promotes accelerated catabolism.

Potential Complications of the Stress Response

The inflammatory response to infection and tissue damage is a desired reaction that is generally self-limiting (Sharma et al., 2019). However, when the response is exaggerated and prolonged, the beneficial response becomes damaging.

- The body mounts an antiinflammatory response to counter the proinflammatory response.
- A disproportionate shift toward an antiinflammatory state can lead to endothelial damage and organ failure, immune suppression, metabolic abnormalities, and loss of body mass.
- The weakened immune system is unable to destroy pathogens, and the host becomes increasingly immunocompromised.

Sepsis

Sepsis
an abnormal systemic host response to infection that causes life-threatening organ dysfunction.

Sepsis is defined as "life-threatening organ dysfunction caused by a dysregulated host response to infection" (Singer et al., 2016, p. 804).

- Sepsis is the primary cause of death from infection (Singer et al., 2016).
- Septic shock is a subset of sepsis in which underlying circulatory and cellular metabolism abnormalities are severe enough to substantially increase the risk of death (Singer et al., 2016).

Malnutrition

Hypermetabolism
higher-than-normal metabolism.

Hypermetabolism and catabolism caused by the inflammatory response can quickly deplete protein stores. It is well understood that inflammation related to critical illness is a potent contributor to malnutrition (Malone & Hamilton, 2013).

- Malnutrition is independently associated with high mortality risk, longer length of hospital stay, and higher cost of hospitalization (Lim et al., 2012).
- Although it is difficult to actually define malnutrition in critically ill clients, it is estimated to affect 39% to 78% of clients with critical illness (Lew et al., 2017).
- Because baseline nutrition status is a strong predictor of clinical outcomes, timely initial screening is imperative to identify clients with malnutrition or high risk for malnutrition who benefit from early nutrition support (Sharma et al., 2019).

NUTRITION SUPPORT

Nutrition plays a key role in modulating inflammatory responses, maintaining immune function, slowing skeletal muscle catabolism, promoting tissue repair, supporting the functional integrity of the gut, and maintaining the pulmonary mucosal barrier (Sharma et al., 2019). However, best practices for providing nutrition care in the ICU remain unclear (Morrissette & Stapleton, 2020). Several factors contribute to the relative lack of strong ICU nutrition research: Sample sizes are small, the surrogate markers (e.g., improved weight) for improved clinical outcomes (e.g., lower infection rates) may not necessarily correlate, ICU clients are a heterogeneous population with different underlying diseases (Sharma et al., 2019), and our understanding of specific nutritional needs during severe physiologic and metabolic stress is poor (Morrissette & Stapleton, 2020).

Nutrition Support Goals

Nutrition Support
the provision of nutrition via enteral feeding tubes or parenteral catheters.

The goal of **nutrition support** is to reduce infectious morbidity, ventilator-dependent days, and length of stay in the ICU (McClave et al., 2016). Additional goals are to minimize body protein catabolism, promote wound healing, and provide the appropriate amount and combination of nutrients to limit or modulate the stress response and complications.

Nutrition Support

An oral diet is preferred over EN or parenteral nutrition (PN) in clients who are able to eat without risk of vomiting or aspiration (Singer et al., 2019). An oral intake that meets 70% of client need from days 3 to 7 is considered adequate.

When oral intake is not adequate, early EN is preferred over early PN (Singer et al., 2019). EN is preferred because it helps maintain gut integrity and has been shown to reduce infectious complications and length of ICU and hospital stay (Singer et al., 2019). It is recommended that EN be initiated as soon as fluid resuscitation is complete and the client is hemodynamically stable, preferably within the first 24 to 48 hours (McClave et al., 2016). When EN is not feasible or adequate, the use of PN is indicated, especially in clients with moderate to severe malnutrition or at risk of malnutrition. Guidelines for nutrition support in critically ill clients are summarized in Box 18.2. Additional points are presented as follows.

Enteral Formula Selection

For most clients, a standard polymeric (intact macronutrients) formula that provides 1.0 to 1.5 cal/mL may be used to initiate nutrition support in the ICU.

- For obese clients, a low-caloric density formula with a reduced nonprotein calorie-to-nitrogen ratio is suggested (proportionately lower in calories from carbohydrates and fats than in protein content).
- For clients in the surgical ICU or with severe trauma, an immune-modulating formula that provides arginine, fish oils, and/or glutamine may be considered.
- No benefit has been shown for routine use of other specialty formulas and disease-specific formulas in the ICU, such as pulmonary formulas for acute respiratory failure and hepatic formulas for critically ill clients with acute or chronic liver disease.

BOX 18.2 Summary of Nutrition Support Guidelines in Critical Illness

Method of Feeding

- An oral diet is recommended if it is feasible.
- EN is strongly recommended over PN when appropriate.
- Either gastric or small bowel feedings are appropriate. Consider small bowel feedings if client is at high risk for aspiration or has intolerance to gastric feedings.

Calories

- It is recommended that IC be used to determine calorie requirements.
- In the absence of IC predictive equations, a simple weight-based formula may be used:
  - 25 to 30 cal/kg/day of *admission weight* for clients with BMI <30
  - 11 to 14 cal/kg/day of *actual body weight* for clients with BMI in the range of 30 to 50
  - 22 to 25 cal/kg/day of *ideal body weight* for clients with BMI >50

Protein

- Positive outcomes in critical illness may be more dependent on adequate protein intake than adequate total calorie intake.
- Protein recommendations are as follows:
  - 1.2 to 2.0 g/kg/day of actual weight for adults with BMI <30; higher amounts may be necessary for certain illnesses, such as burns.
  - at least 2.0 g/kg/day of ideal body weight for clients with BMI of 30 to 40.
  - Up to 2.5 g/kg/day of ideal body weight for clients with BMI ≥40.

Other

- It is recommended that supplemental enteral glutamine *not* be routinely added to an EN regiment in critically ill clients based on randomized controlled trials that showed added glutamine had no significant benefit on mortality, infections, or hospital length of stay.
- Antioxidant vitamins (including vitamins E and C) and trace minerals (including selenium, zinc, and copper) may improve client outcomes, especially in clients with burns, with trauma, and requiring mechanical ventilation.
- Fluid requirements are highly individualized according to losses that occur through exudates, hemorrhage, emesis, diuresis, diarrhea, and fever.
- Clients with persistent diarrhea may benefit from the use of the fiber-containing formula, a semi-elemental formula in place of a standard formula, or a soluble fiber supplement.

Source: McClave, S., Taylor, B., Martindale, R., Warren, M., Johnson, D. R., Braunschweig, C., McCarthy, M., Davanos, E., Rice, T., Cresci, G., Gervasio, J., Sacks, G., Roberts, P., Compher, C., and the Society of Critical Care Medicine and American Society for Parenteral and Enteral Nutrition. (2016). Guidelines for the provision and assessment of nutrition support therapy in the adult critically ill patient: Society of Critical Care Medicine (SCCM) and American Society for Parenteral and Enteral Nutrition (A.S.P.E.N.). *Journal of Parenteral and Enteral Nutrition, 40*(2), 159–211. https://doi.org/10.1177/0148607115621863.

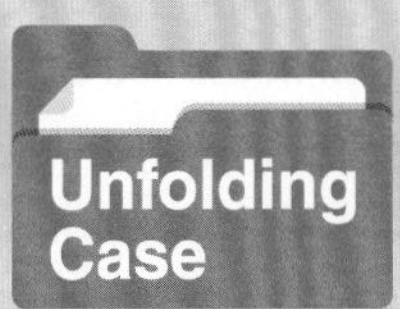

Recall Franny. She was given intravenous (IV) fluids and is hemodynamically stable. A nasoduodenal feeding tube is inserted for EN to begin immediately. Is this the best feeding method and route for Franny?

Calories

Indirect Calorimetry (IC)
an indirect calculation of energy expenditure based on analysis of the oxygen and carbon dioxide of inspired and expired air.

Indirect calorimetry (IC) is considered the gold standard for determining calorie requirements, but it may not be routinely performed due to limited availability, lack of expertise for interpreting results, or costliness of the device.

When IC is not an option, calorie needs can be estimated by either a predictive equation or a simple weight-based equation (see Box 18.2). Although there are more than 200 predictive equations, their accuracy rates range from 40% to 75% when compared to IC and none stand out as being the most accurate for ICU clients (McClave et al., 2016). Regardless of the method used to estimate calorie requirements, calorie expenditure should be reevaluated more than once a week so that intake can be optimized (McClave et al., 2016).

Calorie Targets

Refeeding Syndrome
a potentially fatal complication that occurs from an abrupt change from a catabolic state to an anabolic state and increase in insulin caused by a dramatic increase in carbohydrate intake.

It has been widely debated whether initially limiting the number of calories provided during critical illness may modulate the inflammatory response and thus improve mortality and clinical outcomes. To avoid overfeeding, it is recommended that early full EN and PN not be given to critically ill patients but shall be achieved within 3 to 7 days (Singer et al., 2019). However, clients who are severely malnourished or at high nutrition risk should advance toward goal as quickly as tolerated over 24 to 48 hours and should be monitored for **refeeding syndrome** (Box 18.3) (McClave et al., 2016).

Over the past 10 years, several large randomized controlled trials have studied whether calorie-restricted or full-target enteral feedings are optimal for ICU clients who are relatively well nourished (Morrissette & Stapleton, 2020).

BOX 18.3 Refeeding Syndrome

Refeeding syndrome: Refeeding syndrome is an ill-defined disorder that generally occurs when carbohydrate is reintroduced into the diet of severely malnourished clients, such as clients with

- chronic alcoholism,
- chronic undernutrition or malnutrition of calories and/or protein,
- morbid obesity with recent massive weight loss,
- prolonged fasting,
- long-term use of simple IV hydration, and
- cardiac and cancer cachexia.

It may develop in critically ill clients who receive aggressive nutrition repletion, either via a PN or EN diet or via an oral diet.

Symptoms range from a mild decrease in serum electrolytes that respond quickly to repletion to life-threatening changes in metabolic and organ systems.

- The sudden availability of carbohydrate stimulates insulin secretion and increases the need for thiamin and minerals involved in carbohydrate metabolism.
- Hypophosphatemia, hypokalemia, and hypomagnesemia can occur as cells rapidly remove these minerals from the bloodstream.
- Edema and heart failure can result from sodium and fluid retention.
- Thiamin deficiency can cause acidosis, hyperventilation, and neurologic impairments.
- For mild refeeding syndrome, initiation of EN is not affected as long as electrolyte abnormalities are corrected.
- In severe refeeding syndrome, thiamin supplementation, ongoing electrolyte replacement, and slower advancement of EN may be needed.

- Initial provision of 100% or 70% of calculated calories, or any amount in between, is reasonable in most relatively young and well nourished clients (Morrissette & Stapleton, 2020).
- More research is needed to determine whether (Morrissette & Stapleton, 2020):
    - the short- and long-term outcomes in less well-nourished clients are affected by the number of calories initially provided,
    - briefly delaying the provision of EN would yield different results than instituting early feedings.

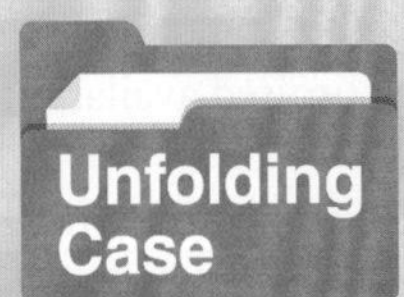

Consider Franny. Calculate her estimated calorie needs. What is an appropriate calorie target for her as the tube feeding begins? What is an appropriate protein intake for her?

Protein

Protein is the most important macronutrient for wound healing, supporting immune function, and maintaining lean body mass (McClave et al., 2016).

- For most critically ill clients, the increased need for protein is proportionately higher than the increased need for calories.
- Optimizing protein intake rather than total calorie intake has been shown to decrease infections, the duration of mechanical ventilation, length of hospitalization, and mortality (Nicolo et al., 2016).
- Study data are lacking on the optimal dose of protein for critically ill clients (Heyland et al., 2018). The recommendations for protein (see Box 18.2) are not universally agreed upon, and there may be more uncertainty over protein requirements than calorie needs.

Micronutrients

It is recommended that a combination of antioxidant micronutrients (e.g., vitamins C and E, selenium, zinc, copper) be provided in safe doses (e.g., 5–10 times the Dietary Reference Intakes) based on trials that showed that antioxidant and trace element supplementation was associated with a significant decrease in overall mortality (McClave et al., 2016). Research is needed to define normal antioxidant status for critically ill clients and determine optimal supplementary dosage, frequency, duration, and route of administration.

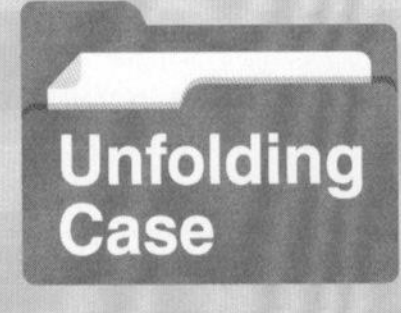

Think of Franny. As her signs and symptoms of inflammation and infection begin to resolve, her appetite improves but only for tea and toast. She wants the feeding tube removed but isn't hungry enough to eat a whole tray of food. What steps will you take to help maximize Franny's oral intake? How many calories should she be consistently consuming before the feeding tube can be removed?

Nutrition during Recovery

Clients are typically transitioned to an oral diet as soon as possible, usually following extubation. The goal of nutrition therapy is to maximize intake to preserve lean body mass.

- Oral intake is commonly inadequate after extubation for a variety of reasons, which may include residual pain after endotracheal tube removal, delays in ordering a diet, restrictive diets, client fatigue, anorexia, gastrointestinal (GI) upset, and nothing-by-mouth orders for tests or procedures.

- Monitoring oral intake and individualizing nutrition therapy are vital to optimize recovery.
- A high-calorie, high-protein diet with small frequent meals may help maximize intake (Box 18.4).
- A nutrient-dense diet provides nutrients important for wound healing and recovery (Table 18.1).
- Oral nutrition supplements can provide significant protein, calories, and nutrients. Supplemental EN may be necessary.

BOX 18.4 A Sample High-Calorie, High-Protein Menu

Breakfast

- orange juice
- cheese and mushroom omelet
- wheat toast with butter and jelly
- milk
- coffee with whipped cream added

Snack

smoothie made with Greek yogurt, instant breakfast mix, whole milk, and strawberries

Lunch

- New England clam chowder
- chicken salad sandwich on a croissant
- milk
- ice cream with chocolate sauce and whipped cream

Snack

Greek yogurt

Dinner

- meat loaf with gravy
- baked potato with sour cream
- broccoli with cheese sauce
- spinach salad with hard-cooked eggs, onions, walnuts, and vinaigrette dressing
- milk
- carrot cake with cream cheese frosting

Snack

melon topped with fruited Greek yogurt

Table 18.1 Nutrients Important for Wound Healing and Recovery

Nutrient	Rationale for Increased Need	Possible Deficiency Outcome
Protein	• to replace lean body mass lost during the catabolic phase after stress • to restore blood volume and plasma proteins lost during exudates, bleeding from the wound, and possible hemorrhage • to replace losses resulting from immobility (increased excretion) • to meet increased needs for tissue repair and resistance to infection	• significant weight loss • impaired/delayed wound healing • shock related to decreased blood volume • edema related to decreased serum albumin • diarrhea related to decreased albumin • anemia • increased risk of infection related to decreased antibodies, impaired tissue integrity • increased mortality
Calories	• to spare protein • to restore normal weight	• signs and symptoms of protein deficiency due to use of protein to meet energy requirements • extensive weight loss
Water	• to replace fluid lost through vomiting, hemorrhage, exudates, fever, drainage, diuresis • to maintain homeostasis	• signs, symptoms, and complications of dehydration such as poor skin turgor, dry mucous membranes, oliguria, anuria, weight loss, increased pulse rate, decreased central venous pressure
Vitamin C	• important for capillary formation, tissue synthesis, and wound healing through collagen formation • needed for antibody formation	• impaired/delayed wound healing related to impaired collagen formation and increased capillary fragility and permeability • increased risk of infection related to decreased antibodies

(continued)

Table 18.1 Nutrients Important for Wound Healing and Recovery (continued)

Nutrient	Rationale for Increased Need	Possible Deficiency Outcome
Thiamin, niacin, riboflavin	• requirements increase with increased metabolic rate	• decreased enzymes available for energy metabolism
Folic acid, vitamin B_{12}	• needed for cell proliferation and, therefore, tissue synthesis • important for maturation of red blood cells • impaired folic acid synthesis related to some antibiotics; impaired vitamin B_{12} absorption related to some antibiotics	• decreased or arrested cell division • megaloblastic anemia
Vitamin A	• important for immune function • plays a role in protein synthesis and cell differentiation; important for epithelial cells	• decreased immune function and increased risk of infectious morbidity and mortality • impaired epithelial cells alter digestion and absorption of nutrients and increase the risk of infections of the respiratory tract, GI tract, urinary tract, vagina, and inner ear
Vitamin K	• important for normal blood clotting • impaired intestinal synthesis related to antibiotics	• prolonged prothrombin time
Iron	• to replace iron lost through blood loss	• signs, symptoms, and complications of iron deficiency anemia such as fatigue, weakness, pallor, anorexia, dizziness, headaches, stomatitis, glossitis, cardiovascular and respiratory changes, possible cardiac failure
Zinc	• needed for protein synthesis and wound healing • needed for normal lymphocyte and phagocyte response	• impaired/delayed wound healing • impaired immune response

BURNS

Extensive burns are a severe form of metabolic stress. The extensive inflammatory response causes rapid fluid shifts and large losses of fluid, electrolytes, protein, and other nutrients from the wound. Fluid and electrolyte replacement to maintain adequate blood volume and blood pressure is the priority of the initial postburn period. Persistent and prolonged increases in metabolism and catabolism can lead to significant loss of lean body mass and weight with increased risks of impaired wound healing, organ dysfunction, and infection. Paralytic ileus, anorexia, pain, infection or other complications, emotional trauma, and medical–surgical procedures may complicate nutrition support.

Although nutrition support is a critical component of burn treatment, there is a lack of consensus regarding the optimal timing, route, amount, and composition of nutritional support (Clark et al., 2017).

Oral Nutrition

For burns covering less than 20% of total body surface area (TBSA), an oral high-protein, high-calorie diet can adequately meet protein and calorie requirements of most clients.

- Small frequent meals of calorie- and protein-dense foods (Box 18.5) and oral nutrition supplements help maximize intake.
- Daily calorie counts may be used to monitor intake.
- When calorie and protein intake is less than 75% of estimated need for greater than 3 days, EN may be indicated for supplemental or total nutrition. Supplemental EN given during the night is useful when nutritional needs are not met through food alone.

Enteral Nutrition

EN is recommended for burn clients who have functional GI tracts but who are unable to orally meet their estimated calorie needs. McClave et al. (2016) recommend

BOX 18.5 Ways to Increase Protein and Calorie Density of Foods

Ways to Increase Protein Density

- Add skim milk powder to milk.
- Substitute milk for water in recipes.
- Melt cheese on sandwiches, casseroles, hot vegetables, or potatoes.
- Spread peanut butter on apples or crackers or mix into hot cereals.
- Sprinkle nuts on cereals, desserts, or salads; mix into casseroles or stir-fry.
- Coat breaded meats with eggs first; add chopped hard-cooked eggs to casseroles.
- Top fruit with yogurt or Greek yogurt.
- Use plain yogurt or plain Greek yogurt in place of sour cream.
- Add commercially available whey protein powder to water, milk, shakes, or smoothies.

Ways to Increase Calorie Density

- Spread cream cheese on hot bread.
- Add butter or olive oil to hot foods: potatoes, vegetables, cooked cereal, rice, pasta, pancakes, and soups.
- Use gravy over potatoes, meat, or vegetables.
- Use mayonnaise in place of salad dressing.
- Use whipped cream on desserts and in coffee and tea.
- Add honey to cooked cereals, fruit, coffee, or tea.
- Add marshmallows to hot chocolate.

- initiating EN within 4 to 6 hours of injury if possible; early initiation is associated with improved structure and function of the GI tract and fewer episodes of infection and may also blunt the hypermetabolic response to burns;
- placing a nasoenteric tube into the small bowel to facilitate early EN; and
- using PN only when EN is not feasible or tolerated.

Nutrient Recommendations

Nutrient needs vary with the TBSA burned, the client's baseline nutritional status, the stage of treatment, and if the client develops complications. Frequent monitoring is necessary to assess the adequacy of nutrition.

Calorie Requirements

IC is recommended as the most accurate method to assess calorie requirements in burn clients. No predictive equations have found to be precise in estimating calorie needs of clients with >20% TBSA burns.

- If IC is not available or feasible, calorie needs may be estimated by the weight-based formula of 25 to 30 cal/kg (Academy of Nutrition and Dietetics, 2020).
- Calorie needs do not immediately decrease with wound closure; hypermetabolism may last for years after the injury (Clark et al., 2017).

Protein

Providing high doses of protein does not reduce the catabolism of body protein stores but does promote protein synthesis and reduces negative nitrogen balance (Clark et al., 2017).

- Recommended protein intake is 1.5 to 2.0 g/kg/day for adults, which is 2 to 2.5 times above the Recommended Dietary Allowances (RDA) for healthy people (McClave et al., 2016).
- Adequacy of protein intake is evaluated by wound healing and adherence of skin grafts.

Micronutrients

Micronutrient supplementation after burns is common practice in order to fight oxidative stress, support the immune system, and promote wound healing. However, research is needed to achieve a consensus on which nutrients, their dosages, and duration of supplementation are optimal for clients with severe burns. McClave et al. (2016) state that antioxidant vitamins (including vitamins E and C) and trace minerals (including selenium, zinc, and copper) may improve client outcomes in burn clients.

Nutrition after Discharge

A high-calorie, high-protein diet is usually recommended for about a year after discharge, even though data on the optimal diet after the acute postburn phase are virtually nonexistent (Clark et al., 2017). Clients should be encouraged to engage in strength training exercise to counter the continued loss of muscle mass and regularly weigh themselves.

ACUTE RESPIRATORY DISTRESS SYNDROME

Acute respiratory distress syndrome (ARDS) is a severe lung disease. Acute lung injury (ALI) is a less severe form of lung disease. Both diseases are characterized by inflammation of the lung parenchyma and increased pulmonary capillary permeability, leading to impaired gas exchange. Pulmonary edema interferes with ventilation and damages the alveoli. Oxygen levels fall in the blood and tissues, leading to impaired cellular function and possibly cell death. Hypercapnia can cause acidosis. Breathing is labored and heart rate increases. Cyanosis, confusion, and drowsiness may develop. Heart arrhythmias and coma may result.

Nutrition Therapy for Clients with Acute Respiratory Distress Syndrome

ARDS and ALI are most often observed as part of systemic inflammatory processes, such as sepsis, pneumonia, trauma, burn, aspiration, and pancreatitis (Academy of Nutrition and Dietetics, 2020). The underlying inflammatory condition increases calorie and protein requirements and the risk for malnutrition.

Enteral Nutrition

EN is used if the GI tract is functional. Intestinal feedings may be preferred because they lower the risk of aspiration.

- EN products specially formulated for clients with pulmonary disorders are high in fat and low in carbohydrate based on the rationale that lesser amounts of carbohydrate reduce CO_2 production.
  - This assumption has been shown to be erroneous; increasing the ratio of fat to carbohydrate only lowers CO_2 production in the client who is overfed (McClave et al., 2016).
  - When the appropriate number of calories is provided, the macronutrient composition of the formula is much less likely to affect CO_2 production (McClave et al., 2016).
  - It is recommended that these high-fat formulas not be used in ICU clients with acute respiratory failure.
- Clients with acute respiratory failure who require fluid restriction may benefit from calorie-dense EN formulas (e.g., those providing 1.5–2.0 cal/mL) that provide more nutrition in less volume than standard formulas (McClave et al., 2016).
- A meta-analysis of studies that examined the effects of omega-3 fatty acids and/or antioxidants in adults with ARDS was unclear as to whether these components improve oxygenation, long-term survival, length of ICU stay, or the number of ventilator-dependent days (Dushianthan et al., 2019).

Calories and Protein

The goal for ARDS is to provide adequate calories and protein to prevent weight loss. However, evidence regarding the calorie needs of clients with ARDS is conflicting (Loi et al., 2017).

- IC is the gold standard for estimating calorie requirements, but it is costly and may not be as accurate in intubated clients with high oxygen requirements (Loi et al., 2017).
- Less accurate methods of estimating calorie requirements include predictive equations or the weight-based formula of 25 to 30 cal/kg.
- Overfeeding is avoided because it increases CO_2 production and may complicate respiratory function and ventilator weaning.
- Either permissive underfeeding or full calorie delivery is appropriate because these two strategies yield similar outcomes over the first week of hospitalization in clients with ARDS (McClave et al., 2016)
  - However, some studies suggest that permissive underfeeding (low calories and protein) or tropic EN (low calories) with slow progression may be more beneficial than aggressive full feeding in clients with ARDS and ALI (Patel et al., 2018; Rice et al., 2011).
- Protein requirements generally range from 1.5 to 2.0 g/kg/day.

NURSING PROCESS Metabolic Stress

Yin is a frail, 74-year-old man admitted to the hospital with multiple serious but non–life-threatening injuries resulting from a car accident. His BMI is 18. A regular diet is ordered with oral nutrition supplements provided 3 times/day. He consumes 25% to 50% of most meals and supplements and states he has no appetite.

Assessment

Medical–Psychosocial History

- current diagnoses and medications
- medical history, including hyperlipidemia, hypertension, cardiovascular disease, renal impairments, diabetes, GI complaints
- medications that affect nutrition, such as lipid-lowering medications, cardiac drugs, antihypertensives
- extent of injuries, significance of GI trauma, if appropriate
- hemodynamic status, signs and symptoms of hemorrhaging
- neurologic status (e.g., confusion, disorientation), ability to eat, ability to self-feed
- GI symptoms, such as distention, complaints of nausea, anorexia
- psychosocial and economic issues prior to injury, such as whether finances, loneliness, or isolation impaired his food intake; determine who does food shopping and preparation and whether the client is a candidate for the Meals on Wheels program

Anthropometric Assessment

- height, current weight, BMI
- recent weight history, usual weight

Biochemical and Physical Assessment

- check abnormal labs for their nutritional significance
- input and output
- clinical symptoms of malnutrition such as wasted appearance

Dietary Assessment

- Do you have any difficulty chewing or swallowing?
- Do you have nausea or any other symptoms that interfere with your ability to eat?
- Are you able to feed yourself?
- Do you follow a special diet at home?
- Do you have enough food to eat at home?
- Do you have any food intolerances or allergies?
- Do you have any cultural, religious, or ethnic food preferences?
- Do you take vitamins, minerals, or supplements? If so, what?
- How much alcohol do you consume?

NURSING PROCESS Metabolic Stress (continued)

Analysis	
Possible Nursing Analysis	Malnutrition risk related to anorexia and underweight status as evidenced by oral intake of 25% to 50% and BMI of 18 on admission.
Planning	
Client Outcomes	The client will • maintain normal fluid and electrolyte balance, • meet 75% of his goal for calories and protein via oral diet with supplements, • describe the principles and rationale of a high-calorie, high-protein diet, and • avoid complications of undernutrition, such as weight loss, poor wound healing, and infections.
Nursing Interventions	
Nutrition Therapy	• Provide regular diet with oral nutrition supplements as ordered. • Encourage the client to eat calorie- and protein-dense foods first during mealtime. • Offer standby menu choices as needed. • Motivate the client to consume oral nutrition supplements.

Client Teaching	Instruct the client on the following:
	• the importance of protein and calories in promoting wound healing and recovery and overall health.
	• the eating plan essentials, including
	  • how to increase calories and protein in the diet,
	  • to eat small frequent meals to maximize intake.

Evaluation	
Evaluate and Monitor	• Monitor fluid and electrolyte balance and other biochemical values. • Monitor percentage of food consumed. • Monitor weight. • Monitor for complications, such as delayed wound healing or infection. • Observe for tolerance to oral diet. • Suggest changes in the meal plan as needed. • Provide periodic feedback and reinforcement.

How Do You Respond?

Do flavored waters marketed to improve immune function really work? There are several flavored waters available on grocery store shelves that feature descriptive terms such as *defend*, *protect*, or *immunity* on the label. All of these products contain added vitamins and/or minerals, such as vitamins A, C, D, E, B vitamins, or zinc. Some provide calories from sweeteners, while others are calorie free. Although certain vitamins and minerals *are* important for normal immune system functioning, it is a huge leap to conclude that any of these products provide health benefits beyond those obtained from a normal mixed diet. In general, consuming more than required of any nutrients necessary for immune system functioning does not boost immune function—unless the immune system was impaired because of a nutrient deficiency. Manufacturers are free to put in whatever nutrients they desire in whatever amounts they choose; scientific evidence of benefit or need is not required to make a function claim.

REVIEW CASE STUDY

Samuel was recently discharged after being hospitalized for burns he had suffered in an industrial accident that covered 18% TBSA. He is 38 years old, 5 ft 9 in. tall, and currently weighs 134 pounds. His pre-burn weight was 150 to 155 pounds. He received three meals a day plus three high-protein shakes while in the hospital. He is motivated to regain weight, but he refuses to drink any more of the shakes—they are too sweet and taste artificial. The dietitian told him he should be eating at least 2000 calories and include protein-dense foods at each meal and snack, but he lives alone and doesn't have the appetite for that amount of food.

His usual pre-burn intake appears in the box on the right.

- Evaluate Samuel's current BMI and usual adult weight. What would be an appropriate goal weight?
- What specific strategies would you recommend that Samuel implement to improve his overall intake?
- Is 2000 calories an appropriate amount of daily calories for Samuel? What sources of protein did he usually consume?
- Devise a sample menu for Samuel that takes into account the calories and protein he needs, living arrangements, and lack of appetite.

Breakfast: coffee with creamer, two doughnuts
Lunch: two hot dogs on buns, french fries, diet soft drink
Dinner: frozen pizza, ice cream, beer

STUDY QUESTIONS

1 When should nutrition support be initiated in a hemodynamically stable, fluid resuscitated, critically ill client?
  a. within 24 hours
  b. within 24 to 48 hours
  c. within 3 to 7 days
  d. within the first week

2 Which of the following strategies will increase protein density?
  a. using whipped cream to replace milk in coffee
  b. spreading cream cheese on hot bread
  c. using plain yogurt to replace sour cream
  d. using mayonnaise to replace salad dressing

3 Why is EN preferred over PN for a client with burns with a functional GI tract?
  a. EN can provide higher amounts of calories and protein.
  b. EN is less likely to interfere with oral intake.
  c. EN is less expensive.
  d. EN has a lower risk of infectious complications.

4 Which of the following strategies will increase calorie density?
  a. using butter instead of margarine on toast
  b. adding brown sugar to cereal instead of white sugar
  c. using gravy over meat
  d. substituting whole wheat bread for white bread

5 What is the primary intervention in the initial postburn period?
  a. PN
  b. supplements of trace elements
  c. fluid and electrolytes
  d. a low-carbohydrate diet to decrease CO_2 production

6 Why may underfeeding critically ill clients be beneficial?
  a. It provides less work for the GI tract to do.
  b. All methods of measuring a person's energy expenditure overestimate calorie requirements, so a lower calorie load is prudent.
  c. It may modulate the inflammatory response.
  d. It provides less strain on the respiratory system.

7 What causes refeeding syndrome in clients who are fed after being in a catabolic state?
  a. a dramatic increase in fluid intake
  b. a dramatic increase protein intake
  c. a dramatic increase in fat intake
  d. a dramatic increase in carbohydrate intake

8 Which of the following metabolic abnormalities is associated with refeeding syndrome?
  a. hyperphosphatemia
  b. thiamin deficiency
  c. hyperkalemia
  d. hypermagnesemia

CHAPTER SUMMARY NUTRITION FOR CLIENTS WITH CRITICAL ILLNESS

Stress Response

Critical illness is any acute, life-threatening illness or injury that requires treatment in the ICU. It is characterized by a systemic inflammatory response and associated with a state of catabolic stress. Stress elicits hormonal and inflammatory responses designed to promote healing and resolve inflammation.

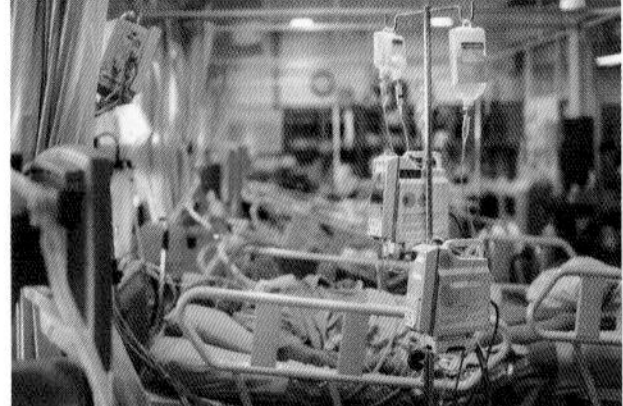

Hormonal Response

This response promotes release of glucose, amino acids, and fatty acids from body reserves to meet increased demands for energy. Other hormones conserve water and sodium to help maintain blood volume.

Inflammatory Response

To destroy infectious agents, this response prevents further tissue damage and promotes changes in acute phase proteins. The inflammatory response is desired and generally self-limiting. Sometimes, this response becomes exaggerated, prolonged, and damaging to the host.

Sepsis

Sepsis is a life-threatening syndrome of abnormal inflammatory response that causes organ dysfunction; the primary cause of death from infection.

Malnutrition

Inflammation of critical illness is a potent contributor to malnutrition. Malnutrition is difficult to diagnose in critically ill people. Baseline nutrition status is a strong predictor of clinical outcomes; nutrition screening is imperative to identify clients with malnutrition or at high risk for malnutrition, who benefit from early nutrition support.

Nutrition Support

EN is the preferred route for feeding critically ill clients if an oral diet is not feasible because it helps maintain gut integrity, modulates stress, and lessens disease severity. PN is indicated when EN is not feasible or inadequate.

Nutrition Support Goals. The goals are to reduce infectious morbidity, ventilator-dependent days, length of stay in ICU, and body protein catabolism.

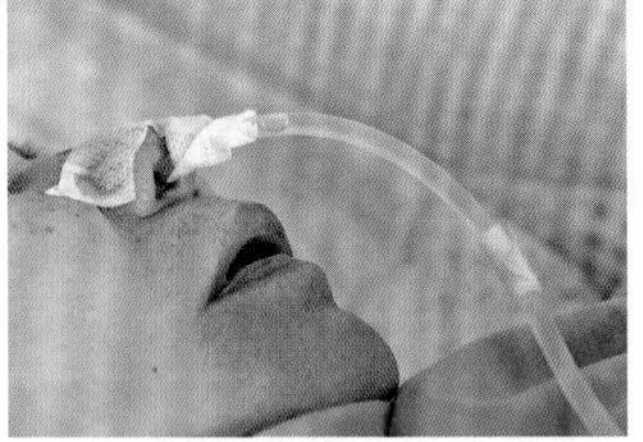

- **Enteral formula selection:** A standard polymeric (intact macronutrients) formula that provides 1.0 to 1.5 cal/mL is generally appropriate.

Calories. Requirements can be determined by indirect calorimetry, predictive equations, or simple weight-based formulas. All methods have disadvantages. Initial provision of 100% or 70% of calculated calorie needs, or any amount in between, is reasonable in most clients.

Protein. Protein requirement increases more than calorie requirement and may be more important than calories. Recommendations are not universally agreed upon.

Micronutrients. Antioxidant micronutrient supplements (e.g., vitamins C and E and selenium, zinc, and copper) are recommended in doses 5 to 10 times the DRI.

Nutrition during Recovery. Oral intake may resume after extubation. A high-calorie, high-protein diet is encouraged. Oral nutrition supplements or supplemental EN may be necessary.

Burns

Severe burns represent the most severe form of metabolic stress. Loss of lean body mass can be significant.

Oral Nutrition. Clients with burns covering <20% TBS may be able to meet their nutrient needs with a high-calorie, high-protein diet with oral nutrition supplements. Supplemental EN may be necessary.

Enteral Nutrition. This should be initiated within 4 to 6 hours after injury if possible. PN is indicated only when EN is not feasible or tolerated.

Nutrient Recommendations

- **Calorie recommendation:** Calorie needs can be estimated by IC, predictive equations, or weight-based formulas.
- **Protein recommendation:** 1.5 to 2.0 g/kg/day.

CHAPTER SUMMARY NUTRITION FOR CLIENTS WITH CRITICAL ILLNESS (continued)

- **Micronutrients:** Antioxidant vitamins (e.g., vitamins C and E) and trace minerals (e.g., selenium, zinc, and copper) may improve outcomes in clients with burns.

Nutrition after Discharge. Increased calorie needs may persist for a year after injury. A high-protein, high-calorie diet with oral nutritional supplements is recommended. Clients should regularly weigh themselves to monitor adequacy of intake.

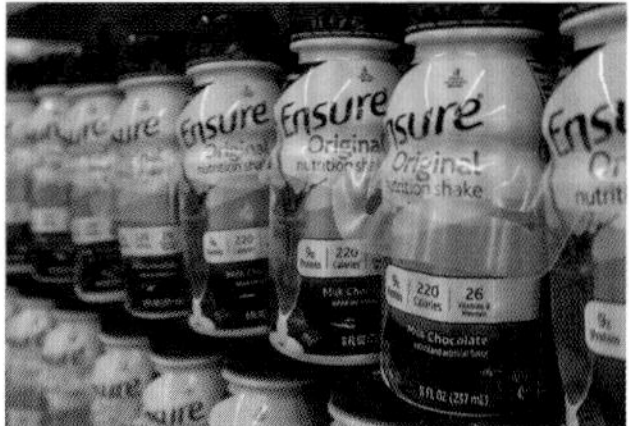

Acute Respiratory Distress Syndrome

ARDS is an inflammatory lung disease often part of systemic inflammatory processes such as sepsis, pneumonia, trauma, burn, and pancreatitis.

Nutrition Therapy. Calorie and protein needs are elevated. Mechanical ventilation makes nutrition support necessary.

- Routine standard formulas are recommended; calorie-dense versions may be appropriate for clients who require a fluid restriction.
- Calorie needs are not easily or accurately determined. The weight-based formula of 25 to 30 cal/kg may be used. Overfeeding should be avoided; permissive underfeeding may be used for the initial feeding period in well-nourished clients.
- Protein recommendation: 1.5 to 2.0 g/kg.
- It is not known if omega-3 fatty acids and/or antioxidants benefit adults with ARDS.

Figure sources: *shutterstock.com/Arne Beruldsen, shutterstock.com/Chaikom, shutterstock.com/nampix*

Student Resources on thePoint®
For additional learning materials, activate the code in the front of this book at https://thePoint.lww.com/activate

Websites

American Association of Critical-Care Nurses at www.aacn.org
American Burn Association at www.ameriburn.org
American Society for Parenteral and Enteral Nutrition at https://www.nutritioncare.org/
Society of Critical Care Medicine at www.sccm.org
Surviving Sepsis Campaign at www.survivingsepsis.org

References

Academy of Nutrition and Dietetics. (2020). *Nutrition care manual.* https://www.nutritioncaremanual.org

Clark, A., Imran, J., Madni, T., & Wolf, S. (2017). Nutrition and metabolism in burn patients. *Burns & Trauma*, *5*, s41038-017-0076-x. https://doi.org/10.1186/s41038-017-0076-x

Dushianthan, A., Cusack, R., Burgess, V. A., Grocott, M., & Calder, P. (2019). Immunonutrition for acute respiratory distress syndrome (ARDS) in adults. *Cochrane Database of Systematic Reviews*, Issue 1. Art. No.: CD012041. https://doi.org/10.1002/14651858.CD012041.pub2

Heyland, D. K., Stapleton, R., & Compher, C. (2018). Should we prescribe more protein to critically ill patients? *Nutrients*, *10*, 462. https://doi.org/10.3390/nu10040462

Lew, C., Yandell, R., Fraser, R., Chua, A., Chong, M., & Miller, M. (2017). Association between malnutrition and clinical outcomes in the intensive care unit: A systematic review. *Journal of Parenteral and Enteral Nutrition*, *41*(5), 744–758. https://doi.org/10.1177/0148607115625638

Lim, S., Ong, K., Chan, Y., Loke, W., Ferguson, M., & Daniels, L. (2012). Malnutrition and its impact on cost of hospitalization, length of stay, readmission and 3-year mortality. *Clinical Nutrition*, *31*(3), 345–350. https://doi.org/10.1016/j.clnu.2011.11.001

Loi, M., Wang, J., Ong, C., & Lee, J. (2017). Nutritional support of critically ill adults and children with acute respiratory distress syndrome: A clinical review. *Clinical Nutrition ESPEN*, *17*, 1–8. https://doi.org/10.1016/j.clnesp.2017.02.005

Malone, A., & Hamilton, C. (2013). The Academy of Nutrition and Dietetics/The American Society for Parenteral and Enteral Nutrition consensus malnutrition characteristics: Application in practice. *Nutrition in Clinical Practice*, *28*(6), 639–650. https://doi.org/10.1177/0884533613508435

McClave, S., Taylor, B., Martindale, R., Warren, M., Johnson, D. R., Braunschweig, C., McCarthy, M., Davanos, E., Rice, T., Cresci, G., Gervasio, J., Sacks, G., Roberts, P., Compher, C. and the Society of Critical Care Medicine and American Society for Parenteral and Enteral Nutrition. (2016). Guidelines for the provision and assessment of nutrition support therapy in the adult critically ill patient: Society of Critical Care Medicine (SCCM) and American Society for Parenteral and Enteral Nutrition (A.S.P.E.N.). *Journal of Parenteral and Enteral Nutrition*, *40*(2), 159–211. https://doi.org/10.1177/0148607115621863

Morrissette, K. M., & Stapleton, R. D. (2020). Mounting clarity on enteral feeding in critically ill patients. *American Journal of Respiratory and Critical Care Medicine, 201*(7), 758–760. https://doi.org/10.1164/rccm.202001-0126ED

Nicolo, M., Heyland, D., Chittams, J., Sammarco, T., & Compher, C. (2016). Clinical outcomes related to protein delivery in a critically ill population: A multicenter, multinational observation study. *Journal of Parenteral and Enteral Nutrition, 40*(1), 45–51. https://doi.org/10.1177/0148607115583675

Patel, J., Martindale, R., & McClave, S. (2018). Controversies surrounding critical care nutrition: An appraisal of permissive underfeeding, protein, and outcomes. *JPEN, 42*(3), 508–515. https://doi.org/10.1177/0148607117721908

Rice, T., Mogan, S., Hays, M., Bernard, G., Jensen, G., & Wheeler, A. (2011). Randomized trial of initial tropic versus full-energy enteral nutrition in mechanically ventilated patients with acute respiratory failure. *Critical Care Medicine, 39*(5), 967–974. https://doi.org/10.1097/CCM.0b013e31820a905a

Sharma, K., Mogensen, K., & Robinson, M. (2019). Pathophysiology of critical illness and role of nutrition. *Nutrition in Clinical Practice, 34*(1), 12–22. https://doi.org/10.1002/ncp.10232

Singer, P., Blaser, A., Berger, M., Alhazzani, W., Clader, P. C., Casaer, M. P., Hiesmayr, M., Mayer, K., Montejo, J. C., Pichard, C., Preiser, J.-C., van Zanten, A. R. H., Oczkowski, S., Szceklik, W., & Bischoff, S. (2019). ESPEN guideline on clinical nutrition in the intensive care unit. *Clinical Nutrition, 38*(1), 48–79. https://doi.org/10.1016/j.clnu.2018.08.037

Singer, M., Deutschman, C. S., Seymour, C. W., Shankar-Hari, M., Annane, D., Bauer, M., Bellomo, R., Bernard, G. R., Chiche, J.-D., Coopersmith, C. M., Hotchkiss, R. S., Levy, M. M., Marshall, J. C., Martin, G. S., Opal, S. M., Rubenfeld, G. D., van der Poll, T., Vincent, J.-L., & Angus, D. C. (2016). The third international consensus definitions for sepsis and septic shock (Sepsis-3). *JAMA, 315*(8), 801–810. https://doi.org/10.1001/jama.2016.0287

Chapter 19

Nutrition for Clients with Upper Gastrointestinal Tract Disorders

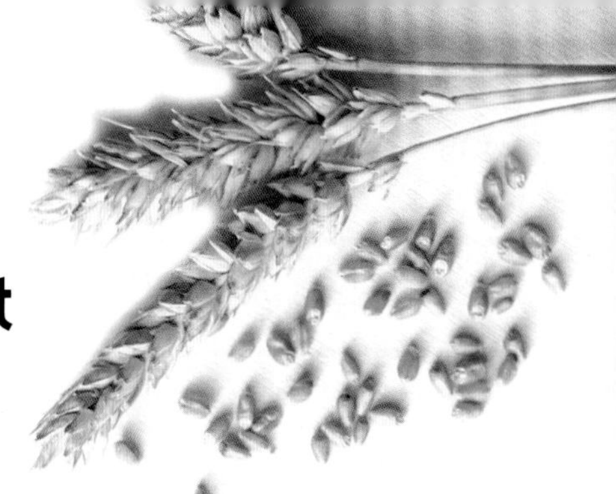

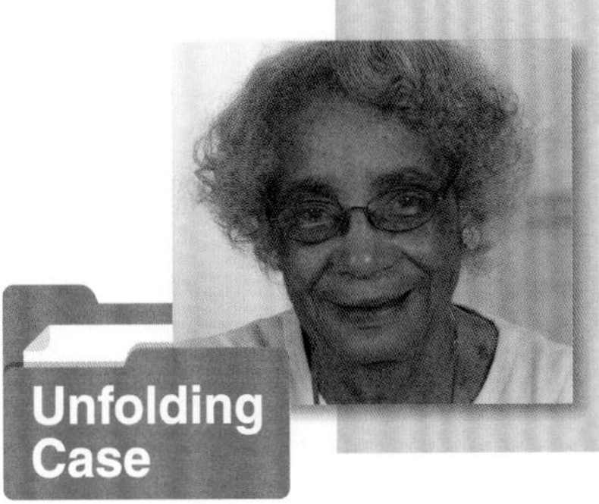

Unfolding Case

Bertha Parker

Bertha is an 84-year-old female who was diagnosed with type 2 diabetes 30 years ago. She has multiple chronic health problems, including mild to moderate dementia and gastroparesis. During a recent hospitalization for uncontrolled diabetes, she was given a swallowing evaluation after nurses observed hoarseness and coughing during and after swallowing.

Learning Objectives

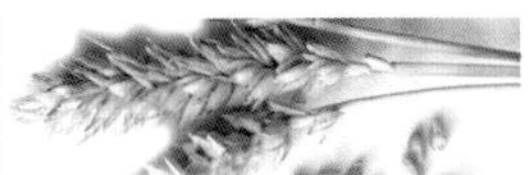

Upon completion of this chapter, you will be able to:

1 Give examples of ways to promote eating in people with anorexia.
2 Describe nutrition interventions that may help maximize intake in people who have nausea.
3 Describe the five levels of food textures in the international dysphagia diet.
4 Describe the five levels of liquid consistencies in the international dysphagia diet.
5 Discuss nutrition and lifestyle recommendations for someone with gastroesophageal reflux disease.
6 Teach a client about the role of nutrition therapy in the treatment of peptic ulcer disease.
7 Summarize nutrition strategies for clients with gastroparesis.
8 Give examples of nutrition therapy recommendations for people experiencing dumping syndrome.

Nutrition therapy is used in treating many digestive system disorders. For many disorders, diet merely plays a supportive role in alleviating symptoms rather than altering the course of the disease. For other gastrointestinal (GI) disorders, nutrition therapy is the cornerstone of treatment. Frequently, nutrition therapy is needed to restore nutritional status that has been compromised by dysfunction or disease.

This chapter begins with disorders that affect eating and covers disorders of the upper GI tract (mouth, esophagus, and stomach) that have nutritional implications. Table 19.1 outlines the roles these sites play in the mechanical and chemical digestion of food. Problems with the upper GI tract affect nutrition mostly by affecting food intake and tolerance to particular foods or textures. Nutrition-focused assessment criteria for upper GI tract disorders are listed in Box 19.1.

Table 19.1 The Role of the Upper Gastrointestinal Tract in the Mechanical and Chemical Digestion of Food

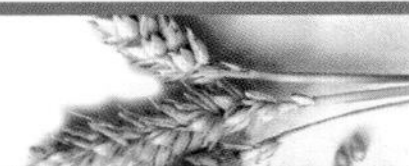

Site	Mechanical Digestion	Chemical Digestion
Mouth	• Chewing breaks down food into smaller particles. • Food mixes with saliva for ease in swallowing.	Saliva contains lingual lipase, which has a limited role in the digestion of fat, and salivary amylase, and begins the process of starch digestion. Food is not held in the mouth long enough for significant digestion to occur there.
Esophagus	• Propels food downward into the stomach. • Lower esophageal sphincter relaxes to move food into stomach.	None.

Stomach	• Churns and mixes food with gastric juices to reduce it to a thin liquid called chyme.
	• Forward and backward mixing motion at the pyloric sphincter pushes small amounts of chyme into the duodenum.
		• Secretes gastric acid (composed of hydrochloric acid, potassium chloride, and sodium chloride), which
		  ◦ denatures protein molecules to make peptide bonds more accessible to enzymes,
		  ◦ activates pepsinogen into the enzyme pepsin, which begins to digest protein into polypeptides,
		  ◦ frees vitamin B_{12} from the protein it is bound to in food, a necessary step for absorption.
		• Enhances the solubility of iron to promote its absorption.
		• Gastric juices (HCl, lipase, pepsin) inactivate swallowed microorganisms to protect against bacterial infections in the GI tract.
		• Secretes gastric lipase, which has a limited role in fat digestion.
		• Secretes intrinsic factor, necessary for the absorption of vitamin B_{12}.
		• Absorbs some water, electrolytes, certain drugs, and alcohol.

BOX 19.1 Nutrition-Focused Assessment for Upper Gastrointestinal Tract Disorders

- GI symptoms that interfere with intake, such as anorexia, early satiety, difficulty chewing and swallowing, nausea and vomiting, heartburn
- Changes in eating made in response to symptoms
- Complications that affect nutritional status, such as weight loss, aspiration pneumonia, diarrhea
- Usual pattern of eating and frequency of meals and snacks
- Use of tobacco, over-the-counter drugs for GI symptoms, and alcohol
- Food allergies or intolerances, such as high-fat foods, citrus fruits, spicy food
- Use of nutritional supplements, including vitamins, minerals, fiber, and herbs
- Client's willingness to change their eating habits

DISORDERS THAT AFFECT EATING

Anorexia

Anorexia
lack of appetite; it differs from anorexia nervosa, a psychological condition characterized by denial of appetite.

Anorexia is a common symptom of many physical conditions and a side effect of certain drugs. Emotional issues, such as fear, anxiety, and depression, frequently cause anorexia. The aim of nutrition therapy is to stimulate the appetite to maintain adequate nutritional intake. The following interventions may help:

- Serve food attractively and season according to individual taste. If decreased ability to taste is contributing to anorexia, enhance food flavors with tart seasonings (e.g., orange juice, lemonade, vinegar, lemon juice) or strong seasonings (e.g., basil, oregano, rosemary, tarragon, mint).
- Schedule procedures and medications when they are least likely to interfere with meals, if possible.

- Control pain, nausea, or depression with medications as ordered.
- Provide small, frequent meals.
- Withhold beverages for 30 minutes before and after meals to avoid displacing the intake of more nutrient-dense foods.
- Offer liquid supplements between meals for additional calories and protein if meal consumption is low.
- Limit fat intake if fat is contributing to early satiety.

Nausea and Vomiting

Nausea and vomiting may be related to a decrease in gastric acid secretion, a decrease in digestive enzyme activity, a decrease in GI motility, gastric irritation, or acidosis. Other causes include bacterial and viral infection; increased intracranial pressure; equilibrium imbalance; liver, pancreatic, and gallbladder disorders; and pyloric or intestinal obstruction. Drugs and certain medical treatments may also contribute to nausea.

The short-term concern of nausea and vomiting is fluid and electrolyte balance, which can be maintained by intravenous administration and/or clear liquids. Dehydration and weight loss are concerns with prolonged or **intractable vomiting**.

Intractable Vomiting vomiting that is difficult to manage or cure.

Nutrition intervention for nausea is a commonsense approach. Food is withheld until nausea subsides.

- When the client is ready to resume an oral intake, clear liquids are offered and intake is progressed to a regular diet as tolerated.
- Small, frequent meals of readily digested carbohydrates are usually best tolerated:
  - dry toast
  - saltine crackers
  - plain rolls
  - pretzels
  - angel food cake
  - oatmeal
  - canned peaches and canned pears
  - banana
- High-fat foods are avoided if they contribute to nausea.
  - fats: nuts, nut butters, oils, margarine, butter, salad dressings, creams (liquid, sour, whipped)
  - fatty meats, including many processed meats (bologna, pastrami, hard salami), bacon, sausage
  - milk and milk products containing whole or 2% milk
  - rich desserts, such as cakes, pies, cookies, pastries
  - many savory snacks, such as potato chips, cheese puffs, and tortilla chips
- Other strategies that may help are to
  - encourage the client to eat slowly and not to eat if they feel nauseated,
  - promote good oral hygiene with mouthwash and ice chips,
  - limit liquids with meals because they can cause a full, bloated feeling,
  - encourage a liberal fluid intake between meals with whatever liquids the client can tolerate, such as clear soup, juice, gelatin, ginger ale, and popsicles,
  - serve foods at room temperature or chilled (hot foods may contribute to nausea),
  - avoid spicy foods if they contribute to nausea,
  - encourage the client to sit up for at least 1 hour after eating, and
  - use ginger (tea, ginger ale, crystallized ginger), anecdotally, which may help relieve nausea.

DISORDERS OF THE ESOPHAGUS

Symptoms of esophageal disorders range from difficulty swallowing and the sensation that something is stuck in the throat to heartburn and reflux. Dysphagia and gastroesophageal reflux disease (GERD) are discussed next.

Dysphagia

Dysphagia
impaired ability to swallow.

Swallowing is a complex series of events characterized by three basic phases (Fig. 19.1). **Dysphagia** is objectively defined as an abnormal delay in the transit of liquids or solid during the oropharyngeal or esophageal phases of swallowing. It can have a profound impact on intake, hydration status, and nutritional status and greatly increases the risk of aspiration and its complications of bacterial pneumonia and bronchial obstruction. The two major types of dysphagia are oropharyngeal dysphagia and esophageal dysphagia; clients can have one or both types.

Oropharyngeal Dysphagia

Oropharyngeal dysphagia occurs when there is difficulty in the initial stage of swallowing that involves transferring food from the mouth into the esophagus. It is most often caused by neurologic or muscular disorders, such as stroke, myasthenia gravis, Parkinson's disease, multiple sclerosis, upper esophageal sphincter dysfunction, muscular dystrophy, radiation injury, amyotrophic lateral sclerosis, and head and neck tumors.

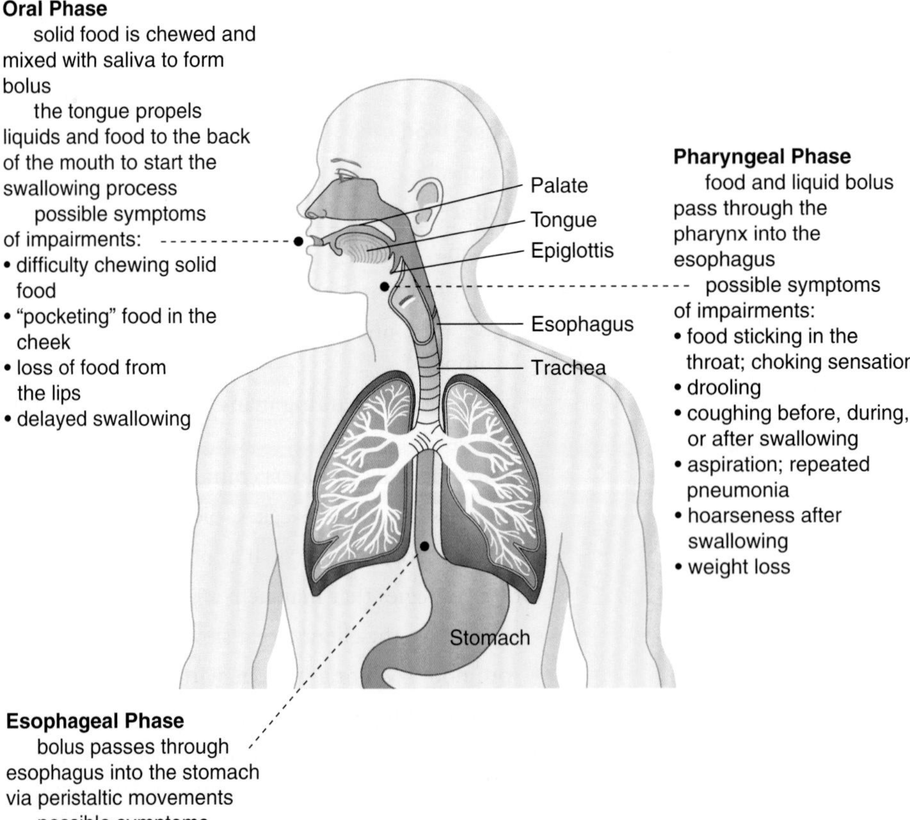
Oral Phase
solid food is chewed and mixed with saliva to form bolus
the tongue propels liquids and food to the back of the mouth to start the swallowing process
possible symptoms of impairments:
• difficulty chewing solid food
• "pocketing" food in the cheek
• loss of food from the lips
• delayed swallowing
Palate
Tongue
Epiglottis
Esophagus
Trachea
Stomach
Pharyngeal Phase
food and liquid bolus pass through the pharynx into the esophagus
possible symptoms of impairments:
• food sticking in the throat; choking sensation
• drooling
• coughing before, during, or after swallowing
• aspiration; repeated pneumonia
• hoarseness after swallowing
• weight loss
Esophageal Phase
bolus passes through esophagus into the stomach via peristaltic movements
possible symptoms of impairments:
• difficulty with solid food (can handle pureed food)
• heartburn
• vomiting
• burping

Figure 19.1 ▶ Swallowing phases and symptoms of impairments.

Esophageal Dysphagia

Esophageal dysphagia is difficulty passing food down the esophagus. It is caused by either a motility disorder (e.g., achalasia, diffuse esophageal spasm) or a mechanical obstruction (e.g., peptic stricture, esophageal cancer, lower esophageal rings). It is characterized by the sensation of food sticking in the throat or in the chest for several seconds after swallowing.

Signs and Symptoms

Signs and symptoms of dysphagia include

- eating meals slowly,
- choking, coughing, or throat clearing while eating or after eating,
- frequent heartburn,
- drooling,
- being hoarse, and
- unintended weight loss.

Texture and Consistency Modification

One of the most common interventions for dysphagia is texture modification (Steele et al., 2015). The appropriate texture modification for dysphagia depends on the particular issue.

- Thickened liquids are generally safer for people with dysphagia because they flow more slowly than thin liquids, allowing the airway time to close.
- However, very thick liquids and solid food may pose a risk for people with diminished tongue strength or pharyngeal muscle strength if food remains in the pharynx after a swallow.
- Pureed food may be appropriate for clients who are unable to bite or chew food or have reduced tongue control.
- People who have some basic chewing ability but are unable to bite off pieces of food safely may benefit from solid food that is minced and moist (International Dysphagia Diet Standardization Initiative [IDDSI], 2019).

A swallow evaluation is done by a speech pathologist, who identifies the appropriate food texture and liquid consistency and recommends feeding techniques based on the client's individual status. Texture and consistency changes are made as the client's ability to swallow improves or deteriorates.

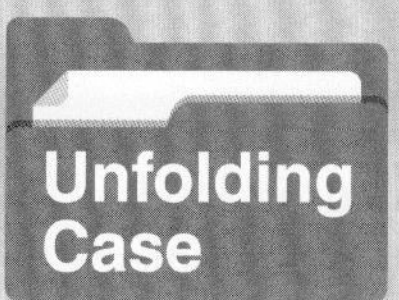

Consider Bertha. Based on her symptoms, which phase of swallowing is impaired? What may be the cause of Bertha's impairment? What other symptoms may she display?

Nutrition Therapy for Dysphagia

Viscosity
the condition of being resistant to flow; having a heavy, gluey quality.

The goal of nutrition therapy for dysphagia is to modify the texture of foods and/or **viscosity** of liquids to promote safe and efficient swallowing, allowing the client to achieve adequate nutrition and hydration while decreasing the risk of aspiration. A new global standardized dysphagia guideline was developed by the International Dysphagia Diet Standardization Initiative board (IDDSI, 2019).

- The guidelines use new standardized terminology and definitions to describe texture-modified foods and thickened liquids for people with dysphagia of all ages, in all care settings, and all cultures.

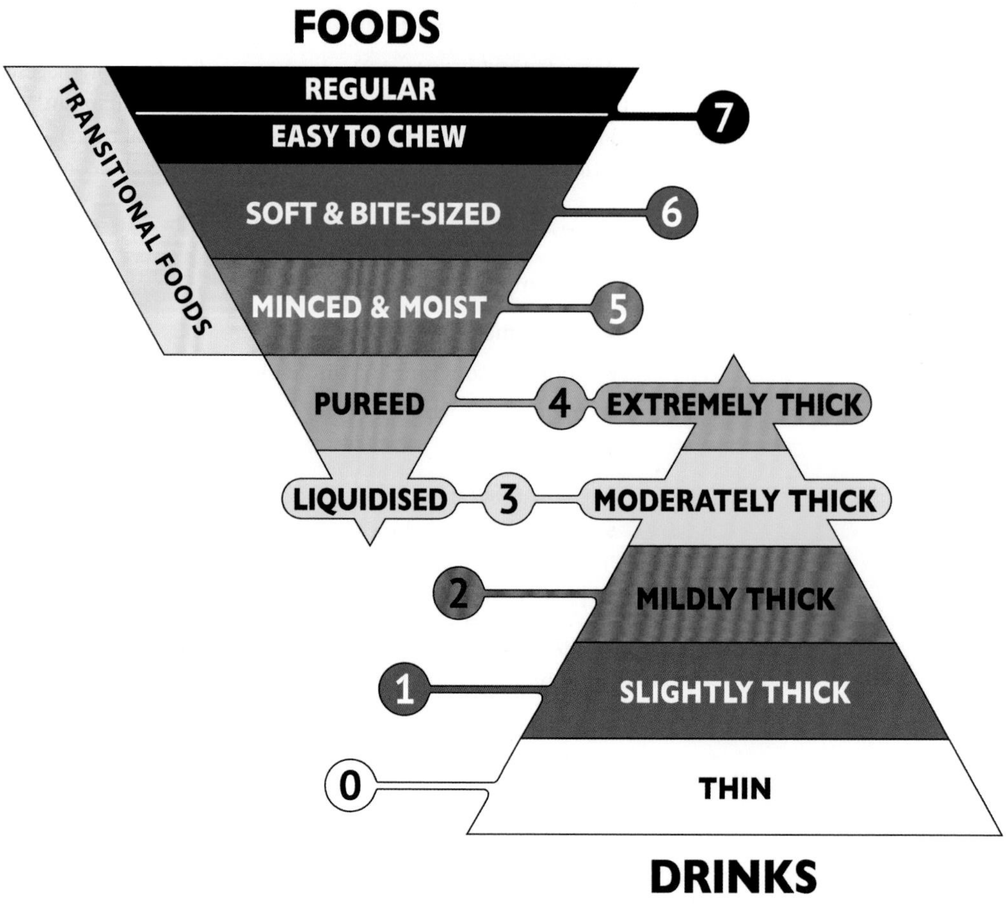

Figure 19.2 ▶ International dysphagia diet: Simplified version of food and liquid levels. (*Source:* The International Dysphagia Diet Standardisation Initiative 2016 https://iddsi.org/framework)

FOODS

TRANSITIONAL FOODS

REGULAR

EASY TO CHEW

7

SOFT & BITE-SIZED

6

MINCED & MOIST

5

PUREED

4

EXTREMELY THICK

LIQUIDISED

3

MODERATELY THICK

2

MILDLY THICK

1

SLIGHTLY THICK

0

THIN

DRINKS

- A continuum of 8 levels is identified by numbers, description titles, and color codes (Fig. 19.2). An upright triangle is used to describe each level of liquids (levels 0–4), and an inverted triangle features food (levels 3–7). Note that the foods and liquids in level 3 and level 4 share the same characteristics; using the same number and color to identify both food and liquid within each of these 2 levels demonstrates this equivalence in texture (IDDSI, 2019). Table 19.2 describes the characteristics of foods in levels 4 to 7 and gives examples of foods included.
- Test instructions are provided to evaluate the consistency or texture for each of the 8 levels.
  - For instance, levels 0 to 4 flow tests provide an objective measurement for liquid thickness based on their rate of flow using a syringe filled to 10 mL of liquid and released over 10 seconds (Fig. 19.3) Videos of the flow test can be found at https://iddsi.org/framework/drink-testing-methods/
  - Tests to evaluate the texture of foods in levels 4 (pureed) to 7 (regular) involve a fork to measure thickness (level 4), size of food pieces (levels 5), or firmness (levels 6 and 7) (Fig. 19.4).
- The standardized terminology will make client transitions from one facility to another safer and easier regarding appropriate texture. However, there is no expectation that every facility will offer all 5 levels of food texture and all 5 levels of liquid levels.

Promoting Intake

Meeting nutrient and fluid needs is a challenge in clients with dysphagia.

- Texture modifications often dilute the nutritional value of the diet and make food and beverages less appealing.
- Emotionally, dysphagia can affect quality of life; clients with dysphagia may feel panic at mealtime, avoid eating with others, and stop eating even when they still feel hungry.

Table 19.2 International Dysphagia Diets 4 to 7: Characteristics and Examples of Foods Included

Level	Characteristics	Examples of Foods Included

4: Pureed	• Usually eaten with a spoon, although eating with a fork is possible.
	• Cannot be drunk from a cup or sucked through a straw.
	• No chewing required.
	• Pureed to smooth.
	• Can be piped, layered, or molded and holds its own shape.
	• Not sticky.
	• Liquid does not separate from solid.
		• Foods pureed in a blender using extra gravy, sauce, or milk, such as
		  • scrambled or baked eggs
		  • soft pasta dishes
		  • meat dishes (e.g., beef stew, chicken curry)
		  • potatoes
		  • vegetables
		  • cooked oatmeal
		  • fruit
		• Smooth soup
		• Smooth yogurt

5: Minced and moist	• Can be eaten with a fork or spoon. • Tender, soft, and moist. • Needs very little chewing. • Small visible lumps are allowed. • Lumps are easy to mash with the tongue. • Usually requires a smooth sauce, gravy, or custard, which should be very thick. • No mixed textures (e.g., thick and thin) such as cereal in milk or separation of liquid from food (e.g., watermelon).	• Smooth soups • Egg (scrambled, poached, boiled) finely mashed with sauce added • Finely minced or chopped meat served in thick, smooth gravy • Mashed potatoes, mashed pasta or rice in a thick sauce • Mashed or finely chopped fruit without excess liquid • Finely mashed or finely chopped cooked vegetables without excess liquid • Thick, smooth cooked cereal • Yogurt, pudding, custard • Soft cheese, hummus
6: Soft and bite sized	• Soft, tender, and moist; requires chewing but not biting. • Can be mashed with a fork; no knife is required for cutting. • Usually requires a smooth sauce, gravy, or custard, which should be very thick. • No mixed textures (e.g., thick and thin) such as cereal in milk or separation of liquid from food (e.g., watermelon).	• Cooked tender and bite-sized pieces of meat and fish or meat and fish finely minced in a thick smooth sauce or gravy • Egg (scrambled, poached, boiled, fried) • Soft and chopped pieces of fruit without excess liquid • Steamed or boiled bite-sized pieces of vegetables that are tender • Cereals that are fully softened with excess liquid drained away • Pancakes with syrup
7: Regular and easy to chew	• Normal foods of soft, tender texture. • May include thin and thick textured food and liquids together (e.g., soup with solids). • Foods may range in size; no size limit or recommendation. • Can be cut or broken apart easily with the side of a fork or spoon. A knife is not required to cut this food. • Can bite off pieces of food. • Eliminates hard, tough, chewy, fibrous, stringy foods with seeds or gristle.	• Tender meats and fish • Fruit soft enough to break apart into smaller pieces • Steamed or boiled vegetables until tender • Cereal with texture softened • Rice
7: Regular	• Normal with various textures. • Size not restricted. • Includes hard, tough, chewy, fibrous, stingy, dry, crispy, crunchy, or crumbly bits. • Includes foods that contain seeds or husks. • Includes mixed consistency foods.	• All foods included

- Acceptability of pureed food is a common concern. Pureed foods can be molded into the appearance of "normal" food by using commercial thickeners and molds designed for pureed foods (Fig. 19.5). Molded food may (Farrer et al., 2016) or may not (Lepore et al., 2014) be preferred over scooped pureed food.
- Various feeding techniques that may facilitate safe swallowing are listed in Box 19.2.

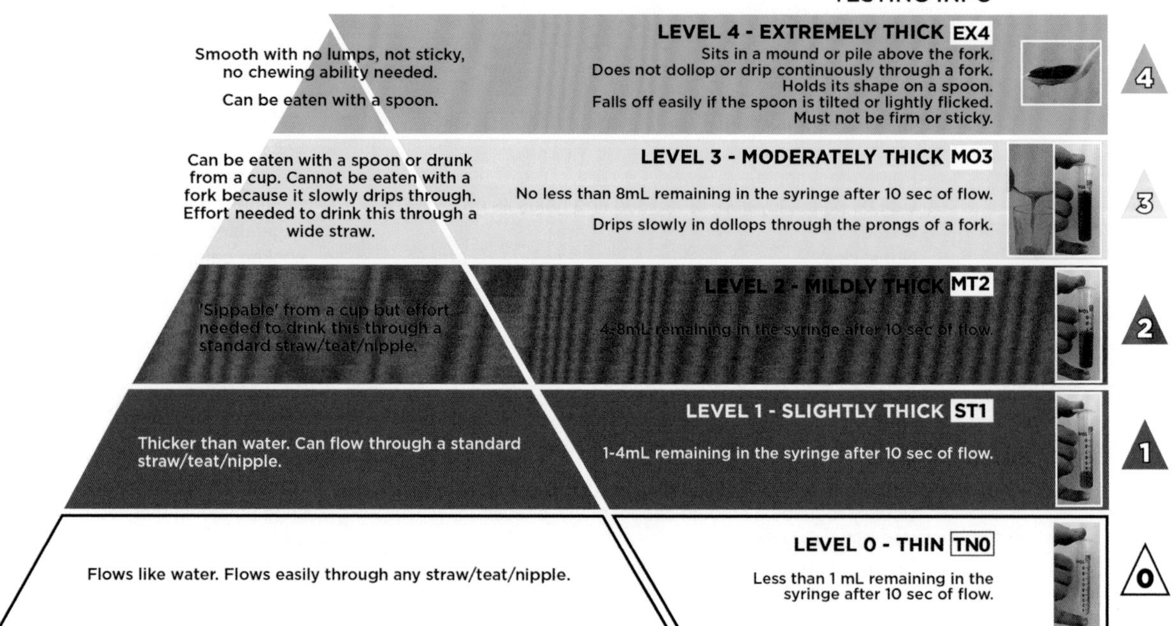
DRINKS / LIQUIDS
TESTING INFO
LEVEL 4 - EXTREMELY THICK EX4
Smooth with no lumps, not sticky, no chewing ability needed.
Can be eaten with a spoon.
Sits in a mound or pile above the fork.
Does not dollop or drip continuously through a fork.
Holds its shape on a spoon.
Falls off easily if the spoon is tilted or lightly flicked.
Must not be firm or sticky.
LEVEL 3 - MODERATELY THICK MO3
Can be eaten with a spoon or drunk from a cup. Cannot be eaten with a fork because it slowly drips through. Effort needed to drink this through a wide straw.
No less than 8mL remaining in the syringe after 10 sec of flow.
Drips slowly in dollops through the prongs of a fork.
LEVEL 2 - MILDLY THICK MT2
'Sippable' from a cup but effort needed to drink this through a standard straw/teat/nipple.
4-8mL remaining in the syringe after 10 sec of flow.
LEVEL 1 - SLIGHTLY THICK ST1
Thicker than water. Can flow through a standard straw/teat/nipple.
1-4mL remaining in the syringe after 10 sec of flow.
LEVEL 0 - THIN TN0
Flows like water. Flows easily through any straw/teat/nipple.
Less than 1 mL remaining in the syringe after 10 sec of flow.
4
3
2
1
0

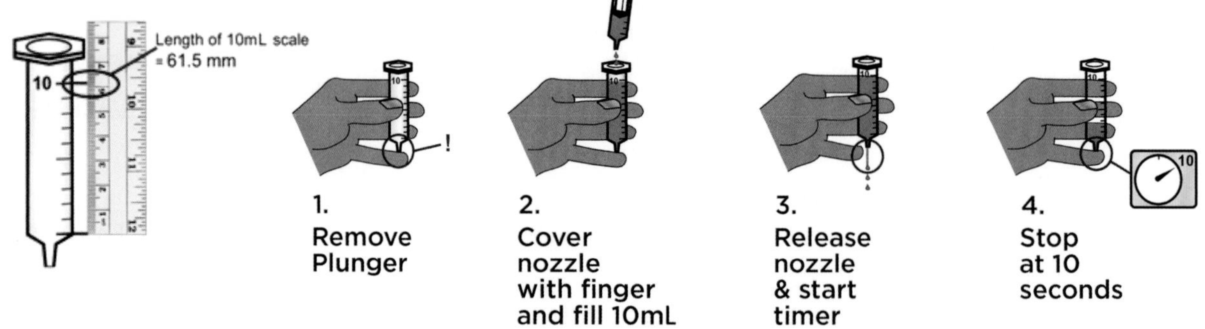
FLOW TEST INSTRUCTIONS
Length of 10mL scale = 61.5 mm
10
1. Remove Plunger
2. Cover nozzle with finger and fill 10mL
3. Release nozzle & start timer
4. Stop at 10 seconds

Figure 19.3 ▲ **International dysphagia diet: Characteristics and testing information for liquids.** (*Source:* The International Dysphagia Diet Standardisation Initiative 2016 https://iddsi.org/framework)

Fluid Intake

Thickened beverages are often poorly accepted, making it difficult to maintain an adequate fluid intake. Potential complications include dehydration, decreased compliance with swallowing guidelines, and decreased quality of life.

The Frazier Free Water Protocol allows certain clients with dysphagia the option to consume water in between meals.

- A recent systematic review of mostly rehabilitation clients with oropharyngeal dysphagia who required thickened liquids or were to remain NPO found that the free water protocol did not result in increased risk of having lung complications and that fluid intake may increase (Gillman et al., 2017).
- Large-scale studies are needed to evaluate the advantages and disadvantages of the free water protocol in the acute care settings (Kenedi et al., 2019).

FOODS

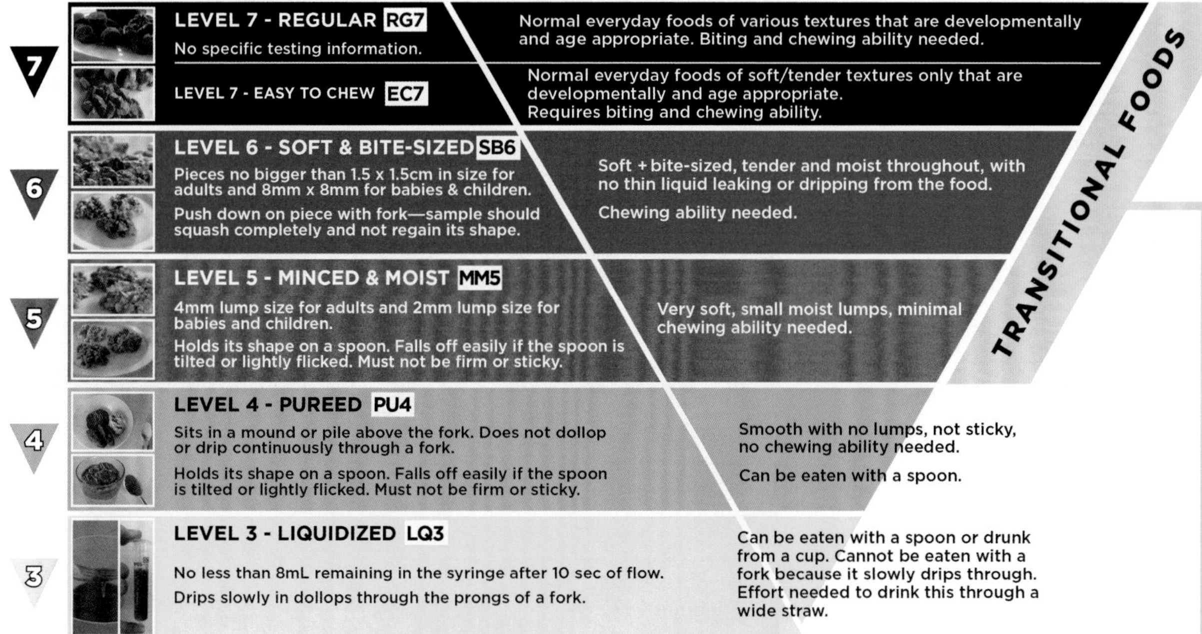

FOOD TEST INSTRUCTIONS

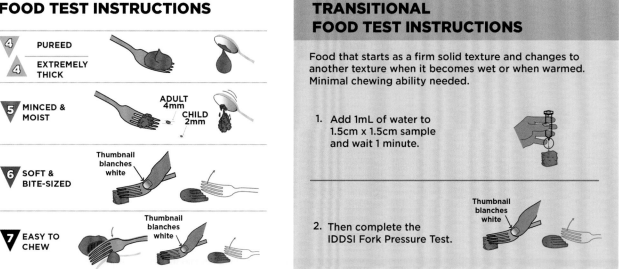

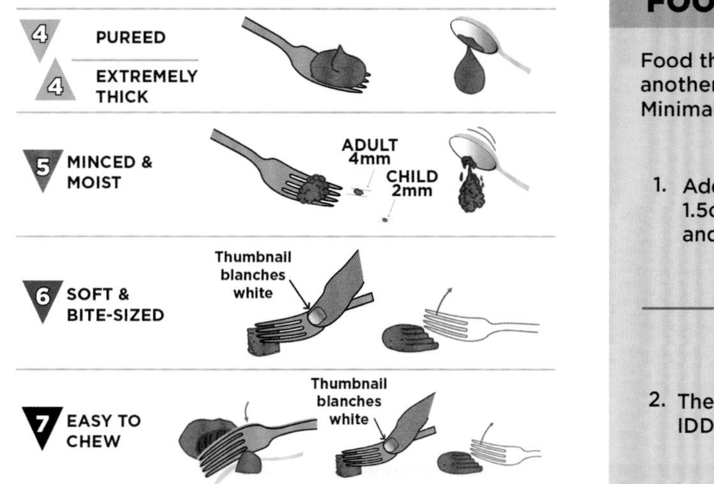

TRANSITIONAL FOOD TEST INSTRUCTIONS

Food that starts as a firm solid texture and changes to another texture when it becomes wet or when warmed. Minimal chewing ability needed.

1. Add 1mL of water to 1.5cm x 1.5cm sample and wait 1 minute.
2. Then complete the IDDSI Fork Pressure Test.

Thumbnail blanches white

Figure 19.4 ▲ **International dysphagia diet: Characteristics and testing information for foods.** (*Source:* The International Dysphagia Diet Standardisation Initiative 2016 https://iddsi.org/framework)

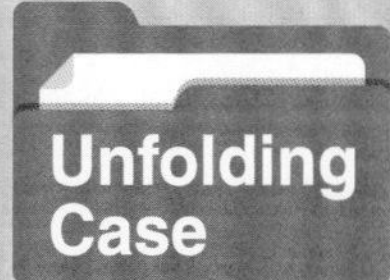

Recall Bertha. The speech-language pathologist has recommended that Bertha be placed on a diet of level 4 pureed foods and level 3 moderately thick liquids. She refuses to eat "baby" food and will not drink thickened liquids. What foods are the appropriate texture in their normal state? Can Bertha meet her nutrient requirements from these foods alone without consuming foods in pureed form? She desperately wants a cup of black tea. How would you respond to her request for tea?

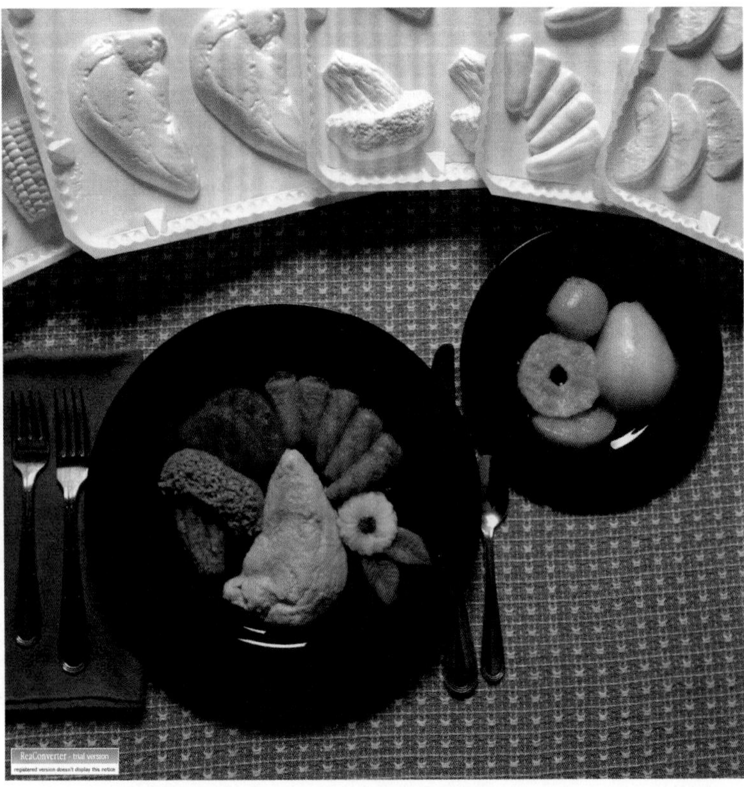

Figure 19.5 ► **Examples of pureed and molded foods.**

BOX 19.2 Various Feeding Techniques to Facilitate Safe Swallowing

Depending on the client's level of impairment, do the following:

- Serve small, frequent meals to help maximize intake.
- Encourage clients to rest before mealtime. Postpone meals if the client is fatigued.
- Position the client in a 90° upright position.
- Give mouth care immediately before meals to enhance the sense of taste.
- Instruct the client to think of a specific food to stimulate salivation. A lemon slice, lemon hard candy, or dill pickles may also help to trigger salivation, as may moderately flavored foods.
- Reduce or eliminate distractions at mealtime.
- Limit disruptions, if possible, and do not rush the client; allow at least 30 minutes for eating.
- If the client has one-sided facial weakness, place the food on the other side of the mouth. Tilt the head forward to facilitate swallowing.
- Use adaptive eating devices, such as built-up utensils and mugs with spouts, if indicated. Syringes should never be used to force liquids into the client's mouth because this can trigger choking or aspiration. Unless otherwise directed, do not allow the client to use a straw.
- Encourage small bites and thorough chewing.
- When possible, offer foods that are naturally at the appropriate texture for the client's ability, such as yogurt, applesauce, and puddings.
- Ensure the client remains sitting upright for 15 to 20 minutes after eating.
- Consider oral nutrition supplements in the appropriate texture, as needed.
- Discourage the client from consuming alcohol because it reduces cough and gag reflexes.

Gastroesophageal Reflux Disease (GERD) the backflow of gastric acid into the esophagus; GERD occurs when symptoms of reflux happen two or more times a week.

Gastroesophageal Reflux Disease

Gastroesophageal reflux disease (GERD) occurs when gastric contents back up into the esophagus or mouth, producing the common symptoms of heartburn, regurgitation, and chest pain. Approximately 20% of American adults experience at least weekly symptoms of GERD, making it the most prevalent GI disorder in the United States (Richter & Rubenstein, 2018). Quality of life is impaired when GERD affects daily functioning and sleep. GERD can lead to dysphagia, bleeding from erosive esophagitis, esophageal adenocarcinoma, and Barrett's esophagus (Richter & Rubenstein, 2018). The frequency and severity of heartburn do not correlate with the degree of esophageal damage (Richter & Rubenstein, 2018).

Proton pump inhibitors (PPIs) are the main drug therapy for GERD, but recent observations associating their use with increased risk of acute and chronic kidney disease, *Clostridium difficile* infection, dementia, rebound gastric acid hypersecretion, and osteoporotic fractures emphasize the importance of nondrug therapies (Sethi & Richter, 2017), namely, lifestyle and nutrition therapy.

Nutrition Therapy for Gastroesophageal Reflux Disease

Clients with GERD are often advised to adhere to the following nutrition therapy and lifestyle recommendations. Box 19.3 features a simplified list.

- Avoid certain items known to trigger symptoms: citrus, alcohol, and carbonated beverages.
- Eliminate any foods not tolerated.
  - Anecdotally, GERD symptoms are linked to eating fat, nonvegetarian foods; fried foods; and chocolate; however, objective studies showing clinical improvement in GERD symptoms from eliminating these foods are lacking (Sethi & Richter, 2017).
  - Although coffee is often blamed for causing GERD symptoms, a meta-analysis found no significant association between coffee intake and GERD symptoms (Kim et al., 2014).
  - Encourage clients to keep a food record to identify particular foods not tolerated.
- Lose weight if overweight.
  - Epidemiologic data show that obesity is an important risk factor for GERD (Chang & Friedenberg, 2014).
  - Clients with increased body mass index (BMI) have been found to have more acid reflux, more severe and more frequent reflux symptoms, and endoscopic findings of erosive esophagitis (Ness-Jensen et al., 2016).
  - Weight gain of as little as 3.5 BMI units is associated with a threefold increase risk of developing reflux symptoms (de Bortoli et al., 2016). Furthermore, a 10% weight loss was associated with significant decrease in reflux symptoms.
- Regular aerobic physical activity may help in the management of GERD (Sethi & Richter, 2017).
- Additional lifestyle interventions that may reduce symptoms are to (Sethi & Richter, 2017)
  - avoid meals within 3 hours of lying down,
  - avoid nighttime snacking, and
  - elevate the head of the bed during sleep.

Concept Mastery Alert

The client with GERD should not lie down for at least 3 hours after eating. Instead, the client should be encouraged to eat small meals as a way to help control their GERD symptoms.

BOX 19.3 Nutrition and Lifestyle Modifications for Gastroesophageal Reflux Disease

- Avoid certain foods known to trigger symptoms: citrus, alcohol, and carbonated beverages.
- Eliminate any foods not tolerated.
- Lose weight if overweight.
- Engage in aerobic physical activity regularly.
- Avoid meals within 3 hours of lying down.
- Avoid nighttime snacking.
- Elevate the head of the bed during sleep.

DISORDERS OF THE STOMACH

Peptic ulcer disease (PUD), gastroparesis, and gastrectomy are disorders of the stomach that use nutrition therapy to help control symptoms.

Peptic Ulcer Disease

Peptic Ulcer
erosion of the GI mucosal layer caused by an excess secretion of, or decreased mucosal resistance to, hydrochloric acid and pepsin.

The majority of **peptic ulcers** occur in the stomach or proximal duodenum. The main risk factors for both gastric and duodenal ulcers are *Helicobacter pylori* infection and the use of nonsteroidal antiinflammatory drugs (NSAIDs). However, most people infected with *H. pylori* or using NSAIDs do not develop the disease, which indicates that individual susceptibility is important (Kuna et al., 2019). *H. pylori* appears to secrete an enzyme that depletes gastric mucus, making the mucosal layer more susceptible to erosion. For these clients, eradicating the bacteria—typically with a combination of antibiotics and acid-suppressing drugs—generally cures the ulcer. Eating spicy food does not cause ulcers.

The most common symptom of peptic ulcers is epigastric pain, which is described as gnawing or burning that is usually worse at night or when the stomach is empty. However, not all people with peptic ulcers experience epigastric pain. Less frequent symptoms include bloating, early satiety, and nausea. The most common and severe complication of PUD is GI bleeding, which can be life threatening. From a nutritional standpoint, pain or early satiety may impair intake and lead to weight loss. Blood loss can lead to iron deficiency. Long-term use of medications to decrease gastric acid production may impair the absorption of calcium, iron, and vitamin B_{12}.

Nutrition Therapy for Peptic Ulcer Disease

Nutrition and diet have not been found to play a role in causing or preventing peptic ulcers (National Institute of Diabetes and Digestive and Kidney Diseases, 2014).

- Although certain foods can increase production of stomach acid, good evidence that they worsen peptic ulcers is lacking.
- As with GERD, clients are advised to avoid any foods not individually tolerated. Commonly avoided foods include black pepper, caffeine, coffee (decaffeinated and regular), tea (decaffeinated and other), mint, chocolate, and tomatoes.
- Probiotics may be a helpful adjunct to antibiotic therapy in eradicating *H. pylori* (Boltin, 2016). However, the optimal species and treatment dosage are not known.
- Alcohol and smoking do contribute to ulcers and should be avoided.

Gastroparesis

Gastroparesis, or delayed gastric emptying, is a chronic motility disorder of the stomach that can cause nausea, vomiting, bloating, early satiety, and upper abdominal pain (Camilleri et al., 2013). Symptoms vary greatly among individuals and can come and go over time. Potentially life-threatening complications include electrolyte imbalances, dehydration, malnutrition, and poor glycemic control. Quality of life can be greatly affected. Although gastroparesis is most commonly associated with diabetes, it may also occur secondary to gastric bypass surgery, neurologic and connective tissue disorders (e.g., Parkinson's disease, multiple sclerosis, scleroderma), post–viral syndrome, or may be idiopathic.

Nutrition Therapy for Gastroparesis

Gastroparesis can lead to poor oral intake, an inadequate calorie intake, and micronutrient deficiencies (Camilleri et al., 2013). The goal of nutrition therapy is to maintain an adequate oral intake. Clients may be advised to do the following (Parrish & McCray, 2011; University of Virginia Digestive Health Center, 2017):

- Consume smaller, more frequent meals. Four to eight meals per day may be necessary to achieve an adequate intake.

- Consume more liquid calories because emptying of liquids is often preserved in gastroparesis even when solid emptying is impaired.
  - Tolerance for solid food may deteriorate as the day progresses, making liquids a better option as the day progresses.
  - Pureed foods (e.g., solid food pureed with milk or broth) or oral nutrition supplements may serve as an important source of calories and protein.
- Consume solid foods that are low in fat if fat in solid food worsens symptoms. Fat in liquids is often well tolerated and can be a valuable source of calories and nutrients. Limit foods high in fibers because they may delay gastric emptying and promote **bezoar** formation, particularly if the client has a history of bezoar formation. Foods to avoid include bran and whole grain cereals, nuts and seeds, fruits (e.g., apples, berries, oranges, kiwi, coconut, figs), dried fruits, certain vegetables (e.g., green beans, peas, broccoli, brussels sprouts, corn, potato peels, sauerkraut, tomato skins), and popcorn.
- Avoid carbonated beverages, which can aggravate gastric distention.
- Chew foods thoroughly, especially meats.
- Sit upright for at least 1 hour after eating.
- Control blood glucose levels if client has diabetes.
- Avoid alcohol and smoking because both can alter gastric emptying.
- Enteral (jejunal feeding) or parenteral nutrition may be necessary in severe gastroparesis.

Bezoar
a solid mass of indigestible material that may become trapped in the stomach, although it can also occur in the small intestine.

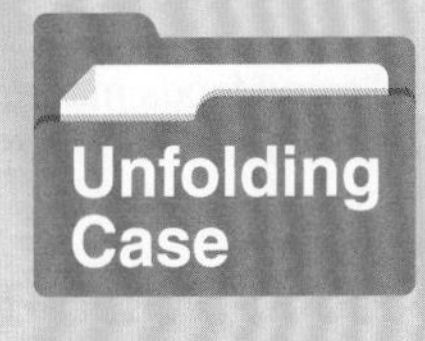

Consider Bertha. She has experienced gastroparesis intermittently for years. Nausea, vomiting, and pain are her most common symptoms. She continues to have symptoms of gastroparesis while on a pureed diet with moderately thick liquids. What other interventions may help reduce Bertha's symptoms? What are nutritional concerns with prolonged vomiting related to gastroparesis?

Gastrectomy

Gastrectomy is the surgical removal of part or all of the stomach, which may be done to treat malignancy, refractory PUD, or GI bleeding. Similar components of gastrectomy surgeries are used in bariatric surgeries, which are surgeries to treat obesity (see Chapter 17). Partial gastrectomies leave a portion of the stomach that is then surgically connected to the duodenum or jejunum. Total gastrectomies remove all of the stomach so that the lower esophagus connects directly to the small intestine. With either type of gastrectomy, a smaller or absent stomach increases the risk of malabsorption due to rapid gastric emptying and shortened transit time.

A common complication after gastric surgery is dumping syndrome. Rapid emptying of stomach contents into the intestine causes fluid from the plasma and extracellular fluid to shift into the intestines to dilute the hyperosmolar bolus. The large volume of hypertonic fluid in the jejunum and an increase in peristalsis lead to cramping, diarrhea, and abdominal pain. Weakness, dizziness, and tachycardia occur as the volume of circulating blood decreases. These symptoms occur within 10 to 20 minutes after eating and characterize the early dumping syndrome.

An intermediate dumping reaction occurs 20 to 30 minutes after eating as undigested food is fermented in the colon, producing gas, abdominal pain, cramping, and diarrhea (Academy of Nutrition and Dietetics, 2020). Malabsorption of calories and nutrients produces weight loss and increases the risk of malnutrition. Malabsorption of micronutrients may lead to iron deficiency anemia, vitamin B_{12} deficiency, and bone disease.

Late dumping syndrome occurs 1 to 3 hours after eating and is especially common after consuming simple sugars (Academy of Nutrition and Dietetics, 2020). The rapid absorption of carbohydrate causes a quick spike in blood glucose levels; the body compensates by oversecreting insulin. Blood glucose levels drop rapidly, and symptoms of hypoglycemia develop, such as shakiness, sweating, confusion, and weakness.

Nutrition Therapy for Clients with Dumping Syndrome

Nutrition intervention can control or prevent symptoms of dumping syndrome. Unlike most initial postoperative feedings, clear liquid diets are not used because sugars contribute to the concentration of particles entering the intestine.

- Clients begin oral feedings with sips of water and broth.
- After tolerance is established, an anti-dumping regimen is followed (Box 19.4).
- Over time, the diet is liberalized as the remaining portion of the stomach or duodenum hypertrophies to hold more food and allows for more normal digestion.
- Liquid multivitamin and mineral supplements are recommended, and vitamin B_{12} injections, nasal gel spray, or oral supplements may be necessary depending on the extent of surgery.
- Clients who are unable to tolerate the normal diet progression may require nutrition support.

BOX 19.4 Anti-Dumping Syndrome Diet Guidelines

Diet Guidelines

- Clients are started on small, frequent meals consisting of only one or two foods per meal or snack, one of which is a protein. Protein is consumed at each feeding because it slows gastric emptying.
- Food must be thoroughly chewed.
- Liquids are provided 30 minutes to 1 hour after consuming solids, not with meals, because they promote quick movement through the GI tract.
- Items avoided include
  - foods containing simple sugars such as sweet desserts, candy, sweetened beverages, canned fruit in heavy syrup, sweetened yogurt, ice cream, sherbet,
  - foods containing sugar alcohols (e.g., sorbitol, xylitol), such as dietetic candy, sugarless gum and mints, and certain fruits (apples, pears, peaches, prunes),
  - gassy vegetables such as broccoli, cauliflower, cabbage, and corn,
  - fried meats, fish, and poultry; high fat luncheon meats, sausage, hot dogs, and bacon; tough or chewy meats; dried peas and beans; nuts,
  - high-fiber foods,
  - carbonated beverages, caffeinated beverages, alcohol, and
  - lactose.
- Clients are advised to lie down after eating.
- Functional fibers, such as pectin and guar gum, may be used to delay gastric emptying and treat diarrhea (Academy of Nutrition and Dietetics, 2020).

Recommended Foods

- **Breads and cereals:** refined plain breads, crackers, rolls, unsweetened cereal, rice, and pasta that provide <2 g fiber per serving.
- **Vegetables:** well-cooked or raw vegetables without seeds or skins, strained vegetable juice, lettuce.
- **Fruits:** banana, soft melons, unsweetened canned fruit.
- **Milk and milk products:** lactose-free and unsweetened 1% or fat-free yogurt, and milk alternatives (e.g., plain soy milk).
- **Meat and meat alternatives:** tender, well-cooked meat, fish, poultry, egg, and soy without added fat; smooth nut butters.
- **Fats:** oils, butter, margarine, cream cheese, mayonnaise.
- **Beverages:** decaffeinated coffee and tea; sugar-free soft drinks.
- **Other:** allowed foods made with artificial sweeteners such as NutraSweet, sucralose, acesulfame potassium.

Sample Menu (When Recovered Enough to Eat Six Times a Day)

Breakfast

1 poached egg
1 slice white toast with butter
1 hour later: 1 cup decaffeinated coffee with half and half

Mid-Morning Snack

1 cup plain lactose-free yogurt
1 hour later: 1 cup plain unsweetened soy milk

Lunch

½ cup lactose-free cottage cheese with two unsweetened, canned peach halves
dinner roll with butter
1 hour later: 8 oz sugar-free ginger ale

Mid-Afternoon Snack

2 oz cheddar cheese
4 saltine crackers

Dinner

3 oz baked chicken
½ cup white rice with butter
½ cup cooked carrots with butter
1 hour later: caffeine-free tea

Bedtime Snack

1 cup lactose-free yogurt without added sugar

NURSING PROCESS Gastroesophageal Reflux Disease

Jason is 28 years old and complains of frequent painful heartburn. He takes antacids on a daily basis and has lost 14 pounds over the past few months. His strategy to avoid pain is to avoid eating. He is 5 ft 8 in. tall, currently weighs 170 pounds, and has an appointment to see his doctor. In the meantime, he has come to you, the corporate nurse on staff where he works, to see what he can do to help control his heartburn.

Assessment

Medical–Psychosocial History

- medical history that would contribute to GERD, such as hiatal hernia
- symptoms that may affect nutrition, such as difficulty swallowing or nausea and vomiting
- use of medications that may decrease lower esophageal sphincter pressure, such as anticholinergic agents, diazepam, or theophylline
- use of medications that may damage the mucosa, such as NSAIDs or aspirin
- history of smoking
- level of activity

Anthropometric Assessment

BMI, weight loss percentage

Biochemical and Physical Assessment

abnormal lab values, if available, especially hemoglobin and hematocrit because low values may indicate bleeding

Dietary Assessment

- How many meals do you eat daily?
- Would you say your meals are small, medium, or large in size?
- Are there any particular foods that cause heartburn, especially alcohol, coffee, tea, caffeine, pepper, mint, chocolate, or fatty foods?
- What foods do you avoid?
- Can you correlate your symptoms to
  - lying down after eating?
  - wearing tight clothes?
  - eating right before bed?
- Do you take vitamins, minerals, herbs, or other supplements?
- Do you have ethnic, religious, or cultural food preferences?

Analysis

Possible Nursing Analysis

Malnutrition risk related to avoidance of eating to avoid post-prandial heartburn, as evidenced by a 14-pound weight loss

Planning

Client Outcomes

The client will

- report relief from symptoms,
- consume adequate calories and nutrients,
- use less medication to control symptoms,
- explain nutrition and lifestyle modifications for controlling GERD symptoms, and
- exhibit normal laboratory values.

Nursing Interventions

Nutrition Therapy

- Eat a balanced eating pattern that promotes healthy weight loss to achieve BMI of <25.
- Avoid items known to trigger symptoms: citrus, alcohol, carbonated beverages.
- Eliminate any foods not tolerated.
- Avoid eating within 3 hours of bedtime.

NURSING PROCESS Gastroesophageal Reflux Disease (continued)

Client Teaching

Instruct the client
- that nutrition interventions may help control symptoms but do not treat the underlying problem,
- to avoid citrus, alcohol, and carbonated beverages,
- to keep a food journal so food intolerances can be identified and avoided,
- to lose weight gradually to achieve a healthy weight of BMI <25,
- on lifestyle modifications that may help improve symptoms, such as elevating the head of the bed, not eating within 3 hours of bedtime, and engaging in regular physical activity.

Evaluation

Evaluate and Monitor

- Monitor for improvement in symptoms.
- Evaluate adequacy and appropriateness of intake.
- Monitor weight.
- Monitor for medication usage.

How Do You Respond?

Are there any foods that can treat heartburn? Evidence linking the use of specific foods with relief of heartburn is largely anecdotal, but as long as the use of natural remedies does not preclude necessary medical treatment, there is little risk in trying unproven food remedies. Such unproven remedies include consuming probiotics, vinegar, coconut water, almonds, and teas such as ginger and persimmon. Clients who are on long-term PPI therapy should not suddenly discontinue drug treatment; gradual tapering and doctor supervision are advised.

REVIEW CASE STUDY

Barbara is a 72-year-old woman with a "type A" personality who was diagnosed with a peptic ulcer more than 40 years ago. At that time, her doctor told her to follow a bland diet and eat three meals per day with three snacks per day of whole milk to "quiet" her stomach. She meticulously complied with the diet to the point of becoming obsessive about not eating anything that may not be "allowed." She lost 15 pounds by following the bland diet because her intake was so restricted. She recently began experiencing ulcer symptoms and has put herself back on the bland diet, convinced it is necessary in order to recover from her ulcer.

Yesterday, she ate the following as shown on the right:

- Barbara's 1600-calorie MyPlate plan calls for 1.5 cups of fruit, 2 cups of vegetables, 5 grains, 5 oz of meat/beans, 3 cups of milk, and 5 teaspoons of oils. How does her intake compare? What food groups is she undereating? Overeating? What are the potential nutritional consequences of her current diet?
- What other information would be helpful for you to know in dealing with Barbara?
- Barbara clearly wants to be on a bland diet. What would you tell her about diet recommendations for PUD? What recommendations would you make to improve her symptoms and meet her nutritional requirements while respecting her need to follow a "diet"?

Breakfast: 1 poached egg, 2 slices dry white toast, 1 cup whole milk
Morning Snack: 1 cup whole milk
Lunch: three fourths cup cottage cheese with one half cup canned peaches
Afternoon snack: 1 cup whole milk
Dinner: 3 oz boiled chicken, one half cup boiled plain potatoes, one half cup boiled green beans, one half cup gelatin
Evening snack: 1 cup whole milk

STUDY QUESTIONS

1 The client asks if coffee is bad for their peptic ulcer. Which of the following is the nurse's best response?
   a. "Coffee does not cause ulcers and drinking it probably does not interfere with ulcer healing. You may try eliminating it from your diet to see what impact it has on your symptoms and then decide whether or not to avoid it."
   b. "Both caffeinated and decaffeinated coffee can cause ulcers and interfere with ulcer healing. You should eliminate both from your diet."
   c. "You need to eliminate caffeinated coffee from your diet, but it is safe to drink decaffeinated coffee."
   d. "You can drink all the coffee you want; it does not affect ulcers."

2 Which of the following statements indicates that the client needs further instruction about GERD?
   a. "I know a bland diet will help prevent the heartburn I get after eating."
   b. "Lying down after eating can make GERD symptoms worse."
   c. "Carbonated beverages can trigger GERD symptoms."
   d. "Losing excess weight can help prevent symptoms of GERD."

3 Which of the following snacks would be best for a client who wants to eat but is experiencing nausea?
   a. cheese
   b. peanuts
   c. banana
   d. a milkshake

4 The nurse knows their instructions have been effective when the client with dumping syndrome verbalizes they should
   a. avoid lying down after eating.
   b. drink liquids between, not with, meals.
   c. consume foods sweetened with sugar alcohols (e.g., sorbitol or xylitol) instead of sugar.
   d. avoid protein.

5 A client with dumping syndrome asks why it is so important to avoid sugars and sweets. Which of the following is the nurse's best response?
   a. "Sugars and sweets provide empty calories, so they should be limited in everyone's diet."
   b. "Sugars draw water into the intestines and cause cramping and diarrhea."
   c. "Sugar should be avoided because it promotes inflammation and delays healing."
   d. "Avoiding sugars and sweets helps ensure that they will not displace the intake of protein, which you need for healing."

6 Which of the following foods is not appropriate for a client on a level 4 pureed diet?
   a. vanilla yogurt
   b. regular scrambled eggs
   c. smooth hummus
   d. chocolate pudding

7 What is the characteristic of level 2 mildly thick liquid?
   a. It is thicker than water but can flow through a standard straw.
   b. It drips slowly in dollops through the prongs of a fork.
   c. It holds its shape on a spoon.
   d. It is "sippable" from a cup but takes effort to drink through a standard straw.

8 The best dessert for a client with gastroparesis is
   a. chocolate cake
   b. strawberry shortcake
   c. blueberry pie
   d. angel food cake

CHAPTER SUMMARY NUTRITION FOR CLIENTS WITH UPPER GASTROINTESTINAL TRACT DISORDERS

Nutrition therapy for GI disorders may help minimize or prevent symptoms. For some GI disorders, nutrition therapy is the cornerstone of treatment.

Disorders That Affect Eating

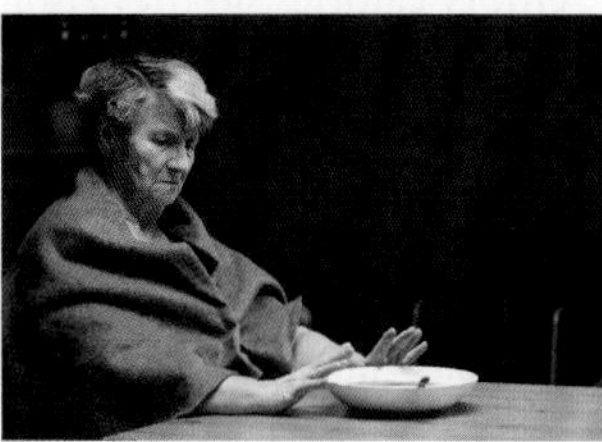

Anorexia is the lack of appetite. Small, frequent meals, limiting fat intake, and seasoning food to taste may help improve appetite.

Nausea and vomiting can cause fluid and electrolyte imbalance in the short term and dehydration and weight loss in the long term. Intake may improve with

- good oral hygiene,
- limiting liquids with meals but otherwise encouraging a liber fluid intake,
- serving room-temperature or cold foods, and
- avoiding high-fat foods.

Disorders of the Esophagus

Dysphagia is an impairment in the swallowing process. Modifying the texture of food and consistency of liquids promotes safe and efficient swallowing. The international dysphagia diet defines the levels of food and liquids and describes objective tests to ensure proper texture and consistency.

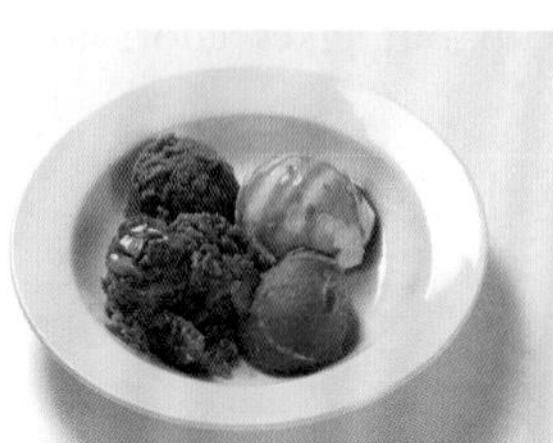

GERD occurs when gastric contents back up into the esophagus.

- Clients should
  - avoid citrus, alcohol, carbonated beverages, and any other food not individually tolerates,
  - lose weight if overweight,
  - engage in regular aerobic physical activity,
  - refrain from eating within 3 hours of bedtime, and
  - elevate the head of the bed during sleep.

Disorders of the Stomach

PUD is caused by *H. pylori* bacteria or nonsteroidal inflammatory medication use, not by food.

- Clients should avoid any foods not tolerated, smoking, and alcohol.
- Probiotics may help, but further research is needed.

Gastroparesis is a chronic motility disorder that can cause nausea, vomiting, early satiety, and pain. Nutrition therapy recommendations include

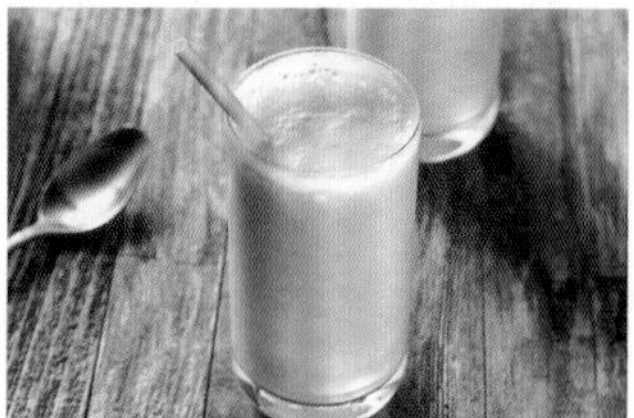

- eating small frequent meals and limiting fat in solid foods if not tolerated,
- consuming more liquid calories because emptying of liquids is often preserved in gastroparesis even when solid emptying is impaired,
- limiting fiber and foods that contribute to bezoar formation,
- chewing foods thoroughly, and
- avoiding alcohol and smoking.

Gastrectomy can cause dumping syndrome after eating. Symptoms may improve by

- eating small meals,
- avoiding liquids with meals and afterward,
- avoiding simple sugars and sugar alcohols, and
- eating protein at each meal.

Figure sources: *shutterstock.com/Photographee.eu, shutterstock.com/zstock, shutterstock.com/Brent Hofacker*

Student Resources on thePoint®
For additional learning materials, activate the code in the front of this book at https://thePoint.lww.com/activate

Websites

American Gastroenterological Association at www.gastro.org
The Helicobacter Foundation at www.helico.com
National Digestive Diseases Information Clearinghouse (NDDIC), a service of the National Institute of Diabetes and Digestive and Kidney Diseases (NIDDK), National Institutes of Health at http://digestive.niddk.nih.gov
Nutrition Issues in Gastroenterology at https://practicalgastro.com/category/disorders/nutrition/

References

Academy of Nutrition and Dietetics. (2020). *Nutrition care manual.* http://www.nutritioncaremanual.org.

Boltin, D. (2016). Probiotics in Helicobacter pylori-induced peptic ulcer disease. *Best Practice & Research Clinical Gastroenterology, 30*(1), 99–109. https://doi.org/10.1016/j.bpg.2015.12.003

Camilleri, M., Parkman, H. P., Shafi, M. A., Abell, T. L., Gerson, L., & American College of Gastroenterology. (2013). Clinical guideline: Management of gastroparesis. *The American Journal of Gastroenterology, 108*(1), 18–38. https://doi.org/10.1038/ajg.2012.373

Chang, P., & Friedenberg, F. (2014). Obesity and GERD. *Gastroenterology Clinics of North America, 43*(1), 161–173. https://doi.org/10.1016/j.gtc.2013.11.009

de Bortoli, N., Guidi, G., Martinucci, I., Savarino, E., Imam, H., Bertani, L., Russo, S., Franchi, R., Macchia, L., Furnari, M., Ceccarelli, L., Savarino, V., & Marchi, S. (2016). Voluntary and controlled weight loss can reduce symptoms and proton pump inhibitor use and dosage in patients with gastroesophageal reflux disease: A comparative study. *Diseases of the Esophagus, 29*(2), 197–204. https://doi.org/10.1111/dote.12319

Farrer, O., Olsen, C., Mousley, K., & Teo, E. (2016). Does presentation of smooth pureed meals improve patients consumption in an acute care setting: A pilot study. *Nutrition & Dietetics 73*(5), 405–409. https://doi.org/10.1111/1747-0080.12198

Gillman, A., Winkler, R., & Taylor, N. (2017). Implementing the free water protocol does not result in aspiration pneumonia in carefully selected patients with dysphagia: A systematic review. *Dysphagia, 3*, 345–361. https://doi.org/10.1007/s00455-016-9761-3

International Dysphagia Diet Standardization Initiative. (2019). Complete IDDSI framework. Detailed definitions. https://ftp.iddsi.org/Documents/Complete_IDDSI_Framework_Final_31July2019.pdf

Kenedi, H., Campbell-Vance, J., Reynolds, J., Foreman, M., Dollaghan, C., Graybeal, D., Warren, A. M., & Bennett, M. (2019). Implementation and analysis of a free water protocol in acute trauma and stroke patients. *Critical Care Nurse, 39*(3), e9–e17. https://doi.org/10.4037/ccn2019238

Kim, J., Oh, S.-W., Myung, S.-K., Kwon, J., Lee, C., Yum, J. M., & Lee, H. K. (2014). Association between coffee intake and gastroesophageal reflux disease: A meta-analysis. *Diseases of the Esophagus, 27*(4), 311–317. https://doi.org/10.1111/dote.12099

Kuna, L., Jakab, J., Smolic, R., Raguz-Lucic, N., Vcev, A., & Smolic, M. (2019). Peptic ulcer disease: A brief review of conventional therapy and herbal treatment options. *Journal of Clinical Medicine, 8*(2), 179. https://doi.org/10.3390/jcm8020179

Lepore, J., Sims, C., Gal, N., & Dahl, W. (2014). Acceptability and identification of scooped versus molded pureed foods. *Canadian Journal Dietetic Practice and Research, 75*(3), 145–147. https://doi.org/10.3148/cjdpr-2014-004

National Institute of Diabetes and Digestive and Kidney Diseases. (2014). *Eating, diet, and nutrition for peptic ulcers (stomach ulcers).* https://www.niddk.nih.gov/health-information/digestive-diseases/peptic-ulcers-stomach-ulcers/eating-diet-nutrition

Ness-Jensen, E., Hveem, K., El-Serag, H., & Lagergren, J. (2016). Lifestyle intervention in gastroesophageal reflux disease. *Clinical Gastroenterology and Hepatology, 14*(2), 175–182. https://doi.org/10.1016/j.cgh.2015.04.176

Parrish, C. R., & McCray, S. (2011). Gastroparesis and nutrition: The art. *Practical Gastroenterology*, series #99. https://https://doi.org/10.1038/ajg.2012.373med.virginia.edu/ginutrition/wp-content/uploads/sites/199/2014/06/ParrishGastroparesisArticle.pdf

Richter, J., & Rubenstein, J. (2018). Presentation and epidemiology of gastroesophageal reflux disease. *Gastroenterology, 154*(2), 267–276. https://doi.org/10.1053/j.gastro.2017.07.045

Sethi, S., & Richter, J. (2017). Diet and gastroesophageal reflux disease: Role in pathogenesis and management. *Current Opinion in Gastroenterology, 33*(2), 107–111.

Steele, C., Alsanei, W., Ayanikalath, S., Barbon, C., Chen, J., Cichero, J., Coutts, K., Dantas, R., Duivenstein, J., Giosa, L., Hanson, B., Lam, P., Lecko, C., Leigh, C., Nagy, A., Namasivayam, A., Nascimento, W., Odendaal, I., Smith, C., & Wang, H. (2015). The influence of food texture and liquid consistency modification on swallowing physiology and function: A systematic review. *Dysphagia, 30*, 2–26. https://doi.org/10.1007/s00455-014-9578-x

University of Virginia Health System, Digestive Health Center. (2017). Diet intervention for gastroparesis. https://med.virginia.edu/ginutrition/wp-content/uploads/sites/199/2014/04/Gastroparesis-Long-Version-02.23.17.pdf

Chapter 20

Nutrition for Clients with Disorders of the Lower Gastrointestinal Tract and Accessory Organs

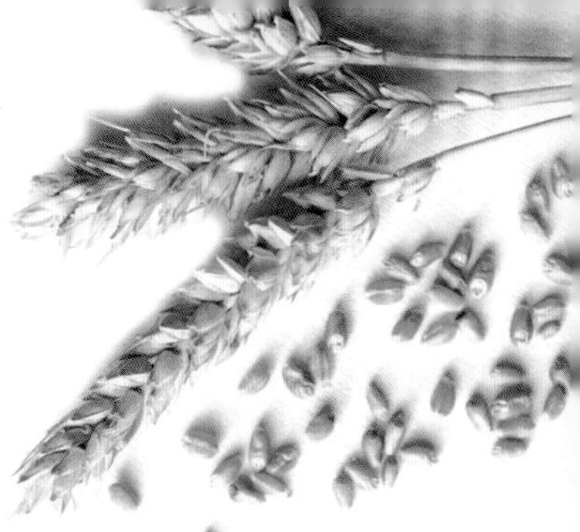

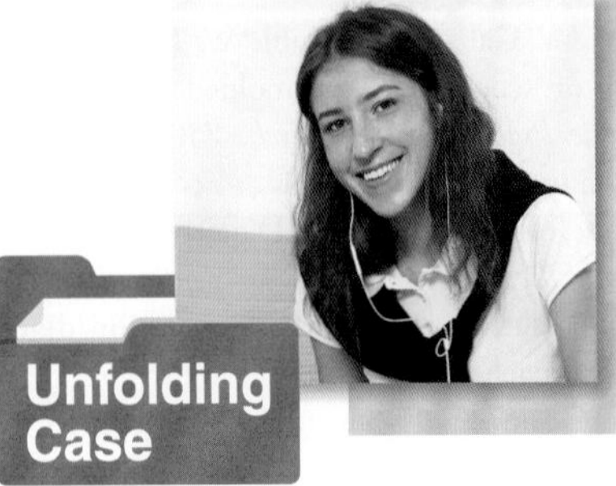

Unfolding Case

Stephanie Schlau

Stephanie is an 18-year-old college freshman who was diagnosed with type 1 diabetes 12 years ago. She has an insulin pump, is of healthy weight, and has no other significant medical history. She went to the student health center on campus with complaints of fatigue, abdominal cramping, and diarrhea.

Learning Objectives

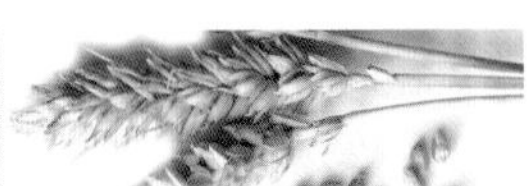

Upon completion of this chapter, you will be able to:

1 Modify a regular diet to be high in fiber.
2 Instruct a client on the nutrition therapy recommendations for diarrhea.
3 Give examples of appropriate nutrition interventions for various symptoms and complications of malabsorption syndrome.
4 Modify a regular diet to be low in lactose.
5 Identify sources of gluten.
6 Discuss nutrition interventions for clients with short bowel syndrome.
7 Describe nutrition interventions for a nonalcoholic liver disease.
8 Summarize nutrition therapy interventions recommended for clients with cirrhosis.
9 Compare a low-fat diet to a regular diet.

The lower gastrointestinal (GI) tract consists of the small and large intestines, rectum, and anus. Most nutrient absorption occurs in the first 100 cm of the jejunum; B_{12} and bile salts are absorbed in the last 100 cm of the ileum; magnesium is absorbed in the terminal ileum and proximal colon; and fluid and sodium absorption occurs throughout the bowel (Fig. 20.1). The large intestine is primarily responsible for water and electrolyte absorption and the elimination of solid wastes. The accessory organs—liver, gallbladder, and pancreas—are involved in nutrient metabolism or digestion. With many disorders of the lower GI tract and accessory organs, nutrition therapy is used to improve or control symptoms; replenish losses; and promote healing, if applicable. For one GI disorder, celiac disease, nutrition therapy is the sole mode of treatment.

This chapter presents nutrition therapy for altered bowel elimination, malabsorption syndromes, disorders of the large intestine, and disorders of the accessory organs. Box 20.1 lists nutrition-focused assessment criteria for lower GI disorders.

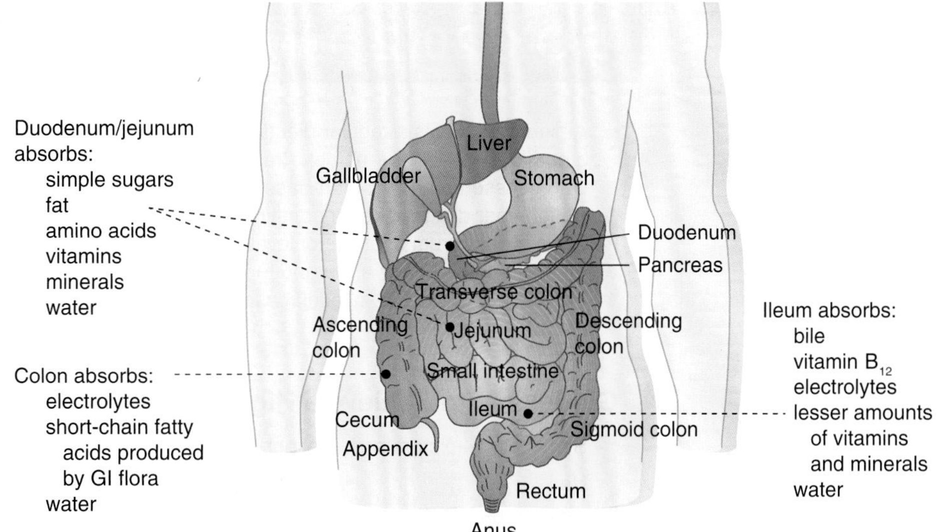

Figure 20.1 ▶ **The sites of nutrient absorption.**

BOX 20.1 Nutrition-Focused Assessment for Lower Gastrointestinal Disorders

- GI symptoms that interfere with intake
  - anorexia
  - early satiety
  - pain
  - abdominal distention
- Changes in eating made in response to symptoms
- Complications that affect nutritional status
  - weight loss
  - diarrhea
  - blood loss
- Usual pattern of eating and frequency of meals and snacks
- Weight, weight stability
- Use of the following:
  - tobacco
  - over-the-counter drugs for GI symptoms
  - alcohol
  - caffeine
- Food allergies or intolerances, such as high-fat foods, milk, and high-fiber foods
- Use of nutritional supplements:
  - vitamins
  - minerals
  - fiber
  - herbs
- Client's willingness to change their eating habits

ALTERED BOWEL ELIMINATION

Constipation

Criteria for diagnosing constipation include having fewer than three bowel movements per week, passing stools that are hard, and excessive straining during defecation. Inadequate fiber intake, physical inactivity, and low food intake increase the risk of constipation. Constipation can occur secondary to irregular bowel habits, psychogenic factors, chronic laxative use, metabolic and endocrine disorders, and bowel abnormalities (e.g., tumors, hernias, strictures). Certain medications, such as analgesics that contain opiates, antidepressants, diuretics, aluminum hydroxide, and iron and calcium supplements, cause constipation. Contrary to popular belief, daily bowel movements are not necessary provided the stools are not hard and dry.

Nutrition Therapy for Constipation

To treat constipation, it is standard practice to recommend that fiber intake be increased (Box 20.2).

BOX 20.2 High-Fiber Diet

- A high-fiber diet is a regular diet that substitutes whole grains for refined grains and is high in other fiber-rich foods—namely, fresh fruits, vegetables, and dried peas and beans.
- Unprocessed bran and bran-based cereals may be added as tolerated.
- A high-fiber diet is used for constipation and diverticulosis. It may also promote weight loss and helps lower serum cholesterol levels and improve glucose tolerance in diabetes.
- All healthy Americans are urged to increase their intake of fiber.
- The diet should not be used in cases of intestinal inflammation or stenosis, postgastrectomy, or pseudo-obstruction.

Guidelines to Achieve a High-Fiber Diet

- Substitute whole grains for refined grains.

Use	In place of
Whole wheat bread	White bread
Brown rice	White rice
Whole wheat pasta	White pasta
Bran or whole-grain cereal	Refined cereals
Whole wheat flour	White flour

- Eat more dried peas or beans.
- Eat more fresh fruit; leave the skin on whenever possible. Apples, blackberries, blueberries, figs, dates, kiwifruit, mango, oranges, pears, prunes, strawberries, and raspberries are high-fiber fruits.
- Eat more vegetables. Cooked asparagus, green beans, broccoli, Brussels sprouts, cabbage, carrots, celery, corn, eggplant, parsnips, peas, snow peas, Swiss chard, and turnips are good choices.
- Other foods with fiber include popcorn, nuts, sunflower seeds, and sesame seeds.

Sample Menu

Breakfast	Lunch	Dinner	Snacks
Prune juice	Split pea soup	Roast chicken	Low-fat popcorn
Bran flakes with milk	Ham sandwich on whole wheat bread with lettuce and tomato	Brown rice	Dried fruits and nuts
Whole wheat toast with jelly	Fresh strawberries	Tossed salad with fresh vegetables	Raw carrots and celery with dip
Fresh orange sections	Date cookie	Steamed broccoli	
	Milk	Whole wheat roll with butter	
		Milk	
		Blueberries over ice cream	

Potential Problems	Recommended Interventions
Flatus, distention, cramping, and osmotic diarrhea related to increasing fiber content of the diet too much or too quickly	Initiate a high-fiber diet gradually to develop the client's tolerance. If symptoms of intolerance persist, reduce fiber content to maximum amount tolerated by the client.

Client Teaching

Instruct the client on the following:

- A variety of foods high in fiber should be eaten; numerous forms of fiber exist, and each performs a different action in the body (see Chapter 3).
- A diet rich in insoluble fiber increases stool bulk and speeds passage of food through intestines.
- Increasing fiber intake gradually may be better tolerated than increasing fiber intake quickly.
- Fiber intake may be increased by making subtle changes in eating and cooking habits such as eating more fresh fruits and vegetables, especially with the skin on.
- Whole wheat bread should be eaten instead of "wheat" bread whenever possible. Ingredient labels that include enriched wheat flour are not 100% whole wheat.
- Wheat bran cereals are not truly "whole wheat" because they contain only the bran portion of the wheat kernel; but they are very high in fiber.

BOX 20.2 High-Fiber Diet (continued)

- Coarse, unprocessed wheat bran, also called Miller's bran, can be incorporated into the diet by mixing it with juice or milk; by adding it to muffins, quick breads, casseroles, and meat loaves before baking; or by sprinkling it over cooked cereals, applesauce, eggs, or other foods.
- Wheat bran should be added to the diet gradually (up to 3 tbsp/day) to decrease the likelihood of developing flatus and distention.
- A meatless main dish made with dried peas and beans is a high-fiber alternative to traditional entrées.
- Snacks of fresh or dried fruits, nuts, and seeds provide fiber.
- Certain foods (in addition to being high in fiber) have laxative effects: prunes and prune juice, figs, and dates.
- At least eight 8 oz glasses of fluid should be consumed daily.

- Fiber increases stool weight, bulk, and fecal water content and stimulates peristalsis to promote a more rapid transit time.
- Insoluble fiber found in whole grains, bran, and the skins and seeds of fruit and vegetables is more effective at treating constipation than soluble fiber.
- Although a goal of 25 to 38 g/day, which is the adequate intake for fiber, may be recommended, those levels are based on the amount of fiber needed to protect against coronary heart disease, not for optimal bowel function. The amount of fiber needed to alleviate constipation varies among individuals and is usually determined by trial and error.
- A gradual increase in fiber is recommended to avoid symptoms of intolerance such as gas, cramping, and diarrhea. If these side effects do occur, they are usually temporary and subside within several days.
- To achieve maximum benefit, fiber intake should be spread throughout the day.
- Fiber supplements, such as Metamucil, Fiberall, and Citrucel, may be necessary if adequate fiber cannot be consumed through food.

Probiotics
live microorganisms found in food that, when consumed in adequate amounts, are beneficial to health.

Prebiotics
nondigestible food components that stimulate the growth of probiotic bacteria within the large intestine.

Other interventions to promote bowel regularity include the following:

- ensuring an adequate fluid intake of at least 64 oz/day; without enough water, a high-fiber diet can worsen constipation, abdominal pain, bloating, and gas (Academy of Nutrition and Dietetics [AND], 2020)
- increasing aerobic exercise
- consuming **probiotics** or **prebiotics** daily, such as yogurt containing live bacterial cultures, acidophilus milk, and kefir

Diarrhea

Diarrhea is a common symptom of many GI disorders, infectious diseases, and antibiotic use (Box 20.3). It is also a frequent side effect of chemotherapy and radiation. Diarrhea is characterized by an increase in the frequency of bowel movements and/or water content of stools, which alters either the consistency or volume of fecal output. A rapid transit time decreases the time available for water, sodium, and potassium to be absorbed through the colon; the result is more water and electrolytes in the stools and the potential for dehydration, hyponatremia, hypokalemia, acid–base imbalance, and metabolic acidosis. Chronic diarrhea can lead to malnutrition related to impaired digestion, absorption, and intake.

Nutrition Therapy for Diarrhea

Nutrition therapy for diarrhea is largely supportive and depends on the severity of diarrhea and the underlying cause.

BOX 20.3 Types of Diarrhea and their causes

Osmotic Diarrhea

Osmotic diarrhea occurs when there is an increase in particles in the intestine, which draws water in to dilute the high concentration.

- Causes include maldigestion of nutrients (e.g., lactose intolerance), excessive intake of sorbitol or fructose, dumping syndrome, tube feedings, and some laxatives.
- Treating the underlying cause cures osmotic diarrhea.

Secretory Diarrhea

Secretory diarrhea is related to an excessive secretion of fluid and electrolytes into the intestines.

- Causes include bacterial, viral, protozoan, and other infections; certain medications; and some GI disorders, such as Crohn's Disease and celiac disease.
- An excessive amount of bile acids or unabsorbed fatty acids in the colon can also cause secretory diarrhea.
- Antibiotics are the primary component of treatment when the cause is infection.
- Symptoms may be treated with medications that decrease GI motility or thicken the consistency of stools, such as the soluble fiber psyllium (Metamucil).

Antibiotic-Acquired Diarrhea

Antibiotic-acquired diarrhea is caused by the disruption in GI microbiota or irritation to the GI mucosa as a side effect of antibiotic therapy.

- Most cases are mild and self-limiting.
- Overgrowth of *Clostridium difficile* is the most clinically significant form; severe cases may cause watery diarrhea of up to 10 to 15 times/day. Pseudomembranous colitis is a severe complication.

- Encourage a liberal fluid intake to replenish losses. Oral rehydration solutions, such as Pedialyte and Speedlyte, may be used.
- Clear liquids are avoided because they have high osmolality related to their high sugar content, which may promote osmotic diarrhea.
- Temporary avoidance of foods that stimulate GI motility may improve diarrhea:
  - alcohol
  - caffeine
  - items high in simple sugars, such as milk (**lactose**), fruit (fructose), and carbonated beverages (sucrose)
  - high-fiber foods, such as whole grains
  - gas-producing foods, such as bran, nuts, beans, corn, broccoli, and cabbage
  - sugar alcohols (e.g., sorbitol in "dietetic" products)
- Probiotics may help lessen diarrhea, especially diarrhea related to use of antibiotics. Because it is not known which strains or doses of probiotics may be most beneficial, it may be prudent to obtain probiotics from food sources, such as yogurt, kefir, and acidophilus milk, instead of supplements.
- Clients with intractable diarrhea may need complete bowel rest (i.e., parenteral nutrition [PN]).

Lactose
the disaccharide (double sugar) in milk composed of glucose and galactose.

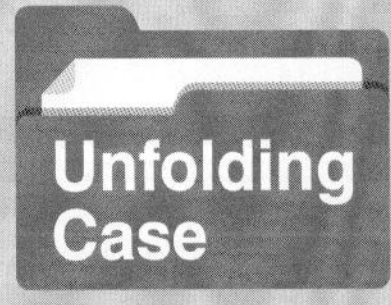

Recall Stephanie. Her vital signs and temperature are within normal limits. The physician assistant diagnoses viral gastritis and advises her to eat a bland diet until her symptoms abate. Is a bland diet the best option for Stephanie? What specific foods would you recommend she consumes? What foods should she avoid?

MALABSORPTION DISORDERS

Malabsorption
a broad term that describes altered or inadequate nutrient absorption from the GI tract.

Steatorrhea
excess fat in the stools that are loose, foamy, and foul smelling.

Malabsorption occurs secondary to nutrient maldigestion or from alterations to the absorptive surface of the intestinal mucosa. Generally, malabsorption related to maldigestion involves one or few nutrients, whereas malabsorption that stems from an altered mucosa is more generalized, resulting in multiple nutrient deficiencies and weight loss. Characteristics of malabsorption vary with the underlying disorder, ranging from minimal to widespread and serious (Box 20.4).

The goal of nutrition therapy for malabsorption syndromes is to control **steatorrhea**, promote normal bowel elimination, restore optimal nutritional status, and promote healing, when applicable. Nutrition therapy is individualized according to symptoms and complications; possible diet modifications appear in Table 20.1. Specific malabsorption syndromes are discussed in the following sections—namely, lactose malabsorption, inflammatory bowel disease (IBD), celiac disease, and short bowel syndrome (SBS).

Lactose Malabsorption

Lactose Malabsorption
incomplete digestion of lactose.

Lactose malabsorption refers to impaired lactose digestion and absorption related to reduced activity of lactase, the enzyme that splits lactose into its component simple sugars glucose and galactose. Without adequate lactase, lactose reaches the large intestine, where microbiota ferment the sugar, which may cause bloating, cramping, flatulence, and diarrhea. Particles of undigested lactose increase the osmolality of intestinal contents, increasing the likelihood of osmotic diarrhea. Symptoms range from mild to severe, depending on the amount of lactase actually produced and the amount of lactose consumed. The occurrence of symptoms in people with lactose malabsorption is known as **lactose intolerance** (Misselwitz et al., 2019). Lactose malabsorption may be caused by the following:

Lactose Intolerance
GI symptoms of lactose malabsorption that occur after a blinded, placebo-controlled lactose challenge.

Lactase Nonpersistence
reduced activity of lactase at the jejunal brush border, which is common in the majority of human adults. Low lactase activity may cause symptoms after lactose is consumed.

Lactase Persistence
persistence of a high level of lactase into adulthood that enables adequate digestion of larger amounts of lactose.

- congenital lactase deficiency, a rare pediatric condition characterized by a complete lack of lactase that results in severe symptoms of failure to thrive in infants (Misselwitz et al., 2019).
- **lactase nonpersistence (LNP)**, a common condition in which lactase activity reaches a peak at birth but decreases during childhood (Misselwitz et al., 2019).
  - Worldwide prevalence is estimated at 68%; it is lowest in Nordic countries (<5% in Denmark) and highest in Korean and Han Chinese populations (approaches 100%) (Misselwitz et al., 2019).
  - LNP is not synonymous with lactose intolerance, which by definition requires evidence of lactose malabsorption and the development of symptoms, which is not currently done in practice (Misselwitz et al., 2019).
  - In comparison to LNP, Caucasians from Northern Europe or Northern European descent retain high lactase levels during adulthood, which is termed **lactase persistence**. Both lactase persistence and nonpersistence are normal human conditions (Misselwitz et al., 2019).

BOX 20.4 General Characteristics of Malabsorption

- Malabsorption may be suspected in clients who have weight loss, growth failure, postprandial abdominal pain, bloating, and flatulence.
- Watery diarrhea and distention are symptoms of malabsorption from carbohydrate maldigestion (e.g., lactose intolerance).
- The passage of less frequent stools that are oily, bulky, and foul smelling is a symptom of malabsorption related to fat maldigestion (e.g., pancreatitis).
- The excretion of fat in the stools means that essential fatty acids, fat-soluble vitamins, and certain minerals are also lost through the stools.
- Nutrient deficiencies can cause metabolic complications, such as osteomalacia and bone pain related to the deficiencies of calcium, vitamin D, and magnesium.
- Appetite may be poor, and nutrient needs may be elevated for healing.
- The risk for malnutrition can be high.

Table 20.1 Nutrition Therapy for Malabsorption Symptoms

Symptoms	Dietary Interventions	Rationale
Anorexia	Small, frequent meals Oral nutrition supplements Enteral nutrition if anorexia is severe and/or prolonged	To maximize intake Liquid supplements are easy to consume, are nutritionally dense, and leave the stomach quickly. To meet calorie and nutrient needs until the client is able to consume an adequate oral intake
Diarrhea	Low-fiber diet Ensure adequate fluid and electrolytes. Avoid lactose	To minimize stimulation to the bowel Increased losses of fluid and electrolytes in the stool Lactase activity may be lost during acute episodes of malabsorption due to altered integrity and function of intestinal villi cells; lactase deficiency may persist into remission.
Nutrient deficiencies	Nutrient-dense diet Vitamin supplements; water-soluble forms of the fat-soluble vitamins may be necessary. Oral, nasal, or parenteral vitamin B_{12} Calcium supplements Other mineral supplements	To replenish losses, facilitate healing, and meet increased needs related to the metabolism of a high-calorie, high-protein diet Dietary sources may not be adequate to meet need. Water-soluble forms do not require normal fat absorption to be absorbed, as do fat-soluble vitamins in their natural form. Bacterial overgrowth, pancreatic insufficiency, and ileal disease or resection impair vitamin B_{12} absorption. Serum calcium may be low related to low serum albumin or calcium malabsorption related to poor vitamin D absorption or the binding of calcium with unabsorbed fats which forms unabsorbable soaps. Magnesium levels are often low in some malabsorption syndromes; losses of zinc are high in clients with fistulas.
Steatorrhea	Limit fat Medium-chain triglyceride (MCT) oil may be used for calories.	To avoid aggravating fat malabsorption MCT oil is absorbed without undergoing digestion.
Tissue damage (e.g., resulting from inflammation or surgery) and/or weight loss	Increase calories (2000–3500 cal/day) Increase protein (1.2–1.5 g/kg/day)	Calories and protein are needed to facilitate healing and restore weight.
Hyperoxaluria (Calcium normally binds with oxalate in the GI tract. Loss of calcium due to fat malabsorption leaves increased amounts of oxalate available for absorption into the blood, resulting in an increased risk of oxalate kidney stones in susceptible people).	Reduce fat If previous history of oxalate kidney stones exists, limit oxalate intake (e.g., tea and fruit).	Lowering fat allows more calcium available to bind with oxalate, rendering it unavailable for absorption

- Secondary lactose malabsorption may occur in people who normally digest lactose but experience a GI condition that alters the integrity and function of intestinal villi cells, where lactase is secreted.
  - The lactase deficiency that results is usually temporary.
  - GI conditions that may cause lactase deficiency include infectious gastroenteritis, IBD, and celiac disease.
  - The loss of lactase may also develop secondary to malnutrition because the rapidly growing intestinal cells that produce lactase are reduced in number and function.
  - Symptoms of secondary lactose malabsorption tend to be more severe and occur more quickly after eating lactose than when lactose malabsorption is caused by LNP.

Nutrition Therapy for Lactose Malabsorption

Nutrition therapy for lactose malabsorption is to reduce lactose to the maximum amount tolerated by the individual, which is dose related (Box 20.5).

- People with lactose nonpersistence may be asymptomatic when they consume doses up to 12 g of lactose (e.g., 1 cup of milk) or more when consumed with food (Misselwitz et al., 2019). Chocolate milk may be better tolerated than plain milk, although the reason is unclear (Heaney, 2013).
- Tolerance to lactose may improve by consuming probiotics that produce lactase in the gut (Heaney, 2013).
- For people who want to consume milk or lactose-containing foods beyond their limit, lactose-reduced milk and lactase enzyme tablets or liquid may be used.
- For clients with secondary lactose malabsorption related to GI disorders, a lactose-restricted diet is indicated at least until the disorder is resolved and sometimes for a prolonged period thereafter. Because lactose is used as an ingredient in many foods and drugs, a lactose-free diet is not realistic.

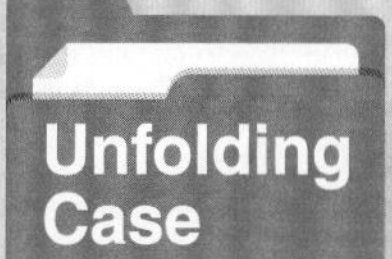

Recall Stephanie. Her symptoms resolved when she limited her intake to chicken broth, Gatorade, and tomato juice, but when she resumed her normal eating pattern, her symptoms returned. She has unintentionally lost a few pounds. She decided to keep a food diary to see if her symptoms correlated to food. She concluded that milk is a problem and has eliminated all milk and dairy products from her eating pattern. What nutrients may she be lacking in by eliminating all dairy? Is it appropriate for her to eliminate all dairy? Does eliminating dairy effectively eliminate all sources of lactose?

BOX 20.5 Low-Lactose Diet

- Lactose is the sugar in milk; limit or avoid milk and foods made with milk.
- Individual tolerance varies; eat dairy foods as tolerance allows.
- Lactose tolerance may improve by introducing a small serving of a lactose-containing food and increasing the amount consumed daily.
- Lactose is better tolerated with meals, not alone. Chocolate milk may be better tolerated than plain milk.
- These ingredients are derived from milk but are lactose-free: casein, lactate, lactalbumin, lactic acid.
- Avoid products whose ingredient list contains butter, cream, milk, milk solids, or whey and products with ingredient lists that state, "May contain milk."
- Consider lactase enzyme supplements.
- Choose nondairy sources of calcium to ensure an adequate intake, such as canned salmon with bones; calcium-fortified tofu, orange juice, and soy milk; shellfish; "greens" such as turnip, collard, and kale; dried peas and beans; broccoli; and almonds.

Lactose-Free Milk and Nondairy Foods	Low-Lactose Dairy Foods	Possible Hidden Sources of Lactose
Milk labeled lactose free	Aged cheese, such as cheddar, Swiss, and parmesan	Bread
Cheese and yogurt labeled lactose free	Cream cheese	Baked goods
Almond, rice, or soy milk	Ricotta cheese	Breakfast cereals
Soy yogurt, soy cheese, soy sour cream	Cottage cheese	Instant potatoes and soups
Almond milk cheese	Yogurt	Margarine
		Lunch meats
		Salad dressings
		Mixes for pancakes, biscuits, and cookies
		Powdered meal-replacement supplements

Inflammatory Bowel Disease

Inflammatory bowel disease (IBD) predominantly refers to Crohn's disease (CD) and ulcerative colitis (UC). Although the exact cause is unknown, a combination of altered immune system functioning, genetics, and environmental factors may be involved. CD and UC are characterized by cycles that alternate between active and quiescent states; they share common symptoms and treatments (Table 20.2).

According to the European Society for Clinical Nutrition and Metabolism (Forbes et al., 2017),

- the increasing incidence of IBD in Western countries supports the hypothesis that lifestyle may play a role in its development;
- smoking, antibiotic use, and diet are potentially reversible risk factors for IBD;
- a diet rich in fruits, vegetables, and omega-3 fatty acids and low in omega-6 fatty acids is associated with a decreased risk of developing IBD and is therefore recommended; and
- vitamin D and zinc may lower the risk of CD but not UC.

Table 20.2 Comparison between Crohn's Disease and Ulcerative Colitis

	Crohn's Disease	Ulcerative Colitis
Area affected	Can occur anywhere along the GI tract but most commonly occurs in the ileum and colon.	Confined to the rectum and colon
Disease pattern	Inflammation is discontinuous, with normal tissue between patches of inflamed tissue. All layers of the bowel are affected.	Inflammation is continuous, beginning at rectum and usually extending into the colon. Affects only the mucosal layer.
Main symptoms	Diarrhea, abdominal pain, weight loss	Diarrhea, abdominal pain, rectal bleeding Weight loss, fever, and weakness are common when most of the colon is involved.
Complications	Fistulas, abscesses Stricture of the ileum Bowel perforation Bowel obstructions may occur from scar tissue formation. Toxic megacolon Increased risk of intestinal cancer	Tissue erosion and ulceration Toxic megacolon Greatly increased risk of: cancer
Nutritional complications	Impaired bile acid reabsorption may cause malabsorption of fat, fat-soluble vitamins, calcium, magnesium, and zinc. Malnutrition may occur from nutrient malabsorption, decreased intake, or intestinal resections. Anemia related to blood loss or malabsorption Vitamin B_{12} deficiency related to B_{12} malabsorption from the ileum due to inflammation	Anemia related to blood loss Dehydration and electrolyte imbalances related to diarrhea Protein depletion from losses through inflamed tissue
Medical treatment	Antidiarrheals, immunosuppressants, immunomodulators, biologic therapies, and anti-inflammatory agents	Antidiarrheals, immunosuppressants, and anti-inflammatory agents
Surgical intervention	Most common procedure is ileostomy; disease often recurs in the remaining intestine.	Most common procedure is total colectomy; surgery prevents recurrence.

IBD increases the risk of malnutrition, more so in clients with CD than UC (Forbes et al., 2017).

- Malnutrition may be caused by poor intake, increased nutrient excretion, drug–nutrient interactions, and, in clients with CD, previous surgical resection of the bowel.
- Because malnutrition worsens client prognosis, complication rates, and quality of life, malnutrition screening should occur at the time of diagnosis and regularly thereafter (Forbes et al., 2017).

Nutrition Therapy for Active Inflammatory Bowel Disease

Currently, evidence is lacking on the effects of experimental diets, such as specific carbohydrate, gluten-free, paleolithic, and the Fermentable Oligo-, Di-, and Monosaccharides, and Polyols (FODMAP) diet, on promoting remission in clients with active disease (Forbes et al., 2017).

- Actual nutrient needs vary among individuals and with the presence and severity of symptoms, the presence of complications, and the nutritional status of the client. Table 20.1 outlines dietary interventions that may be appropriate based on symptoms.
- Restrictions are kept to a minimum to encourage an adequate intake. Diets should be modified according to individual tolerance.
- Low-fiber diets are frequently recommended to reduce the volume and bulk of stool and slow intestinal transit time (Box 20.6).
- Calorie expenditure does not increase as a direct result of IBD, therefore calorie needs are not elevated above normal (Forbes et al., 2017). However, many clients with CD are malnourished and underweight and require additional calories for repletion.
- During active disease, protein needs increase to 1.2 to 1.5 g/kg. Protein need returns to normal during remission.
- Micronutrient deficiencies are common. A multivitamin may correct most deficiencies but additional iron, zinc, and vitamin D may be needed (Forbes et al., 2017).
- Enteral nutrition (EN) is considered when oral intake is inadequate. A routine polymeric is recommended. Disease-specific modified formulas (e.g., fortified with glutamine or omega-3 fatty acids) are not recommended.
- PN is considered only when enteral feeding is contraindicated.
- Any dietary restrictions followed during active disease are liberalized to tolerance during periods of remission.

Nutrition Therapy during Remission of Inflammatory Bowel Disease

No specific diet is routinely recommended for maintaining remission of IBD. Of note (Forbes et al., 2017):

- IBD patients tend to choose a diet low in fiber and vegetables.
- A lactose-restricted diet is recommended for patients with secondary lactose malabsorption, which is mainly prevalent in clients with proximal CD.
- Limited, controlled data suggest clients with CD eliminate the following items but *only* when they are poorly tolerated: lactose, dairy products, spices, herbs, fried foods, and gassy and high-fiber products.
- Cohort studies in clients with UC suggest those who habitually consume more meat and alcohol have a higher rate of relapse.
- General advice may be to follow a Mediterranean-Style Eating Pattern rich in fruit and vegetables, unless there are known strictures.

BOX 20.6 Low-Fiber Diet

- This diet restricts fiber to decrease the volume and frequency of stools.
- This diet is a short-term diet to be used when the bowel is inflamed, such as in the acute stages of diverticulitis, UC, and CD. It may also be used for esophageal and intestinal stenosis, in preparation for or after bowel surgery, or for new colostomy or ileostomy.

General Guidelines to Achieve a Low-Fiber Diet

- Choose refined white flour products with less than 2 g fiber/serving such as white bread and rolls, white pasta, white rice, refined, low-fiber cereals.
- Eat only well-cooked vegetables that do not have skins or seeds.
- Choose fresh ripe banana or melon; canned or cooked fruit except pineapple; fruit juices without pulp (except prune juice).
- Eat plain desserts made without nuts or coconut, such as plain cakes, puddings (rice, bread, and plain), cookies, and ice cream.
- Avoid foods high in fiber:
  - whole-grain breads and cereals
  - most raw vegetables, vegetables with seeds, gassy vegetables, cooked greens or spinach
  - all fresh fruits except banana and melons; fruit juice with pulp, prune juice, any fruits sweetened with sorbitol
  - dried peas and beans
  - anything containing nuts, seeds, or coconut; popcorn

Additional Recommendations

- Avoid milk and milk products that contain lactose if lactose intolerance is suspected. Low-lactose and lactose-free alternatives include acidophilus milk, yogurt, soy milk, and almond milk.
- Avoid high-fat protein foods (sausage, bacon, many cold cuts).
- Avoid items that stimulate GI motility: alcohol, caffeine, sorbitol, and xylitol.
- Probiotic foods may help, such as yogurt with live bacterial cultures, acidophilus milk, and kefir.

Sample Menu

Breakfast	Lunch	Dinner	Snacks
Pulp-free orange juice	Chicken noodle soup	Roast chicken	Saltine crackers
Poached egg	Tuna sandwich on white bread with mayonnaise	White rice	Rice cakes
White toast with jelly	Canned peach halves	Cooked carrots	Tomato juice
	Milk if tolerated	Italian bread with olive oil	Fresh banana
		Frozen yogurt	Soy milk

Potential Problems	Recommended Interventions
Constipation related to low fiber content of diet; insufficient fiber intake causes decrease in stool bulk and slowing of intestinal transit time.	Liberalize diet to allow more fiber; this diet is intended to be short term.
Persistent diarrhea related to poor tolerance of even small amounts of fiber contained in a low-fiber diet; tolerance of fiber varies among clients and conditions.	Further reduce fiber content by eliminating all fruits and vegetables except strained fruit juice.

Client Teaching

Instruct the client on the following:

- Reducing fiber slows passage of food through the bowel.
- Fiber is a component of plants and, therefore, is found in fruits, vegetables, whole grains, dried peas and beans, and nuts.
- This diet is intended to be short term.
- Food preparation techniques to reduce fiber include removing skins, seeds, and membranes of fruits and vegetables that are high in fiber and cooking allowed vegetables until they are very tender.

Celiac Disease

Celiac disease is a chronic, genetic autoimmune disorder characterized by chronic inflammation of the proximal small intestine mucosa related to a permanent intolerance to certain gluten-forming proteins found in wheat, barley, and rye. When ingested, these proteins trigger an immune response that damages the villi that line the mucosa of the small intestine.

- Once thought to be a pediatric disease, improved diagnostic testing has helped establish celiac disease as a systemic autoimmune disease that can develop at any age (Leonard et al., 2017).
- People at risk of celiac disease are those who have an autoimmune disease (e.g., type 1 diabetes), Down syndrome, or a first-degree relative with celiac disease.

The significant variation in presenting symptoms in clients makes the diagnosis of celiac disease challenging (Caio et al., 2019).

- Clients may present with GI symptoms, extraintestinal symptoms, or both (Box 20.7).
- The gold standard for diagnosis is a combination of mucosal changes identified by duodenal biopsy and positive serological tests; biopsy remains necessary, because no antibody test currently available is 100% sensitive or specific (Caio et al., 2019).
- Testing for celiac disease needs to occur *before* a gluten-free diet is implemented because once the diet is initiated, testing for celiac disease is no longer accurate (Leonard et al., 2017).

Complications of celiac disease include hyposplenism, intestinal lymphoma, small bowel adenocarcinoma, and ulcerative jejunoileitis (Caio et al., 2019). Complications are suspected when symptoms (e.g., diarrhea, abdominal pain, weight loss, fever) persist or return despite adherence to a gluten-free diet.

Nutrition Therapy for Celiac Disease

The only effective treatment for celiac disease is a lifelong gluten-free diet (Box 20.8). The gluten-free diet has been shown to promote mucosal healing, reduce serum levels of celiac antibodies, improve nutrient deficiencies and bone health, and increase body fat, although it is not successful in all clients (Cichewicz et al., 2019). The response to the diet may be slow, particularly in people diagnosed in adulthood.

Gluten
a general name for the storage proteins gliadin (in wheat), secalin (in rye), and hordein (in barley).

- **Gluten** occurs naturally in barley, wheat, and rye. Wheat products are the predominant complex carbohydrate in the typical American diet.
- Oats is considered a source of gluten in the United States due to possible contamination with other grains, unless it is specifically labeled as gluten free.
- The diet is difficult to comply with because of the pervasiveness of gluten in processed foods and medications and confusion over identifying sources of gluten on food labels.
- Special gluten-free products (e.g., breads, pastry) made with rice, corn, or potato flour have different textures and tastes than "normal" products and may not be well accepted. They may also cost more than similar gluten-containing products.
- It is difficult to actually achieve a gluten-free diet because minute amounts of gluten may be present in gluten-free foods. As defined by the Food and Drug Administration (FDA), foods labeled as "gluten-free" must contain <20 ppm of gluten (U.S. Food and Drug Administration [FDA], 2018). According to the FDA (2018), this is the lowest level that can be consistently detected in foods using valid scientific analytical tools.

The crucial benefits of adhering to a gluten-free diet are accompanied by some disadvantages, such as the following (Caio et al., 2019):

- Impaired quality of life: This diet requires a major lifestyle change: it is very restrictive, necessitates conscientious label reading, and is difficult to adhere to while eating out.

BOX 20.7 Types of Clinical Presentations in Celiac Disease

Intestinal Presentation

- More common in children younger than 3 years of age. Symptoms include diarrhea, anorexia, abdominal distention, and failure to thrive.
- Older children and adults may experience diarrhea, bloating, constipation, abdominal pain, or weight loss. However, malabsorption syndrome is rare. When it does occur, it can cause weight loss, sarcopenia, and electrolyte abnormalities.
- More frequently, adults present with symptoms of IBS or nausea with occasional vomiting.

Extraintestinal presentation: attributed to a combination of chronic inflammation, nutrient deficiencies, and possibly an adaptive immune response spreading from the intestinal mucosa to other tissues and organs (Leonard et al., 2017).

- Common in children and adults.
- Symptoms include iron deficiency anemia, bone disease, dermatitis herpetiformis, neurologic disorders, fatigue, and reproductive alterations (e.g., late menarche, amenorrhea, recurrent miscarriages, early menopause).

Subclinical Form

- Clients have symptoms below the clinical threshold for identification.
- Often only recognized after adherence to a gluten-free diet produces beneficial effects.

Potential Form

- It is characterized by positive serological and genetic markers but with normal intestinal mucosa and minimal signs of inflammation.
- It can manifest with classic and non-classic symptoms or be entirely asymptomatic.
- It is not known if a gluten-free diet should be prescribed.

Refractory Celiac Disease

- It is characterized by persistent malabsorption symptoms and atrophy of intestinal villi despite strict adherence to a gluten-free diet for at least 6 to 12 months.

Nonceliac Gluten Sensitivity

- Clinical symptoms occur after eating gluten and disappear or improve when gluten is eliminated from the diet.
- Symptoms include abdominal pain, bloating, bowel irregularity (diarrhea, constipation, or both).
- Extraintestinal symptoms include "foggy brain," headache, joint and muscle pain, fatigue, depression, leg or arm numbness, dermatitis, and anemia (Leonard et al., 2017).

Source: Caio, G., Volta, U., Sapone, A., Leffler, D., DeGiorgio, R., Catassi, C., & Fasano, A. (2019). Celiac disease: A comprehensive current review. *BMC Medicine, 17*, 142. https://doi.org/10.1186/s12916-019-1380-z; Leonard, M., Sapone, A., Catassi, C., & Fasano, A. (2017). Celiac disease and nonceliac gluten sensitivity: A review. *Journal of the American Medical Association, 318*(7), 647–656. https://doi.org/10.1001/jama.2017.9730

- Psychological problems, which may include fear of involuntary or inadvertent gluten consumption.
- Nutrient deficiencies: Adults diagnosed with celiac disease are likely to have a nutrient deficiency, such as folate, B_{12}, zinc, and iron (Leonard et al., 2017).
- Increased risk of metabolic syndrome and cardiovascular disease.
- Possible severe constipation related to elimination of wheat, specifically whole wheat. Other allowed grains and starchy foods that provide fiber are less commonly consumed.

Nonceliac Gluten Sensitivity

Nonceliac gluten sensitivity (NCGS) is a condition in which people do not have the diagnostic features of celiac disease but develop celiac-like symptoms in response to eating gluten and experience improvement or disappearance of symptoms when gluten is eliminated from the diet.

- No specific biomarkers have been identified and validated for NCGS, and symptoms alone cannot reliably differentiate celiac disease from NCGS because symptoms overlap between the two conditions (Leonard et al., 2017).

BOX 20.8 Gluten-Free Diet

- Celiac disease and NCGS are the only indications for a gluten-free diet. There is no evidence that a gluten-free diet is part of a healthier lifestyle or is helpful in treating overweight or obesity (Leonard et al., 2017).
- Gluten, a protein fraction found in wheat, rye, and barley, is eliminated. All products made from these grains or their flours are eliminated. Oats are at high risk of gluten contamination, so only oats labeled gluten free are suitable.
- Many foods are naturally gluten free: milk, butter, cheese; fresh, frozen, and canned fruits and vegetables; fresh meat, fish, poultry, eggs; dried peas and beans; nuts; corn; and rice.

Naturally Gluten-Free Grains and Other Starch-Containing Foods

Amaranth
Arrowroot Buckwheat
Cassava
Chia
Corn, cornstarch
Flax
Gums
- Acacia (gum Arabic)
- Carob bean gum
- Carrageenan
- Cellulose
- Guar
- Locust bean
- Xanthan

Legumes, legume flours
Millet
Nut flours
Certified gluten-free oats
Potatoes, potato flour
Quinoa
Rice, all plain; wild rice; rice flour
Soy
Sorghum
Tapioca
Teff
Yucca

Gluten-Containing Grains to Eliminate

Wheat—all forms, including wheat flours, such as bread flour, bromated flour, cake flour, durum flour, enriched flour, graham flour, pastry flour, phosphated flour, plain flour, self-rising flour, semolina, white flour
Wheat starch, wheat bran, wheat germ, cracked wheat, hydrolyzed wheat protein, farina, matzo
Wheat sources of
- Dextrin
- Caramel color
- Maltodextrin
- Modified food starch

"Ancient" types of wheat: Einkorn, emmer, spelt, kamut

Barley
Rye
Malt
Triticale (a cross between wheat and rye)
Oats not certified gluten-free

Foods Not Recommended (May Contain Wheat, Barley, or Rye)

Beer
Bouillon cubes
Brown rice syrup
Chips/potato chips
Candy
Cold cuts, hot dogs, salami, sausage
Communion wafer
Flavored or herbal coffee
Flavored or herbal tea
French fries
Gravy
Imitation fish
Licorice
Malt, malted syrup, malt beverages, malt vinegar
Meat substitutes
Rice and corn cereals (may contain barley malt)
Rice mixes
Sauces
Seasoned or dry-roasted nuts
Seasoned tortilla chips
Self-basting poultry
Soups
Soy sauce
Vegetables in sauce

Sample Menu

Breakfast

Orange juice
Gluten-free cornflakes
Milk
Coffee

Lunch

Cuban black beans with brown rice
Pure corn tortilla
Milk
Plain yogurt topped with chopped almonds
Coffee/tea

Dinner

Tomato juice
Roast chicken
Quinoa pilaf
Steamed broccoli
Corn bread made without wheat flour
Blueberries over ice cream made without gluten stabilizers

Snacks

Plain nuts
Rice cake
Banana
Apple slices with peanut butter

Additional Considerations

- Clients may be discouraged and overwhelmed when faced with a lifelong restricted diet. Provide support, encouragement, and thorough diet instructions.
- The client may have temporary lactose malabsorption and may require a lactose-restricted diet.

BOX 20.8 Gluten-Free Diet (continued)

Potential Problems	Recommended Interventions
Increased expense related to buying special gluten-free foods	Encourage the client to use as many "normal" items as possible such as corn, grits, quinoa, rice, and rice cereals; they are easy to obtain and less expensive than special products.
Inadequate intake of several nutrients (B vitamins, calcium, zinc, and iron) related to the lower content of these nutrients in gluten-free products compared to the enriched and fortified grains and cereals they replace	Encourage a varied diet of allowed foods and enriched gluten-free products over non-enriched; recommend a gluten-free, age-appropriate multivitamin and mineral supplement.
Inadequate intake of fiber related to the absence of whole wheat products	Encourage fiber from legumes, nuts, fruits, vegetables, and gluten-free whole grains such as flax seed, millet, uncontaminated oats, quinoa, brown rice, and amaranth.

Client Teaching

Instruct the client on the importance of adhering to the diet even when no symptoms are present. "Cheating" on the diet can damage intestinal villi even if no symptoms develop.

To permanently eliminate all flours and products containing wheat, rye, barley, triticale, and malt, the client should do the following:

- Read labels. By law, foods labeled gluten free must contain <20 ppm of gluten.
- Check with the manufacturer *before* using products of questionable composition. While all food products must be clearly labeled to indicate the presence of wheat, other sources of gluten are less obvious (e.g., malt flavorings and extracts from barley).
- Use corn, potato, rice, arrowroot, and soybean flours and their products.
- Use the following as thickening agents: arrowroot starch, cornstarch, tapioca starch, rice starch, and sweet rice flour.
- Eat an otherwise normal, well-balanced diet adequate in nutrients and calories. Lactose is restricted only if not tolerated. Weight gain may be slowly achieved.

Provide the client with the following aids:

- A detailed list of foods allowed and not allowed.
- Information regarding support groups; see "Websites" section at the end of this chapter.
- Gluten-free recipes.

- Treatment is a gluten-free diet, although it is not known if long-term strict avoidance of all gluten is necessary, because NCGS may be transient (Fasano et al., 2015).
- It is recommended that a gluten-free diet be followed for 12 to 24 months before repeating testing for gluten tolerance (Leonard et al., 2017).
- Some clients with NCGS choose to follow a gluten-free diet indefinitely.

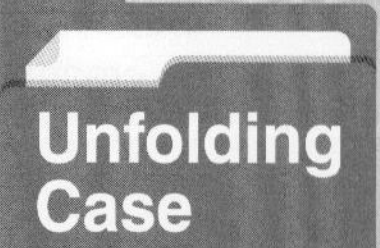

Think of Stephanie. Despite conscientiously following a low-lactose eating pattern, her symptoms persisted, and her weight loss continued. She is eventually seen by a gastroenterologist who diagnoses celiac disease and iron deficiency anemia. Is there a connection between type 1 diabetes and celiac disease? Should she continue to restrict lactose from her eating pattern? How will nutrition counseling for a college student who lives in a dorm differ from counseling for an adult living in her own home? Stephanie knows she should eat fiber to help regulate her blood glucose levels; what sources of fiber would be appropriate on a gluten-free diet?

Short Bowel Syndrome

Short Bowel Syndrome (SBS)
a complex condition resulting from extensive surgical resection of the intestinal tract resulting in an inadequate absorptive surface that may lead to maldigestion and malabsorption.

Short bowel syndrome (SBS), the most frequent cause of intestinal failure, is intestinal malabsorption related to a functional small intestine length of less than 200 cm (Pironi, 2016). This functional definition is necessary due to the variations in the length of small bowel remaining and the ability of the remaining small bowel to compensate for the shortened length (Parrish & DeBaise, 2017). There are three anatomical types of SBS depending on the portion and length of bowel that remains (Box 20.9).

SBS is a challenging and often disabling malabsorptive disorder associated with significant morbidity and mortality and decreased quality of life (Parrish & DeBaise, 2017). Loss of the ileum, especially the terminal ileum, is more detrimental than loss of jejunum, because it is the only site for absorption of intrinsic factor–bound vitamin B_{12} and bile salts. Disruption of enterohepatic circulation of bile salts leads to severe fat malabsorption and steatorrhea. Clients with a small bowel <100 cm that ends in a jejunostomy may need permanent PN and hydration to survive.

The most common causes of SBS in adults are complications from abdominal surgery (e.g., bariatric surgery), radiation enteritis, CD, ischemia, or trauma (Parrish & DeBaise, 2017). The complications, prognosis, and treatment depend on the length, health, and area of the remaining bowel. Symptoms include diarrhea/malabsorption, steatorrhea, electrolyte imbalances, weight loss, dehydration, fat-soluble vitamin deficiencies, oxalate kidney stones, metabolic acidosis, metabolic bone disease, and impaired wound healing related to malnutrition (Pironi, 2016).

Advances in the treatment of SBS have led to the reduction or elimination of PN in many formerly PN-dependent clients (Parrish & DeBaise, 2017). Early initiation of EN therapy postsurgically is critical for promoting optimal intestinal adaptation (the process whereby the absorptive capacity of the small bowel increases), which occurs mainly during the first 2 years after surgery. Strategies that may promote independence from PN include (Parrish & DeBaise, 2017)

- early introduction of enteral and oral feedings to stimulate intestinal adaptation and optimize absorption,
- the use of medications to control symptoms and improve quality of life,

BOX 20.9 Characteristics of the Anatomical Types of Short Bowel Syndrome

End jejunostomy

- Ileum and colon are completely removed; losses of sodium and fluid are large.
- Malabsorption of macronutrients, vitamin B_{12}, and bile salts occurs.
- Acid hypersecretion.
- Rapid gastric and intestinal transit.
- Long-term PN is usually required depending on the length of small bowel remaining.

Jejunocolic anastomosis

- Ileum and part of the colon are removed; the benefits of having even a part of the colon remain are related to its ability to absorb fluid, electrolytes, and fatty acids; slow transit time; and stimulate intestinal adaptation.
- Vitamin B_{12} and bile salt malabsorption occurs because the ileum is removed.
- Rapid intestinal transit.
- Long-term PN may be required depending on the length of small bowel remaining.

Jejunoileal anastomosis

- Part of the small intestine is removed but the colon remains intact; rarest type.
- Vitamin B_{12} and bile salt absorption are preserved.
- Transit is normal.
- Long-term PN may not be required.

- intestinal growth factors (e.g., somatropin and teduglutide), and
- surgery when appropriate (e.g., to relieve obstruction or add bowel into continuity).

Course of Nutrition Therapy

- Initially after surgery, most clients with SBS require PN.
- As soon as possible in the early post-op period, an intact EN formula should be added to the treatment regimen for maximum bowel stimulation and adaptation (Matarese, 2013). However, PN remains the major source of nutrition and hydration.
- As adaptation occurs, EN combined with oral feedings may promote weaning off PN.
- When the client can consume oral nutrition without excessive stool or ostomy output and can maintain or gain weight, the amount of PN is gradually decreased.

Nutrition Therapy Interventions

Nutrition interventions are highly individualized. Few comparative studies on diet composition are available due to the complexity of SBS and the heterogenous sample (AND, 2020). Diet recommendations are typically based on clinical experience and observational studies. General eating and nutrition guidelines are summarized in Box 20.10.

BOX 20.10 General Eating and Nutrition Guidelines for Short Bowel Syndrome

Eating Guidelines

- Eat 6 to 8 small meals or snacks.
- Chew food thoroughly.
- Avoid liquids with solids and for 30 minutes after eating to help reduce diarrhea.
  - If coffee, tea, and iced tea are allowed, limit intake to less than 4 ounces per day.
- Avoid the following:
  - Food and beverages containing simple sugars, such as desserts, sugar-sweetened beverages, fruit juices, fruit drinks, oral nutrition supplements, and sweetened cereals.
  - Food and beverages containing sugar alcohols (sorbitol, xylitol, mannitol). Artificial sweeteners, such as Splenda, Equal, and Stevia, may be used.
  - Alcohol.
  - Lactose if not tolerated.

General Nutrition Guidelines

- Consume a high-quality protein at each meal and snack. Protein should supply approximately 20% of total calories.
- The percent contribution of carbohydrate and fat is based on whether or not the colon is present.
  - For clients with any remaining colon, a low-fat, high-carbohydrate diet is recommended. Excess fat can promote steatorrhea and increase oxalate absorption, which may increase the risk of oxalate kidney stones. Oxalate intake may need to be limited.
  - For clients without a colon (end jejunostomy or ileostomy), a diet low in carbohydrates and higher in salt is recommended. Fat intake does not increase stoma output and can help meet calorie needs.
- Oral rehydration solutions may be more beneficial than water, especially in clients with an end jejunostomy.
- Clients not receiving PN may need oral vitamin and mineral supplements, possibly 2 to 3 times/day to compensate for malabsorption. Depending on the extent of small and large bowel, remaining micronutrients of greatest concern are calcium, fat-soluble vitamins, vitamin B_{12}, zinc, and selenium.

Source: Parrish, C., & DiBaise, J. (2017). Managing the adult client with short bowel syndrome. *Gastroenterology & Hepatology*, *13*(10), 600–608; Academy of Nutrition and Dietetics. (2020). *Nutrition care manual*. https://www.nutritioncaremanual.org/

CONDITIONS OF THE LARGE INTESTINE

Irritable Bowel Syndrome

Irritable bowel syndrome (IBS), one of the most frequently diagnosed GI conditions, is a chronic functional disorder characterized by abdominal pain with diarrhea, constipation, or both in the absence of any other disease that may cause these symptoms (Chey et al., 2015). Bloating and distention are other common complaints. IBS can greatly impair quality of life and work productivity.

The cause of IBS is unclear and not likely to be singular. Factors that may contribute to its pathogenesis include disruption of the brain–gut axis, gut dysmotility, visceral hypersensitivity, low-grade mucosal inflammation, increased intestinal permeability, and altered microbiota (Hayes et al., 2014). Life stressors (changes in employment, relocation, etc.) can trigger or worsen symptoms as can excessive use of laxatives or antidiarrheal drugs, lack of regular sleep, and inadequate fluid intake (University of Virginia Nutrition, 2016). Over 80% of IBS clients report food-related symptoms (Böhn et al., 2013).

Nutrition Therapy for Irritable Bowel Syndrome

FODMAP is an acronym for Fermentable Oligo-, Di-, and Monosaccharides, and Polyols, which are carbohydrates that are poorly absorbed and rapidly fermented, resulting in diarrhea, gas, and abdominal pain in susceptible individuals (Staudacher et al., 2014).

- Dietary restriction of FODMAPs has been shown to be an effective treatment for IBS symptoms, with 50% to 76% of clients experiencing clinical benefits (Böhn et al., 2013).
- It is recommended that high-FODMAP foods are restricted for 4 to 6 weeks (Box 20.11).
- After symptom improvement is achieved, reintroduction of individual FODMAPs is encouraged to keep restrictions to a minimum and increase the likelihood of nutritional adequacy.
- A long-term FODMAP diet (6–18 months) has been shown to be not only effective for IBS management but also nutritionally adequate and generally well accepted by clients (O'Keeffe et al., 2018).

Anecdotally, the following interventions may help reduce symptoms (University of Virginia Nutrition, 2016):

- Eat smaller, more frequent meals.
- Reduce fat intake, which can be achieved by selecting lean meats, avoiding fried foods, choosing low-fat or nonfat dairy products, and avoiding high-fat snacks and sweets.
- Avoid caffeine, chocolate, and alcohol.
- Slowly increase soluble fiber intake (e.g., oatmeal, lima beans, peas, sweet potato) while consuming adequate fluid.

Other nutrition therapy interventions are often used for IBS with varying effectiveness.

- Probiotics may be effective in improving overall IBS symptoms and quality of life, but more studies are needed to determine what type, strain, dose, and treatment duration are optimal (Zhang et al., 2016).
- Peppermint oil improves cramping but may cause GERD or constipation (Chey et al., 2015).
- Other unproven but safe supplements often used include chamomile tea, evening primrose oil, and fennel seeds (University of Virginia Nutrition, 2016).

Diverticular Disease

Diverticular disease (DD) is characterized by the presence of **diverticula** and includes the conditions of **diverticulosis** and **diverticulitis**. Diverticulitis can be uncomplicated (inflammation of ≥1 diverticula) or complicated if abscess, perforation, fistula formation, or obstruction occurs (Pearlman & Akpotaire, 2019).

Diverticula
pouches that protrude outward from the muscular wall of the intestine usually in the sigmoid colon.

Diverticulosis
the presence of colonic diverticula, without inflammation or symptoms.

Diverticulitis
macroscopic inflammation of diverticula with related acute or chronic complications.

BOX 20.11 Low–Fermentable Oligo-, Di-, and Monosaccharides, and Polyols Diet

Incomplete digestion of fructose and other short-chain carbohydrates distends the bowel via osmotic effects and rapid fermentation and leads to the production of short-chain fatty acids and gas. In some people with IBS, FODMAPs may result in IBS symptoms (Staudacher et al., 2011). However, because there are no defined cutoff values for high- and low-FODMAP foods, there are discrepancies in identifying foods to avoid.

FODMAPs are found in the following:

- Honey and certain fruits that are high in free fructose. These items cause symptoms.
- Fruits that contain equal or greater amounts of glucose compared to fructose may be tolerated in measured amounts because glucose promotes the absorption of fructose. That is why fructose from white sugar and high-fructose corn syrup (HFCS), which are composed of equal parts of glucose and fructose, is generally completely absorbed. In contrast, fructose from a pear, which contains approximately 4 times more fructose than glucose, is poorly absorbed.
- Wheat, onions, leeks, garlic asparagus, artichokes, and inulin (fructans)
- Milk, yogurt, and ice cream (lactose)
- Legumes (galacto-oligosaccharides)
- Certain fruits and sugarless gums, mints, and dietetic foods that contain sugar alcohols such as sorbitol, mannitol, or xylitol

Guidelines to Achieve a Low–FODMAP Diet

- Keep a record of the amount and types of food and beverages consumed and the type, severity, and onset of symptoms to help identify intolerances.
- Avoid products that list fructose, crystalline fructose (not HFCS), honey, and sorbitol on the label.
- Avoid sugar alcohols found in "diet" or "dietetic" foods.
- Limit beverages with HFCS to ≤12 oz/day. Consume with food for improved tolerance.
- Fresh or frozen fruit may be better tolerated than canned fruit.
- Cooked vegetables may be better tolerated than raw.
- Fructose and sorbitol may be ingredients in medications. Check with the pharmacist.
- Tolerance is dose related; whereas small amounts of FODMAPs may be tolerated, eating beyond a person's threshold causes symptoms to develop.
- Keep in mind that not all FODMAP-containing foods worsen IBS symptoms in all clients.
- After a period of 6 to 8 weeks, clients who are able to control their symptoms with complete exclusion of FODMAPs are encouraged to gradually reintroduce eliminated foods, to keep restrictions to a minimum.

	Foods Low in FODMAP	High-FODMAP Foods to Avoid	Questionable Foods/Foods to Limit
Fruit	Bananas, blackberries, blueberry, grapefruit, honeydew, kiwifruit, lemons, limes, mandarin orange, melons (except watermelon), oranges, passion fruit, pineapple, raspberries, rhubarb, strawberries, tangelos	Fruit: apples, pear, guava, honeydew melon, mango, Asian pear, papaya, quince, star fruit, watermelon Stone fruit: apricots, peaches, cherries, plums, nectarines Fruits high in sugar: grapes, persimmon, lychee Dried fruit Fruit juice Dried fruit bars Fruit pastes and sauces: tomato paste, chutney, plum sauce, sweet and sour sauce, barbecue sauce Fruit juice concentrate	Fruit canned in heavy syrup, other fruits

(continued)

BOX 20.11 Low–Fermentable Oligo-, Di-, and Monosaccharides, and Polyols Diet (continued)

	Foods Low in FODMAP	High-FODMAP Foods to Avoid	Questionable Foods/Foods to Limit
Vegetables	Bamboo shoots, bok choy, carrots, cauliflower[a], celery, cucumber[a], eggplant[a], green beans[a], green peppers[a], leafy greens, parsnip, pumpkin, spinach, sweet potatoes, white potatoes, other root vegetables	Onion, leek, garlic, shallots, asparagus, artichokes, cabbage, Brussels sprouts, cauliflower, mushrooms, sugar snap peas, snow peas Legumes and lentils	Avocado, corn, mushrooms, tomatoes, other beans
Other	All meats All fats Oats Rice Lactose-free yogurt and hard cheeses Eggs Aspartame (Equal, NutraSweet) Saccharin (Sweet'N Low) Sugar Glucose Maple syrup	Wheat and wheat products (e.g., wheat pasta, cereals, cakes cookies, and crackers) Rye and rye products Milk, ice cream, yogurt containing lactose, and other sources of lactose Fortified wines: sherry, port, etc. Chicory-based coffee substitute Honey, agave nectar Certain additives identified on food labels, such as inulin (often labeled as chicory root extract), fructo-oligosaccharides, sorbitol, mannitol, xylitol, maltitol, isomalt Desserts sweetened with fructose or sorbitol (e.g., ice cream, cookies, popsicles)	Items containing HFCS if not tolerated

[a]Possible gas-forming foods that may need to be avoided.

It was a long-standing belief that low-fiber diets caused DD by increasing pressure within the intestinal lumen leading to mucosal herniation and the formation of diverticula. However, there is a lack of evidence to support this idea (Pearlman & Akpotaire, 2019). Dietary factors that have been shown to increase the risk of diverticulitis include red meat intake, particularly unprocessed red meat (Cao et al., 2018), and obesity and weight gain in adulthood (Ma et al., 2018).

Nutrition Therapy for Diverticular Disease

Some evidence suggests a high-fiber diet may decrease the risk of diverticulitis recurrence and/or symptomatic DD (Dahl et al., 2018). Based on very low evidence, the American Gastroenterology Association suggests a high-fiber diet or fiber supplements in clients with a history of acute diverticulitis (Stollman et al., 2015).

- Even though the certainty and magnitude of benefit are difficult to determine, a high-fiber diet or supplements are unlikely to pose a substantial risk (Stollman et al., 2015).
- A "prudent diet" (cholesterol-lowering diet rich in fruits, vegetables, whole grains, legumes, poultry, and fish) may decrease the risk of diverticulitis. Interestingly, recent intake seems

to be as effective as past intake, suggesting that it is not too late to adopt a prudent diet (Stollman, 2017).

- It is common practice for clients to be told to avoid nuts, seeds, and popcorn based on the theory that these can become trapped in diverticula and cause diverticulitis. However, there is no scientific evidence that proves nuts and seeds cause flares of diverticulitis (Kim, 2019).
- The efficacy of probiotics in different phases of DD is not fully understood (Ojetti et al., 2018).

Ileostomies and Colostomies

Ileostomy
a surgically created opening (stoma) on the surface of the abdomen from the ileum.

Colostomy
a surgically created opening on the surface of the abdomen from the colon.

The surgical creation of a stoma causes temporary or permanent alteration in the transit of food and/or elimination of stool (de Oliveira et al., 2018). Medical conditions that may necessitate an **ileostomy** or **colostomy** include colorectal cancer, congenital disorders, trauma, IBD, intestinal obstruction, and diverticulitis. The process of nutrient absorption is interrupted at the point of the stoma.

- Ileostomies are created in the small intestine, the site of nutrient absorption. Nutrients that may be lost include calcium, magnesium, iron, vitamins B_{12}, the fat-soluble vitamins, folic acid, water, protein, fat, and bile salts. A normal, mature ileostomy should only make about 1200 mL of output each day (Bridges et al., 2019). Stools are liquid to semiliquid.
- Colostomies are created in the colon; there is little or no nutrient loss. Colostomies usually only put out 200 to 600 mL/day (Bridges et al., 2019). Stools range from semiliquid to hard.

Nutrition Therapy for Ileostomies and Colostomies

Specific dietary guidelines for people with a stoma are lacking. Restrictions should be kept to a minimum. Common sense eating strategies that may be beneficial include the following (Bridges et al., 2019):

- Eat 4 to 6 small meals per day.
- Chew food thoroughly.
- Eat food you normally eat, but avoid mushrooms, nuts, corn, coconut, celery, and dried fruit for the first 2 weeks after surgery. Slowly reintroduce these foods, as desired, in moderation.
- Eat a source of protein at each meal and snack.
- Use salt liberally.
- Consume adequate fluid. At least 80 oz/day may be needed to protect kidney function.

High Output Stomas

An estimated 16% of stomas will suffer from a high output (Arenas Villafranca et al., 2015), which is generally defined as ≥1500 mL/day.

- Causes of high output stoma include SBS, intra-abdominal sepsis, enteritis, paralytic ileus, and medications.
- Clients with prolonged high output are at greater risk of dehydration, acute kidney injury, and malnutrition (Ahmad et al., 2019).
- A diet similar to that recommended for SBS may be indicated, at least until the output is under control (see Box 20.10).
- Fluid requirement is individualized to ensure a urine output of at least 1200 mL/day (Bridges et al., 2019).

DISORDERS OF THE ACCESSORY GASTROINTESTINAL ORGANS

The liver, pancreas, and gallbladder are known as accessory organs of the GI tract. Although food does not come in direct contact with these organs, they play vital roles in the digestion of macronutrients. Liver disease, pancreatitis, and gallbladder disease are discussed next.

Liver Disease

The liver is a highly active organ involved in the metabolism of almost all nutrients. After absorption, almost all nutrients are transported to the liver, where they are "processed" before being distributed to other tissues. The liver synthesizes plasma proteins, blood clotting factors, and nonessential amino acids and forms urea from the nitrogenous wastes of protein. Triglycerides, phospholipids, and cholesterol are synthesized in the liver, as is bile, an important factor in the digestion of fat. Glucose is synthesized, and glycogen is formed, stored, and broken down as needed. Vitamins and minerals are metabolized, and several are stored in the liver. Finally, the liver is vital for detoxifying drugs, alcohol, ammonia, and other poisonous substances.

Liver damage can have profound and devastating effects on the metabolism of almost all nutrients. It can range from mild and reversible (e.g., fatty liver) to severe and terminal (e.g., hepatic coma). Liver failure can occur from chronic liver disease or secondary to critical illnesses.

The objectives of nutrition therapy for liver disease are to avoid or minimize permanent liver damage, restore optimal nutritional status, alleviate symptoms, and avoid complications. Adequate protein and calories are needed to promote liver cell regeneration. However, regeneration may not be possible if liver damage is extensive.

Fatty Liver Disease

Fatty liver disease is characterized by abnormal fat deposition in the liver. Fatty liver occurs in the majority of clients with alcoholic liver disease. Nonalcoholic fatty liver disease (NAFLD) is a spectrum of diseases ranging in severity from simple hepatic steatosis, which is often asymptomatic and benign, to nonalcoholic **steatohepatitis** (NASH), its progressive subtype, characterized by inflammation and liver cell damage. Complications such as advanced fibrosis, **cirrhosis**, and hepatocellular carcinoma may result.

Steatohepatitis
fat accumulation in the liver with inflammation.

Cirrhosis
irreversible liver disease that occurs when damaged liver cells are replaced by functionless scar tissue, seriously impairing liver function and disrupting normal blood circulation through the liver.

First described in 1980, NAFLD is estimated to be the most common cause of chronic liver disease, affecting 80 to 100 million American adults, among whom nearly 25% will progress to NASH (Perumpail et al., 2017).

- NASH has been recognized as one of the leading causes of cirrhosis in American adults, and NASH-related cirrhosis is the second indication for liver transplants in the United States (Younossi et al., 2016).
- NAFLD is strongly associated with obesity and metabolic syndrome—a cluster of symptoms that include central obesity, insulin resistance, type 2 diabetes, hypertension, and abnormal blood lipid levels.
- Clients with NAFLD are twice as likely to die of cardiovascular disease as liver disease, largely because of their shared risk factors such as diabetes, hypertension, and obesity (Friedman et al., 2018).
- A high intake of calories, saturated fat, refined carbohydrates, sugar-sweetened beverages, and fructose have all been associated with weight gain, obesity, and NAFLD (EASL-EASD-EASO, 2016).

Treatment of NAFLD focuses on controlling the underlying risk factors, such as obesity, diabetes, and hyperlipidemia (Romero-Gómez et al., 2017).

- Lifestyle interventions, such as a healthy eating plan and physical activity, are well-established treatment strategies for these conditions.
- Sustained weight loss is the most effective treatment for NAFLD and should serve as the cornerstone of treatment.

Nutrition Therapy for Nonalcoholic Fatty Liver Disease

Clinical Practice Guidelines for the treatment of NAFLD suggest the following lifestyle interventions (EASL-EASD-EASO, 2016):

- Reduce calories by 500 to 1000/day to promote gradual weight loss.
- A target weight loss of 7% to 10% is recommended.
- A Mediterranean diet has been shown to reduce liver fat even when weight loss is not achieved. It is the most recommended dietary pattern for NAFLD.
- Avoid fructose (e.g., high fructose corn syrup) in beverages and food.
- Limit alcohol.
- Coffee exerts a protective effect in NAFLD; there are no liver-related restrictions on coffee intake.
- Both aerobic and resistance training reduce liver fat. One hundred fifty to 200 minutes/week of moderate-intensity aerobic physical activities is recommended. Benefits are dose related. Resistance straining is encouraged.
- Clients who are unable to achieve weight loss and metabolic improvements with lifestyle modification and drug therapy may consider bariatric surgery.

Hepatitis

Hepatitis
inflammation of the liver that may be caused by viral infections, alcohol abuse, and hepatotoxic chemicals such as chloroform and carbon tetrachloride.

Although fatty liver and alcohol toxicity can cause **hepatitis**, the most frequent causes are infection from hepatitis viruses A, B, and C. Early symptoms of hepatitis include anorexia, nausea and vomiting, fever, fatigue, headache, and weight loss. Later, symptoms such as dark-colored urine, jaundice, liver tenderness, and, possibly, liver enlargement may develop. In many cases, particularly those caused by hepatitis A, liver cell damage that occurs from acute hepatitis is reversible with proper rest and adequate nutrition.

Nutrition Therapy for Hepatitis

A healthy diet adequate in calories, protein, and micronutrients is recommended for clients with acute hepatitis (first 6 months of illness). Food restrictions are usually not necessary. For clients with chronic hepatitis (illness that persists beyond 6 months), diet modifications are based on symptoms (AND, 2020).

- Limit sodium to 2 g/day if there is fluid retention.
- Consume 4 to 6 small meals and/or snacks to promote an adequate intake.
- Consume 1.0 to 1.2 g protein/kg.
- Follow a carbohydrate-controlled eating pattern appropriate for diabetes if hyperglycemia develops.
- Limit fat to <30% of total calories if steatorrhea develops.

Cirrhosis

Scarring from chronic hepatitis can lead to cirrhosis. Liver damage progresses slowly, and some clients are asymptomatic. Early nonspecific symptoms include fever, anorexia, weight loss, and fatigue. Glucose intolerance is common. Later, portal hypertension, dyspepsia, diarrhea or constipation, jaundice, esophageal varices, hemorrhoids, ascites, edema, bleeding tendencies, anemia, hepatomegaly, and splenomegaly may develop.

Malnutrition affects an estimated 20% of clients with compensated cirrhosis and >50% of clients with decompensated liver disease (European Association for the Study of the Liver [EASL], 2019).

Hepatic Encephalopathy
the CNS manifestations of advanced liver disease characterized by irritability, short-term memory loss, and impaired ability to concentrate.

- Malnutrition is associated with the progression of liver failure and with a higher rate of complications such as infection, **hepatic encephalopathy**, and ascites.
- Whether malnutrition can be reversed in cirrhotic clients is controversial.

- Although commonly assumed to mean "undernutrition," overweight and obesity are increasingly seen in cirrhotic clients due to the increase in NAFLD (EASL, 2019).
- Obesity and sarcopenic obesity may worsen the prognosis of clients with cirrhosis.

Nutrition Therapy for Cirrhosis

According to the EASL (2019), a varied healthy eating pattern is recommended for all clients with cirrhosis. Fruit and vegetables to tolerance are encouraged. Other points are as follows (EASL, 2019):

- Other than alcohol, no food is contraindicated because no food actually damages the liver.
- Emphasis should be placed on consuming appropriate calories and adequate protein:
  - Nonobese clients should consume 35 cal/kg/day of actual body weight and at least 1.2 to 1.5 g protein/kg.
  - Clients with obesity should consume a hypocaloric diet that is 500 to 800 cal/day less than their estimated need to promote gradual weight loss of greater than 5% to 10% of body weight. Protein intake should not fall below 1.5 g/kg/ideal body weight to preserve body protein stores.
- Three meals plus 3 snacks daily are recommended. The last snack should be substantial because of overnight fasting.
- Oral nutrition supplements can help achieve an adequate intake.
- Clients with ascites should limit sodium intake to 2 g/day. Effort should be made to ensure overall calorie intake is not reduced due to lower diet palatability.
- Micronutrient supplements may be necessary.

Following are additional considerations for clients with hepatic encephalopathy (EASL, 2019):

- Optimal calorie and protein intake should not be lower than the recommendations for clients with cirrhosis.
- Protein restriction is generally considered detrimental.
- Protein in plants and dairy products may be better tolerated than meats.
- Supplements of branch-chain amino acids may provide neuropsychiatric benefits.
- Clients who are unable to consume an adequate oral intake need EN or PN.

Nutrition Therapy for Liver Transplantation

Liver transplantation is a treatment option for clients with severe and irreversible liver disease. Many clients awaiting a transplant are malnourished. Moderate-to-severe malnutrition increases the risk of complications and death after transplantation. Whenever possible, nutrient deficiencies and imbalances are corrected before the transplantation to promote a positive outcome.

Following are the presurgical recommendations (EASL, 2019):

- Provide 30 cal/kg/day and 1.2 g protein/kg body weight/day for clients with adequate nutritional status. Increase calories to 35 cal/kg and protein to 1.5 g/kg in clients who need nutritional repletion.
- Use standard nutritional regimens because specialized nutrition formulas (e.g., branch-chain amino acid–enriched or immune-enhancing formulas) have not been shown to improve morbidity or morality.

Following are the postsurgical recommendations (EASL, 2019):

- Initiate oral or EN within 12 to 24 hours after surgery, or as soon as possible. PN is used if EN is contraindicated or impractical.
- Provide 35 cal/kg body weight and 1.5 g protein/kg body weight after the acute post-op period.

- Provide 25 cal/kg/day and 2.0 g protein/kg/day for patients with obesity receiving EN or PN.
- Be aware that long-term survivors of liver transplant are at high risk of overweight or obesity and comorbidities of metabolic syndrome.

Pancreatitis
inflammation of the pancreas.

Pancreatitis

The pancreas is responsible for secreting enzymes needed to digest dietary carbohydrates, protein, and fat. Until they are needed, these enzymes are held in the pancreas in their inactive form. Inflammation of the pancreas causes digestive enzymes to be retained in the pancreas and converted to their active form, where they literally begin to digest the pancreas. Because the pancreas also produces insulin, people with pancreatitis may also develop hyperglycemia related to insufficient insulin secretion.

Acute Pancreatitis

Pathobiome
the set of host-associated microbial organisms associated with impaired or potentially impaired health due to interactions between microbial members and the host.

Commensal Microbiome
a living relationship in which one organism derives food or other benefits from the host organism without helping or hurting it.

Severe acute pancreatitis can be triggered by drugs, alcohol, gallstones, or hypertriglyceridemia (McClave, 2019). Inflammation and a subsequent series of events can injure the intestinal mucosa, causing a breakdown of barrier defenses, impaired immune function, development of a virulent **pathobiome**, gut-derived sepsis, and multiple organ failures (McClave, 2019). Innovative treatment strategies have emerged from a better understanding of intestinal failure and the loss of the **commensal microbiome** (McClave, 2019). For instance, shorter use of antibiotics and minimal use of narcotics are suggested because both of these drugs may stimulate virulent pathogen activity.

Nutrition Therapy for Acute Pancreatitis

Current approaches in nutrition therapy are intended to help mitigate disease severity and reduce complications (McClave, 2019). Recommendations for clients with mild-to-moderate acute pancreatitis are as follows (McClave, 2019):

- Encourage an oral diet. Allowing the client to decide when to advance to an oral diet reduces hospital length of stay. Clear liquid diets are not necessary.
- Emulsifying agents found in processed food, such as carboxymethylcellulose or polysorbate 80, should be avoided because they have been shown to reduce the mucus layer of the intestinal tract and promote low-grade virulence of microbiota.

Recommendations for clients with severe acute pancreatitis necessitating intensive care unit (ICU) admission are as follows (McClave, 2019):

- Early initiation of EN via nasogastric route is recommended. EN initiated within 24 to 48 hours is more likely to reduce infection, length of hospital stay, and multiple organ failure than delayed feedings.
- After tolerance to a polymeric formula is established and goal rate is achieved, it is recommended that a whole food formula be used instead. Whole food formulas may reduce systemic infection, decrease growth of pathogens, and lead to greater bacterial diversity in the colon.
- The provision of prebiotics and probiotics may be considered.

Chronic Pancreatitis

Acute pancreatitis that is not resolved or recurs frequently can lead to chronic pancreatitis (CP), an inflammatory disorder that causes irreversible pancreatic damage, resulting in both exocrine and endocrine dysfunction.

- Diabetes, steatorrhea, and malabsorption can result.
- Diarrhea may occur in up to 70% of clients with CP (Sikkens et al., 2012).

- Malnutrition is common and multifactorial and may be due to altered endocrine and exocrine function, significant abdominal pain, delayed gastric emptying, increased metabolism, and often continued alcohol consumption (O'Brien & Omer, 2019).
- Malnutrition significantly affects quality of life and is a component of client disability.

Nutrition Therapy for Chronic Pancreatitis

The commonly experienced problems of inadequate intake and maldigestion/malabsorption contribute to the challenge of nutrition therapy for CP (O'Brien & Omer, 2019).

- Most clients can be managed with an oral diet and pancreatic enzyme replacement.
- Low-fat diets are often recommended to reduce abdominal pain but consideration should be given to the long-term impact this can have on calorie intake and the client's weight.
- A carbohydrate-controlled diet is indicated for clients with diabetes.
- Oral nutrition supplements can help promote an adequate intake of protein and calories.

Gallbladder Disease

The gallbladder plays an important but not vital role in digestion in that it stores and releases bile, which prepares fat for digestion. As bile is held in the gallbladder, water is slowly removed, making it more concentrated and increasing the likelihood that solids (either cholesterol crystals or bilirubin) will precipitate out into hard clumps known as gallstones. Incomplete emptying of the gallbladder may also be involved in gallstone formation. Interestingly, data show that people with obesity who follow a very low-fat diet to achieve weight loss are at higher risk of gallstones and that diets higher in fat may help reduce the risk of gallstones in people trying to lose weight (Stokes et al., 2014).

Cholelithiasis formation of gallstones.

Cholecystitis inflammation of the gallbladder.

- While some people with **cholelithiasis** are asymptomatic, others experience severe abdominal pain, nausea, and vomiting.
- For some people, eating a fatty meal precipitates symptoms; for others, symptoms develop during sleep.
- Gallstones that obstruct the cystic duct can lead to **cholecystitis**, and less commonly, obstructive jaundice, cholangitis, acute pancreatitis, and gangrene of the gallbladder (Madden et al., 2017).

Surgical removal of the gallbladder is the only definitive therapy for acute cholecystitis and the gold standard for treating symptomatic gallstones (Altomare et al., 2017).

- After the gallbladder is removed, secondary bile acids are continuously secreted directly into the small bowel, leading to diarrhea and probably changes in the gut microflora (Altomare et al., 2017).
- A postcholecystectomy syndrome characterized by nausea, bloating, diarrhea, and abdominal pain has been reported to occur in 5% to 40% of people who have had a cholecystectomy (Sagar et al., 2015).

Nutrition Therapy

Clients with symptomatic gallstones are often advised to consume a low-fat diet (<30% total calories from fat) based on the rationale that limiting fat intake reduces stimulation to the gallbladder and minimizes pain. However, there is no published evidence of the benefits of a low-fat diet compared to a regular diet (Madden et al., 2017).

Likewise, there are no evidence-based nutrition therapy recommendations for clients who have had a cholecystectomy. The following advice is commonly given:

- Consume a low-fat diet and reduce the amount of fat at each meal to allow the body time to adapt to the gallbladder's absence (Box 20.12).
- Increase soluble fiber intake, which may help normalize bowel function. Soluble fiber is found in canned fruit; fresh fruit without skins, peels, membranes, and/or seeds; oatmeal; and barley.

- Consider prebiotics and probiotics, especially if the client has diarrhea.
- Consume small meals if reflux is a problem.
- Avoid any foods not tolerated, which may or may not include spicy foods and caffeine.
- Consider micronutrient supplements, particularly of fat-soluble vitamins, to replenish nutrients malabsorbed due to diarrhea.

BOX 20.12 Low-Fat Diet

- Total fat is limited to reduce symptoms of steatorrhea and pain in clients who are intolerant to fat, such as for people with cholecystitis, chronic pancreatitis, radiation enteritis, and SBS.

Guidelines to Achieve a Low-Fat Diet

- Select only very lean meats, fish, and skinless poultry; egg whites; and low-fat egg substitutes.
- Bake, broil, or boil foods instead of frying.
- Use milk and dairy products that provide less than 1 g fat/serving and use low-fat cheese with not more than 3 g fat/serving.
- Enjoy all fruits and vegetables that are prepared without added fat.
- Choose grain products that are prepared without added fat (e.g., avoid muffins, waffles, biscuits, cakes, cookies, doughnuts, pastries, other baked goods, chips, cheese crackers).
- Choose low-fat and fat-free desserts: sherbet, fruit ices, gelatin, angel food cake, vanilla wafers, graham crackers, nonfat ice cream and frozen yogurt, and fruit whips with gelatin.
- Use fats and oils sparingly, including oils, soft margarines, salad dressings, and avocados.

Sample Menu

Breakfast	Lunch	Dinner	Snacks
Orange juice	Fat-free vegetable soup	2 oz broiled lean chicken	Pretzels
Oatmeal with fat-free milk	2 oz of fat-free ham on whole wheat bread with lettuce and fat-free mayonnaise	Brown rice	Fat-free yogurt
Whole wheat toast with jelly	Fresh strawberries	Tossed salad with vegetables and fat-free dressing	Fresh fruit
	Fat-free milk	Steamed broccoli	
		Whole wheat roll with 1 tsp butter	
		Blueberries	
		Fat-free milk	

Potential Problems	Recommended Interventions
Noncompliance related to decreased palatability and satiety from the reduction in fat intake	Encourage the client to eat a variety of foods and to use nonfat and fat-free versions of familiar foods. Encourage use of butter-flavored sprinkles and sprays to season hot vegetables and potatoes.
Persistent symptoms of steatorrhea or pain after eating that are related to fat intolerance	Decrease fat content by eliminating fats and oils and reducing the amount of low-fat meat allowed.
Inadequate intake of iron related to the limited allowance of meat (red meat is the best absorbed source of iron in the diet)	Monitor Hgb and Hct; recommend iron supplements as needed. Encourage a liberal intake of high-iron foods such as fortified cereals and grains and dried peas and beans; advise the client to consume a rich source of vitamin C at each meal to maximize iron absorption.

Client Teaching

Ensure that the client understands the following:

- The total amount of dietary fat must be reduced regardless of the source.
- Sources of fat may be visible (e.g., butter, margarine, shortening, fat on meat, salad dressings) or invisible (e.g., marbled meat, whole milk and whole-milk products, egg yolks, nuts).

(continued)

BOX 20.12 Low-Fat Diet (continued)

- Careful selections when eating out can greatly reduce fat intake.
  - Choose juice or broth-based soup instead of cream soup as an appetizer.
  - Use lemon, vinegar, low-calorie dressing (if available), or fresh-ground pepper on salad, or request that the dressing be brought on the side.
  - Order plain baked or broiled foods.
  - Avoid warm bread and rolls, which absorb more butter than those at room temperature.
  - Order fresh fruit, gelatin, or sherbet for dessert.
  - Request milk for coffee or tea in place of cream and nondairy creamers.
- Various food preparation techniques reduce fat content
  - Trim fat from meat and remove skin from chicken before cooking.
  - Place meats to be baked or roasted on a rack to allow the fat to drain.
  - Rinse oil-packed tuna and salmon.
  - Bake, broil, steam, or sauté foods in a vegetable cooking spray or allowed fats.
  - Cook with bouillon, lemon, vinegar, wine, herbs, and spices instead of adding fat.
  - Make fat-free soup stock and gravies by preparing the stock a day ahead and refrigerating it overnight. The fat will harden and can easily be removed from the surface.
  - Purchase "select" grade meats because they are lower in fat than "choice" and "prime" grades.

NURSING PROCESS Crohn's Disease

Andrew is a 20-year-old man who is admitted to the hospital for suspected CD. His chief complaints are crampy abdominal pain, diarrhea, weight loss, fatigue, and anorexia. He has unintentionally lost 15 pounds since his symptoms began 2 weeks ago. He is prescribed IV fluids, sulfasalazine, prednisone, an antidiarrheal medication, and a diet as tolerated.

Assessment

Medical–Psychosocial History
- Medical and surgical history
- Use of prescribed and over-the-counter medications
- Support system

Anthropometric Assessment
- Height, current weight, usual weight; percentage weight loss; body mass index

Biochemical and Physical Assessment
- Hemoglobin (Hgb), hematocrit (Hct)
- Serum electrolyte levels
- Blood pressure
- Signs of dehydration (poor skin turgor, dry mucous membranes, etc.)

Dietary Assessment
- How has your intake changed since you began experiencing symptoms?
- Do you know if any particular foods cause problems? Did you have any food intolerances or allergies before your symptoms began?
- How many meals per day are you eating?
- How much fluid are you drinking in a day?
- Have you ever followed any kind of diet before?
- Do you take vitamins, minerals, or other supplements?
- Do you use alcohol?
- Who prepares your meals?

Analysis

Possible Nursing Analysis
Malnutrition risk related to anorexia and diarrhea as evidenced by unintentional 15-pound weight loss in 2 weeks

NURSING PROCESS Crohn's Disease (continued)

Planning

Client Outcomes

The client will
- consume adequate calories and protein to restore normal weight,
- experience improvement in symptoms (diarrhea, abdominal pain, fatigue, anorexia),
- maintain normal fluid balance, and
- describe the principles and rationale of nutrition therapy for CD and implement the appropriate interventions.

Nursing Interventions

Nutrition Therapy

- Provide a low-fiber, high-protein, lactose-restricted diet as tolerated.
- Provide lactose-free commercial supplements between meals to enhance protein and calorie intake.
- Encourage high fluid intake, especially of fluids high in potassium such as tomato juice, apricot nectar, and orange juice.
- Promote gradual return to normal diet as tolerated.

Client Teaching

Instruct the client
- on the purpose and rationale of a low-fiber, lactose-restricted diet; advise the client that after the disease goes into remission, dietary restrictions are limited only to items not individually tolerated,
- on the importance of consuming adequate protein, calories, and fluid to promote healing and recovery,
- to maximize intake by eating small, frequent meals,
- to avoid colas and other sources of caffeine because they stimulate peristalsis,
- to eliminate individual intolerances, and
- to communicate any side effects he experiences from the medications.

Evaluation

Evaluate and Monitor

- Percentage of food consumed
- Weight
- Symptoms (diarrhea, abdominal pain, fatigue, anorexia). If client does not tolerate an oral diet, determine whether a defined formula EN feeding is appropriate.
- Fluid and electrolyte balance
- Client knowledge of principles and rationale of nutrition therapy for CD

How Do You Respond?

Is it a good idea to detox or cleanse the gut? Not only is it unnecessary to detox or cleanse the gut, it is also potentially harmful based on the regimen used, such as consuming only juices or water for several days, fasting, taking specific supplements, irrigating the colon, or using enemas or laxatives. The body naturally eliminates toxins through the lungs, kidneys, colon, lymph system, and the liver. There is no convincing evidence that detox or cleansing actually removes toxins from the body or improves health.

Are "live active cultures" the same thing as probiotics? Live active cultures are microorganisms associated with foods that are often used to ferment food. For instance, live active cultures in yogurt refer to the mixture of bacterial species, such as *Lactobacillus acidophilus*, *Lactobacillus bulgaricus*, and *Lactobacillus casei*, that ferment milk into yogurt. Some live active cultures do not survive the fermentation process and therefore do not provide health benefits when consumed. In contrast, probiotics are live microorganisms in foods that have been shown to benefit health when consumed in adequate amounts. Some yogurts contain therapeutic doses of probiotics to provide a health benefit, such as to prevent or treat acute diarrhea.

REVIEW CASE STUDY

Brittany is a 33-year-old woman who was recently diagnosed with IBS. She alternates between episodes of diarrhea and constipation and complains of distention and abdominal pain. Her doctor suggested she eat more fiber and take Metamucil. She dislikes whole wheat bread. She is reluctant to take a fiber supplement; she knows fiber helps people with constipation, and because she also has diarrhea, she believes it will only make her problem worse. She is thinking about adding yogurt to her usual diet to see if that helps. She drinks an "irritable bowel syndrome–friendly tea" that is supposed to help, but she hasn't noticed any improvement.

Her usual intake is as follows:

Breakfast: orange juice, white toast with peanut butter, coffee
Snacks: small bag of chips from the vending machine
Lunch: fast-food hamburger on a bun, small French fries, and diet coke
Snacks: cheese and crackers, glass of wine
Dinner: beef or chicken, mashed potatoes, broccoli, tossed salad with Italian dressing, ice cream, coffee
Snacks: milk and cookies, apples

- What does Brittany need to know about fiber and bowel function? What would you say to her about eating more fiber? About taking a fiber supplement? About yogurt? And about "irritable bowel syndrome–friendly tea?"
- What else do you need to know about Brittany to help relieve her symptoms?
- What other diet interventions could she implement to try to improve her symptoms?
- What foods does Brittany consume that are high in FODMAPs?

STUDY QUESTIONS

1 When developing a teaching plan for a client who has chronic diarrhea, which of the following items would the nurse suggest the client avoid?
   a. tomato juice
   b. whole wheat pasta
   c. saltine crackers
   d. soy milk

2 Which statement indicates the client with cirrhosis needs further instruction about what to eat?
   a. "As with alcohol, certain foods, such as white sugar and white bread, must be avoided because they damage the liver."
   b. "I should eat 3 meals/day and 3 snacks, especially a bedtime snack."
   c. "I may need to limit sodium due to fluid retention."
   d. "I need to be sure I eat enough protein."

3 Which statement indicates the client following a low FODMAP understands instruction about the diet?
   a. "A low-FODMAP diet is the same thing as a gluten-free diet."
   b. "I understand that I can eventually try adding sources of FODMAPs into my diet to test for tolerance."
   c. "The low-FODMAP diet effectively controls symptoms of IBS in all people who adhere to the diet."
   d. "FODMAPs are only found in certain fruits and vegetables so as long as I am careful in choosing those, I can eat items from all other food groups without concern."

4 The nurse knows their instructions have been effective when the client with celiac disease verbalizes that an appropriate breakfast is
   a. eggs and toast
   b. grits with berries
   c. bran flakes cereal with milk
   d. buttermilk pancakes with syrup

5 Which of the following would be most effective in modifying a regular diet to a high-fiber diet?
   a. romaine in place of ice berg lettuce
   b. bran cereal in place of cornflakes
   c. rice in place of mashed potatoes
   d. black beans in place of garbanzo beans

6 Which of the following may be the best tolerated source of calcium for a client who is lactose intolerant?
   a. calcium-fortified orange juice
   b. pudding
   c. cottage cheese
   d. refined breads and cereals

7 A client with fat malabsorption is at risk for which of the following?
   a. calcium oxalate kidney stones
   b. constipation
   c. fatty liver disease
   d. type 2 diabetes

8 Which of the following strategies would help a client achieve a low-fat diet?
   a. Substitute margarine for butter.
   b. Eat nonfat frozen yogurt in place of nonfat frozen ice cream.
   c. Substitute whole wheat bread for white bread.
   d. Prepare chicken by roasting instead of frying.

CHAPTER SUMMARY NUTRITION FOR CLIENTS WITH DISORDERS OF THE LOWER GASTROINTESTINAL TRACT AND ACCESSORY ORGANS

Most nutrient absorption occurs in the first half of the small intestine. Conditions that affect the small intestine can impair the absorption of one or many nutrients. The large intestine absorbs water and electrolytes. Disorders of the colon can cause problems with fluid and electrolyte balance.

Altered Bowel Elimination

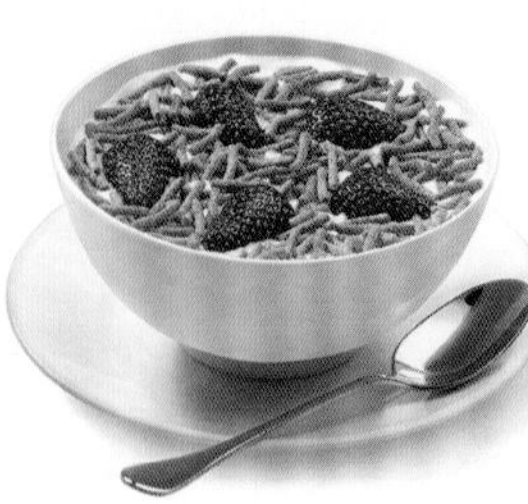

Constipation. Increasing fiber, particularly insoluble fiber in whole grains and bran, can alleviate or prevent most cases of constipation. The amount of fiber needed to promote bowel regularity varies among people.

Diarrhea. Short-term acute diarrhea usually does not require nutrition therapy.

- Avoid clear liquids.
- Avoid items that stimulate peristalsis, such as caffeine, alcohol, high-fiber foods, gassy foods, and sugar alcohols.

Malabsorption Disorders

Lactose Malabsorption. A deficiency or lack of the enzyme lactase causes symptoms of lactose intolerance: cramping, bloating, and diarrhea after consuming lactose.

- Lactose is the naturally occurring sugar in milk.
- Lactase decreases after childhood in many populations.
- Secondary lactose malabsorption occurs secondary to other GI disorders.
- Lactose is restricted to the amount individually tolerated.

Inflammatory Bowel Disease. A group of chronic immune disorders characterized by alternating periods of exacerbation and remission.

- Nutrition may be impacted by poor intake, malabsorption, increased requirements related to systemic inflammation, drug–nutrient interactions, and previous surgeries.
- **During exacerbation:** no specific diet is recommended. Low fiber, high protein, increased calories for weight restoration, if appropriate, and supplemental micronutrients may be advised. EN or PN is used if oral intake is inadequate or contraindicated. Restrictions are liberalized as symptoms improve.
- **During remission:** no specific diet is known to help maintain remission. Many clients consume a low-fiber, low vegetable intake. A Mediterranean diet may be recommended.

Celiac Disease. Chronic autoimmune disorder characterized by inflammation of the proximal small bowel from permanent intolerance to the gluten-containing proteins. Malabsorption of macro- and micronutrients occurs.

- The only treatment is a lifelong gluten-free diet. Gluten is found in wheat, barley, rye, and oats and products made from these grains.
- The diet is highly restrictive, can be difficult to follow, and may cause constipation and nutrient deficiencies.

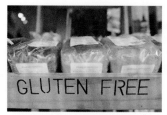

- NCGS causes celiac-like symptoms but without other diagnostic features of celiac disease. It is not known if permanent elimination of gluten from the diet is necessary.

Short Bowel Syndrome. Occurs when the small bowel is surgically shortened to the extent that nutrient absorption is not adequate to meet the client's needs.

- Symptoms include diarrhea, steatorrhea, electrolyte imbalances, dehydration, weight loss, and malnutrition.

CHAPTER SUMMARY NUTRITION FOR CLIENTS WITH DISORDERS OF THE LOWER GASTROINTESTINAL TRACT AND ACCESSORY ORGANS (continued)

- Adaptation occurs during the first 2 years after surgery. Adaptation is promoted with early EN.
- Some clients need PN indefinitely.
- Dietary tolerance varies with the length of small bowel remaining and the health of the remaining bowel.
- An oral diet limits fluid with meals, simple sugars, sugar alcohols, and possibly lactose. Oral rehydration solutions, small frequent meals, and liberal intake of sodium are encouraged. Clients should chew food thoroughly.

Conditions of the Large Intestine

Irritable Bowel Syndrome. A functional disorder characterized by diarrhea, constipation, or alternating periods of each.

- A low-FODMAP diet improves symptoms in many people. After 4 to 6 weeks on the diet, sources of FODMAPs are reintroduced to keep dietary restrictions to a minimum. High-FODMAP foods are not objectively defined or universally agreed upon.

FERMENTABLE
OLIGO–
DI–
MONOSACCHARIDES
AND
POLYOLS

- Other strategies that may help include eating small frequent meals; limiting fat intake; avoiding caffeine, chocolate, and alcohol; and increasing soluble fiber intake gradually.

Diverticular Disease. A spectrum of conditions related to diverticula.

- There is no evidence to support the idea that a low-fiber diet causes DD.
- Some evidence suggests a high-fiber diet may decrease the risk of diverticulitis or its reoccurrence.
- Red meat intake and obesity and weight gain during adulthood increase the risk of diverticulitis.
- A prudent diet may help prevent diverticulitis.
- It is not necessary for clients to avoid nuts, seeds, or popcorn.
- The value of using probiotics has not been determined.

Ileostomies and Colostomies. Surgical creation of a stoma in the small intestine or colon. Ileostomies have a greater impact on nutritional status than do colostomies.

- There are no dietary guidelines for after an ileostomy or colostomy.
- General recommendations include eating small frequent meals and snacks that contain a source of protein; chewing food thoroughly; avoiding foods that may cause a blockage, such as mushrooms, nuts, corn, celery, and dried fruit; and consuming adequate fluid and sodium.
- Output ≥1500 mL/day is considered high output. Following the diet for SBS may be beneficial.

Disorders of the Accessory Gastrointestinal Organs

Liver Disease

Fatty liver disease: occurs from alcohol abuse or secondary to obesity/metabolic syndrome.

- Sustained weight loss is the most effective treatment for NAFLD.
- Alcohol is avoided.
- A Mediterranean diet may help reduce fat in the liver even if weight loss does not occur. It is the most recommended dietary pattern for NAFLD.

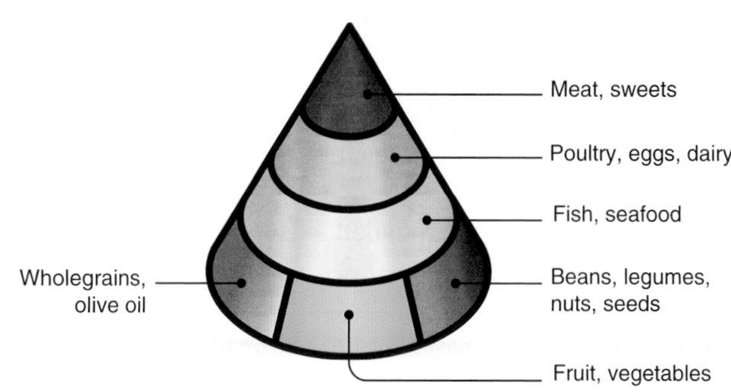

- Coffee exerts a protective effect in NAFLD and is not restricted.
- Bariatric surgery may be considered if lifestyle therapy fails to achieve healthy weight.

Hepatitis: inflammation of the liver frequently caused by certain viruses.

- **Acute hepatitis:** A healthy diet is recommended.
- **Chronic hepatitis:** Small frequent meals and an increased protein intake is recommended. Additional

(continued)

CHAPTER SUMMARY NUTRITION FOR CLIENTS WITH DISORDERS OF THE LOWER GASTROINTESTINAL TRACT AND ACCESSORY ORGANS (continued)

diet modifications are based on symptoms, such as a low-sodium diet for ascites, carbohydrate controlled for diabetes, and low-fat diet for steatorrhea.

Cirrhosis: an irreversible late stage of liver disease characterized by scarring secondary to hepatitis or alcohol abuse.

- Other than alcohol, no food is contraindicated because no food actually damages the liver.
- Adequate calories and protein are emphasized. Clients with obesity should gradually lose weight.
- Three meals plus 3 snacks daily are recommended with a substantial late night snack.
- Oral nutrition supplements can help achieve an adequate intake.
- Sodium is limited if necessary and if it does not compromise adequate intake.
- Micronutrient supplements may be necessary.

Following are considerations for clients with hepatic encephalopathy:

- Calorie and protein intake should not be lower than the recommendations for clients with cirrhosis.
  - Protein restriction is detrimental; however, plant and dairy proteins may be better tolerated than meats.
  - Supplements of branch-chain amino acids may provide neuropsychiatric benefits.
  - EN or PN may be necessary.

Pancreatitis

Acute pancreatitis: inflammation of the pancreas that may be caused by drugs, alcohol, gallstones, or hypertriglyceridemia.

- An oral diet is recommended as soon as the client is able to eat.
- Emulsifiers in processed food should be avoided because they reduce the mucus layer of the GI tract.
- Clients in ICU should be placed on EN within 24 to 48 hours. After tolerance and goal rate are achieved, the polymeric formula should be replaced by a whole food formula.
- Probiotics may be considered.

Chronic pancreatitis: results from recurring or unresolved acute pancreatitis characterized by irreversible anatomical changes and damage.

- Most clients can be managed with an oral diet and pancreatic enzyme replacement.
- Low-fat diets may be used to reduce abdominal pain but may detrimentally impact calorie intake and the client's weight.
- A carbohydrate-controlled diet is indicated for clients with diabetes.
- Oral nutrition supplements may be used.

Gallbladder disease: includes cholelithiasis, cholecystitis, and cholecystectomy.

- Clients with symptomatic gallstones may be advised to consume a low-fat diet (less than 30% total calories from fat) based on the rationale that limiting fat intake reduces stimulation to the gallbladder and minimizes pain. This is not supported by evidence.
- There are no evidence-based nutrition therapy recommendations for clients who have had a cholecystectomy. Strategies that may be recommended include a low-fat diet, an increased intake of soluble fiber, the use of pre- and probiotics, small meals, and eliminating individual food intolerances.

Figure sources: *shutterstock.com/PERLA BERANT WILDER, shutterstock.com/ChameleonsEye, shutterstock.com/mkldesigns, and shutterstock.com/Zern Liew*

Student Resources on thePoint®
For additional learning materials, activate the code in the front of this book at https://thePoint.lww.com/activate

Websites

Celiac Disease Foundation at www.celiac.org
Crohn's and Colitis Foundation of America at www.ccfa.org
Gluten Intolerance Group at www.gluten.net
National Digestive Diseases Information Clearinghouse at http://digestive.niddk.nih.gov
United Ostomy Associations of America, Inc. at www.uoa.org

References

Academy of Nutrition and Dietetics. (2020). *Nutrition care manual.* https://www.nutritioncaremanual.org/

Ahmad, S., Khan, A., Madhotra, R., Exadaktylos, A., Milioto, M., Macfaul, G., & Rostami, K. (2019). Semi-elemental diet is effective in managing high output ileostomy; a case report. *Gastroenterology and Hepatology from Bed to Bench, 12*(2), 169–173.

Altomare, D., Rotelli, M., & Palasciano, N. (2017). Diet after cholecystectomy. *Current Medicinal Chemistry, 24*(00), 1–4. https://doi.org/10.2174/0929867324666170518100053

Arenas Villafranca, J., López-Rodríguez, C., Abilés, J., Rivera, R., Adan, N., & Navarro, P. (2015). Protocol for the detection and nutritional management of high-output stomas. *Nutrition Journal, 14,* 45. https://doi.org/10.1186/s12937-015-0034-z

Böhn, L., Störsrud, S., Törnblom, H., Bengtsson, U., & Simrén, M. (2013). Self-reported food-related gastrointestinal symptoms in IBS are common and associated with more severe symptoms and reduced quality of life. *American Journal of Gastroenterologists, 108*(5), 634–641. https://doi.org/10.1038/ajg.2013.105

Bridges, M., Nasser, R., & Parrish, C. (2019). High output ileostomies: The stakes are higher than the output. *Practical Gastroenterology, XLIII*(9), 20–33. https://med.virginia.edu/ginutrition/wp-content/uploads/sites/199/2019/09/High-Output-Ostomies-September-2019.pdf

Caio, G., Volta, U., Sapone, A., Leffler, D., De Giogio, R., Catassi, C., & Fasano, A. (2019). Celiac disease: A comprehensive current review. *BMC Medicine 17,* 142. https://doi.org/10.1186/s12916-019-1380-z

Cao, Y., Strate, L. L., Keeley, B. R., Tam, I., Wu, K., Giovannucci, E. L., & Chan, A. T. (2018). Meat intake and risk of diverticulitis among men. *Gut, 67*(3), 466–472. https://doi.org/10.1136/gutjnl-2016-313082

Chey, W., Kurlander, J., & Eswaran, S. (2015). Irritable bowel syndrome: A clinical review. *Journal of the American Medical Association, 313*(9), 949–958. https://soi.org/10.1001/jama.2015.0954

Cichewicz, A., Mearns, E., Taylor, A., Boulanger, T., Gerber, M., Leffler, D., Drahos, J., Sanders, D., Craig, K., & Lebwohl, B. (2019). Diagnosis and treatment patterns in celiac disease. *Digestive Diseases and Sciences, 64,* 2095–2106. https://doi.org/10.1007/s10620-019-05528-3

Dahl, C., Crichton, M., Jenkins, J., Nucera, R., Hamoney, S., Marx, W., & Marshall, S. (2018). Evidence for dietary fibre modification in the recovery and prevention of reoccurrence of acute, uncomplicated diverticulitis: A systematic literature review. *Nutrients, 10,* 137. https://doi.org/10.3390/nu10020137

de Oliveira, A., Moreira, A., Netto, M., & Leite, I. (2018). A cross-sectional study of nutritional status, diet, and dietary restrictions among persons with an ileostomy or colostomy. *Ostomy Wound Management, 64,* 18–20. https://doi.org/10.25270/owm.2018.5.1829

European Association for the Study of the Liver. (2019). EASL Clinical practice guidelines on nutrition in chronic liver disease. *Journal of Hepatology, 70,* 172–193. https://doi.org/10.1016/j.jhep.2018.06.024

European Association for the Study of the Liver (EASL), European Association for the Study of Diabetes (EASD), European Association for the Study of Obesity (EASO). (2016). EASL-EASD-EASO Clinical practice guidelines for the management of non-alcoholic fatty liver disease. *Obesity Facts, 9,* 65–90. https://doi.org/10.1159/000443344

Fasano, A., Sapone, A., Zevallos, V., & Schuppan, D. (2015). Nonceliac gluten sensitivity. *Gastroenterology, 148*(6), 1195–1204. https://doi.org/10.1053/j.gastro.2014.12.049

Forbes, A., Escher, J., Hébuterne, X., Klek, S., Krznaric, Z., Schneider, S., Shamir, R., Stardelova, K., Wierdsma, N., Wiskin, A., & Bischoff, S. (2017). ESPEN guideline: Clinical nutrition in inflammatory bowel disease. *Clinical Nutrition, 36*(2), 321–347. https://doi.org/10.1016/j.clnu.2016.12.027

Friedman, S. L., Neuschwander-Tetri, B. A., Rinella, M., & Sanyal, A. J. (2018). Mechanisms of NAFLD development and therapeutic strategies. *Nature Medicine, 24*(7), 908–922. https://doi.org/10.1038/s41591-018-0104-9

Hayes, P., Fraher, M., & Quigley, E. (2014). Irritable bowel syndromes: The role of food in pathogenesis and management. *Gastroenterology & Hepatology, 10*(3), 164–174.

Heaney, R. (2013). Dairy intake, dietary adequacy, and lactose intolerance. *Advances in Nutrition, 4*(2), 151–156. https://doi.org/10.3945/an.112.003368

Kim, S.-E. (2019). Importance of nutritional therapy in the management of intestinal diseases: Beyond energy and nutrient supply. *Intestinal Research, 17*(4), 443–454. https://doi.org/10.5217/ir.2019.00075

Leonard, M., Sapone, A., Catassi, C., & Fasano, A. (2017). Celiac disease and nonceliac gluten sensitivity. A review. *Journal of the American Medical Association, 318*(7), 647–656. https://doi.org/10.1001/jama.2017.9730

Ma, W., Jovani, M., Liu, P.-H., Nguyen, L., Cao, Y., Tam, I., Wu, K., Giovannucci, E., Strate, L., & Chan, A. (2018). Association between obesity and weight change and risk of diverticulitis in women. *Gastroenterology, 155*(1), 58–66. https://doi.org/10.1053/j.gastro.2018.03.057

Madden, A., Trivedi, D., Smeeton, N., & Culkin, A. (2017). Modified dietary fat intake for treatment of gallstone disease. *The Cochrane Database of Systematic Reviews, 2017*(3), CD012608. https://doi.org/10.1002/14651858.CD012608

Matarese, L. (2013). Nutrition and fluid optimization for patients with short bowel syndrome. *Journal of Parenteral and Enteral Nutrition, 37*(2), 161–170. https://doi.org/10.1177/0148607112469818

McClave, S. (2019). Factors that worsen disease severity in acute pancreatitis: Implications for more innovative nutrition therapy. *Nutrition in Clinical Practice, 34*(S1), S43–S48. https://doi.org/10.1002/ncp.10371

Misselwitz, B., Butter, M., Verbeke, K., & Fox, M. (2019). Update on lactose malabsorption and intolerance: Pathogenesis, diagnosis and clinical management. *Gut, 68,* 2080–2091. https://doi.org/10.1136/gutjnl-2019-318404

O'Brien, S., & Omer, E. (2019). Chronic pancreatitis and nutrition therapy. *Nutrition in Clinical Practice, 34*(S1), S13–S26. https://doi.org/10.1002/ncp.10379

Ojetti, V., Petruzziello, C., Cardone, S., Saviano, L., Migneco, A., Santarelli, L., Gabrielli, M., Zaccaria, R., Lopetuso, L., Covino, M., Candelli, M., Gasbarrini, A., & Franceschi, F. (2018). The use of probiotics in different phases of diverticular disease. *Reviews on Recent Clinical Trials, 13*(2), 89–96. https://doi.org/10.2174/1574887113666180402143140

O'Keeffe, M., Jansen, C., Martin, L, Williams, M., Seamark, L., Staudacher, H., Irving, P., Whelan, K., & Lomer, M. (2018). Long-term impact of the low-FODMAP diet on gastrointestinal symptoms, dietary intake, patient acceptability, and healthcare utilization in irritable bowel syndrome. *Neurogastroenterology & Motility, 30*(1), e13154. https://doi.org/10.1111/nmo.13154

Parrish, C., & DiBaise, J. (2017). Managing the adult patient with short bowel syndrome. *Gastroenterology & Hepatology, 13*(10), 600–608.

Pearlman, M., & Akpotaire, A. (2019). Diet and the role of food in common gastrointestinal diseases. *Medical Clinics of North America, 103*(1), 101–110. https://doi.org/10.1016/j.mcna.2018.08.008

Perumpail, B., Khan, M., Yoo, R., Cholankeril, G., Kim, D., & Ahmed, A. (2017). Clinical epidemiology and disease burden of nonalcoholic fatty liver disease. *World Journal of Gastroenterology, 23*(47), 8263–8276. https://doi.org/10.3748/wjg.v23.i47.8263

Pironi, L. (2016). Definitions of intestinal failure and the short bowel syndrome. *Best Practice & Research Clinical Gastroenterology, 30*(2), 175–185. https://doi.org/10.1016/j.bpg.2016.02.011

Romero-Gómez, M., Zelber-Sagi, S., & Trenell, M. (2017). Treatment of NAFLD with diet, physical activity and exercise. *Journal of Hepatology, 67*(4), 829–846. https://doi.org/10.1016/j.jhep.2017.05.016

Sagar, N., Cree, I., Covington, J., & Arasaradnam, R. (2015). The interplay of the gut microbiome, bile acids, and volatile organic compounds. *Gastroenterology Research and Practice*, 2015, Article ID 398585. https://doi.org/10.1155/2015/398585

Sikkens, E., Cahen, D., van Eijck, C., Kuipers, E. J., & Bruno, M. J. (2012). Patients with exocrine insufficiency due to chronic pancreatitis are undertreated: A Dutch national survey. *Pancreatology, 12*, 71–73. https://doi.org/10.1016/j.pan.2011.12.010

Staudacher, H., Irving, P., Lomer, M., & Whelan, K. (2014). Mechanisms and efficacy of dietary FODMAP restriction in IBS. *Nature Reviews Gastroenterology and Hepatology, 11*, 256–266. https://doi.org/10.1038/nrgastro.2013.259

Staudacher, H., Whelan, K., Irving, P., & Lomer, M. (2011). Comparison of symptom response following advice for a diet low in fermentable carbohydrates (FODMAPs) versus standard dietary advice in patients with irritable bowel syndrome. *Journal of Human Nutrition and Dietetics, 24*(5), 487–495. https://doi.org/10.1111/j.1365-277X.2011.01162.x

Stokes, C., Gluud, L., Casper, M., & Lammert, F. (2014). Ursodeoxycholic acid and diets higher in fat prevent gallbladder stones during weight loss: A meta-analysis of randomized controlled trials. *Clinical Gastroenterology and Hepatology, 12*(7), 1090–1100. https://doi.org/10.1016/j.cgh.2013.11.031

Stollman, N. (2017). The importance of being (dietarily) prudent. *Gastroenterology, 152*(5), 934–936. https://doi.org/10.1053/j.gastro.2017.02.025

Stollman, N., Smalley, W., Hirano, I., & American Gastroenterological Association Institute Clinical Guidelines Committee. (2015). American Gastroenterological Association Institute guideline on the management of acute diverticulitis. *Gastroenterology, 149*(7), 1944–1949. https://doi.org/10.1053/j.gastro.2015.10.003

U.S. Food and Drug Administration. (2018). *'Gluten-Free' means what it says.* https://www.fda.gov/consumers/consumer-updates/gluten-free-means-what-it-says

University of Virginia Nutrition, University of Virginia Health System. (2016). *Irritable bowel syndrome.* https://med.virginia.edu/ginutrition/wp-content/uploads/sites/199/2014/04/IBS-Diet-12-2016.pdf

Younossi, Z., Koenig, A., Abdelatif, D., Fazel, Y., Henry, L., & Wymer, M. (2016). Global epidemiology of nonalcoholic fatty liver disease—meta-analytic assessment of prevalence, incidence, and outcomes. *Hepatology, 64*(1), 73–84. https://doi.org/10.1002/hep.28431

Zhang, Y., Li, L., Guo, C., Mu, D., Feng, B., Zuo, X., & Li, Y. (2016). Effects of probiotic type, dose and treatment duration on irritable bowel syndrome diagnosed by Rome III criteria: A meta-analysis. *BMC Gastroenterology, 16*, 62. https://doi.org/10.1186/s12876-016-0470-z

Chapter 21

Nutrition for Clients with Diabetes Mellitus

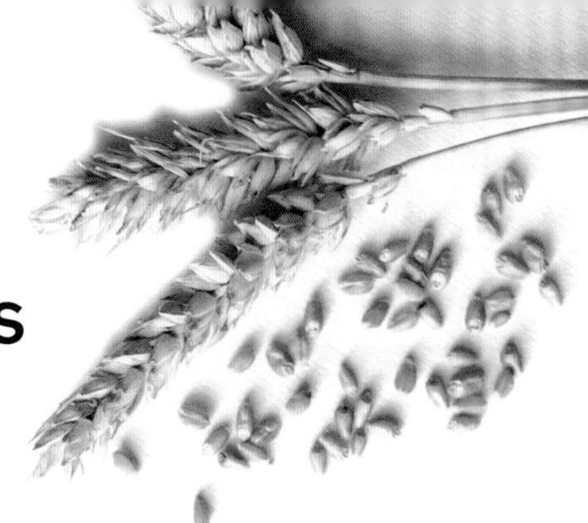

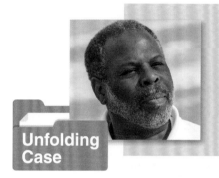

Unfolding Case

Darius Jackson

Darius is the first man in his family to reach the age of 60 years without having a stroke or myocardial infarction. He has had hypertension for decades and was recently diagnosed with type 2 diabetes with a hemoglobin A1c of 9.2%. He was immediately prescribed metformin and a basal insulin regimen of 10 units/day and told to lose weight.

Learning Objectives

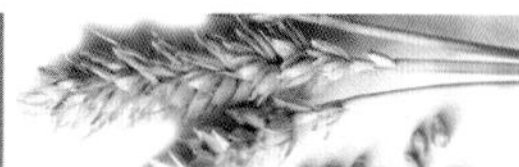

Upon completion of this chapter, you will be able to:

1 Discuss strategies recommended to prevent diabetes.
2 Describe the nutrient and dietary recommendations for managing diabetes.
3 Name eating patterns that are associated with a decrease in A1c levels.
4 Explain meal-planning approach recommendations for adults based on pharmacological therapy.
5 List the characteristics of a consistent carbohydrate diet.
6 Explain carbohydrate choice lists.
7 Describe the plate method of meal planning.
8 Determine the number of carbohydrate choices a serving of food provides by using the "Nutrition Facts" label.
9 Discuss diabetes nutrition therapy in youth and older adults.

Diabetes is one of the most costly and burdensome chronic diseases of our time and is expected to increase in prevalence due at least in part to an aging population, increasing prevalence of overweight and obesity, and growing minority populations that are at higher risk of diabetes. Nutrition therapy is a vital component of diabetes prevention and management. Although medical nutrition therapy is the domain of the registered dietitian nutritionist, all health-care team members need to be knowledgeable in the basic principles of diabetes nutrition therapy so they can facilitate basic meal planning, dispel misconceptions, and reinforce diabetes nutrition education.

This chapter describes nutrition therapy for the treatment of type 1 and type 2 diabetes and also the prevention and treatment of type 2 diabetes. Gestational diabetes is presented in Chapter 12.

DIABETES

Diabetes mellitus is a heterogeneous group of metabolic disorders characterized by hyperglycemia and abnormal insulin metabolism. Absent or ineffective insulin impairs the metabolism of all three macronutrients, resulting in high blood glucose levels, increased levels of fatty acids and triglycerides in the blood, and muscle wasting (Table 21.1). Diagnostic criteria for diabetes appear in Table 21.2.

Table 21.1 Actions of Insulin and Effects of Its Insufficiency

Nutrient	Action of Insulin	Results of Insulin Insufficiency
Glucose	Promotes uptake of glucose into cells Promotes formation of glycogen in the liver and muscle Promotes conversion of excess glucose into triglycerides for storage	Decreases uptake of glucose into muscle and adipose Decreases glycogen formation in liver and muscle Increases glycogen breakdown in liver and muscle Increases gluconeogenesis (the formation of glucose from a noncarbohydrate source, such as amino acids or glycerol) Hyperglycemia
Protein	Promotes uptake of amino acids into tissue protein	Decreases uptake of amino acids into muscle Decreases protein synthesis Increases protein breakdown
Fat	Promotes formation of adipose from excess fat	Increases production of ketones in the liver Decreases formation of triglycerides in adipose Increases triglyceride breakdown in adipose Increases serum triglyceride and fatty acid levels

Table 21.2 Diagnostic Criteria for Diabetes and Prediabetes

	Fasting Plasma Glucose		Oral Glucose Tolerance		A1c Blood Test
Prediabetes	100–120 mg/dL	or	140–100 mg/dL	or	5.7%–6.4%
Diabetes	≥126 mg/dL	or	≥200 mg/dL	or	≥6.5%

Source: American Diabetes Association. (2020a). Classification and diagnosis of diabetes: Standards of Medical Care in Diabetes—2020. *Diabetes Care*, *43*(Suppl. 1), S14–S31. https://doi.org/10.2337/dc20-S002

The statistics of diabetes prevalence are staggering (Centers for Disease Control and Prevention [CDC], 2020a, 2020b). Crude estimates for 2018 were as follows:

- 34.1 million Americans aged 18 or older had diabetes (13% of all U.S. adults).
- 7.3 million adults aged 18 or older who met laboratory criteria for diabetes were not aware of or did not report having diabetes.
- 88 million adults aged 18 or older had prediabetes.

Type 1 Diabetes
diabetes characterized by the absence of insulin secretion.

Polyuria
excessive urine excretion.

Polydipsia
excessive thirst.

Polyphagia
excessive appetite.

Ketoacidosis
the accumulation of ketone bodies leading to acidosis related to incomplete breakdown of fatty acids from carbohydrate deficiency or inadequate carbohydrate utilization.

Type 1 Diabetes

Type 1 diabetes, formerly known as insulin-dependent diabetes mellitus, is characterized by the absence of insulin. It accounts for 5% to 10% of diabetes cases. Although type 1 can occur at any age, it is most often diagnosed before the age of 18 years. Type 1 diabetes occurs from an autoimmune response that damages or destroys pancreatic beta cells, leaving them unable to produce insulin. Interaction between genetic susceptibility and environmental factors, such as viral infection, is thought to be responsible. The classic symptoms of **polyuria**, **polydipsia**, and **polyphagia** appear abruptly. Sometimes, the first sign of the disease is **ketoacidosis**. There is no known way to prevent type 1 diabetes. All people with type 1 diabetes require exogenous insulin.

Insulin Resistance
decreased cellular response to insulin.

Type 2 Diabetes

Type 2 diabetes, previously referred to as non–insulin-dependent diabetes, accounts for 90% to 95% of diagnosed cases of diabetes. Although it is most often diagnosed after the age of 45 years, the rising prevalence of obesity in youth has led to an increase in type 2 diabetes in young adults and adolescents (Sattar et al., 2019).

Unlike type 1 diabetes, in which there is a relatively abrupt and absolute end to insulin production, type 2 diabetes is a slowly progressive disease characterized by a combination of peripheral **insulin resistance** and relative insulin deficiency. When cells do not respond to

Impaired Fasting Glucose fasting plasma glucose levels of 100 to 125 mg/dL.

Impaired Glucose Tolerance 2-hour values in the oral glucose tolerance test of 140 to 199 mg/dL.

Hyperinsulinemia elevated blood levels of insulin.

Metabolic Syndrome (MetS) a clustering of interrelated risk factors that includes hypertension, low high-density lipoprotein (HDL) cholesterol, high triglycerides levels, elevated serum glucose, and central or abdominal obesity, as indicated by waist circumference.

insulin as they should, the pancreas compensates by secreting higher than normal levels of insulin but not high enough to lower serum glucose to normal levels. **Impaired fasting glucose** and **impaired glucose tolerance** occur despite high levels of circulating insulin. Over time, chronic **hyperinsulinemia** leads to a decrease in the number of insulin receptors on the cells and a further reduction in tissue sensitivity to insulin. Insulin production progressively falls to a deficient level, and frank type 2 diabetes develops. Because hyperglycemia develops gradually in type 2 diabetes and is often not severe enough for clients to recognize any of the classic diabetes symptoms, type 2 diabetes may go undiagnosed for years. Undiagnosed clients are at increased risk of developing microvascular and macrovascular complications (American Diabetes Association [ADA], 2020a).

Although the exact cause of type 2 diabetes is unknown, genetic and environmental factors, such as being 45 years of age or older; overweight; physically inactive; or a member of a high-risk racial or ethnic group, such as people who are African American, Latino, Native American, Asian American, or Pacific Islander; and having a history of gestational diabetes, are contributing factors (ADA, 2020a). **Metabolic syndrome (MetS)** is a cluster of risk factors, such as central obesity, insulin resistance, dyslipidemia, and hypertension that, when combined, increases the risk of type 2 diabetes fivefold and cardiovascular disease (CVD) threefold (O'Neill & O'Driscoll, 2015).

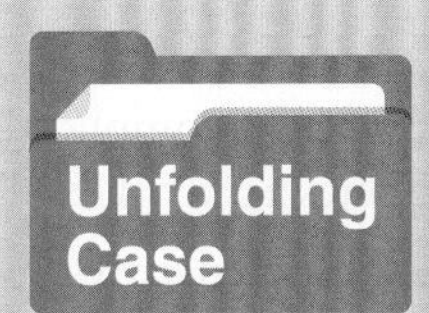

Consider Darius. He is 5 ft 10 in. tall. At the time of diagnosis, he weighed 205 pounds. He wants to lose weight to get off insulin. What is his body mass index (BMI)? What risk factors does he have for type 2 diabetes? How much weight should he initially lose? Is it possible for him to manage his diabetes without insulin?

Prediabetes

Prediabetes describes the condition where glucose levels are not high enough to reach the criteria for diabetes but are too high to be considered normal (Table 21.2). Rather than viewed as a clinical entity, prediabetes should be considered an increased risk for diabetes and CVD (ADA, 2020a). Prediabetes is associated with MetS.

Because of the strong link between excess weight and insulin resistance/type 2 diabetes, modest weight loss is the primary focus of diabetes prevention. Several major randomized controlled trials show that lifestyle and behavioral therapy that includes an individualized hypocaloric meal plan, a healthy eating pattern (e.g., Mediterranean-style, Dietary Approaches to Stop Hypertension [DASH] diet, or vegetarian diet), and physical activity is highly effective in preventing type 2 diabetes and improving cardiometabolic markers such as blood pressure, lipid levels, and inflammation (ADA, 2020b). One such trial is the Diabetes Prevention Program that is summarized in Box 21.1.

Long-Term Diabetes Complications

Sustained hyperglycemia, regardless of what type of diabetes causes it, alters glucose metabolism in virtually every tissue. Damage to small vessels (microvascular) can lead to retinopathy, nephropathy, and neuropathy. Large blood vessel (macrovascular) damage increases the risk of CVD. In fact, atherosclerotic cardiovascular disease (ASCVD) (coronary heart disease, cerebrovascular disease, or peripheral arterial disease) is the leading cause of morbidity and mortality for people with diabetes (ADA, 2020c). Other diabetes complications include impaired wound healing, gangrene, periodontal disease, and increased susceptibility to other illnesses.

Intensive glucose control has been shown to

- significantly lower the rates of development and progression of microvascular complications in clients with type 1 diabetes (Diabetes Control and Complications Trial Research Group, 1993),

BOX 21.1 The Diabetes Prevention Program: What It Was and What It Showed

What it was: It was a major, multicenter, randomized controlled trial in a diverse group of overweight people with impaired glucose tolerance.

- The 2 major goals of the intensive, behavioral lifestyle intervention were to achieve a minimum weight loss of 7% at a rate of 1 to 2 pounds/week and 150 minutes/week of physical activity of the intensity of brisk walking.
- All participants were given the same goals.
- The program was individual based, not group based.
- The core curriculum was 16 sessions completed in 24 weeks.

What is showed:

- The program lowered the incidence of type 2 diabetes by 58% over 3 years (Knowler et al., 2002).
- Average weight loss among study participants was a modest 5% to 7% of initial weight.
- Participants were also benefited from improvements in their lipid profiles, blood pressure, and markers of inflammation (Haffner et al., 2005; Ratner et al., 2005).
- A 10-year follow-up on the original participants showed that the lifestyle intervention group maintained a decreased risk of diabetes over time (Diabetes Prevention Program Research Group, 2009).

- significantly lower the rates of microvascular complications in clients with short-duration type 2 diabetes (UK Prospective Diabetes Study [UKPDS] Group, 1998), and
- provide a cardiovascular benefit when initiated early the course of type 1 diabetes (Nathan et al., 2005).

LIFESTYLE MANAGEMENT

Diabetes is a progressive disease that requires lifelong treatment. Lifestyle management, encompassing effective behavior management and psychological well-being, is fundamental to achieving treatment goals for people with diabetes (ADA, 2020d). Lifestyle management components discussed in the following section are **diabetes self-management education and support (DSMES)**, medical nutrition therapy, and physical activity. Lifestyle strategies not discussed here are smoking cessation and psychosocial care (ADA, 2020d).

Diabetes Self-Management Education and Support (DSMES)
the process of facilitating the knowledge, skill, and ability needed to self-manage diabetes and the support needed to implement and maintain skills on an ongoing basis.

Diabetes Self-Management Education and Support

It is recommended that all people with diabetes participate in DSMES at diagnosis and thereafter as needed to learn and sustain the knowledge, skills, and ability needed to manage diabetes self-care (ADA, 2020d). Examples of self-care behaviors include healthy eating, being active, monitoring glucose and eating, taking medication, problem-solving, and healthy coping. Critical times to assess, provide, and fine-tune DSMES are at diagnosis, annually, when new complicating factors arise (e.g., a change in health or physical ability), and during transitions (e.g., changes in living situation or insurance coverage) (ADA, 2020d).

Although DSMES has been shown to lower A1c, improve quality of life, reduce all-cause mortality risk, and reduce health-care costs, only 5% to 7% of people eligible for DSMES through Medicare or a private insurance plan actually receive it (ADA, 2020d). Initial and ongoing diabetes education is vital to empowering clients with the tools necessary to optimize self-care.

Medical Nutrition Therapy

Individualized medical nutrition therapy is recommended for all people with type 1 or type 2 diabetes and prediabetes whether or not medication is used and regardless of weight status.

Atherosclerotic Cardiovascular Disease (ASCVD)
diseases of the cardiovascular system caused by atherosclerosis, which is the accumulation of plague within arteries. ASCVD includes acute coronary syndromes, myocardial infarction, stable or unstable angina, coronary or other arterial revascularization, stroke, transient ischemic attack, or peripheral arterial disease.

Because **atherosclerotic cardiovascular disease (ASCVD)** is the most common cause of death among adults with diabetes, nutrition therapy for diabetes includes strategies to reduce the risk of ASCVD. The goals of nutrition therapy for adults with diabetes are to (ADA, 2020d)

- Promote and support healthful eating patterns to
  - improve overall health;
  - attain and maintain body weight goals;
  - achieve individualized goals for glucose, lipids, and blood pressure;
  - delay or prevent diabetes complications;
- individualize a nutrition plan consistent with the clients' preferences and culture, health literacy, access to healthy foods, willingness and ability to change, and barriers to change;
- preserve pleasure in eating; and
- provide practical tools for developing healthy eating patterns rather than concentrating on individual macronutrients, micronutrients, or single foods.

Weight Management

Losing and maintaining weight are recommended for all overweight and obese people with type 1, type 2, or prediabetes. There is strong evidence that weight loss is highly effective in preventing the progression from prediabetes to type 2 diabetes and in managing cardiometabolic health in type 2 diabetes (Evert et al., 2019). Overweight and obesity are also becoming increasingly prevalent in people with type 1 diabetes.

- For people with prediabetes: A weight loss goal of 7% to 10% of body weight is recommended to prevent the progression to type 2 diabetes (ADA, 2020d).
- For people with type 1 diabetes who are overweight or obese: Improvements in A1c and lipid levels are benefits of sustained weight loss. The use of insulin complicates weight loss efforts (ADA, 2020d).
- For many overweight and obese people with type 2 diabetes: A modest weight loss of 5% of body weight is recommended to achieve clinical improvements in glycemic control, blood pressure, and/or blood lipid levels (Macleod et al., 2017).
  - Weight loss benefits are dose related; more intense weight loss goals (e.g., >15%) may be indicated (ADA, 2020d).
  - A deficit of 500 to 750 cal/day or total calorie intake of 1200 to 1500 cal/day for women and 1500 to 1800 cal/day for men is appropriate for most people.
  - The "best" weight-loss eating pattern is one the client will be able to maintain.
  - Additional strategies may be appropriate in carefully selected patients (ADA, 2020e):
    - Very low-calorie diets (<800 cal/day) and meal replacements used for a short term.
    - Adjunct use of weight loss medications (see Chapter 17).
    - Metabolic surgery may be an option of adults who do not achieve durable weight loss and improvement in comorbidities (see Chapter 17).

Nutrients and Dietary Recommendations

- People with diabetes generally have the same nutritional requirements as the general population, and dietary recommendations to promote health and well-being in the general public—lose weight if overweight, eat a variety of nutrient-dense foods; limit saturated fat, trans fat, sodium, and added sugars; eat more fiber—are also appropriate for people with diabetes. An ideal macronutrient composition for all people with diabetes has not been determined, nor is there a universal "diabetic diet" that is recommended for all people with diabetes (ADA, 2020d).
- The ADA's nutrition therapy recommendations are summarized in Box 21.2.

BOX 21.2 Nutrition Therapy Recommendations for People with Diabetes

Carbohydrate

- Although the rise in glucose that occurs after eating is primarily determined by the amount of carbohydrates consumed (and the amount of available insulin), the ideal amount of carbohydrate intake for people with diabetes is unknown (ADA, 2020d).
- Growing evidence shows that lowering overall carbohydrate intake improves glycemic control for people with diabetes and prediabetes; however, "low carb" is not definitively defined (Evert et al., 2019).
- Consistent with recommendations for the general population, nutrient-dense and high-fiber sources of carbohydrate should be chosen whenever possible over refined or processed carbohydrates with added sodium, fat, and sugar.
- The majority of carbohydrate calories should come from fruit, vegetables, whole grains, and legumes.
- Study results are mixed on whether using low-glycemic index eating patterns improves glucose levels.

Fiber

- Fiber intake should be at least as much as the amount recommended for the general population (14 g fiber/1000 calories) with at least ½ of all grain choices being whole grains.

Added Sugar

- Sugar-sweetened beverages, including fruit juices, should be avoided to help control glucose levels and weight and reduce the risk of CVD and fatty liver.
- The intake of foods with added sugar should be minimized to avoid displacing the intake of nutrient-dense foods.

Protein

- Usual protein intake (typically 1.0–1.5 g/kg/day or 15%–20% of total calorie intake) seems to be appropriate for clients who do not have diabetic kidney disease.
- For people with diabetic kidney disease, the RDA for protein (0.8 g/kg) should be maintained. Lowering protein intake beyond this amount does not improve glycemic control, CVD risk factors, or the rate of glomerular filtration rate decline (ADA, 2020d).

Fat

- The ideal total fat intake for people with diabetes is not known; the type of fat consumed is more important than the total amount.
- A Mediterranean-Style Eating Pattern that is rich in polyunsaturated and monounsaturated fats can improve glucose control and lower CVD risks and may be an effective alternative to a low-fat, high-carbohydrate eating pattern (ADA, 2020d).
- Recommendations to eat less saturated fat and trans fat are appropriate for the general population, including people with diabetes.
- Eating omega-3 fatty acids in fatty fish (DHA and EPA) and nuts and seeds (ALA) is recommended to prevent or treat CVD. The routine use of omega-3 supplements is not supported by evidence.

Sodium

- The general population, including people with diabetes, is advised to limit sodium intake to <2300 mg/day (Evert et al., 2019).
- Limiting intake to <1500 mg is generally not recommended, even for those with hypertension (ADA, 2020d).

Micronutrients and Herbal Supplements

- Unless there is an underlying nutrient deficiency, there is no clear evidence that taking supplements of micronutrients (e.g., vitamins and minerals) or herbal supplements provides benefits for people with diabetes (ADA, 2020d).

Alcohol

- Moderate alcohol intake has minimal long-term detrimental effects on blood glucose control in people with diabetes (ADA, 2020d).
- Adults with diabetes who choose to drink alcohol should follow the same guidelines as for those people who do not have diabetes: limit intake to one drink per day or less for women and two drinks per day or less for men.
- Delayed hypoglycemia is a risk, especially in people who take insulin or insulin secretagogues.
- Consuming alcohol with food can minimize the risk of nocturnal hypoglycemia (Evert et al., 2019).

BOX 21.2 Nutrition Therapy Recommendations for People with Diabetes (continued)

Nonnutritive Sweeteners

- Nonnutritive sweeteners, such as saccharin, aspartame, acesulfame potassium, and sucralose, may be acceptable alternatives to caloric sweeteners for people with diabetes when used in moderation (ADA, 2020d).
- Using them does not guarantee weight loss.
- People are encouraged to consume water in place of sugar-sweetened and nonnutritive-sweetened beverages.

Source: American Diabetes Association. (2020d). Facilitating behavior change and well-being to improve health outcomes: Standards of medical care in diabetes—2020. *Diabetes Care*, *43*(suppl 1), S48–S65. https://doi.org/10.2337/dc20-S005; Evert, A., Dennison, M., Gardner, C., Garvey, W. T., Lau, K. H., MacLeod, J., Mitri, J., *Pereira*, R. F., Rawlings, K., Robinson, S., Saslow, L., Uelmen, S., Urbanski, P. B., & Yancy, W. S. (2019). Nutrition therapy for adults with diabetes or prediabetes: A consensus report. *Diabetes Care*, *42*(5), 731–754. https://doi.org/10.2337/dci19-0014

Eating Patterns

Personal preferences (e.g., culture, religion, economics), health status, metabolic goals, and ability to sustain the eating pattern should be used to determine the best eating pattern for the individual.

- No single eating pattern has been proven to be consistently better than any other.
- Eating patterns associated with a decrease in A1c include the Mediterranean diet, vegetarian and vegan diets, DASH diet, and low-carb and very low-carb diets (Evert et al., 2019).
- Total calorie intake is important regardless of the type of eating pattern selected.
- Regardless of the specific eating pattern chosen,
  - nutrient-dense foods are emphasized: fruit, vegetables, legumes, lean proteins, nuts, and whole grains;
  - added sugars and refined grains are minimized; and
  - whole foods are chosen over highly processed foods.

Meal-Planning Approaches

Managing carbohydrate intake is a primary strategy for achieving glycemic control (MacLeod et al., 2017). Meal-planning approaches to manage carbohydrate intake include carbohydrate counting, the plate method, and food lists. Any of these approaches can be used to implement a healthy eating pattern, such as Mediterranean-style, DASH, vegetarian or vegan, or low-carbohydrate eating patterns. Meal-planning approach recommendations are based on the client's pharmacological treatment (Table 21.3) and consider the client's literacy and numeracy abilities, preferences, and management goals (Evert et al., 2019; McLeod et al., 2017).

Carbohydrate Counting

Carbohydrate counting has become a mainstay meal-planning approach and is fundamental to diabetes self-management in clients on insulin. In clients with type 1 diabetes, it has been shown to significantly decrease A1c concentration compared to other meal-planning approaches (Fu et al., 2016).

- Foods containing carbohydrates are counted as carbohydrate choices. One carbohydrate choice provides 15 g of carbohydrate per specified serving size.
- Clients are given a meal plan based on their calorie needs that specifies the number of carbohydrate choices to consume at each meal and snack.
- Clients choose whatever carbohydrate sources they want (Box 21.3) as long as they adhere to their choice allotment.

Table 21.3 Meal-Planning Approach Recommendations for Adults Based on Pharmacological Therapy

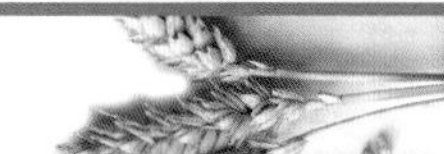

Pharmacological Therapy	Meal-Planning Approach Recommendation	Rationale for Recommendation
Multiple daily injections of insulin or insulin pump therapy	Carbohydrate counting using insulin-to-carbohydrate ratios	Shown to result in significant decreases in A1c and significant increases in quality of life with continued maintenance of these improvements for up to 44 months with no significant change in weight using this approach
Fixed insulin doses or insulin secretagogues	Emphasis on consistency in the timing and amount of carbohydrate intake using any of the following: Carbohydrate counting Plate method with portion control and a simplified meal plan Food lists and carbohydrate choices	In people using fixed insulin doses or insulin secretagogues, consistent carbohydrate intake can improve glycemic control and lower the risk of hypoglycemia
No diabetes medication (e.g., treated with lifestyle alone) or medications other than secretagogues	Any of the following: Carbohydrate counting Plate method with portion control and a simplified meal plan Food lists and carbohydrate choices	Monitoring carbohydrate intake remains vital for glycemic control A simple healthful eating plan approach may be best suited for clients with type 2 diabetes who have low health literacy or numeracy skills

Source: MacLeod, J., Franz, M., Handu, D., Gradwell, E., Brown, C., Evert, A., Reppert, A., & Robinson, M. (2017). Academy of Nutrition and Dietetics Nutrition Practice Guidelines for type 1 and type 2 diabetes in adults: Nutrition intervention evidence reviews and recommendations. *Journal of the Academy of Nutrition and Dietetics*, *117*(10), 1637–1658. https://doi.org/10.1016/j.jand.2017.03.022

- Clients are taught how to estimate portion sizes and how to use the "Nutrition Facts" label for an accurate estimation of carbohydrate content when available (Fig. 21.1).
- Box 21.4 features characteristics of a consistent carbohydrate diet and the number of carbohydrate choices recommended based on total calorie allotment.
- Guidance is provided on the amount and types of protein foods and fat to consume. Although only carbohydrates are "counted," patients are encouraged to maintain a consistent intake of protein and fat because they also require insulin for metabolism, provide calories, and are essential nutrients.
- The two levels of carbohydrate counting are basic and advanced.

BOX 21.3 Sources of Carbohydrates

Carbohydrates that count as 1 carbohydrate choice (15 g carbohydrate) when consumed in a specified amount. Amounts vary by item.

- Bread, rolls, crackers
- Grains (e.g., rice) and cereals (cooked and ready to eat)
- Pasta
- Starchy vegetables (e.g., corn, peas, potatoes)
- Fruit—fresh, frozen, canned, or juice
- Milk and yogurt
- Sweets and desserts (e.g., brownie, ice cream, granola bar)

Nonstarchy vegetables provide 5 g carbohydrate in a typical serving. Three servings are counted as 1 carbohydrate choice.

- Fresh, canned, or frozen varieties of nonstarchy vegetables such as asparagus, carrots, green beans, summer squash, and tomatoes
- Vegetable juice
- Salad greens

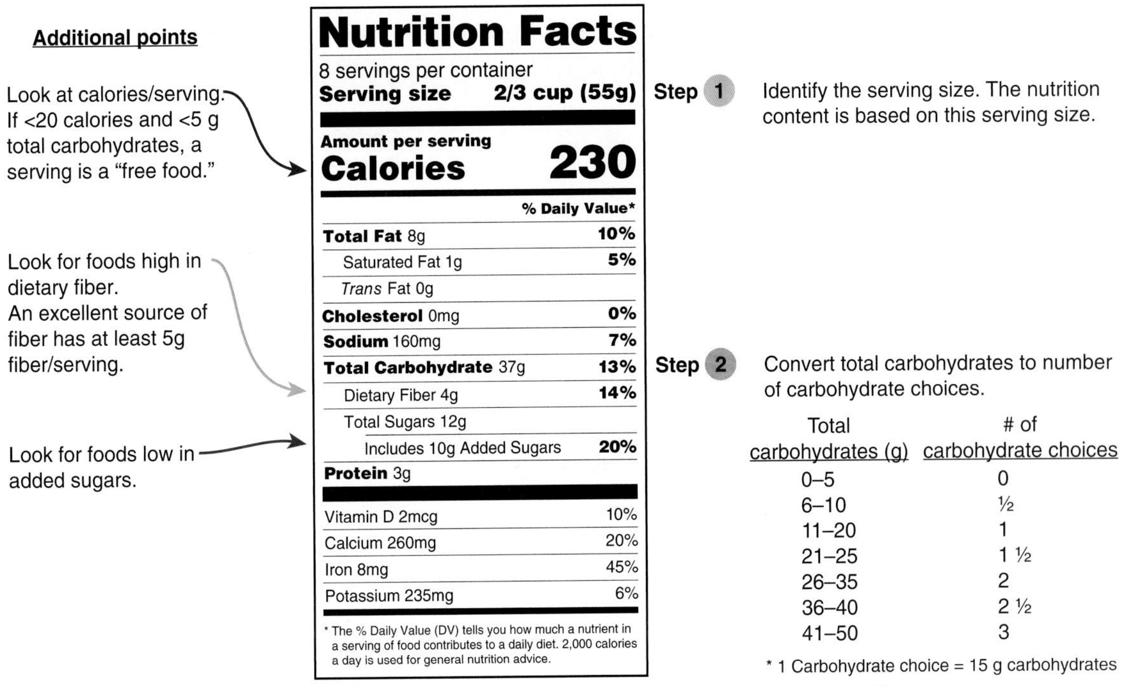

Figure 21.1 ▲ **Label reading for carbohydrate counting.**

BOX 21.4 Consistent Carbohydrate Diet

Characteristics

- Total calorie intake is individualized.
- The number of carbohydrate choices may differ between meals (e.g., more for dinner than for breakfast) but should be consistent from day to day.
- No foods are omitted. If sugar-sweetened foods are used, the serving size is based on carbohydrate content of the item and the grams of carbohydrate allotted.
- Clients should consume a variety of carbohydrate sources (e.g., starches, vegetables, fruit, milk) and variety within each food group to ensure an adequate nutritional intake.
- Typical ranges of carbohydrate choices for meals and snacks are as follows:

Total Calories/Day	Carbohydrate Choices/Meal	Carbohydrate Choices/Snack (If Desired)
1200–1500 (for weight loss)	3 (45 g)	1 (15 g)
1600–2000 (for weight control)	4 (60 g)	1–2 (15–30 g)
2100–2400 (for active people)	5 (75 g)	1–2 (15–30 g)

Basic Carbohydrate Counting

Basic carbohydrate counting is a structured approach with a focus on consistency in the timing and amount of carbohydrates consumed.

- This approach is recommended for clients who take fixed doses of insulin, take oral diabetes medications, or manage their diabetes with lifestyle changes alone.
- Clients use a meal pattern that is consistent from day to day.
- Although the daily amount and timing of carbohydrate consumption remain constant, there should be variety in the type of carbohydrates chosen.
- Two sample menus that count carbohydrates in an 1800-calorie meal pattern are featured in Box 21.5.

BOX 21.5 Carbohydrate Counting: Samples of 1800-Calorie Menus

Sample Menu	Carbohydrate Choices	Sample Menu	Carbohydrate Choices
Breakfast			
½ cup orange juice	1	A parfait consisting of	
1 low-fat waffle	1	1¼ cup whole strawberries	1
Topped with ¾ cup blueberries	1	½ cup granola	2
1 cup nonfat milk	1	6 oz artificially sweetened vanilla Greek yogurt	1
1 tsp light margarine		Coffee	
Lunch			
6-in. submarine with 2 oz meat and light mayonnaise	3	Hamburger on a hamburger bun	2
1 apple	1	1 cup oven-baked French fries	1
Calorie-free soft drink		Lettuce and tomato	
		Light mayonnaise	
		1 cup nonfat milk	1
Dinner			
2 taco shells (each 5 in diameter)	1	⅔ cup spaghetti noodles	2
		2 meatballs	
3 oz taco meat		½ cup spaghetti sauce	1
2 cups combined lettuce, tomato, onion	1	Tossed salad	
		1 slice Italian bread	
⅓ cup rice	1	1 tsp butter	1
1 cup cubed papaya	1	Calorie-free soft drink	
Bedtime Snack			
½ cup shredded wheat	1	3 cups added popcorn	1
1 cup nonfat milk	1	Calorie-free flavored seltzer water	
Total carbohydrate choices/day	14		13

Note. 4 carbohydrate choices/meal, 1–2 carbohydrate choices per snack.

Basal Insulin
insulin injected once or twice a day to regulate glucose levels between meals. Types include the intermediate-acting insulin NPH (e.g., Humulin N, Novolin N), long-acting insulin (e.g., glargine/Lantus), and ultra-long–acting insulin (e.g., degludec/Tresiba).

Bolus Insulin
the rapid-acting insulin injected, such as aspart (Novolog), lispro (Humalog), and glulisine (Apidra), at mealtimes to counteract the rise in blood glucose after eating.

Insulin-to-Carbohydrate Ratio (ICR)
the number of units of rapid-acting insulin needed to handle a specific number of grams of carbohydrate consumed. An ICR of 1:15 means that 1 unit of rapid-acting insulin is needed for each 15 g of carbohydrate consumed.

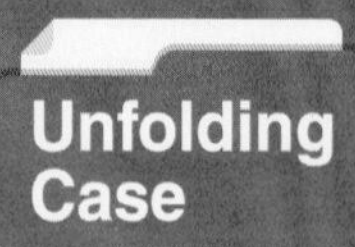

Think of Darius. He has been counseled on basic carbohydrate counting and has a meal pattern that allows him four carbohydrate choices per meal and two for a bedtime snack. His usual dinner is 4 pieces of thick crust cheese and pepperoni pizza and a sugar-free soft drink. He was shocked to learn that each piece of pizza counts as 2½ carbohydrate choices. How can Darius continue to enjoy pizza and still adhere to his meal plan?

Advanced Carbohydrate Counting

Advanced carbohydrate counting is more flexible than basic carbohydrate counting in that it gives the client the freedom to choose how much carbohydrate they want to eat at each meal and the responsibility to calculate the corresponding insulin dose.

- Advanced carbohydrate counting is best suited to clients who take multiple daily injections of insulin (e.g., **basal insulin** 1 to 2 times/day and **bolus insulin** at meals) or use an insulin pump.
- Clients are taught how to determine their bolus insulin dose according to the amount of carbohydrate consumed based on a given **insulin-to-carbohydrate ratio (ICR)**. For instance, if a meal provides 45 g of carbohydrate and the individual's ICR is 1:15, the amount of bolus insulin needed is 3 units of rapid-acting insulin (45 divided by 15 = 3).

- Insulin pumps are programmed with the individual's ICR; the client simply inputs the amount of carbohydrates they will eat, and the pump calculates and secretes the appropriate bolus dose.
- Patients are able to adjust the bolus insulin dose to compensate for deviations in preprandial glucose levels.

Plate Method for Meal Planning

The plate method for meal planning with portion control serves as a simple approach to meal planning.

- This approach is suited to people who have difficulty understanding health and math concepts. It may also be an effective strategy for older adults.
- A 9" dinner plate is used to illustrate healthy balance and portion control (Fig. 21.2).
- Additional guidance is provided on healthy foods to emphasize (e.g., whole grains, lean meats) and nutrients to limit (e.g., salt, added sugar, saturated fat).
- Accurate estimation of portion sizes is stressed (see sections Food Lists for Diabetes and Estimating Portion Size).

Food Lists for Diabetes

The *Choose Your Foods: Food Lists for Diabetes* is a meal-planning approach that groups foods into lists that, per serving size given, are similar in carbohydrate, protein, fat, and calories based on rounded averages (ADA & Academy of Nutrition and Dietetics, 2019).

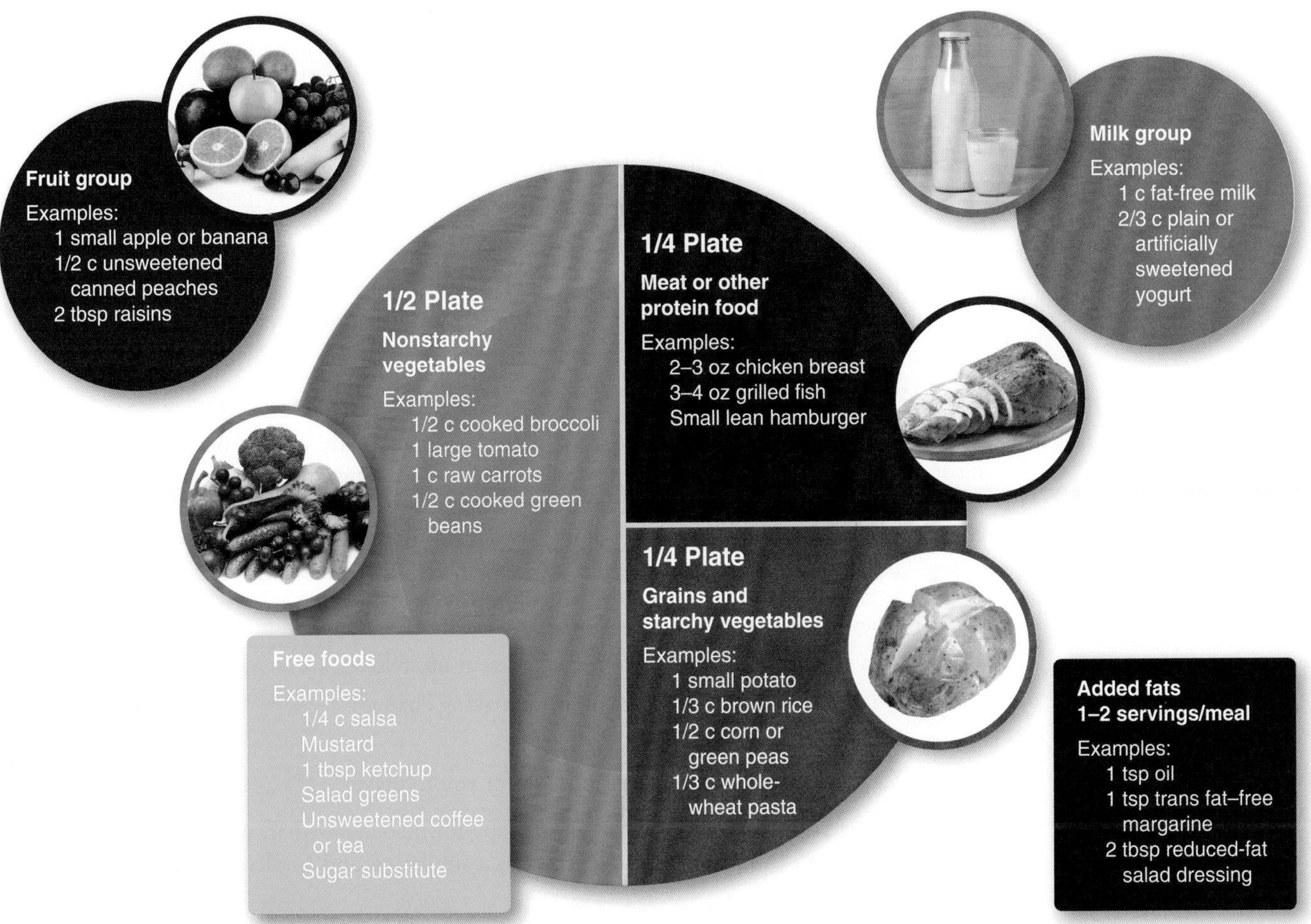

Figure 21.2 ▲ **The plate method of meal planning.**

- Its three major categories are carbohydrates, protein, and fats.
  - The carbohydrate list includes sub-lists for starch, fruit, milk, nonstarchy vegetables, and sweets/desserts/other carbohydrates.
  - The protein list has sub-lists for lean, medium-fat, high-fat, and plant-based proteins.
  - The fat list is divided into 3 sub-lists based on whether they predominately provide saturated, monounsaturated, or saturated fat.
- An individualized meal plan specifies the number of servings allowed from each list for each meal and snack.
- Any food (in the serving size specified) can be exchanged for any other within each list.
- Information is provided on the serving sizes, calories, and number of carbohydrate choices per serving of various alcohol beverages; so clients who choose to drink alcohol know how to count it in their meal plan.
- As with carbohydrate counting, accurate portion sizes are vital to maintaining a consistent carbohydrate and calorie intake.
- The food lists can be helpful for people who want, or need, structured meal-planning guidance and are able to understand complex details.
- The food list approach is not better than carbohydrate counting for maintaining glycemic control, is less flexible, and may not be appropriate or acceptable for all age, ethnic, and cultural groups.

Estimating Portion Sizes

Correctly estimating portion sizes is a crucial component of all meal-planning approaches, especially carbohydrate counting. Inaccurate portion size estimates have the potential to cause weight gain or loss and hypo- or hyperglycemia. Food models or measuring cups can help teach appropriate portion sizes to patients. Other strategies that may help include urging patients to

- measure foods once per week to reinforce serving sizes and correct quantification;
- note how a portion size looks on the plate or where it comes to in their bowls or cups;
- create a cheat sheet of the carbohydrate content of foods they usually eat;
- check the nutritional content of restaurant items online before ordering food out; and
- use standard household items to approximate size; for instance, the size of a baseball is approximately 1 cup and the size of a deck of cards is approximately 3 oz of meat.

Promoting Behavior Change

The diagnosis of diabetes often triggers anxiety and uncertainty. People often see "diet" as the most difficult part of treatment. Even people with healthy eating patterns may need to adjust their intake to improve glycemic control. Giving someone a list of dos and don'ts can add to a resentful client's frustration. Before recommending changes, it is useful to ask the following:

- What are your goals?
- What behaviors do you want to change?
- What changes can you make in your present lifestyle?
- What obstacles may prevent you from making changes?
- What changes can you make right now?
- What changes would be most difficult for you to make?

Mastering the intricacies of nutrition therapy for diabetes—what, when, and why—occurs over a continuum, from learning basic facts to assimilating and implementing more advanced information (Fig. 21.3).

- Individuals differ in how much information they want or need to know and in how motivated they are to improve their eating behaviors.

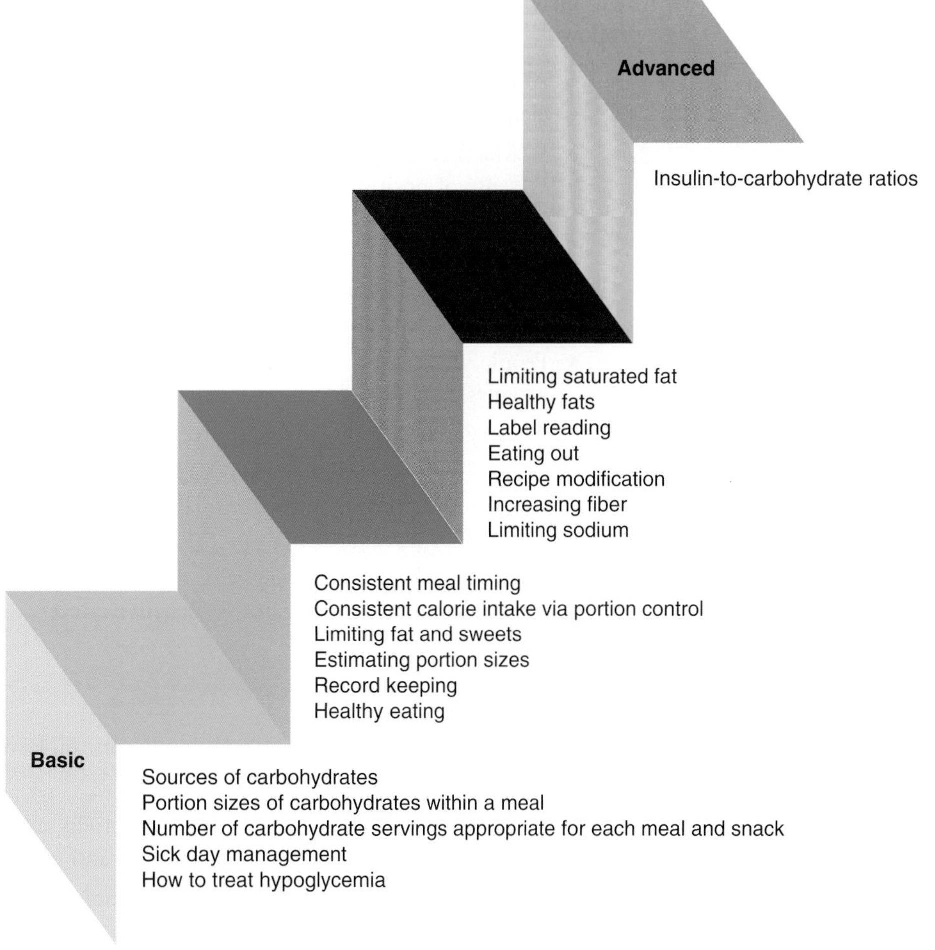

Figure 21.3 ▶
An illustration of knowledge and skills attained in stepwise fashion. Actual progression and concepts learned vary among individuals.

- Ideally, positive changes occur progressively over time in stepwise fashion with the client actively involved in goal setting, self-monitoring, and record keeping.
- In reality, motivation to change eating behaviors may be initially high but commitment and diligence may wane when clients realize that "cheating" does not cause immediate illness.
- Periodic and ongoing follow-up is necessary.

Diabetes Medications

People with type 1 diabetes require exogenous insulin. Most people with type 1 diabetes should be treated with multiple daily injections of prandial and basal insulin, or continuous subcutaneous insulin infusion (ADA, 2020f). Rapid-acting insulin analogs are recommended for most people with type 1 diabetes to reduce the risk of hypoglycemia.

For people with type 2 diabetes, metformin is recommended at the time of diagnosis, along with lifestyle modifications, unless there are contraindications (ADA, 2020f).

- It is recommended that metformin be continued as long as it is tolerated and that other agents, including insulin, should be added to metformin as needed.
- Clients who continue to lose weight, who have persistent symptoms of hyperglycemia, or whose A1c or blood glucose levels are very high may be candidates for early introduction of insulin.
- Because of the progressive nature of the disease, it is common for most people with type 2 diabetes to eventually need the greater potency of injectable medications (ADA, 2020f).

General nutrition-related considerations regarding the use of antidiabetic medications are as follows:

- Although the exact cause is unknown, metformin is associated with vitamin B12 deficiency.
  - Macrocytic anemia, neurologic changes (e.g., paresthesia of the hands and feet, decreased sense of position, depression), and gastrointestinal (GI) changes (e.g., anorexia, indigestion, diarrhea or constipation) may develop. Neurological impairments can be permanent without adequate vitamin B_{12} supplementation.
  - Annual testing of vitamin B_{12} levels should be considered in people taking metformin, especially in those with anemia or peripheral neuropathy (Evert et al., 2019).
- People who take medications that can cause hypoglycemia (e.g., insulin, insulin secretagogues) should
  - carry a readily absorbable source of carbohydrate with them at all times to treat hypoglycemia (see section Hypoglycemia);
  - keep an appropriate source of carbohydrate on the nightstand in case hypoglycemia develops during the night.
- In people who are overweight or obese, a side effect of weight loss may be considered positive whereas weight gain is a negative effect.

Physical Activity

Exercise
a specific form of physical activity that is structured and intended to improve physical fitness.

Physical Activity
all movement that increases calorie expenditure.

Exercise has been shown to improve glycemic control, lower ASCVD risk factors, contribute to weight loss, and improve well-being (ADA, 2020d).

- Moderate-to-high amounts of aerobic activity are associated with lower cardiovascular and overall mortality risks in both type 1 and type 2 diabetes (ADA, 2020d).
- **Physical activity** is as important for people for type 1 diabetes as it is for the general population, but its role in preventing diabetes complications and managing glucose levels is not as clear as it is for those with type 2 diabetes (ADA, 2020d).
- Physical activity recommendations for adults with diabetes are similar to those of the general population (ADA, 2020d) (Box 21.6).

BOX 21.6 Physical Activity Suggestions and Considerations for Adults with Diabetes

Activity Suggestions

- Engage in 150 minutes or more per week of moderate-intensity physical activity. One way to achieve this goal is to exercise at least 20 to 25 minutes every day.
- Engage in activities that work all major muscle groups (e.g., legs, hips, back, abdomen, chest, shoulders, and arms) on 2 or more days a week.
- Stretching exercises promote flexibility and balance.

Additional Considerations

- Consume adequate fluid during activity to avoid dehydration.
- Wear cotton socks and properly fitting athletic shoes. Check feet for blisters and other injuries after exercising.
- Check blood glucose level before engaging in physical activity, especially if insulin is used.
  - If serum glucose is <100 mg/dL, consuming an extra 15 to 30 g of carbohydrate may be necessary to avoid hypoglycemia.
  - If serum glucose is >240 mg/dL, it may not be safe to engage in physical activity, particularly if ketones are present in the urine because ketoacidosis may occur during activity.
- Check blood glucose levels after exercising.

Source: Centers for Disease Control and Prevention. (2018, April 24). *Get active!* https://www.cdc.gov/diabetes/managing/active.html

ACUTE DIABETES COMPLICATIONS

Untreated or poorly controlled diabetes can lead to acute life-threatening complications related to high blood glucose concentrations. Conversely, hypoglycemia caused by overuse of medication, too little food, or too much exercise can also be life threatening.

Diabetic Ketoacidosis

People with type 1 diabetes are susceptible to diabetic ketoacidosis (DKA), characterized by hyperglycemia (glucose levels >250 mg/dL) and ketonemia.

- DKA is caused by a severe deficiency of insulin or from physiologic stress, such as illness or infection.
- It is sometimes the presenting symptom when type 1 diabetes is diagnosed.
- Hyperventilation, diabetic coma, and death are possible.
- DKA rarely develops in people with type 2 diabetes because only very little insulin is needed to prevent ketosis. If DKA does occur in people with type 2 diabetes, infection or illness is usually to blame.

Hyperosmolar Hyperglycemic State

Hyperosmolar hyperglycemic state (HHS) is characterized by hyperglycemia (>600 mg/dL) without significant ketonemia.

- HHS occurs most commonly in people with type 2 diabetes because they have enough insulin to prevent ketosis.
- Dehydration and heat exposure increase the risk; illness or infection is usually the precipitating factor.
- Older people may be particularly vulnerable because they have a diminished sense of thirst or may be unable to replenish fluid losses due to illness or physical impairments.
- HHS develops relatively slowly over a period of days to weeks.
- The best protection against HHS is regular glucose monitoring.

Hypoglycemia

Hypoglycemia (blood glucose level <70 mg/dL) occurs from taking too much insulin or some oral medications and inadequate food intake, delayed or skipped meals, extra physical activity, or consumption of alcohol without food.

- Symptoms include weakness, shakiness, dizziness, cold sweat, clammy feeling, headache, confusion, irritability, and light-headedness.
- Readily absorbable forms of carbohydrate, such as pure sugars, are used to quickly raise blood glucose levels; items like chocolate candy bars, which contain fat that slows gastric emptying time and delays the rise in blood glucose, are not recommended.
- Mild hypoglycemia is treated with the "15–15 Rule" (Box 21.7)
- Regular blood glucose monitoring and exercising with someone are recommended.
- Frequent bouts of hypoglycemia may mean the care plan needs to be revised or further education is needed.
- Clients with long-standing diabetes may develop hypoglycemic unawareness. This occurs because the body no longer signals hypoglycemia. Consistent monitoring of blood glucose is especially important for people who are not cognizant of hypoglycemic symptoms.

BOX 21.7 The "15-15 Rule"

Eat 15 g of readily absorbable carbohydrate if blood glucose is <70 mg/day.
Wait 15 minutes. If glucose level is still <70 mg/dL, repeat the process.
When glucose is back to normal, eat a meal or snack.

Each of the following provides approximately 10 to 15 g of readily absorbable sugar:

4 glucose tablets
½ cup fruit juice
4 to 6 oz regular soft drink (not diet)
1 tbsp sugar, honey, or corn syrup
5 to 6 Life Savers
8 SweeTARTS
16 Skittles
1 fruit roll-up
2 tbsp raisins
1 tube (0.68 oz) of Cake Mate decorator gel

SICK-DAY MANAGEMENT

Acute illnesses, even mild ones such as a cold or flu, can significantly raise blood glucose levels. Unless otherwise instructed by the physician, clients should maintain their normal medication schedule, monitor their blood glucose levels every 2 to 4 hours, maintain an adequate fluid intake, and continue with their normal meal plan. Softer foods such as soup, crackers, applesauce, and fruit juice may help maintain an adequate intake. If the client cannot tolerate solids, carbohydrate targets can be met by consuming sweetened liquids, which are generally a well-tolerated source of carbohydrates and fluid. A daily intake of 150 to 200 g of carbohydrates, approximately 50 g (approximately three carbohydrate choices) every 3 to 4 hours, is recommended. Examples of items that may be best tolerated during illness are as follows (each serving specified provides approximately one carbohydrate choice [15 g of carbohydrate]):

- 6 oz regularly sweetened ginger ale
- 8 oz sports drink
- ½ cup ice cream
- ½ cup apple juice
- 1 frozen 100% juice bar
- ¼ cup sherbet or sorbet
- ½ cup gelatin
- 1 cup cream soup made with water

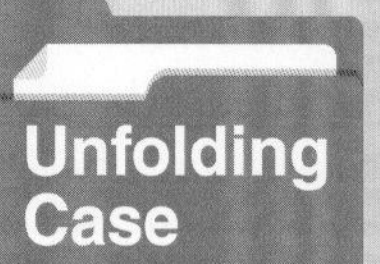

Consider Darius. He developed the flu and was advised to drink plenty of fluids; continue with his four carbohydrates per meal pattern by using regular ginger ale, fruit juice, and ice cream; and increase his monitoring of blood glucose and ketones. He is reluctant to consume regular ginger ale and ice cream because he knows sugar is bad for him. How do you respond?

Diabetes in the Hospital

Consistent carbohydrate meal plans are used by many hospitals; these menus also typically feature heart-healthy selections that limit saturated fat, trans fat, and sodium.

- The American Diabetes Association does not endorse any single meal plan or specified percentages of macronutrients (ADA, 2020g).

- The following hospital diets previously designated for clients with diabetes are obsolete: "no concentrated sweets," "no sugar added," "low sugar," and "liberal diabetic" diets. These diets do not reflect the current nutrient recommendations for diabetes, are unnecessarily restrictive in sugar, and may give clients the false impression that glycemic control is achieved by limiting sugar.
- Enteral formulas designed for clients with diabetes appear to be superior to standard formulas in controlling postprandial glucose, A1c, and the insulin response (ADA, 2020g).

Recall Darius. He is admitted to the hospital with pneumonia and uncontrolled diabetes. He is ordered a soft diet without any carbohydrate restrictions. He is confused by the lack of restriction and announces he is no longer going to count carbohydrates because it is too confusing and difficult. What strategies are available to help Darius eat a hypocaloric meal plan to promote weight loss and manage diabetes?

LIFE-CYCLE CONSIDERATIONS

There are unique nutrition therapy challenges for managing diabetes in children and adolescents as well as in older adults. Special considerations for these groups are presented in the following sections.

Children and Adolescents

Diabetes management in children and adolescents is complicated by the impact of growth on nutrient needs, irregular eating patterns, and erratic activity levels. Other unique challenges include the ability to provide self-care, supervision in childcare and school settings, neurological vulnerability to hypoglycemia and hyperglycemia in young children, and possible adverse neurocognitive effects of diabetic ketoacidosis (ADA, 2020h). Young children are unable to recognize or articulate hypoglycemia. Psychosocial issues and family stresses can impact diabetes management.

Youth with type 1 diabetes may have subclinical CVD within the first decade of diagnosis (ADA, 2020h). Current standards for diabetes management reflect the need to lower glucose as safely as possible (ADA, 2020h). Lower A1c in adolescence and young adulthood is associated with lower risk and rate of microvascular and macrovascular complications (ADA, 2020h). Individualized nutrition therapy for youth is an essential component of diabetes management.

Nutrition Therapy Recommendations and Considerations for Type 1 Diabetes

- Family habits, food preferences, religious or cultural preferences, schedules, physical activity, and the youth's and family's literacy and numeracy skills are all considered when determining the nutrition plan of care.
- Either carbohydrate counting or experience-based estimation can be used to monitor carbohydrate intake (ADA, 2020h).
- Failure to provide adequate calories and nutrients results in poor growth, as do poor glycemic control and inadequate insulin administration.
- Excessive weight gain occurs from excessive calorie intake, overtreatment of hypoglycemia, or excess insulin administration.
- Neither withholding food nor having a child eat when not hungry is an appropriate strategy to manage glucose levels.
    - Increased use of basal-bolus regimens, insulin pumps, frequent blood glucose monitoring, goal setting, and improved client education in youth are associated with more children achieving blood glucose targets (ADA, 2020h).
    - Advanced carbohydrate counting and intensive insulin regimens can provide flexibility for erratic eating, activity, and growth.

Type 2 Diabetes in Youth

Type 2 diabetes in youth has increased over the past 20 years and estimates suggest an incidence of ~5000 new cases per year in the United States (ADA, 2020h). Nutrition-related considerations are as follows (ADA, 2020h):

- Evidence suggests type 2 diabetes in youth differs not only from type 1 but also from type 2 diabetes in adults in that there is a faster decline in beta-cell function and accelerated development of diabetes complications (ADA, 2020h).
- Risk factors for type 2 diabetes in youth include adiposity, family history of diabetes, female sex, low socioeconomic status, and certain ethnicities and racial minorities.
- Youth who are overweight or obese should participate with their families in a comprehensive lifestyle program with the goal of losing 7% to 10% of excess weight.
- Lifestyle intervention focuses on an increase in physical activity and healthy eating patterns that emphasize nutrient-dense foods and minimize calorie-dense foods, especially sugar-sweetened beverages.
- Distinguishing between type 1 and type 2 diabetes can be difficult due to the increasing prevalence of overweight and obesity among youth, including those with type 1 diabetes.

Diabetes in Later Life

In general, older adults are at greater nutritional risk than younger adults due to a variety of changes that may occur with aging, such as oral and GI changes (e.g., difficulty chewing, decreased nutrient absorption), CNS changes (e.g., cognitive impairments, depression), sensory losses (e.g., decreased sense of smell and taste), reliance on medications, social isolation, and decreased appetite. Older adults with diabetes may be at even greater nutritional risk than the general older population related to the following:

- Higher rates of comorbidities: hypertension, coronary heart disease, and stroke.
- Higher risk of reduced muscle strength, poor muscle quality, and accelerated loss of muscle mass, resulting in sarcopenia (ADA, 2020i).
- Frailty because diabetes is also an independent risk factor for frailty. Frailty impairs physical functioning and increases the risk of poor health outcomes (ADA, 2020i).

An optimal nutrient and protein intake, along with aerobic physical activity and resistance training, is encouraged for all older adults who can safely engage in such activities (ADA, 2020i). Glycemic goals may be based on the health of the client, including their remaining life expectancy.

NURSING PROCESS Type 2 Diabetes

Mark is 52 years old and is sedentary. His doctor has been monitoring his fasting blood glucose and cholesterol levels for several years, urging Mark to eat better and exercise or he would eventually need medications to bring down both his glucose and cholesterol levels. Mark was unmotivated to change until he was recently diagnosed with type 2 diabetes. His mother went blind from type 2 diabetes, and he now realizes he must make lifestyle changes to manage his diabetes. He admits to knowing little about diabetes management and is seeking nutrition information. He is 5 ft 9 in. tall and weighs 190 pounds.

Assessment

Medical–Psychosocial History

- Medical history and comorbidities, including hyperlipidemia, hypertension, ASCVD, renal impairments, neuropathy, and GI complaints.
- Use of prescribed and over-the-counter medications that may affect nutrition.
- Psychosocial and economic issues such as the living situation, cooking facilities, adequacy of food budget, education, need for food assistance, and level of family and social support.
- Usual activity patterns.

NURSING PROCESS

Type 2 Diabetes (continued)

Anthropometric Assessment

- Height, current weight, usual weight; recent weight history.
- BMI.
- Waist circumference to identify abdominal obesity.

Biochemical and Physical Assessment

- Hemoglobin A1c, fasting glucose levels, glucose tolerance results.
- Lipid profile.
- Measures of renal function, if available.
- Blood pressure.

Dietary Assessment

- How many meals and snacks do you usually eat in a day? Do you ever skip meals? Do you eat at regular intervals? When do you eat snacks?
- What is a typical day's intake?
- Have you ever tried to follow a diet or improve your eating habits?
- What changes can you make in your present lifestyle?
- What obstacles may prevent you from making changes?
- What changes would be difficult to make?
- What questions do you have about nutrition for diabetes?
- How is your appetite?
- Do you have any food intolerances or allergies? Do you ever have GI symptoms that affect what you eat?
- How do you feel about your weight?
- Do you have any cultural, religious, or ethnic food preferences?
- Who prepares your meals?
- Do you take vitamins, minerals, or other supplements?
- Do you use alcohol?

Analysis

Possible Nursing Analysis

Food- and nutrition-related knowledge deficit related to a new diagnosis of type 2 diabetes as evidenced by request for information.

Planning

Client Outcomes

Short term

The client will do the following:

- Explain carbohydrate counting.
- Begin strategies to shift toward a nutritionally adequate, balanced, and varied diet that has the following:
  - Four carbohydrate choices at each meal and two at a bedtime snack that are composed of a variety of fruits, vegetables, whole grains, and low-fat or nonfat milk
  - 4 to 6 oz of protein/day
  - Small amounts of healthy fats
  - Little saturated fat and minimal trans fats
- Lose 1 to 2 pounds/week.
- Eat three meals plus a bedtime snack at approximately the same times every day.
- Keep periodic food records that include the timing of meals and snacks and type and amount of food eaten.
- Walk 10 minutes three times a day at least 3 days a week.

Long term

The client will do the following:

- Lose 13 pounds in 6 months (7% of initial weight).
- Sustain his lower weight.
- Achieve hemoglobin A1c and preprandial and postprandial blood glucose levels within target levels established by his physician.
- Improve lipid profile.
- Prevent or delay chronic complications.
- Increase physical activity to at least 30 minutes daily five times per week.

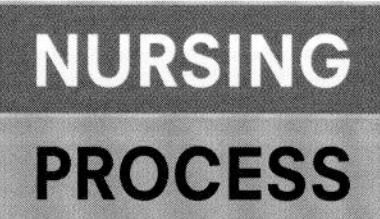

Type 2 Diabetes (continued)

Nursing Interventions

Nutrition Therapy

Introduce basic concepts: characteristics of a healthy eating pattern, sources of carbohydrates, appropriate serving sizes for carbohydrates, and how many carbohydrate choices are prescribed for each meal and snack.

Client Teaching

Instruct the client on the following:
The role of nutrition therapy in managing blood glucose levels, including the following:

- Nutrition therapy is essential and nutrition is important even when no symptoms are apparent.
- Modest weight loss can achieve glycemic goals.
- If medication is prescribed, it is used in addition to nutrition therapy, not as a substitute.
- Ongoing or follow-up counseling is necessary to make adjustments and expand skills and knowledge to optimize diabetes management.

Eating plan essentials, including the importance of the following:

- Eating meals and snacks at regular times every day.
- Eating a varied, nutrient-dense eating pattern that limits refined foods and foods processed with added sugar, fat, or sodium.
- Eating approximately the same amount of food every day, especially the same amount of carbohydrates.
- Eating enough high-fiber foods such as whole-wheat bread, whole-grain ready-to-eat cereals, whole-wheat pasta, brown rice, oats, vegetables, fruit, and dried peas and beans.
- Avoiding sugar-sweetened beverages and limiting empty calorie foods

Behavioral matters, including the following:

- How to read labels to determine the amount of carbohydrate choices a serving of food provides.
- Not skipping meals or snacks.
- How to order from a restaurant menu.
- Physical activity goals.
- Having a source of glucose handy at all times.
- The importance of monitoring food intake.
- Where to get additional information.

Evaluation

Evaluate and Monitor

- Food intake records for consistency in meal timing, the number and quality of carbohydrate choices per meals and snacks, and overall quality and adequacy of food choices made.
- Appetite/satiety.
- Weight.
- Laboratory data as available.
- Need for nutritional counseling.
- Progress toward physical activity goals.

How Do You Respond?

Are "dietetic" products like candy and cookies worth the added expense? Dietetic products are not necessarily calorie free or specifically intended for people with diabetes. Foods that are labeled "dietetic" may be made without sugar, without salt, with a particular type of fat, or for particular food allergies. Read the ingredient label and check with a nutrition counselor before adding a dietetic food to the diet—or avoid dietetic foods altogether because they are expensive and usually do not taste as good as the foods they are intended to replace.

Can I save some carbs from breakfast and lunch for a special dinner? Carbohydrate intake should stay relatively consistent, not light for 2 meals so it can be heavier at the other. This is particularly true for people on fixed insulin regimens or who take insulin secretagogues. Instead of skimping during the day to add carbs at dinner, on occasion it is fine to forgo some healthy carb dinner choices (e.g., fruit, grains, milk) for a small portion of special dessert. It is better to make reasonable adjustments on occasion than to just add extra carbs.

REVIEW CASE STUDY

Keisha is a 42-year-old black woman with a BMI of 29. She was recently diagnosed with diabetes and hypertension. Her mother and two sisters also have type 2 diabetes. She is the mother of three children and had gestational diabetes with her last two pregnancies. Although she knows she should exercise, she doesn't have time in her busy schedule.

The doctor gave her a 1500-calorie diet and told her if her glucose does not improve, she will have to go on medication and possibly insulin. She has tried the "diet" but finds it too restrictive: It tells her to eat things she doesn't like (such as milk) and won't let her eat the things she loves (like sweetened tea and fast foods). She is scared of the potential for needing insulin and the complications associated with diabetes.

- What risk factors does Keisha have for type 2 diabetes?
- Is a 1500-calorie diet appropriate for her? Should it promote weight loss or maintain her current weight?
- What would you tell Keisha about weight and diabetes management?
- What would you tell her about drinking milk? What about sweetened tea and fast foods?
- What approaches would you take to improve compliance yet increase her satisfaction with eating?
- What other lifestyle changes would you propose to Keisha to manage diabetes and reduce the risk of complications?

STUDY QUESTIONS

1 Which statement indicates the client understands nutrition recommendations regarding carbohydrate intake?
   a. "People with diabetes should not eat sugars and foods that contain sugars."
   b. "It is important to consume the proper balance of starch, sugar, and fiber at each meal."
   c. "It is important to consume the correct amount of carbohydrate at each meal and snack."
   d. "People with diabetes should avoid starchy foods."

2 The client with type 1 diabetes asks if they can have a glass of wine with dinner on the weekends. Which of the following would be the nurse's best response?
   a. "It is better to have wine between meals than with meals so that it doesn't interfere with your normal food intake."
   b. "People with diabetes cannot have alcohol because it raises blood glucose levels very quickly."
   c. "A mixed drink would be better than wine because the mixer will help slow the absorption of the alcohol."
   d. "An occasional glass of wine with dinner will not cause problems. Be sure to limit yourself to one serving."

3 When developing a teaching plan for a client who is taking insulin, which of the following foods would the nurse suggest the client carry with him to treat mild hypoglycemia?
   a. Crackers
   b. Peanuts
   c. Chocolate drops
   d. Life Savers

4 The best approach for monitoring carbohydrate intake is to use
a. the food list system
b. carbohydrate counting
c. the plate method
d. the approach that best helps the individual control blood glucose levels

5 How many carbohydrate choices are provided in a serving of food that supplies 19 g of carbohydrate?
a. 1
b. 2
c. 3
d. 4

6 The nurse knows her instructions about label reading have been effective when the client verbalizes that to determine the amount of carbohydrate in a serving you must
a. use only the grams of added sugars
b. use only the grams of total carbohydrate
c. add the grams of total carbohydrate and grams of added sugars together
d. add the grams of total carbohydrate, grams of added sugars, and grams of dietary fiber together

7 What is the priority for preventing diabetes in people who are at high risk?
a. Eat a low-carbohydrate diet.
b. Consume a consistent amount of carbohydrate at every meal.
c. Achieve moderate weight loss through increased activity and lowered calorie intake.
d. Eat a low-sugar diet.

8 Which types of food provide carbohydrates? (Select all that apply.)
a. Vegetables
b. Fruit
c. Milk
d. Animal proteins

CHAPTER SUMMARY NUTRITION FOR CLIENTS WITH DIABETES MELLITUS

Diabetes is a group of diseases characterized by hyperglycemia related to an absent or ineffective secretion of insulin. The metabolism of all three macronutrients is affected, resulting in high blood glucose levels, increased levels of fatty acids and triglycerides in the blood, and muscle wasting. The prevalence is increasing.

Type 1 Diabetes. Characterized by an absolute absence of insulin.

- 5% to 10% of diabetes cases are type 1.
- Most often diagnosed before the age of 18 years.
- Caused by an autoimmune response that damages or destroys pancreatic beta cells. Interaction between genetic and environmental factors (e.g., viral infection) may be responsible.

Type 2 Diabetes. Characterized by defective insulin secretion and insulin resistance.

- 90% to 95% of diabetes cases are type 2.
- Most often diagnosed after age 45; prevalence among younger people is increasing.
- Exact cause is unknown, but genetic and environmental factors, such as overweight and inactivity, are contributing factors.

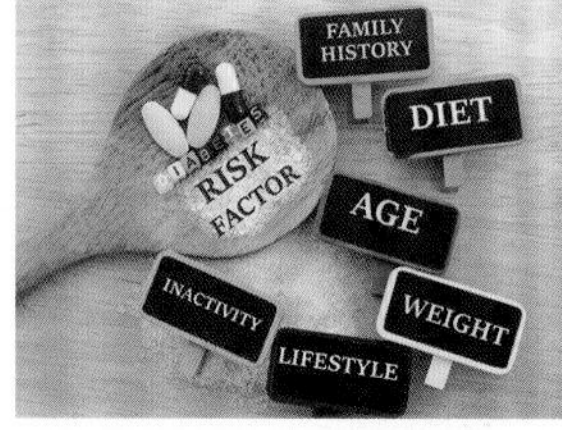

Prediabetes. Characterized by glucose levels that are not high enough to reach the criteria for diabetes but are above normal.

- Almost 40% of people >18 years of age have prediabetes.
- Rather than viewed as a clinical entity, it should be considered an increased risk for diabetes and CVD.
- Strongly associated with obesity, especially central obesity, dyslipidemia with high triglycerides and/or low HDL cholesterol, and hypertension.
- Lifestyle and behavioral therapy, including an individualized hypocaloric meal plan, is highly effective in preventing type 2 diabetes and improving cardiometabolic markers.

Long-Term Diabetes Complications. Sustained hyperglycemia alters glucose metabolism in virtually every cell.

- Damage occurs in micro- (e.g., retinopathy, nephropathy, neuropathy) and macro- (e.g., cardiovascular) vessels.
- Other complications include impaired wound healing, gangrene, periodontal disease, and increased susceptibility to other illnesses.

Lifestyle Management

Diabetes is a progressive disease that requires lifelong treatment. Lifestyle management, which includes DSMES, medical nutrition therapy, and physical activity, is the cornerstone of diabetes management.

Diabetes Self-Management Education and Support. Imparts the skills and knowledge necessary for clients to manage their diabetes.

- Recommended for all people at the time of diabetes diagnosis.
- Support is ongoing and necessary in response to changes in health, age, or life circumstances.
- Only a small percentage of clients participate in DSMES.

CHAPTER SUMMARY NUTRITION FOR CLIENTS WITH DIABETES MELLITUS (continued)

Medical Nutrition Therapy. Individualized nutrition therapy is recommended for all people with type 1 or type 2 diabetes and prediabetes.

- A major goal is to promote healthy eating to improve overall health; manage weight; achieve glucose, lipid, and blood pressure goals; and prevent/delay diabetes complications.
  - **Weight Management.** Losing and maintaining weight are important for overweight and obese people with type 1, type 2, or prediabetes. Weight loss can prevent the progression of prediabetes to type 2 diabetes. Five to ten percent weight loss leads to improvements in glycemic control, blood pressure, and blood lipid levels.
  - **Nutrient and Dietary Recommendations.** Nutrient needs of people who have diabetes are not different from the general population. There is no "diabetic diet" with prescribed percentages of calories for each macronutrient.
  - **Eating patterns.** No single eating pattern has been proven to be consistently better than any other. Patterns associated with a decrease in A1c include the Mediterranean diet, vegetarian and vegan diets, DASH diet, and low-carb and very low-carb diets.

Mediterranean Diet

Meat, sweets
Poultry, eggs, dairy
Fish, seafood
Beans, legumes, nuts, seeds
Whole grains, olive oil
Fruit, vegetables

  - **Carbohydrates.** Low-carb eating patterns are beneficial for people with diabetes and prediabetes; however, "low carb" is not definitively defined. High-fiber sources are recommended; added sugar intake should be minimized.
  - **Protein.** Usual protein intake is appropriate unless the client has diabetic kidney disease, in which case intake should be lowered to the recommended dietary allowance (RDA) of 0.8 g/kg body weight.
  - **Fat.** The type of fat is more important than the total amount. Unsaturated fats are encouraged; saturated and trans fats are restricted.
  - **Sodium.** People with diabetes have the same guideline as the general population—limit intake to 2300 mg/day.
  - **Micronutrient and herbal supplements.** Micronutrient supplements are not helpful except if the client has a deficiency. No herbal supplements are recommended to improve glycemic control.
  - **Alcohol.** Moderate alcohol has minimal acute or long-term effects on blood glucose. If consumed, it should be accompanied by food to decrease the risk of hypoglycemia.

Meal-Planning Approaches

- **Carbohydrate counting**
  - 15 g of carbohydrates equal one carbohydrate "choice."
  - Clients follow a meal plan that specifies the number of carbohydrate choices per meal and snack.
  - Clients choose how to satisfy their choice allotment.
  - Basic carb counting uses a consistent daily meal plan; advanced counting adjusts the carbohydrate allotment based on premeal glucose and insulin dosage.
- **Plate method:** Uses a dinner plate to illustrate proportion and balance.

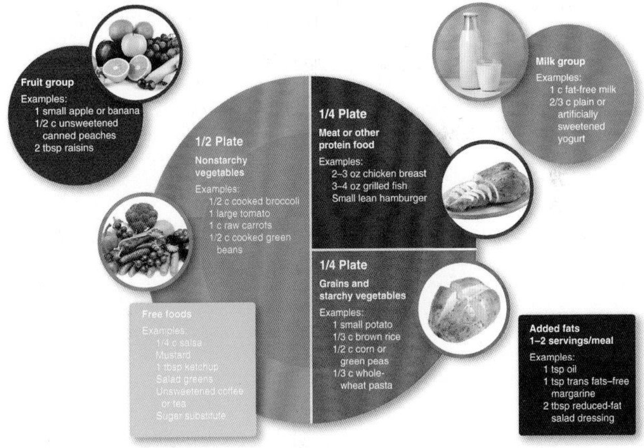

- **Food lists for diabetes:** Similar to carbohydrate counting but the meal plan also includes servings of protein and fat.
- **Estimating portion sizes:** Accuracy in portion sizes is vital to avoid undesirable weight changes or hypo- and hyperglycemia.

Promoting Behavior Change. "Diet" is often considered the most difficult part of managing diabetes. Behavior change should occur over a continuum based on how much information the client needs or wants to know.

Physical Activity. Physical activity guidelines for people with diabetes are similar to those of the general public. Aerobic exercise, resistance training, and a decrease in sedentary time are recommended.

(continued)

CHAPTER SUMMARY NUTRITION FOR CLIENTS WITH DIABETES MELLITUS (continued)

Acute Diabetes Complications

Diabetic ketoacidosis. Characterized by glucose >250 mg/dL and ketonemia; usually occurs in only people with type 1 diabetes.

Hyperosmolar hyperglycemic state. Characterized by glucose >600 mg/dL without significant ketonemia; occurs most commonly in people with type 2 diabetes. Regular glucose monitoring helps to prevent it.

Hypoglycemia. Characterized by glucose < 70 mg/dL that occurs from too much insulin/medication, inadequate food intake, extra physical activity, or alcohol consumed without food. A quickly absorbed simple sugar is needed to raise glucose.

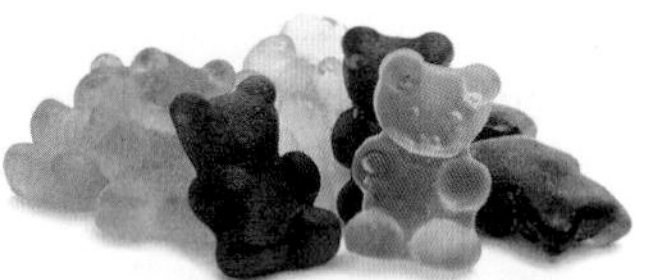

Sick-Day Management

General advice during acute illness: Maintain the usual medication schedule, monitor blood glucose levels closely, consume adequate fluids, eat the usual amount of carbohydrate, and use sugar-sweetened fluids (e.g., sugar-sweetened soft drinks, ice cream, sherbet) if liquids are tolerated over solids.

Life-Cycle Considerations

Children and Adolescents. Diabetes management is complicated by growth needs, irregular eating patterns, emotional immaturity, and erratic activity levels. Glycemic goals are set by balancing the long-term benefits of lowering A1c against the risks of hypoglycemia and the burdens of intensive regimens.

Nutrition recommendations:

- Individualize the meal plan.
- Use carbohydrate counting/experience-based portion estimation to achieve consistency in intake.
- Overweight and obese youth with type 2 diabetes should participate with their families in a lifestyle intervention program with the goal of losing 7% to 10% of body weight.

Older adults. Aging increases nutritional risk; diabetes adds to the risk. An adequate nutrient intake, especially of protein, along with aerobic physical activity and resistance training, is recommended, especially for older adults who are frail.

Figure sources: *shutterstock.com/Raihana Asral, shutterstock.com/Zern Liew, shutterstock.com/oksana2010*

Student Resources on thePoint®
For additional learning materials, activate the code in the front of this book at https://thePoint.lww.com/activate

Websites

American Diabetes Association at www.diabetes.org
Joslin Diabetes Center at www.joslin.org
National Institute of Diabetes and Digestive and Kidney Diseases at www.niddk.nih.gov

References

American Diabetes Association. (2020a). Classification and diagnosis of diabetes: Standards of Medical Care in Diabetes—2020. *Diabetes Care*, *43*(suppl 1), S14–S31. https://doi.org/10.2337/dc20-S002

American Diabetes Association. (2020b). Prevention or delay of type 2 diabetes: Standards of medical care in diabetes—2020. Classification and diagnosis of diabetes: Standards of Medical Care in Diabetes. *Diabetes Care*, *43*(suppl 1), S32–S36. https://doi.org/10.2337/dc20-S003

American Diabetes Association. (2020c). Cardiovascular disease and risk management: Standards of medical care in diabetes—2020. *Diabetes Care*, *43*(suppl 1), S111–S134. https://doi.org/10.2337/dc20-S010

American Diabetes Association. (2020d). Facilitating behavior change and well-being to improve health outcomes: Standards of medical care in diabetes—2020. *Diabetes Care*, *43*(suppl 1), S48–S65. https://doi.org/10.2337/dc20-S005

American Diabetes Association. (2020e). Obesity management for the treatment of type 2 diabetes: Standards of medical care in diabetes—2020. *Diabetes Care*, *43*(suppl 1), S89–S97. https://doi.org/10.2337/dc20-S008

American Diabetes Association. (2020f). Pharmacologic approaches to glycemic treatment: Standards of medical care in diabetes—2020. *Diabetes Care*, *43*(suppl 1), S98–S110. https://doi.org/10.2337/dc20-S009

American Diabetes Association. (2020g). Diabetes care in the hospital: Standards of medical care in diabetes—2020. *Diabetes Care*, *43*(suppl 1), S193–S202. https://doi.org/10.2337/dc20-S015

American Diabetes Association. (2020h). Children and adolescents: Standards of medical care in diabetes—2020. *Diabetes Care*, *43*(suppl 1), S163–S182. https://doi.org/10.2337/dc20-S013

American Diabetes Association. (2020i). Older adults: Standards of medical care in diabetes—2020. *Diabetes Care, 43*(suppl 1), S152–S162. https://doi.org/10.2337/dc20-S012

American Diabetes Association & Academy of Nutrition and Dietetics. (2019). Choose your foods: Food lists for diabetes. American Diabetes Association; Academy of Nutrition and Dietetics.

Centers for Disease Control and Prevention. (2020a, June 24). *Prevalence of both diagnosed and undiagnosed diabetes.* https://www.cdc.gov/diabetes/data/statistics-report/diagnosed-undiagnosed-diabetes.html

Centers for Disease Control and Prevention. (2020b, June 30). *Prevalence of prediabetes among adults.* https://www.cdc.gov/diabetes/data/statistics-report/prevalence-of-prediabetes.html

Diabetes Control and Complications Trial Research Group. (1993). The effect of intensive treatment of diabetes on the development and progression of long-term complications in insulin-dependent diabetes mellitus. *New England Journal of Medicine, 329,* 977–986. https://doi.org/10.1056/NEJM199309303291401

Diabetes Prevention Program Research Group, Knowler, W. C., Fowler, S. E., Hamman, R. F., Christophi, C. A., Hoffman, H. J., Brenneman, A. T., Brown-Friday, J. O., Goldberg, R., Venditti, E., & Nathan, D. M. (2009). 10-year follow-up of diabetes incidence and weight loss in the Diabetes Prevention Program Outcomes Study. *Lancet, 374*(9702), 1677–1686. https://doi.org/10.1016/S0140-6736(09)61457-4

Evert, A., Dennison, M., Gardner, C., Garvey, W. T., Lau, K.H., MacLeod, J., Mitri, J., Pereira, R. F., Rawlings, K., Robinson, S., Saslow, L., Uelmen, S., Urbanski, P. B., & Yancy, W. S. (2019). Nutrition therapy for adults with diabetes or prediabetes: A consensus report. *Diabetes Care, 42*(5), 731–754. https://doi.org/10.2337/dci19-0014

Fu, S., Li, L., Deng, S., Zan, L., & Liu, Z. (2016). Effectiveness of advanced carbohydrate counting in type 1 diabetes mellitus: A systematic review and meta-analysis. *Scientific Reports, 6,* 37067. https://doi.org/10.1038/srep37067

Haffner, S., Temprosa, M., Crandall, J., Fowler, S., Goldberg, R., Horton, Marcovina, S., Mather, K., Orchard, T., Ratner, R., & Barrett-Connor, E. (2005). Intensive lifestyle intervention or metformin on inflammation and coagulation in participants with impaired glucose tolerance. *Diabetes, 54*(5), 1566–1572. https://doi.org/10.2337/diabetes.54.5.1566

Knowler, W., Barrett-Connor, E., Fowler, S. E., Hamman, R. F., Lachin, J. M., Walker, E. A., & Nathan, D. M. (2002). Reduction in the incidence of type 2 diabetes with lifestyle intervention or metformin. *The New England Journal of Medicine, 346*(6), 393–403. https://doi.org/10.1056/nejmoa012512.

Nathan, D. M., Cleary, P. A., Backlund, J.-Y. C., Genuth, S. M., Lachin, J. M., Orchard, T. J., Raskin, P., Zinman, B. for Diabetes Control and Complications Trial/ Epidemiology of Diabetes Interventions and Complications (DCCT/EDIC) Study Research Group. (2005). Intensive diabetes treatment and cardiovascular disease in patients with type 1 diabetes. *New England Journal of Medicine, 353,* 2643–2653. https://doi.org/10.1056/NEJMoa052187

O'Neill, S., & O'Driscoll, L. (2015). Metabolic syndrome: A closer look at the growing epidemic and its associated pathologies. *Obesity Reviews, 16*(1), 1–12. https://doi.org/10.1111/obr.12229

Ratner, R., Goldberg, R., Haffner, S., Marcovina, S., Orchard, T., Fowler, S., & Temprosa, M. for the Diabetes Prevention Program Research Group. (2005). Impact of intensive lifestyle and metformin therapy on cardiovascular disease risk factors in the Diabetes Prevention Program. *Diabetes Care, 28*(4), 888–894. https://doi.org/10.2337/diacare.28.4.888

Sattar, N., Rawshani, Z., Franzen, S., Rawshani, A., Svensson, A.-M., Rosengren, A., McGuire, D. K., Eliasson, B., & Gudbjornsdottir, S. (2019). Age at diagnosis of type 2 diabetes mellitus and associations with cardiovascular and mortality risks. *Circulation, 139*(19), 2228–2237. https://doi.org/10.1161/CIRCULATIONAHA.118.037885

UK Prospective Diabetes Study (UKPDS) Group. (1998). Effect of intensive blood-glucose control with metformin on complications in overweight patients with type 2 diabetes (UKPDS34). *Lancet, 352*(9139), 854–865. https://doi.org/10.1016/S0140-6736(98)07037-8

Chapter 22

Nutrition for Clients with Cardiovascular Disorders

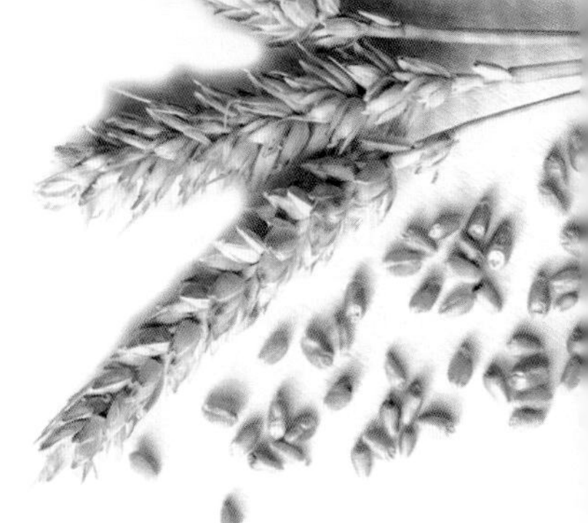

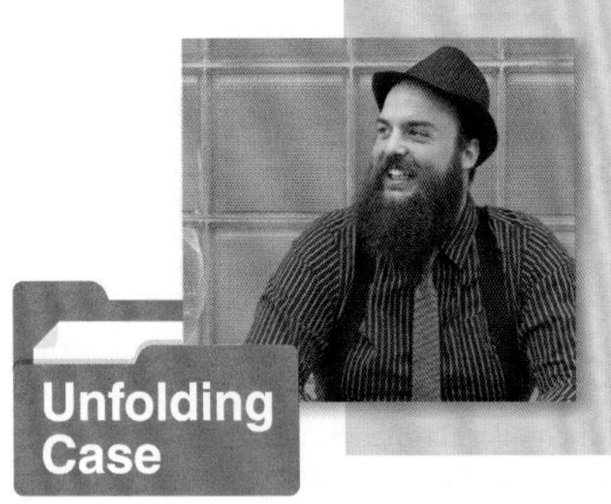

Unfolding Case

Jacob Holzhausen

Jacob is 49 years old and wants to eat healthier and lose weight. He is 6 ft 1 in. tall, weighs 298 pounds, and does not exercise. His physician advised him to get down to 250 pounds and told him to follow a 2000-calorie diet. He has prediabetes, hypertension, and hypercholesterolemia. He lives alone and doesn't cook. Instead, he normally eats fast-food meals. He admits to being a heavy beer drinker.

Learning Objectives

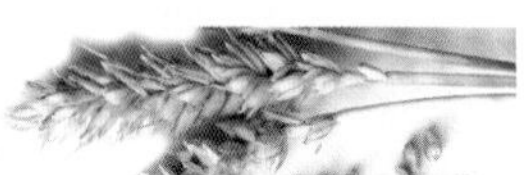

Upon completion of this chapter, you will be able to:

1 List the metrics that define cardiovascular health.
2 Discuss the characteristics that define an optimal healthy diet score.
3 Summarize the characteristics of a Dietary Approaches to Stop Hypertension (DASH) diet.
4 Describe the characteristics of a Mediterranean-style eating pattern.
5 Compare the DASH diet with the traditional Mediterranean-style eating pattern.
6 Summarize nutrition interventions recommended for the primary and secondary prevention of hypertension.
7 Discuss diet-related recommendations for hypercholesterolemia.
8 Discuss diet-related recommendations for metabolic syndrome.
9 List the top six sources of sodium in the U.S. diet.

Cardiovascular disease (CVD) is a general term that refers to heart and blood vessel conditions such as coronary heart disease (CHD), stroke, hypertension, and heart failure (HF). Atherosclerotic cardiovascular disease (ASCVD) refers to cardiac conditions caused by atherosclerosis, a progressive disease characterized by the buildup of fatty plaques that can develop in the arteries that supply blood to the heart, brain, kidneys, and extremities. The majority of CVD, including CHD and stroke, are ASCVD.

ASCVD is the leading cause of morbidity and mortality worldwide (Arnett et al., 2019). In the United States, heart disease remains the leading cause of death as it has been for decades (Heron, 2019). ASCVD is largely a result of modifiable risk factors, including lifestyle (Lachman et al., 2016). A healthy lifestyle throughout life, namely, a healthy eating pattern, adequate physical activity, and avoidance of tobacco, is the most important way to prevent atherosclerotic vascular disease, HF, and atrial fibrillation (Arnett et al., 2019) and is vital to the secondary prevention of CVD and its risk factors, including obesity, hypercholesterolemia, hypertension, and diabetes.

This chapter discusses cardiovascular health, healthy eating patterns recommended for cardiovascular health, and nutrition therapy for primary and secondary CVD and its nutrition-related risk factors.

CARDIOVASCULAR HEALTH

In 2010, the American Heart Association introduced a new concept of cardiovascular health based on 7 metrics, commonly referred to "Life's Simple 7" (Virani et al., 2020). These metrics include four health behaviors (diet quality, physical activity, tobacco use, body mass index [BMI]) and three health factors (blood cholesterol, blood pressure, blood glucose). Because cardiovascular health occurs along a continuum and an **ideal cardiovascular health** profile is rare, a range of values are used to score each metric as ideal, intermediate, and poor. (Table 22.1 lists the ideal for each metric and the percentage of adults who achieve each ideal.)

Ideal Cardiovascular Health the absence of clinically evident CVD and the simultaneous presence of optimal levels of all 7 metrics without the use of medication to control blood glucose, blood cholesterol, and blood pressure.

Multiple independent studies show a strong protective association between cardiovascular health metrics and many conditions, including premature all-cause mortality, CVD mortality, and HF; subclinical measures of atherosclerosis such as carotid arterial wall stiffness; impaired physical function and frailty; and cognitive decline and depression (Virani et al., 2020). Research shows that even a moderately unhealthy lifestyle is associated with a significantly lower risk of CVD events compared to those with a very unhealthy lifestyle, suggesting that even small improvements may result in a substantial reduction in the risk of CVD (Lachman et al., 2016).

Cardiovascular Health Among American Adults

Among American adults aged 20 and older (Virani et al., 2020),

- less than 20% met the criteria for 5 or more ideal metrics;
- ideal score prevalence improved from 1999–2000 to 2015–2016 for smoking, total cholesterol, blood pressure, and physical activity
- ideal score prevalence during that same period declined for BMI and diabetes.

As indicated in Table 22.1, the metric scored as ideal by the lowest percentage of Americans is in achieving a healthy eating pattern (0.3%), and achieving a low sodium intake is the primary dietary characteristic least often attained (Virani et al., 2020).

Table 22.1 "Life's Simple 7": Definition of Ideal Cardiovascular Health Metrics and Prevalence of Each Metric of for Adults ≥20 Years Old

	Ideal	% of Adults Who Achieve Ideal
Health Behaviors		
Current smoking	Never or quit >12 months	78.8
BMI	<25	28.7
Physical activity	≥150 minutes/week moderate or ≥75 minutes/week vigorous or ≥150 minutes/week moderate + 2x vigorous	41.5
Healthy diet pattern:	4–5 primary components	0.3
≥4.5 c/day fruits and vegetables		10.2
≥2 servings/week of fish		18.0
≥3 servings/day of whole grains		7.1
≤36 oz/week sugar-sweetened beverages		53.3
≤1500 mg/day sodium		0.7
Health Factors		
Total cholesterol	<200 mg/dL	49.4
Blood pressure	<120/<80 mm Hg	41.0
Fasting plasma glucose	<100 mg/dL	58.4

Source: Virani, S. S., Alonso, A., Benjamin, E. J., Bittencourt, M. S., Callaway, C. W., Carson, A. P., Chamberlain, A. M., Chang, A. R., Cheng, S., Delling, F. N., Djousse, L., Elkind. M. S. V., Ferguson, J. F., Fornage, M., Khan, S. S., Kissela, B. M., Knutson, K. L., Kwan, T. W., Lackland, D. T., ... Tsao, C. W. on behalf of the American Heart Association Council on Epidemiology and Prevention Statistics Committee and Stroke Statistics Subcommittee. (2020). Heart disease and stroke statistics—2020 update: A report from the American Heart Association. *Circulation*, *141*(9), e139–e596. https://doi.org/10.1161/CIR.0000000000000757

The "ideal" eating pattern, scaled to 2000 calories and a Dietary Approaches to Stop Hypertension (DASH)—type eating pattern, is defined as achieving 4 of the 5 primary characteristics of

- ≥4.5 cups fruit and vegetables/day
- ≥2 servings of fish/week
- <1500 mg sodium/day
- <36 oz sugar-sweetened beverages/week
- ≥3 servings of whole grains/day

Secondary diet metrics include

- ≥4 servings/week of nuts/legumes/seeds
- ≤2 servings/week of processed meats
- <7% total calories from **saturated fat**

Saturated Fat or Fatty Acids
fatty acids in which all the carbon atoms are bonded to as many hydrogen atoms as they can hold, so no double bonds exist between carbon atoms; animal fats (meat and dairy), coconut oil, palm oil, and palm kernel oil are the biggest sources.

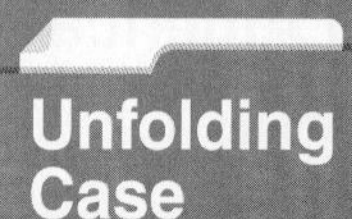

Recall Jacob. A diet history reveals that his typical first meal of the day is two egg-and-sausage breakfast sandwiches along with coffee, cream, and sugar. Lunch is two peanut butter and jelly sandwiches on white bread with chips and soda. Dinner is a submarine sandwich, pizza, or tacos. During the evening, he eats chips and salsa while drinking three to four beers. How does his usual intake compare to the ideal diet metrics? What specific suggestions would you make to improve his usual intake?

Heart-Healthy Eating Patterns

Historically, nutrients, not eating patterns, were the focus of dietary recommendations, such as lowering sodium to prevent or treat hypertension and lowering cholesterol and saturated fat to treat hypercholesterolemia. Currently, the emphasis is on healthy eating patterns to promote overall health and reduce the risk of all chronic diseases, including CVD, CVD risk factors, certain cancers, and age-related decline.

While "Life's Simple 7" uses a DASH-type diet as the ideal, plant-based and Mediterranean-style eating patterns are also linked to lower risk of ASCVD (Arnett et al., 2019). Both the DASH diet and Mediterranean-style eating pattern have the characteristics recommended for the primary prevention of CVD (Arnett et al., 2019). Both patterns

- emphasize the intake of vegetables, fruit, legumes, nuts, whole grains, vegetable oils, and fish
- limit the intake of red and processed meat, refined grains, added sugars, butter, high sodium foods, and commercial **trans fat**
- are higher in fiber, vitamins, antioxidants, minerals, phytonutrients, and **unsaturated fat** and lower in glycemic index, glycemic load, salt, and trans fat than the typical Western diet (Mozaffarian, 2016).

Trans Fats
fatty acids with hydrogen atoms on opposite sides of the double bond. Most trans fats in the diet come from partially hydrogenated fats.

Unsaturated Fat or Fatty Acids
fatty acids in which one or more double bonds exist between carbon atoms. A fatty acid with one double bond is classified as a monounsaturated fat. Polyunsaturated fats have two or more double bonds between carbon atoms.

With attention to cultural considerations, as appropriate (Box 22.1), the DASH diet and Mediterranean-style eating pattern come close to being "one size fits all." Although the DASH diet is most often recommended for hypertension and the Mediterranean-style eating pattern is often recommended for CVD and diabetes, the "best" diet for an individual is the one the client can adhere to. Table 22.2 summarizes the DASH diet and Mediterranean-style eating pattern. A sample menu comparison of DASH diet and Mediterranean-style eating pattern menus appears in Table 22.3. Additional points appear in the following section.

Dietary Approaches to Stop Hypertension Diet

DASH was a multicenter feeding study that set out to test whether eating whole "real" foods rather than individual nutrients would lower blood pressure as a result of some combination of nutrients, interactions among individual nutrients, or other food factors (Appel et al., 1997).

- The results clearly showed that the eating pattern substantially lowers both systolic and diastolic blood pressures as well as low-density lipoprotein cholesterol (LDL-C).

BOX 22.1 Cultural Considerations

For all cultural groups, emphasize the positive aspects of their eating styles and suggest ways to lower saturated fat and sodium content of traditional foods.

African American Tradition

Traditional soul foods tend to be high in saturated fat and sodium. On the positive side, there is a heavy emphasis on vegetables and complex carbohydrates.

Suggested changes in cooking techniques include the following:

- Using nonstick skillets sprayed with cooking spray when pan-frying eggs, fish, and vegetables
- Using small amounts of liquid smoke flavoring in place of bacon, salt pork, or ham
- Using more seasonings, such as onion, garlic, and pepper, in place of some of the salt
- Using turkey ham or turkey sausage in place of bacon
- Using "lite" or sugar-free syrups

Mexican American Tradition

The traditional diet is primarily vegetarian with a heavy emphasis on fruits, vegetables, rice, and dried peas and beans. Processed foods are used infrequently.

Cooking techniques rely on frying and stewing with liberal amounts of oil or lard. An alternative is to sauté or stew with small amounts of canola or olive oil.

High-fat meats and lard are commonly used. Using less meat, choosing lower-fat varieties, trimming visible fat, and substituting oil for lard are heart-healthy alternatives.

Chinese American Tradition

Traditional Chinese cooking relies heavily on vegetables and rice with plants providing the majority of calories. Meat is used more as a condiment than an entrée. Cooking techniques tend to preserve nutrients. Sauces add little fat.

Sodium intake is highly related to heavy use of soy sauce, monosodium glutamate (MSG), and salted pickles. Reduced-sodium soy sauce is available, but it is still high in sodium. Because of the difficulty in eliminating the use of soy sauce, a more practical approach is to gradually use less.

Native North American/Indigenous People of Alaska Traditions

Widely diverse eating styles make useful generalizations difficult.

In general,

- Encourage traditional cooking methods such as baking, roasting, boiling, and broiling.
- Encourage the use of traditional meats, such as fish, deer, and caribou.
- Remove fat from canned meats.
- Use vegetable oil for frying instead of lard or shortening.

Jewish Tradition

Many traditional foods are high in sodium such as *kosher* meats (salt is used in the koshering process), herring, lox, pickles, canned chicken broth or soups, and delicatessen meats (e.g., corned beef, pickled tongue, pastrami).

Pareve (neutral) nondairy creamers are often used as a dairy substitute in meals containing meat, but they are high in saturated fat. Encourage light and fat-free versions.

Encourage methods to lower fat in traditional recipes such as the following:

- Baking instead of frying potato pancakes
- Limiting the amount of schmaltz (chicken fat) used in cooking
- Using reduced-fat or fat-free cream cheese on bagels
- Using low-fat or nonfat cottage cheese, sour cream, and yogurt in kugels and blintzes

Table 22.2 A Summary of the DASH Diet and Mediterranean-Style Eating Pattern

	DASH Diet	Mediterranean Diet
Origin	Designed to see if a healthy eating pattern, not specifically individual nutrients, could lower high blood pressure.	Traditional eating pattern of people living in countries that border the Mediterranean Sea. As an eating pattern of the poor, it consisted of locally grown, seasonally fresh foods.
Most notable health benefits	Primary and secondary prevention of hypertension (Appel et al., 1997).	Lower risk of CVD (Estruch et al., 2018). Lower risk of recurrent CHD events and all-cause mortality (Shikany et al., 2018). Improvements in hemoglobin A1c, fasting glucose, and fasting insulin (Huo et al., 2014).
Characteristics	High in fruit, vegetables, whole grains, lean protein, and low-fat dairy products. Moderate in whole grains, poultry, fish, and nuts. Low in saturated fat, red meat, sweets, and sugar-sweetened beverages	A uniform definition does not exist. In general, the traditional diet: (Boucher, 2017; Estruch et al., 2018) Is rich in olive oil, fruit, nuts, vegetables, legumes, and grains (mostly whole grains) Includes the liberal use of herbs and spices (e.g., sofrito) instead of salt to flavor foods Includes the frequent intake of fish and seafood Includes poultry and eggs in moderation and red wine with meals Is lower in dairy products, red meat, processed meats, and sweets
Most salient nutritional attributes	Low in fat and saturated fat. High content of potassium, calcium, and magnesium.	High in fat (e.g., up to 40% of total calories predominately from olive oil, fish, and nuts). Relatively low in saturated fat.
Selected U.S. News & World Report 2020 Rankings[a]		
Best diets overall	#2 (tie with Flexitarian diet)	#1
Best diets for healthy eating	#1 (ties with Mediterranean diet)	#1 (ties with DASH diet)
Best plant-based diets	#2 (tie with Flexitarian diet)	#1
Best diabetes diets	#2 (tie with Flexitarian diet)	#1
Easiest to follow	#6	#1
Best heart-healthy diets	#3	#2

[a]U.S. News & World Report. (2020). *Best diets overall*. https://health.usnews.com/best-diet/best-diets-overall

Table 22.3 A Comparison of Dietary Approaches to Stop Hypertension Diet and Mediterranean-Style Eating Pattern Menus

	DASH Diet (Approximately 2000 calories)	Mediterranean-Style Eating Pattern
Breakfast	2 slices whole-wheat toast 2 tbsp peanut butter 1 banana 1 cup fat-free milk	½ cup cooked oatmeal topped with Greek yogurt, dates, ground flax seed, and almonds Banana
Lunch	3 oz turkey on 2 slices of whole-wheat bread with mustard Large salad made of lettuce, tomato, onions, cucumber, carrots, and mushrooms with 1 T low-fat salad dressing 1 orange 1 cup fat-free milk	Sautéed white beans and zucchini, tomatoes, onions, and garlic on a bed of greens drizzled with olive oil 1 slice whole-wheat bread dipped in olive oil Orange slices
Dinner	3 oz grilled chicken breast ½ cup brown rice ½ cup roasted winter squash 1 small corn bread muffin 1 tsp soft margarine 1 medium pear 1 cup fat-free milk	3 oz pan-seared trout Tabouli (bulgur, parsley, tomatoes, green onions, and cucumbers with a splash of fresh lemon juice and olive oil) Roasted eggplant Red wine Pear
Snacks	Walnuts Fruit Fresh vegetables with hummus	Walnuts Fruit Fresh vegetables with hummus
Comparison	Compared to Mediterranean-style eating pattern Higher in dairy and grains Lower in fat	Compared to DASH diet Higher in olive oil, nuts, legumes, wine Lower in dairy and grains

- Reductions in blood pressure were similar in men and women and similar in magnitude to the effects seen with drug monotherapy for mild hypertension. It is likely that several aspects of the diet, not just one nutrient or food, lowered blood pressure (Appel et al., 2006).
- Especially noteworthy is that the decrease in blood pressure occurred without lowering sodium intake and without lowering calories to produce weight loss.
- A second study, DASH-sodium, was designed to test whether limiting sodium on a DASH diet would yield even better results. It showed that at each sodium level, blood pressure was lower on the DASH diet than on the control diet and that the greatest blood pressure reductions occurred in Black Americans; middle-aged and older people; and people with hypertension, diabetes, or chronic kidney disease (Sacks et al., 2001).

Mediterranean-Style Eating Pattern

Arguably, the healthiest and best-studied eating pattern is a Mediterranean-style pattern (Fig. 22.1). A large, strong, plausible, and consistent body of prospective evidence confirms the benefits of the Mediterranean-style eating pattern on cardiovascular health (Martinez-González et al., 2019).

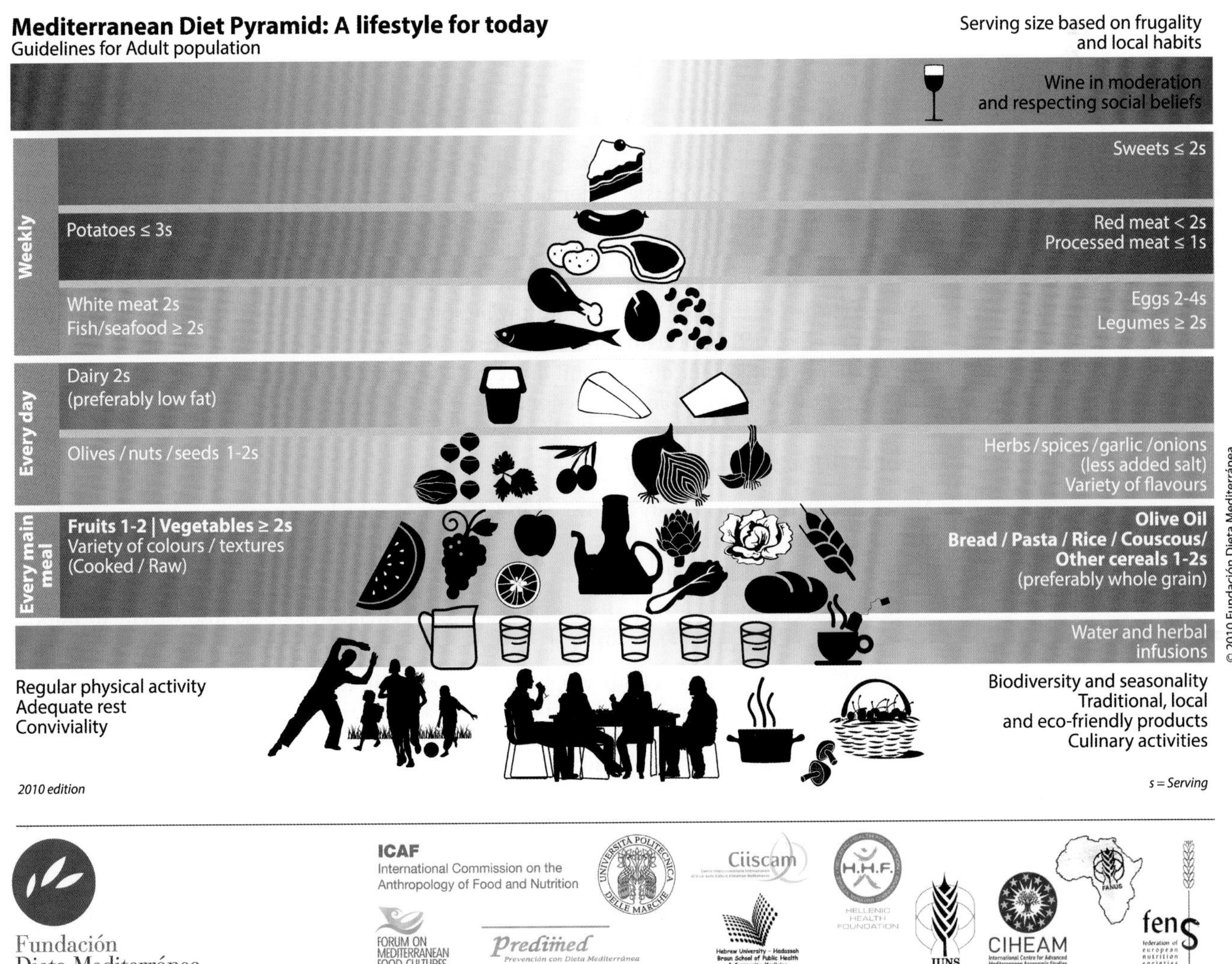

Figure 22.1 ▲ **Mediterranean Diet Pyramid: A lifestyle for today.** (©2010 Foundacion dieta mediterranea. The use and promotion of the pyramid is recommended without any restriction.)

- The PREDIMED study showed that in people at high cardiovascular risk, the incidence of major cardiovascular events was lower among those who consumed a non-calorie–restricted Mediterranean diet supplemented with extra-virgin olive oil or nuts than among those assigned to a low-fat diet (Estruch et al., 2018).
- A large meta-analysis shows that the Mediterranean-style eating pattern is associated with lower risks of CVD incidence and mortality, including CHD and myocardial infarction (MI) (Grosso et al., 2017). The protective effects of the diet appeared to be most attributable to olive oil, fruits, vegetables, and legumes.
- The Mediterranean-style eating pattern is associated with lower risk of all-cause mortality than standard diets (Arnett et al., 2019), a lower risk of Metabolic Syndrome (MetS) (Godos et al., 2016), and with improved glycemic control and CVD risk factors in people with type 2 diabetes (Esposito et al., 2017).

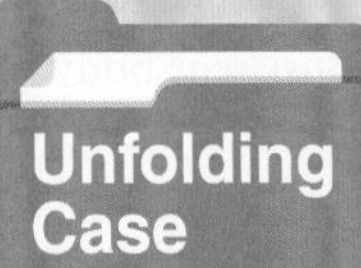

Think of Jacob. Is 2000 calories an appropriate weight loss diet for a male? What factors should be considered when deciding whether Jacob should be counseled to adhere to a DASH diet or a Mediterranean-style eating pattern? Can either pattern be adjusted to the appropriate calorie level? Jacob says he prefers a Mediterranean-style eating pattern because it includes wine, which he will drink in place of beer. What does Jacob need to know about alcohol and his CVD risks?

Nutrition for Cardiovascular Disease Risks

Diet has traditionally been considered a main determinant of cardiovascular health (Martinez-González et al., 2019) and is a major factor in the development or treatment of several other cardiovascular health metrics, namely, hypertension, hypercholesterolemia, obesity (Chapter 17), and diabetes (Chapter 21). These risk factors are often interrelated. For instance, poor diet increases the risk of obesity, which increases the risk of hypertension, type 2 diabetes, and ASCVD (Arnett et al., 2019). A heart-healthy lifestyle is the foundation of ASCVD risk reduction (Grundy et al., 2019). A heart-healthy lifestyle is also recommended for the secondary prevention of ASCVD, hypertension, obesity, and diabetes. Nutrition recommendations for selected CVD risks are presented in the following section.

Overweight and Obesity

Although nutrition for obesity is covered in Chapter 17, the high prevalence of overweight and obesity and its association with heart disease and its risks (e.g., diabetes, hypertension, MetS) warrant inclusion of the topic here.

- It is recommended that all people who are overweight or obese lose weight to improve ASCVD risk profile (Arnett et al., 2019).
- Although a 5% loss of body weight may not result in ideal BMI range, it is associated with moderate improvement in blood pressure, LDL-C, triglyceride levels, and glucose levels in people who are overweight or obese and lowers or delays the development of type 2 diabetes (Arnett et al., 2019).
- Comprehensive weight loss programs are recommended to attain and maintain weight loss. They consist of the following:
  - A hypocaloric diet, such as 1200–1500 cal/day for women and 1500–1800 cal/day for men.
  - At least 150 minutes/week of aerobic physical activity (e.g., brisk walking) for initial weight loss. Higher levels of activity are recommended long term.
  - Self-monitoring of intake, weight, and physical activity.
- BMI should be calculated annually or more frequently to identify who may benefit from weight loss.
- Measuring waist circumference may be useful to identify clients who are at greater cardiometabolic risk.

Hypertension

Hypertension is a major risk factor for CVD and stroke (Virani et al., 2020). The ideal blood pressure metric used in "Life's Simple 7" is defined as less than 120/ less than 80 for adults aged 20 and older. The 2017 Hypertension Clinical Practice Guidelines defines hypertension as systolic blood pressure 130 mm Hg or more or diastolic blood pressure 80 mm Hg or more (Carey et al., 2018).

Some of the diet-related components that have been associated with hypertension include overweight and obesity, excess intake of sodium, and inadequate intakes of potassium, calcium, magnesium, protein (particularly from vegetables), fiber, and fish fats (Whelton et al., 2018). Because poor diet, physical inactivity, and excessive alcohol intake, alone or in combination, are the underlying cause of a large proportion of hypertension, correcting these behaviors is an important approach to preventing and managing hypertension (Whelton et al., 2018).

Recommended interventions for the prevention and treatment of hypertension are as follows (Carey et al., 2018):

- Lose weight if overweight.
- Consume a heart-healthy eating pattern (e.g., DASH diet) (Tables 22.2 and 22.3)
- Limit sodium intake.
    - The top six sources of sodium in a typical American eating pattern are identified as (American Heart Association, 2020):
        - Bread and rolls
        - Pizza
        - Sandwiches
        - Cold cuts and cured meats
        - Soup
        - Burritos and tacos
    - Given that more than 75% of the sodium in a typical American diet comes from processed foods (Box 22.2), it is difficult for people who regularly consume processed, prepackaged, and restaurant foods to lower their sodium intake.
    - Box 22.3 outlines strategies to lower sodium intake and client teaching points.
- Increase potassium intake unless otherwise contraindicated (e.g., use of medications that reduce potassium excretion). High potassium foods include:
    - Dried apricots, raisins, and prunes
    - Potatoes, both sweet and white (especially when baked with the skin on)
    - Leafy greens
    - Lentils and legumes
    - Certain fruit and vegetable juices: prune juice, tomato puree or juice, carrot juice, orange juice, and vegetable juice
    - Milk and yogurt
    - Seafood
- Abstinence from or moderation in alcohol intake (≤2 drinks/day for men, ≤1 drink/day for women).

Hypercholesterolemia

Serum cholesterol and the lipoproteins that carry it (low-density lipoprotein [LDL], very-low-density lipoprotein [VLDL], and high-density lipoprotein [HDL]) are known to be related to ASCVD (Grundy et al., 2019).

- The ideal total cholesterol metric is defined as less than 200 mg/dL.
- LDL and VLDL are atherogenic. Optimal LDL level is less than 100 mg/dL.
- HDL is seemingly not atherogenic (Grundy et al., 2019). Recommended HDL level is at least 40 mg/dL for men and at least 50 mg/dL for women.

BOX 22.2 The Effect of Food Processing on Sodium Content

Examples of the Impact Food Processing Has on Sodium Intake

Food Groups	Sodium (mg)
Whole and other grains and grain products	
Cooked cereal, rice, pasta, unsalted, ½ cup	0–5
Ready-to-eat cereal, 1 cup	0–360
Bread, 1 slice	110–175
Vegetables	
Fresh or frozen, cooked without salt, ½ cup	1–70
Canned or frozen with sauce, ½ cup	140–460
Tomato juice, canned, ½ cup	330
Low-fat or fat-free milk and milk products	
Milk, 1 cup	107
Yogurt, 1 cup	175
Natural cheeses, 1½ oz	110–450
Processed cheeses, 2 oz	600
Nuts, seeds, and legumes	
Peanuts, unsalted, ½ cup	0–5
Peanuts, salted, ½ cup	120
Beans, cooked from dried or frozen, without salt, ½ cup	0–5
Beans, canned, ½ cup	400
Lean meats, fish, and poultry	
Fresh meat, fish, poultry, 3 oz	30–90
Ham, lean, roasted, 3 oz	1020
Tuna (canned water pack), no salt added, 3 oz	35–45
Tuna-canned water pack, 3 oz	230–350
Convenience and Fast Foods	**Sodium (mg)**
1 packet dry onion soup mix	3132
1 tsp salt	2325
1 fast-food single cheeseburger with condiments and bacon	1314
One 6-in., fast-food tuna salad sub	1293
1 large fast-food taco	1233
2 fast-food pancakes with syrup	1104
1 cup canned macaroni and cheese	1061
1 fast-food beef chimichanga	910
1 cup canned soup	800+
1 slice of 14" pizza	640

Historically, nutrition recommendations for reducing CVD risk are dietary cholesterol restriction (U.S. Department of Health and Human Services [USDHHS] & U.S. Department of Agriculture [USDA], 2010). Newer guidelines, including the 2020–2025 Dietary Guidelines for Americans (U.S. Department of Agriculture [USDA] & U.S. Department of Health and Human Services [USDHHS], 2020) and the American Heart Association/American College of Cardiology (AHA/ACC) guideline on the management of blood cholesterol (Grundy et al., 2019), do not make specific recommendations regarding cholesterol intake. The National Academies recommends that dietary cholesterol intake be as low as possible without compromising the nutritional adequacy of the diet (National Research Council, 2005). The issue is cloudy (Carson et al., 2020).

- Observational studies from several countries generally do not indicate a significant association between cholesterol intake and CVD risk.
- Most meta-analysis of intervention studies shows cholesterol intakes that exceed the current average levels of intake are associated with elevated total cholesterol or LDL-C.

BOX 22.3 Strategies to Lower Sodium Intake and Client Teaching Points

In General

- Eat more meals at home. Cook in batches and freeze for use on busy days.
- Avoid or limit convenience foods, such as boxed mixes, frozen dinners, and canned goods.
- Compare labels to find items lowest in sodium.
- Don't add salt when cooking.
- Making changes gradually may be easier.

Grains and Cereals

- Find lower-sodium varieties by comparing labels.
- Cook rice and pasta without adding salt.
- Eat cereals without added salt, such as oatmeal, shredded wheat, and puffed whole-grain cereal.
- Avoid instant flavored rice, pasta, and cereal mixes.

Vegetables

- Eat more fresh or frozen vegetables without salt added.
- Rinse canned vegetables before using.
- Switch to pasta sauce without added salt or dilute regular bottled pasta sauce with equal parts of no-salt-added tomato sauce.
- Substitute fresh vegetables for pickles and other pickled foods.

Fruits

- Fresh, frozen, and canned fruits are salt free; enjoy.

Milk and Milk Products

- Use cheese sparingly, especially processed cheeses.

Protein Foods

- Choose fresh poultry, fish, and lean meat instead of canned, smoked, deli, or other processed varieties.
- Limit frozen dinners.
- Limit cured meat intake, such as sausages and hot dogs. Compare labels to find lower-sodium varieties.
- Limit imitation crab and lobster products.
- Limit soy substitutes, such as imitation ground beef or chicken.
- Use no-salt-added nut butters.

Fats and Oils

- Use homemade vinegar and oil dressings instead of bottled salad dressings.

Miscellaneous

- Use herbs and spices instead of salt to season foods.
- Replace garlic and onion salts with garlic and onion powders.
- Use reduced-salt or no-salt-added condiments such as ketchup, soy sauce, and mayonnaise.
- Use no-salt-added broth to make soup instead of using canned soup.

When Eating Out

- Request that food not be salted, if possible.
- Avoid fast-food restaurant meals, which usually are high in sodium. If you have to go, order a child-sized meal.
- Order sandwiches without mayonnaise, sauces, or condiments; load with lettuce, tomato, and onion.

Client Teaching

Provide general information:

- Reducing sodium intake will help the body rid itself of excess fluid and help lower high blood pressure.
- Sodium appears in the diet in the form of salt and, to some degree, in almost all foods and beverages.
  - Most unprocessed, unsalted foods are low in sodium.
  - The majority of the sodium in a typical American diet comes from processed foods.
  - Sodium-containing compounds are used extensively as preservatives (sodium propionate, sodium sulfite, and sodium benzoate), leavening agents (sodium bicarbonate, baking soda, and baking powder), and flavor enhancers (e.g., salt, MSG) and are found in foods that may not taste salty.
- Salt substitutes replace sodium with potassium or other minerals. "Low-sodium" salt substitutes are not sodium free and may contain half as much sodium as regular table salt. Use neither type without a physician's approval.
- The preference for salty taste eventually will decrease.
- When an occasional food containing ≥300 mg/serving is eaten, balance it out with low-sodium foods the rest of the day.

Teach the client food preparation techniques to minimize sodium intake:

- Prepare foods from "scratch" whenever possible.
- Experiment with sodium-free seasonings, such as herbs, spices, lemon juice, vinegar, and wine. Fresh ingredients are more flavorful than dried ones.
- Try a commercial "salt alternative" for sodium-free flavor enhancement.
- Consult a low-sodium cookbook or online low-sodium recipes.

Teach the client how to read labels:

- Salt, MSG, baking soda, and baking powder contain significant amounts of sodium. Other sodium compounds such as sodium nitrite, benzoate of soda, sodium saccharin, and sodium propionate add less sodium to the diet.
- Sodium labeling terms are reliable:
  - "Sodium-free" and "salt-free" foods provide <5 mg sodium/serving.
  - "Very low sodium" provides <35 mg sodium/serving.
  - "Low sodium" provides <140 mg sodium/serving.
- A variety of low- and reduced-sodium products are available, such as bread and bread products, cereal, crackers, cakes, cookies, pastries, soups, bouillon, canned vegetables, tomato products, meats, entrées, processed meats, hard and soft cheeses, condiments, nuts and peanut butter, butter, margarine, salad dressings, and snack foods. The difference in flavor between some low-sodium products and their high-sodium counterparts is barely noticeable; others taste flat and may need to have herbs or spices added.

- It is difficult to study the relationship between cholesterol intake and CVD because most sources of cholesterol are usually high in saturated fat.

The evidence-based diet-related recommendations featured in the 2013 AHA/ACC guidelines on lifestyle management to lower cardiovascular risk (Eckel et al., 2014) are still supported for the general public and for clients at risk for ASCVD (Grundy et al., 2019).

- Dietary guidance should focus on heart-healthy eating patterns, such as the DASH diet and the Mediterranean-style eating pattern (Carson et al., 2020). These patterns are inherently low in cholesterol.
- The emphasis on vegetables, fruit, whole grains, legumes, healthy protein sources (low-fat dairy, low-fat poultry, fish, seafood, and nuts), and nontropical vegetable oils provides a relatively high ratio of polyunsaturated fatty acids to saturated fatty acids.
- Because egg yolks are relatively high in cholesterol, it is advisable to limit intake in healthy individuals to up to a whole egg daily (Carson et al., 2020).
  - Lacto-ovo vegetarians may include more eggs.
  - Because of the nutritional benefits and convenience of eating eggs, older clients with normal cholesterol may include up to 2 eggs/day within the context of a heart-healthy eating pattern.
  - People with diabetes should be cautious about consuming high-cholesterol foods.

Metabolic Syndrome

Metabolic syndrome (MetS) is a multicomponent risk factor for CVD and type 2 diabetes (Virani et al., 2020).

- MetS consists of a cluster of metabolic abnormalities, namely, elevated triglycerides, low HDL-C, high blood pressure, high fasting blood glucose levels, and central obesity (Alberti et al., 2009).
- Although multiple definitions for MetS have been proposed, generally three abnormal findings out of five qualify a person for MetS (Table 22.4).
- Because MetS is closely linked to excess weight and particularly to central obesity, the prevalence has increased sharply among adults and children in tandem with the increase in overweight and obesity (Grundy et al., 2019).

In all age groups, lifestyle therapy is the main intervention for the primary and secondary prevention of MetS.

- A Mediterranean-style eating pattern is recommended (Table 22.2):
  - A meta-analysis of epidemiological studies and clinical trials indicates that adherence to the Mediterranean-style eating pattern is associated with lower MetS prevalence and progression and has a beneficial effect on the components of MetS, namely, abdominal obesity, lipid levels, glucose metabolism, and blood pressure (Kastorini et al., 2011).
- Calories should be appropriate to maintain weight or lose weight if overweight or obese.

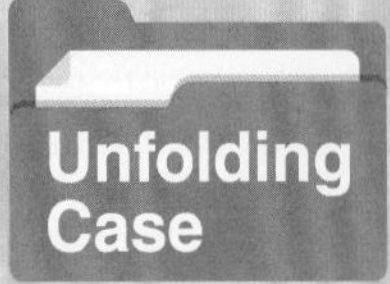

Consider Jacob. Does he meet the criteria for having MetS? Does his diet contribute to his risk of MetS? What should be Jacob's highest dietary priority? How would you respond when he asks if he can use meal replacements for two meals a day so he doesn't have to think about what to eat?

Table 22.4 Diagnostic Criteria for Metabolic Syndrome

Risk Factor	Defining Level
Metabolic syndrome is confirmed by the presence of any three of the following five risks:	
Central obesity	
Men	>40-in. waist
Women	>35-in. waist Or population- and country-specific definitions, especially Asians and non-Europeans who have predominantly lived outside the United States
Elevated triglycerides	≥150 mg/dL Or taking medication for high triglyceride levels
Low HDL-C	
Men	<40 mg/dL in men
Women	<50 mg/dL in women Or taking medication for low HDL-C
Elevated blood pressure	≥130 mm Hg systolic blood pressure ≥85 mm Hg diastolic blood pressure Or taking antihypertensive medication with a history of hypertension
Elevated fasting glucose	≥100 mg/dL Or taking medication to control blood sugar level

Note. HDL-C = high-density lipoprotein cholesterol.
Source: Alberti, K., Eckel, R., Grundy, S., Zimmet, P. Z., Cleeman, J. I., Donato, K. A., Fruchart, J.-C., James, W. P. T., Loria, C. M., & Smith, S. C., Jr. (2009). Harmonizing the metabolic syndrome: A joint interim statement of the International Diabetes Federation Task Force on Epidemiology and Prevention; National Heart, Lung, and Blood Institute: American Heart Association; World Heart Federation: International Atherosclerosis Society; and International Association for the Study of Obesity. *Circulation*, *120*, 1640–1645.

SECONDARY PREVENTION OF CARDIOVASCULAR DISEASES

Secondary prevention of CVD focuses on the management of care for clients who have a history of ASCVD, such as a history of myocardial infarction, angina, prior stenting or bypass surgery, stroke or transient ischemic attack, or symptomatic peripheral arterial disease. The goal is to prevent recurrent events, improve symptoms, and improve quality of life. Treatment approaches include drug therapy (e.g., lipid-lowering medications, antihypertensives, antiplatelets), cardiac rehabilitation, and lifestyle intervention, including a healthy eating pattern.

Healthy Eating Pattern

Yet again, evidence points to the benefits of a Mediterranean-style eating pattern. The Lyon Diet Heart Study, a secondary prevention trial in clients with recent MI, showed rates of CHD events and death were reduced for up to 4 years after an initial event in those assigned a Mediterranean-style eating pattern (de Lorgeril et al., 1999). Likewise, Lopez-Garcia et al. (2014) found an inverse relationship between adherence to a Mediterranean-style eating pattern and all-cause mortality in men and women with CVD, showing that a healthy eating pattern can still be beneficial at an advanced stage of the atherosclerotic process. However, individual preference should determine whether a DASH diet or Mediterranean-style eating pattern is used because both patterns are heart healthy and can be adjusted for appropriate calories and sodium content.

Heart Failure

Cachexia
a wasting syndrome characterized by loss of lean tissue, muscle mass, and bone mass.

Heart failure (HF) is a complex progressive syndrome characterized by specific symptoms—particularly dyspnea, fatigue, and fluid retention—that result from any structural or functional impairment of the heart's ability to adequately pump blood. Malnutrition among clients with advanced HF, known as cardiac **cachexia**, may occur from decreased sensation of hunger, diet restrictions, fatigue, shortness of breath, nausea, anxiety, or malabsorption related to gastrointestinal edema. Sarcopenia, characterized by progressive and generalized loss of skeletal muscle mass and strength, can also be common in clients with HF (Someya et al., 2016).

HF is treated with drug therapy and lifestyle modifications including a healthy eating pattern, weight management, physical activity, and smoking cessation. High adherence to a Mediterranean-style diet has been associated with a lower risk of HF and mortality from HF in men (Tektonidis et al., 2016).

Nutrition Therapy for Heart Failure

Evidence-based nutrition therapy guidelines from the Academy of Nutrition and Dietetics (Kuehneman et al., 2018) includes the following:

- Calorie intake is individualized according to the client's weight and health status.
  - In stable clients, weight loss may be recommended to improve quality of life or comorbidities such as diabetes or hypertension.
- Protein intake should be at least 1.1 g/kg of actual body weight to prevent catabolism. Clients who are malnourished may need 1.1 to 1.4 g/kg actual body weight/day.
- Sodium and fluid intake are individualized within the ranges of 2000 to 3000 mg sodium/day and 1 to 2 L fluid/day.
  - These levels of sodium and fluid intake are associated with improvements in renal function, lab values, symptoms, and quality measures (e.g., readmission rate, length of stay, mortality rate).
  - This level of sodium intake exceeds the current DRI of 1500 mg/day for adults although is less than the typical American intake.
  - There is a lack of evidence to support or refute sodium restriction for HF clients (Mahtani et al., 2018).
- Due to interactions between supplements and medications, it is unclear whether certain supplements, such as coenzyme Q10, n-3 fatty acids, vitamin D, iron, and thiamin, are appropriate for clients with HF.

NURSING PROCESS Heart Failure

Mrs. Gigante is a 79-year-old widow admitted with moderate-to-severe HF, with a long-standing history of hypertension and one previous MI. She lives alone and complains of poor appetite and fatigue. She appears frail and has experienced progressive unintentional weight loss despite significant lower extremity edema. She is diagnosed with cardiac cachexia.

Assessment

Medical–Psychosocial History

- Medical history and comorbidities including diabetes, hypertension, MI, alcohol abuse, and other CHD risk factors
- Use of medications that affect nutrition, such as diuretics, antihypertensives, antidiabetics, and lipid-lowering medications; adherence to prescribed drug therapy
- Additional symptoms that interfere with intake, such as shortness of breath or nausea
- Psychosocial and economic issues, such as living situation, ability to cook and shop, financial status, education, and eligibility for the Meals on Wheels program

Anthropometric Assessment

- Height, weight; BMI
- Recent weight history, especially rapid weight gain

NURSING PROCESS — Heart Failure (continued)

Biochemical and Physical Assessment

- General appearance; signs of muscle wasting
- Blood pressure
- Measure of edema
- Laboratory values related to comorbidities, such as total cholesterol, LDL, HDL, and triglyceride levels
- Intake and output
- Lung sounds respirations for breathing effort

Dietary Assessment

- How many meals and snacks do you usually eat?
- What is your usual 24-hour food intake like?
- What foods are most appealing to you?
- Are there certain times of the day when your appetite is best?
- What symptoms interfere with eating?
- Do you have any cultural, religious, or ethnic influences on your food preferences or eating habits?
- Do you take any vitamins, minerals, and nutritional supplements? If so, what are the reasons?
- Do you use alcohol or caffeine?

Analysis

Possible Nursing Analysis

Evident malnutrition related to poor appetite, eating alone, and fatigue as evidenced by progressive unintentional weight loss and muscle wasting.

Planning

Client Outcomes

The client will do the following:

- Consume a varied and nutritious diet with adequate calories and protein. Eat small, frequent meals to maximize intake.
- Consume appropriate amounts of fluid and sodium.

Nursing Interventions

Nutrition Therapy

- Provide regular diet with in-between meal oral nutrition supplements as ordered.
- Encourage the client to eat calorie- and protein-dense foods first during mealtime.
- Monitor intake.

Client Teaching

Instruct the client on the following:

- The importance of protein and calories to improve nutritional status and overall health.
- The eating plan essentials, including
  - how to increase calories and protein in the diet
  - the benefits of consuming oral nutrition supplements between meals to maximize intake, especially when fatigued
  - to rest before meals
  - to avoid excessive sodium
- The availability of a Meals on Wheels–type program. Explain that Meals on Wheels can provide her with the appropriate diet after discharge to ensure that she gets the proper foods that can be supplemented with oral nutrition supplements as needed. (Notify the discharge planner that the client may be a candidate for Meals on Wheels.)

Evaluation

Evaluate and Monitor

- Monitor percentage of food consumed.
- Monitor weight daily for rapid weight gain.
- Monitor edema and other signs of fluid retention.
- Monitor tolerance to oral diet.
- Suggest changes in the meal plan as needed.
- Provide periodic feedback and reinforcement.

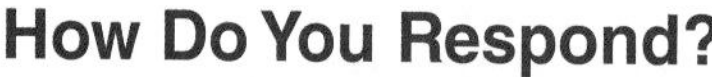

How Do You Respond?

Are there any supplements that lower the risk of heart disease? There is a lack of convincing evidence to support the use of supplements to lower CVD risk; however, it is difficult to study the effects of supplements because people who use supplements generally have a healthier lifestyle and eating pattern and randomized studies are rarely performed (Bronzato & Durante, 2018). Results of the Physician's Healthy Study II showed that taking a daily multivitamin did not reduce major cardiovascular events, MI, stroke, or CVD mortality in male physicians after more than a decade of treatment and follow-up (Sesso et al., 2012). The U.S. Preventive Services Task Force (U.S. Preventive Services Task Force [USPSTF], 2014) states that there is not enough evidence to determine whether taking multivitamins, paired vitamin and mineral supplements, or most single vitamins or minerals will help prevent CVD. Evidence from most randomized controlled trials does not support the use of vitamin E supplementation for the primary or secondary prevention of CVD (Wang & Xu, 2019). More research is needed to clarify the following (Bronzato & Durante, 2018):

- Low–vitamin D levels have been linked to coronary artery disease (CAD), HF, and arterial fibrillation.
- CoQ10 deficiency has been associated with myocardial dysfunction and to statin myopathies.
- Probiotics may be involved in lowering blood pressure and lipid levels

Because hard evidence on the benefits of supplements is lacking at this time, it is safer to obtain nutrients and phytonutrients from food instead of supplements. The DASH diet and Mediterranean-style eating patterns fit the bill once again.

Why should I eat less sodium if my blood pressure is normal? Even for people who are normotensive, lowering sodium intake will blunt the rise in blood pressure that occurs with aging (Appel et al., 2011). In addition to its effect on blood pressure, a high sodium intake also increases the risk of fibrosis in the heart, kidneys, and arteries; kidney damage, gastric cancer, and possibly osteoporosis by increasing the excretion of calcium. Reducing sodium intake is considered an important public health effort to prevent CVD, stroke, and kidney disease (Appel et al., 2011).

REVIEW CASE STUDY

Matt is 34 years old. His waist circumference is 42 and BMI is 30; both have steadily increased over the last few years when he accepted a position with his company that requires frequent travel. It is hard for him to exercise, and he eats out often. He is a "steak and potatoes" kind of guy who wouldn't dream of eating lunch or dinner without meat as the centerpiece of the meal. At his most recent annual employee physical, Matt's total cholesterol level was 245 mg/dL, his HDL level was 33, fasting glucose level was 92, and his blood pressure was 154/85 mm Hg. His father died of a heart attack at age 49 years. Matt feels doomed by genetics and is resistant to going on medication because of the potential side effects. He is willing to try to change his diet and lifestyle but is skeptical that it will help.

- What risks does Matt have for heart disease? What criteria does he have for MetS?
- Knowing that he is willing to change his diet and lifestyle, what additional information would you ask of Matt before devising a teaching plan?
- What diet recommendations would you prioritize in helping Matt initiate a healthy eating pattern? What suggestions could you offer him to help him meet these recommendations?
- How would you respond to Matt's skepticism that lifestyle factors will probably not lower his risk of heart disease?

STUDY QUESTIONS

1 Which statement indicates the client understands the instruction about a DASH-style diet?
a. "The most important thing about a DASH diet is to eat less cholesterol. No egg yolks for me."
b. "I need to eat more fruits, vegetables, and low-fat dairy products."
c. "As long as I don't add salt to my food while cooking or at the table, I will be able to achieve a low-sodium diet."
d. "I need to use olive oil liberally in food preparation and eat nuts every day."

2 The client asks if he can use butter on a heart-healthy diet. Which of the following would be the nurse's best response?
a. "No, butter does not fit into a heart-healthy diet."
b. "Butter is not limited in a heart-healthy diet because most people only use small amounts."
c. "You can fit in small amounts of butter if you are willing to reduce saturated fat elsewhere, such as eating red meat less often.
d. "Butter is considered a dairy product and you can have up to 3 servings/day. "

3 When developing a teaching plan for a client on a low-sodium diet, which of the following foods would the nurse advise the client to limit?
a. Cold cuts
b. Canned fruit
c. Eggs
d. Milk

4 The nurse knows that instructions for a Mediterranean-style eating pattern have been effective when the client expresses a need to eat more
a. fish and nuts
b. lean red and deli meats
c. dairy products
d. sweets that are fat free instead of full fat

5 Which of the following are characteristics of an "ideal" healthy eating pattern for someone consuming 2000 cal/day. Select all that apply.
a. ≥4.5 cups of fruits and vegetables/day
b. ≥3 servings of whole grains/day
c. ≥2 servings of fish/week
d. <1500 mg sodium/day

6 A client asks how to alter a diet to lower high cholesterol levels. Which of the following is the nurse's best response?
a. "Alcohol lowers serum cholesterol, but limit consumption to a moderate intake."
b. "Eliminate egg yolks and butter."
c. "Eat less processed foods."
d. "The issue of reducing cholesterol intake to lower serum cholesterol is murky. Eat a DASH diet or Mediterranean-style eating pattern to lower your risk of ASCVD."

7 The client understands that lifestyle therapy is the cornerstone of primary and secondary prevention of MetS. What does the client need to know about nutrition therapy for MetS?
a. Because the primary goal is to lose weight, it doesn't matter what kind of hypocaloric diet is chosen.
b. The DASH diet has been shown to be most effective at improving MetS risk factors.
c. A Mediterranean-style eating pattern has been shown to be most effective at improving MetS risk factors.
d. Low-fat diets are the best for MetS because it is beneficial to eat less of all types of fat in the diet.

8 Which statement indicates the client does not understand the nutrition recommendations for hypertension?
a. "Weight loss will help lower my blood pressure."
b. "Sodium restriction is not necessary as long as I eat enough potassium in fruits and vegetables."
c. "Alcohol intake should be limited to 1 drink/day for women and 2 drinks/day for men."
d. "The DASH diet is probably better for high blood pressure than the Mediterranean-style eating pattern."

CHAPTER SUMMARY NUTRITION FOR CLIENTS WITH CARDIOVASCULAR DISORDERS

The American Heart Association defines cardiovascular health with seven metrics: eating pattern, physical activity, tobacco use, BMI, blood cholesterol, blood pressure, and blood glucose.

Cardiovascular health among American adults: Americans achieve the ideal most often for tobacco use and least often for eating pattern.

Healthy eating pattern: The "ideal" intake is to achieve 4 of the 5 primary characteristics of a healthy pattern:

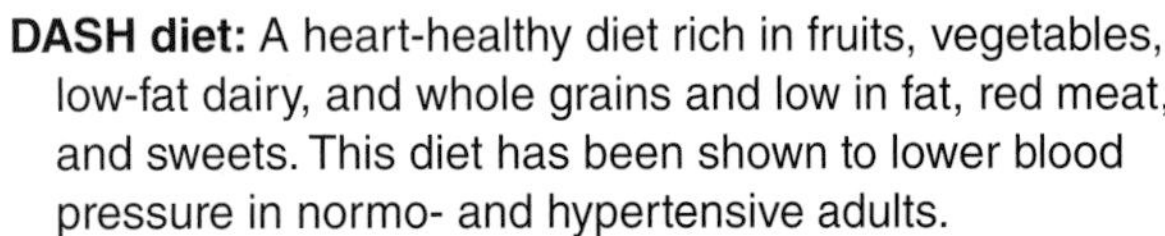

- ≥4.5 cups fruit and vegetables per day
- ≥2 servings of fish/week
- <1500 mg sodium/day
- <36 oz sugar-sweetened beverages/week
- ≥3 servings of whole grains/day

DASH diet: A heart-healthy diet rich in fruits, vegetables, low-fat dairy, and whole grains and low in fat, red meat, and sweets. This diet has been shown to lower blood pressure in normo- and hypertensive adults.

Mediterranean-style eating pattern: The traditional eating pattern of populations living along the Mediterranean basin. It is high in olive oil, fruit, nuts, vegetables, and grains; moderate in fish and poultry; low in dairy, red meat, processed meats, and sweets; and moderate in wine consumed with meals. This heart-healthy eating pattern is associated with reduced risks of CVD and diabetes.

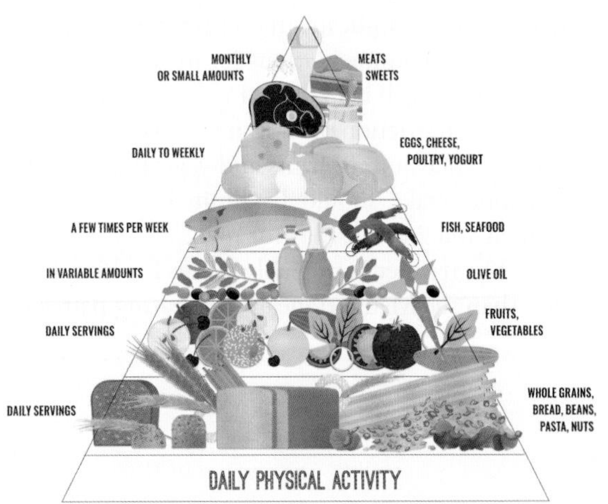

MEDITERRANEAN DIET

Nutrition for CVD risks: Diet is a primary determinant of cardiovascular health and a major factor in the development or treatment of all the other cardiovascular health metrics, namely, hypertension, hypercholesterolemia, obesity, and diabetes.

Overweight and obesity: To reduce the risk of CVD, weight loss is recommended for all people who are overweight or obese. A 5% loss of body weight may result in moderate improvements in blood pressure, LDL-C, triglyceride, and glucose levels. Central obesity indicates greater cardiometabolic risks.

Hypertension: Diet-related lifestyle recommendations for the primary or secondary prevention of hypertension include losing weight if overweight, following a DASH diet, reducing sodium intake, consuming adequate potassium, and using alcohol in moderation, if at all.

Hypercholesterolemia: Previously, the general public and clients with high cholesterol levels were advised to restrict their intake of cholesterol. Currently, the recommendation is to eat a heart-healthy diet (e.g., DASH or Mediterranean style) because they are inherently low in cholesterol and saturated fat. For most people, eating an egg a day is acceptable.

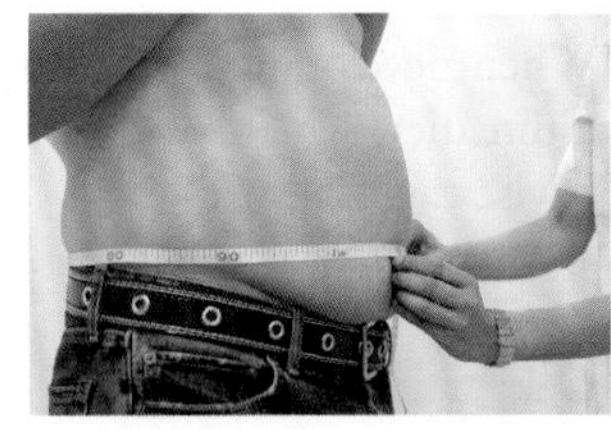

Metabolic syndrome: A multicomponent risk factor for both ASCVD and type 2 diabetes characterized by at least three of the following: high triglycerides, low HDL cholesterol, high blood pressure, elevated fasting glucose, and central obesity. Lifestyle therapy is the cornerstone of treatment. A Mediterranean-style eating pattern with appropriate calories for weight loss is recommended.

Secondary Prevention of Cardiovascular Diseases

Lifestyle modifications, including regular physical activity and weight management, are fundamental to treating existing CHD.

Healthy eating pattern: Both the Mediterranean-style eating pattern and DASH diet are heart healthy. The "best" pattern is the one the client can adhere to. Calories should be adjusted to promote weight loss, if overweight or obese.

Heart failure: HF is treated with drug therapy and lifestyle modifications including a healthy eating pattern, weight management, physical activity, and smoking cessation. Greater adherence to a Mediterranean-style eating pattern is associated with a lower risk of HF. Calories are adjusted for weight status; higher amounts of protein are indicated. The ideal intake of sodium is controversial; 2000 to 3000 mg/day may be appropriate with a fluid restriction, if necessary.

Figure sources: *shutterstock.com/Alexander Raths, shutterstock.com/Double Brain, shutterstock.com/JenJ_Payless*

Student Resources on thePoint®
For additional learning materials, activate the code in the front of this book at https://thePoint.lww.com/activate

Websites

American Heart Association at www.americanheart.org
Heart and Stroke Foundation of Canada at www.hsf.ca
Mediterranean-style eating pattern at https://oldwayspt.org/
National Heart, Lung and Blood Institute at www.nhlbi.nih.gov
To estimate your risk of heart disease, go to http://cvdrisk.nhlbi.nih.gov/

References

Alberti, K., Eckel, R., Grundy, S., Zimmet, P. Z., Cleeman, J. I., Donato, K. A., Fruchart, J.-C., James, W. P. T., Loria, C. M., & Smith, S. C., Jr. (2009). Harmonizing the metabolic syndrome: A joint interim statement of the International Diabetes Federation Task Force on Epidemiology and Prevention; National Heart, Lung, and Blood Institute: American Heart Association; World Heart Federation: International Atherosclerosis Society; and International Association for the Study of Obesity. *Circulation*, *120*(16), 1640–1645. https://doi.org/10.1161/CIRCULATIONAHA.109.192644

American Heart Association. (2020). The salty six infographic. https://www.heart.org/en/healthy-living/healthy-eating/eat-smart/sodium/salty-six-infographic

Appel, L. J., Brands, M. W., Daniels, S. R., Karanja, N., Elmer, P. J., & Sacks, F. M. (2006). Dietary approaches to prevent and treat hypertension: A scientific statement from the American Heart Association. *Hypertension*, *47*(2), 296–308. https://doi.org/10.1161/01.HYP.0000202568.01167.B6

Appel, L. J., Frohlich, E. D., Hall, J. E., Pearson, T. A., Sacco, R. L., Seals, D. R., Sacks, F. M., Smith, S. C., Jr., Vafiadis, D. K., & Van Horn, L. V. (2011). The importance of population-wide sodium reduction as a means to prevent cardiovascular disease and stroke. *Circulation*, *123*(10), 1138–1143. https://doi.org/10.1161/CIR.0b013e31820d0793

Appel, L. J., Moore, T. J., Obarzanek, E., Vollmer, W. M., Svetkey, L. P., Sacks, F. M., Bray, G. A., Vogt, T. M., Cutler, J. A., Windhauser, M. M., Lin, P.-H., Karanja, N., Simons-Morton, D., McCullough, M., Swain, J., Steele, P., Evans, M., Miller, E. R., & Harsha, D. W. for the DASH Collaborative Research Group. (1997). A clinical trial of the effects of dietary patterns on blood pressure. *The New England Journal of Medicine*, *336*, 1117–1124. https://doi.org/10.1056/NEJM199704173361601

Arnett, D. K., Blumenthal, R. S., Albert, M. A., Buroker, A. B., Goldberger, Z. D., Hahn, E. J., Himmelfarb, C. D., Khera, A., Lloyd-Jones, D., McEvoy, J. W., Michos, E. D., Miedema, M. D., Muñoz, D., Smith, S. C., Jr., Virani, S. S., Williams, K. A., Sr., Yeboah, J., & Ziaeian, B. (2019). 2019 ACC/AHA guideline on the primary prevention of cardiovascular disease: A report of the American College of Cardiology/American Heart Association Task Force on Clinical Practice Guidelines. *Circulation*, *140*, e596–e646. https://doi.org/10.1161/CIR.0000000000000678

Boucher, J. (2017). Mediterranean eating pattern. *Diabetes Spectrum*, *30*(2), 72–76. https://doi.org/10.2337/ds16-0074

Bronzato, S., & Durante, A. (2018). Dietary supplements and cardiovascular diseases. *International Journal of Preventive Medicine*, *9*, 80. https://doi.org/10.4103/ijpvm.IJPVM_179_17

Carey, R. M., & Whelton, P. K. for the 2017 ACC/AHA Hypertension Guideline Writing Committee. (2018). Prevention, detection, evaluation, and management of high blood pressure in adults: Synopsis of the 2017 American College of Cardiology/American Heart Association Hypertension Guideline. *Annals of Internal Medicine*, *168*(5), 351–358. https://doi.org/10.7326/M17-3203

Carson, J. A., Lichtenstein, A. H., Anderson, C. A. M., Appel, L. J., Kris-Etherton, P. M., Meyer, K. A., Petersen, K., Polonsky, T., Van Horn, L., and on behalf of the American Heart Association Nutrition Committee of the Council on Lifestyle and Cardiometabolic Health; Council on Arteriosclerosis, Thrombosis and Vascular Biology; Council on Cardiovascular and Stroke Nursing; Council on Clinical Cardiology; Council on Peripheral Vascular Disease; and Stroke Council. (2020). Dietary cholesterol and cardiovascular risk: A science advisory from the American Heart Association. *Circulation*, *141*(3), e39–e53. https://doi.org/10.1161/CIR.0000000000000743

de Lorgeril, M., Salen, P., Martin, J.-L., Monjaud, I., Delaye, J., & Mamelle, N. (1999). Mediterranean diet, traditional risk factors, and the rate of cardiovascular complications after myocardial infarction: Final report of the Lyon Diet Heart Study. *Circulation*, *99*(6), 779–785. https://doi.org/10.1161/01.CIR.99.6.779

Eckel, R. H., Jakicic, J. M., Ard, J. D., de Jesus, J. M., Miller, N. H., Hubbard, V. S., Lee, I.-M., Lichtenstein, A. H., Loria, C. M., Millen, B. E., Nonas, C. A., Sacks, F. M., Smith, S. C., Jr., Svetkey, L. P., Wadden, T. A., & Yanovski, S. Z. (2014). 2013 AHA/ACC guideline on lifestyle management to reduce cardiovascular risk: A report of the American College of Cardiology/American Heart Association Task Force on Practice Guidelines. *Circulation*, *129*(25, suppl 2), S76–S99. https://doi.org/10.1161/01.cir.0000437740.48606.d1

Esposito, K., Maiorino, M., Bellastella, G., ePanagiotakos, D. B., & Giugliano, D. (2017). Mediterranean diet for type 2 diabetes: Cardiometabolic benefits. *Endocrine*, *56*, 27–32. https://doi.org/10.1007/s12020-016-1018-2

Estruch, R., Ros, E., Salas-Salvadó, J., Covas, M.-I., Corella, D., Aros, F., Gomez-Garcia, E., Ruiz-Gutierrez, V., Fiol, M., Lapetra, J., Lamuela-Raventos, R. M., Serra-Majem, L., Pinto, X., Basora, J., Munoz, M. A., Sorli, J.-V., Martinez, J. A., Fito, M., Gea, A., … Martinez-Gonzalez, M. A. for the PREDIMED Study Investigators. (2018). Primary prevention of cardiovascular disease with a Mediterranean diet supplemented with extra-virgin olive oil or nuts. *The New England Journal of Medicine*, *378*, e34. https://doi.org/10.1056/NEJMoa1800389

Godos, J., Zappalà, G., Bernardini, S., Giambini, I., Bes-Rastrollo, M., & Martinez-Gonzalea, M. (2016). Adherence to the Mediterranean diet is inversely associated with metabolic syndrome occurrence: A meta-analysis of observational studies. *International Journal of Food Sciences and Nutrition*, *68*(2), 138–148. https://doi.org/10.1080/09637486.2016.1221900

Grosso, G., Marventano, S., Yang, J., Micek, A., Pajak, A., Scalfi, L., Galvano, F., & Kales, S. N. (2017). A comprehensive meta-analysis on evidence of Mediterranean diet and cardiovascular disease: Are individual components equal? *Critical Reviews in Food Science and Nutrition*, *57*(15), 3218–3232. https://doi.org/10.1080/10408398.2015.1107021

Grundy, S. M., Stone, N. J., Bailey, A. L., Beam, C., Birtcher, K. K., Blumenthal, R. S., Braun, L. T., de Ferranti, S., Faiella-Tommasino, J., Forman, D. E., Goldberg, R., Heidenreich, P. A., Hlatky, M. A., Jones, D. W., Lloyd-Jones, D., Lopez-Pajares, N., Ndumele, C. E., Orringer, C. E., Peralta, C. A., … Yeboah, J. (2019). 2018 AHA/ACC/AACVPR/AAPA/ABC/ACPM/ADA/AGS/APhA/ASPC/NLA/PCNA guideline on the management of blood cholesterol: A report of the American College of Cardiology/American Heart Association Task Force on Clinical Practice Guidelines. *Circulation, 139*, e1082–e1143. https://doi.org/10.1161/CIR.0000000000000625

Heron, M. (2019). Deaths: Leading causes for 2017. *National Vital Statistics Reports, 68*(6), 8. Hyattsville, MD: National Center for Health Statistics.

Huo, T., Du, T., Xu, Y., Xu, W., Chen, X., Sun, D., & Yu, X. (2014). Effects of Mediterranean-style diet on glycemic control, weight loss and cardiovascular risk factors among type 2 diabetes individuals: A meta-analysis. *European Journal of Clinical Nutrition, 69*, 1200–1208. https://doi.org/10.1038/ejcn.2014.243

Kastorini, C.-M., Milionis, H. J., Esposito, K., Guigliano, D., Goudevenos, J. A., & Panagiotakos, D. B. (2011). The effect of Mediterranean diet on metabolic syndrome and its components. A meta-analysis of 50 studies and 534,906 individuals. *Journal of the American College of Cardiology, 57*(11), 1299–1313. https://doi.org/10.1016/j.jacc.2010.09.073

Kuehneman, T., Gregory, M., de Waal, D., Davidson, P., Frickel, R., King, C., Gradwell, E., & Handu, D. (2018). Academy of Nutrition and Dietetics Evidence-based practice guideline for the management of heart failure in adults. *Journal of the Academy of Nutrition and Dietetics, 118*(12), 2331–2345. https://doi.org/10.1016/j.jand.2018.03.004

Lachman, S., Peters, R. J. G., Lentjes, M. A. H., Mulligan, A. A., Luben, R. N., Wareham, N. J., Khaw, K.-T., & Boekholdt, S. M. (2016). Ideal cardiovascular health and risk of cardiovascular events in the EPIC-Norfolk prospective population study. *European Journal of Preventive Cardiology, 23*(9), 986–994. https://doi.org/10.1177/2047487315602015

Lopez-Garcia, E., Rodriguez-Artalejo, F., Li, T. Y., Fung, T. T., Li, S., Willett, W. C., Rimm, E. B., & Hu, F. B. (2014). The Mediterranean-style dietary pattern and mortality among men and women with cardiovascular disease. *The American Journal of Clinical Nutrition, 99*(1), 172–180. https://doi.org/10.3945/ajcn.113.068106

Mahtani, K., Heneghan, C., Onakpoya, I., Tierney, S., Aronson, J. K., Roberts, N., Hobbs, F. D. R., & Nunan, D. (2018). Reduced salt intake for heart failure: A systematic review. *JAMA Internal Medicine, 178*(12), 1693–1700. https://doi.org/10.1001/jamainternmed.2018.4673

Martinez-González, M., Gea, A., & Ruiz-Canela, M. (2019). The Mediterranean diet and cardiovascular health: A critical review. *Circulation Research, 124*(5), 779–798. https://doi.org/10.1161/CIRCRESAHA.118.313348

Mozaffarian, D. (2016). Dietary and policy priorities for cardiovascular disease, diabetes, and obesity: A comprehensive review. *Circulation, 133*(2), 187–225. https://doi.org/10.1161/CIRCULATIONAHA.115.018585

National Research Council. (2005). *Dietary reference intakes for energy, carbohydrate, fiber, fat, fatty acids, cholesterol, protein, and amino acids (macronutrients)*. The National Academies Press.

Sacks, F. M., Svetkey, L. P., Vollmer, W. M., Appel, L. J., Bray, G. A., Harsha, D., Obarzanek, E., Conlin, P. R., Miller, D. R., Simons-Morton, D. G., Karanja, N., Lin, P.-H., Aiken, M., Most-Windhauser, M. M., Moore, T. J., Proschan, M. A., & Cutler, J. A. for the DASH-Sodium Collaborative Research Group. (2001). Effects on blood pressure of reduced dietary sodium and the Dietary Approaches to Stop Hypertension (DASH) diet. *The New England Journal of Medicine, 344*, 3–10. https://doi.org/10.1056/NEJM200101043440101

Sesso, H., Christen, W., Bubes, V., Smith, J. P., MacFadyen, J., Schvartz, M., Manson, J. E., Glynn, R. J., Buring, J. E., & Gaziano, J. M. (2012). Multivitamins in the prevention of cardiovascular disease in men: The Physicians' Health Study II randomized controlled trial. *The Journal of the American Medical Association, 308*(17), 1751–1760. https://doi.org/10.1001/jama.2012.14805

Shikany, J., Safford, M., Bryan, J., Newby, P. K., Richman, J. S., Durant, R. W., Brown, T. M., & Judd, S. E. (2018). Dietary patterns and Mediterranean Diet Score and hazard of recurrent coronary heart disease events and all-cause mortality in the REGARDS Study. *Journal of the American Heart Association, 7*(14), e008078, https://doi.org/10.1161/JAHA.117.008078

Someya, R., Wakabayashi, H., Hayashi, K., Akiyama, E., & Kimura, K. (2016). Rehabilitation nutrition for acute heart failure on inotropes with malnutrition, sarcopenia, and cachexia: A case report. *Journal of the Academy of Nutrition and Dietetics, 116*(5), 765–767. https://doi.org/10.1016/j.jand.2015.11.002

Tektonidis, T. G., Akesson, A., Gigante, B., Wolk, A., & Larsson, S. (2016). Adherence to a Mediterranean diet is associated with reduced risk of heart failure in men. *European Journal of Heart Failure, 18*(3), 253–259. https://doi.org/10.1002/ejhf.481

U.S. Department of Agriculture & U.S. Department of Health and Human Services. (2020, December). *Dietary guidelines for Americans, 2020–2025*. https://www.dietaryguidelines.gov

U.S. Department of Health and Human Services & U.S. Department of Agriculture. (2010). *Dietary Guidelines for Americans, 2010* (7th ed.). https://health.gov/sites/default/files/2020-01/DietaryGuidelines2010.pdf

U.S. News & World Report. (2020). *Best diets overall*. https://health.usnews.com/best-diet/best-diets-overall

U.S. Preventive Services Task Force. (2014). Vitamin supplementation to prevent cancer and CVD: Preventive medication. https://www.uspreventiveservicestaskforce.org/Page/Document/UpdateSummaryFinal/vitamin-supplementation-to-prevent-cancer-and-cvd-counseling

Virani, S. S., Alonso, A., Benjamin, E. J., Bittencourt, M. S., Callaway, C. W., Carson, A. P., Chamberlain, A. M., Chang, A. R., Cheng, S., Delling, F. N., Djousse, L., Elkind, M. S. V., Ferguson, J. F., Fornage, M., Khan, S. S., Kissela, B. M., Knutson, K. L., Kwan, T. W., Lackland, D. T., … Tsao, C. W. on behalf of the American Heart Association Council on Epidemiology and Prevention Statistics Committee and Stroke Statistics Subcommittee. (2020). Heart disease and stroke statistics—2020 update: A report from the American Heart Association. *Circulation, 141*(9), e139–e596. https://doi.org/10.1161/CIR.0000000000000757

Wang, T., & Xu, L. (2019). Circulating vitamin E levels and risk of coronary artery disease and myocardial infarction: A Mendelian randomization study. *Nutrients, 11*(9), 2153. https://doi.org/10.3390/nu11092153

Whelton, P. K., Carey, R. M., Aronow, W. S., Casey, D. E., Jr., Collins, K. J., Himmelfarb, C. D., DePalma, S. M., Gidding, S., Jamerson, K. A., Jones, D. W., McLaughlin, E. J., Munter, P., Ovbiagele, B., Smith, S. C., Spencer, C. C., Stafford, R. S., Taler, S. J., Thomas, R. J., Williams, K. A., … Wright, J. T., Jr. (2018). 2017 ACC/AHA/AAPA/ABC/ACPM/AGS/APhA/ASH/ASPC/NMA/ PCNA Guideline for the prevention, detection, evaluation, and management of high blood pressure in adults: executive summary—A report of the American College of Cardiology/American Heart Association Task Force on Clinical Practice Guidelines. *Hypertension, 71*(6), 1269–1324. https://doi.org/10.1161/hyp.0000000000000066

Chapter 23

Nutrition for Clients with Kidney Disorders

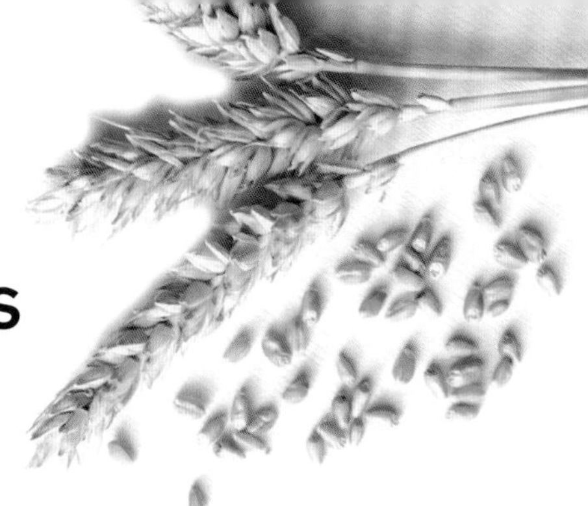

Unfolding Case

Sonja Fern

Sonja is 46 years old, is 6 ft 1 in. tall, and weighs 218 pounds. She has intentionally lost 25 pounds in the last month after donating one of her kidneys. She was extremely moved by the significance of being healthy enough to help a friend through organ donation and recognizes that she must proactively protect her remaining kidney to preserve her own health. She had borderline hypertension before the surgery, is a previous heavy smoker, but has no other medical history. She has adopted a lacto-ovo vegetarian eating pattern and occasionally eats fish.

Learning Objectives

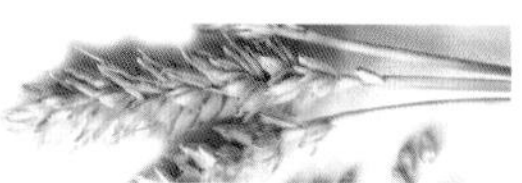

Upon completion of this chapter, you will be able to:

1 Explain general nutrition recommendations for nephrotic syndrome.
2 Discuss nutrition and lifestyle interventions that may help prevent chronic kidney disease (CKD).
3 Explain why sodium, protein, phosphorus, and potassium are restricted as kidney disease progresses.
4 Summarize the importance of consuming adequate calories when protein intake is restricted.
5 Give examples of foods to eat or avoid when sodium, protein, phosphorus, and potassium are restricted.
6 Review characteristics of the Mediterranean-Style Eating Pattern that may benefit clients with CKD.
7 Explain how nutrient recommendations differ for clients with CKD after renal replacement therapy begins.
8 Explain nutrient recommendations for posttransplant clients.
9 Summarize nutrition and lifestyle strategies that may help prevent kidney stones from forming.

Chronic Kidney Disease (CKD)
an estimated GFR <60 mL/min/1.73 m^2 for ≥3 months with evidence of kidney damage as indicated by albuminuria.

The kidneys play many vital roles in maintaining overall health (Box 23.1); impairments in kidney function can cause widespread disruptions in metabolism, bone health, fluid balance, nutritional status, and nutrient requirements. Kidney diseases are the ninth leading cause of death in the United States (Kochanek et al., 2019). Fifteen percent of U.S. adults are estimated to have **chronic kidney disease (CKD)** and 9 out of 10 adults with CKD do not know they have it (Centers for Disease Control and Prevention [CDC], 2019). Kidney diseases vary in severity, chronicity, and etiology.

BOX 23.1 Kidney Functions

Filter blood and form urine to

- regulate extracellular fluid volume and osmolarity, electrolyte concentration, and acid–base balance;
- excrete nitrogenous wastes from protein metabolism (e.g., urea, creatinine), toxic substances, and drugs;

Help regulate blood pressure by secreting renin, an enzyme that activates the precursor of angiotensin, a hormone involved in blood pressure regulation
Stimulate the production of RBC in the bone marrow by producing the hormone erythropoietin
Help regulate calcium balance and bone formation by converting vitamin D to its active form

Nutrition is implicated in several of the chronic disease risk factors for CKD and is an integral component of kidney disease management. This chapter presents the role of nutrition in maintaining kidney health and nutrition therapy for the treatment of nephrotic syndrome, CKD, acute kidney injury (AKI), and urolithiasis.

NUTRITION IN MAINTAINING KIDNEY HEALTH

The typical American diet, characterized by a high intake of red meat, saturated fat, trans fat, added sugar, and processed foods and a low intake of fruits, vegetables, whole grains, and fish, increases the risk of several chronic diseases, such as obesity, diabetes, hypertension, and cardiovascular disease (CVD). Each of these chronic diseases increases the risk of kidney disease. Furthermore, the Nurse's Health Study showed that people who consume a typical American-Style Eating Pattern are more likely to have moderate to severely increased levels of urinary albumin excretion and are more likely to have a rapid decline in **glomerular filtration rate (GFR)** compared to people who do not eat a western diet (Lin et al., 2011).

Glomerular Filtration Rate (GFR)
the rate at which the kidneys form filtrate estimated from the amount of creatinine excreted per 24 hours. Normal GFR is about 120 to 130 mL/min.

Preventing CKD and its complications is possible by managing risk factors to slow its progression (CDC, 2017). Given their shared risks, general suggestions to reduce the risk of CKD are consistent with recommendations for promoting cardiovascular health (Chapter 22).

- Lose weight if overweight.
- Consume a healthy eating pattern, such as a Dietary Approaches to Stop Hypertension (DASH) diet or Mediterranean-Style Eating Pattern.
- Be physically active.
- Do not use tobacco.
- Control blood glucose levels.
- Maintain normal blood pressure.
- Maintain normal serum cholesterol.

Healthy Eating Pattern

Known to reduce the risk of CVD, the DASH diet and Mediterranean-Style Eating Patterns have also been shown to reduce the incidence of CKD disease (Huang et al., 2013b; Rebholz et al., 2016). Both patterns are inherently low in cholesterol, saturated fat, and processed foods (e.g., sodium) and can be adjusted to provide the appropriate number of calories for achieving or maintaining healthy weight. Unlike recommendations for cardiovascular health, a healthy eating pattern for healthy kidneys also includes avoiding an excessive intake of protein. Protein metabolism generates **nitrogenous wastes** that the kidney must excrete. Increasing the proportion of plant sources of protein is recommended (Kalantar-Zadek & Fougue, 2017).

Nitrogenous Wastes
wastes produced from nitrogen—namely, ammonia, urea, uric acid, and creatinine.

DASH Diet

A prospective cohort study has found that participants who consumed an eating pattern similar to the Dietary Approaches to Stop Hypertension (DASH) diet had a lower risk for kidney disease, independent of demographic characteristics, kidney disease risk factors, and baseline kidney function (Rebholz et al., 2016).

- The DASH diet is high in fruits, vegetables, whole grains, nuts and legumes, and low-fat dairy products and low in red and processed meats, sugar-sweetened beverages, and sweets (see Chapter 22).
- Benefits may be attributed to its effect on lowering blood pressure and reducing inflammation.
- In addition, researchers specifically found that high intakes of nuts, legumes, and low-fat dairy products were associated with a lower risk for kidney disease, whereas high red and processed meat intake was associated with a higher kidney disease risk.

Mediterranean-Style Eating Pattern

Strong adherence to a Mediterranean-Style Eating Pattern is associated with lower prevalence of CKD and lower mortality risk (Huang et al., 2013b).

- The Mediterranean-Style Eating Pattern is a plant-based pattern that emphasizes whole grains, fruit, vegetables, nuts, legumes, and olive oil; frequent intake of fish; limited amounts of red meat, processed meats, and sweets; and wine in moderation with meals.
- The Mediterranean-Style Eating Pattern may help preserve kidney function through favorable effects on endothelial function, inflammation, lipid levels, and blood pressure (Chauveau et al., 2018).
- Strong adherence to a Mediterranean-Style Eating Pattern has also been shown to lower the risk of two major risk factors for CKD, namely, CVD (Estruch et al., 2018) and type 2 diabetes (Salas-Salvado et al., 2016).

NEPHROTIC SYNDROME

Nephrotic Syndrome
a collection of symptoms that occur when increased capillary permeability in the glomeruli allows serum proteins to leak into the urine.

Hypoalbuminemia
low blood levels of albumin, the most abundant plasma protein.

Proteinuria
protein in the urine; also known as albuminuria.

Hyperlipidemia
abnormally high level of lipids in the blood, such as low-density lipoprotein cholesterol and triglycerides.

Nephrotic syndrome refers to a collection of symptoms caused by alterations in the kidney's glomerular basement membrane that result in large urinary losses of albumin and other plasma proteins. It can arise from any kidney disease that damages the glomeruli, such as diabetes, autoimmune diseases (e.g., lupus, IgA nephropathy), infection, and certain chemicals.

- **Hypoalbuminemia**, **proteinuria**, **hyperlipidemia**, and edema are major features of nephrotic syndrome.
- The majority of the urinary protein excreted is albumin; hypoalbuminemia, along with sodium and fluid retention, leads to edema.
- Possible complications related to the loss of other plasma proteins include anemia (loss of transferrin), increased risk of infection (loss of immunoglobulins), vitamin D deficiency (loss of vitamin D–binding protein), and increased blood clotting (loss of anti–blood clotting proteins).
- Hyperlipidemia (elevated serum levels of cholesterol and triglycerides) increases the risk of atherosclerosis, myocardial infarction, and stroke and may play a role in the increased risk of thrombosis associated with nephrotic syndrome (Agrawal et al., 2018). The dyslipidemia of nephrotic syndrome also causes kidney injury and may contribute to the development of CKD.
- Protein–calorie malnutrition may develop.
- In some cases, treating the underlying disorder corrects nephrotic syndrome. In others, especially diabetes, nephrotic syndrome may be the beginning of CKD.

Nutrition Therapy for Nephrotic Syndrome

The primary objective of nutrition therapy for nephrotic syndrome is to reduce proteinuria (Academy of Nutrition and Dietetics, 2020).

- The recommended protein intake for nephrotic syndrome in adults is 0.8 to 1.0 g/kg/day (adult Recommended Dietary Allowance [RDA] is 0.8 g/kg/day.) (Cadnapaphornchai et al., 2014). Although nephrotic syndrome is characterized by increased urinary losses of plasma proteins, a high-protein diet is contraindicated because it exacerbates urinary protein losses, promoting further kidney damage.
- Sodium intake should be restricted to ≤2 g/day to help control edema and blood pressure (Cadnapaphornchai et al., 2014).
- A low-fat, low-cholesterol diet is recommended because it improves dyslipidemia. However, no study has proven that this intervention improves prognosis (Nishi et al., 2016).
- Adequate calories, such as 35 cal/kg, are required to spare protein and maintain weight.
- Supplements of vitamin D are provided when vitamin D deficiency is diagnosed.

CHRONIC KIDNEY DISEASE

Estimated Glomerular Filtration Rate (eGFR) determined through an equation that takes into account serum creatinine level, age, gender, and race; used interchangeably with the term glomerular filtration rate (GFR).

Normal kidney function is defined as an **estimated glomerular filtration rate (eGFR)** of at least 90 mL/min 1.73 m^2, although 60 to 89 may be normal for some people, including adults over the age of 60. CKD is diagnosed when eGFR is <60 for 3 months or longer.

CKD, a generally progressive and irreversible loss of kidney function, is categorized into five stages based on eGFR. Stages 1 and 2 are the mildest stages, whereas stage 5 represents advanced CKD. The decision to begin dialysis or perform a transplant is made not only on the basis of residual kidney function, but also on the basis of symptoms of uremia (e.g., anorexia, hyperazotemia, hyperphosphatemia, metabolic acidosis, malnutrition, etc.) that are no longer manageable (Cupisti et al., 2018).

Chronic Kidney Disease Risk Factors

Diabetes (Chapter 21) and hypertension (Chapter 22) are responsible for 3 out of 4 of new cases of kidney failure (CDC, 2020). Other risk factors include CVD, obesity, advancing age, and a family history of CKD. Individuals of African-American, Native American, or Hispanic ethnicities are at increased risk for CKD. CKD increases the risk of early death, heart disease, and stroke. Not all clients with CKD progress to kidney failure. Control of risk factors, annual testing, lifestyle changes, and medication may help prevent CKD and lower the risk of kidney failure (CDC, 2020).

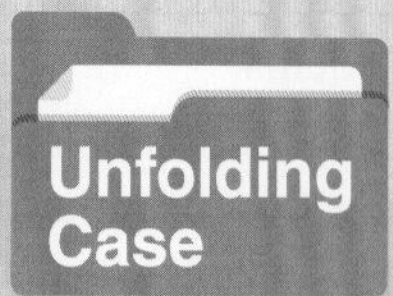

Think of Sonja. What is her body mass index (BMI)? What risk factors for CKD did she have or currently has? What interventions would you suggest to help her maintain kidney health? Is a lacto-ovo eating pattern adequate and appropriate?

Disease Progression

CKD and its progression are closely linked to increased inflammatory response of the body (Pluta et al., 2017). As kidney function deteriorates, especially in advanced stages, the ability to excrete adequate amounts of nitrogenous wastes, sodium, fluid, potassium, phosphorus, and hydrogen

BOX 23.2 Complications of Chronic Kidney Disease

- Sodium and fluid retention → hypertension, edema, shortness of breath, heart failure, and oxidative stress.
- Impaired synthesis of renin contributes to hypertension.
- Phosphorus retention → secondary hyperparathyroidism → renal bone disease, vascular calcification, accelerated progression of kidney disease due to vascular injury, and increased risk of cardiovascular mortality.
- Decreased excretion of the **fixed acid** load → metabolic acidosis.
- Metabolic acidosis → anorexia, nausea, and vomiting; it also stimulates protein and muscle catabolism, bone demineralization, insulin resistance, and hyperkalemia. Associated with more rapid kidney disease progression and increase in overall risk of death.
- Impaired synthesis of erythropoietin → anemia; GI absorption of iron is also impaired and iron intake may be inadequate.
- Alterations in carbohydrate, protein, and fat metabolism may contribute to hypoglycemia, cachexia, and CVD (de Boer & Utzschneider, 2017).
- Accumulation of nitrogenous wastes (from food intake and muscle protein catabolism) → uremic syndrome, characterized by anemia, bone disease, hormonal imbalances, bleeding impairment, impaired immunity, fatigue, decreased mental acuity, muscle twitches, cramps, anorexia, nausea, vomiting, diarrhea, itchy skin, and gastritis.
- Uremic syndrome → PEW → decreased physical activity, onset of a micro-inflammatory state, and higher rates of hospitalization and mortality.
- Inflammation, oxidative stress, and vascular calcification contribute to accelerated onset of cardiovascular risk.
- Cardiovascular death is 2 to 3 times higher in clients with CKD compared with the general population (Saglimbene et al., 2020).

Source: Cupisti, A., Brunori, G., Di Iorio, B. R., D'Alessandro, C., Pasticci, F., Cosola, C., Bellizzi, V., Bolasco, P., Capitanini, A., Fantuzzi, A. L., Gennari, A., Piccoli, G. B., Quintaliani, G., Salomone, M., Sandrini, M., Santoro, D., Babini, P., Fiaccadori, E., Gambaro, G., ... Gesualdo, L. (2018). Nutritional treatment of advanced CKD: Twenty consensus statements. *Journal of Nephrology*, *31*(4), 457–473. https://doi.org/10.1007/s40620-018-0497-z

Fixed Acid
Acid produced in the body from sources other than carbon dioxide that are not excreted by the lungs. These acids are mostly produced from the metabolism of sulfur in dietary protein; plant foods yield bicarbonate. Dietary acid load must be excreted by the kidney to maintain acid–base balance.

ions becomes increasingly impaired. Interrelated and multifactorial metabolic and clinical complications develop, and the disruption to homeostasis is profound (Box 23.2).

- Complications increase in frequency and severity as CKD progresses; however, complications can occur at any stage and can lead to death before CKD progresses to end-stage renal disease (ESRD).
- Complications may arise not only from diminishing kidney function, but also from CVD or treatments.
- Significant weight loss relatively early in the course of CKD is associated with a substantially higher risk for death after dialysis is initiated (Ku et al., 2018). More studies are needed to determine if optimizing weight and nutritional status before the initiation of dialysis will improve ESRD outcomes.
- Protein energy wasting (PEW), similar to cachexia, has a prevalence of 11% to 54% among clients during Stages 3 to 5 of CKD (Carrero et al., 2018): However, there is a lack of consensus on how to define PEW in this population and how to measure proposed criteria, such as skeletal muscle depletion, reduced food intake, and abnormal lab values (e.g., serum albumin) (Koppe et al., 2019).
- CKD is associated with an increase in atherosclerosis from its early stages and the progression of CKD is associated with the progression of atherosclerosis
  - Among the emerging risk factors for atherosclerosis in CKD are altered bone mineral metabolism, vascular calcification, uremic toxins, inflammation, oxidative stress, and endothelial dysfunction (Valdivielso et al., 2019).

Nutrition Therapy

The goal of nutrition therapy in CKD is to promote optimal nutritional status; prevent and or improve signs, symptoms, and complications of CKD; and possibly delay the initiation of dialysis (Cupisti et al., 2018). Indeed, nutrition therapy can help manage uremia, electrolyte and acid–base imbalances, water and sodium retention, mineral and bone disorders, and protein–energy malnutrition (Kalantar-Zadek & Fougue, 2017). Control of blood pressure and glucose levels remains the crucial strategy in all stages of kidney disease.

Although the potential benefits of nutrition therapy in CKD are recognized, there is lack of consensus on actual nutrient recommendations; variations exist among experts, the level of existing kidney function, and comorbidities. Generally, all clients with CKD are urged to eat a heart-healthy eating pattern and to avoid excessive intakes of protein and sodium; additional restrictions for phosphorus and potassium are added as necessary (Table 23.1). Salient points about these and other nutrients of concern are presented in the following section. As restrictions become more numerous and severe, overall diet quality may be compromised (Campbell & Carrero, 2016). Box 23.3 provides a general guide for food selection.

Table 23.1 General Nutrient Recommendations for Chronic Kidney Disease

Nutrient	Adult DRI	Average Adult American Intake	General Recommendations for Normal Kidney Function with Increased CKD Risk (e.g., Due to Diabetes, Hypertension, Polycystic Kidney Disease, or Only Having One Kidney)	General Recommendations for Mild/Moderate-to-Severe CKD (Not on Dialysis)
Protein	0.8 g/kg	1.35 g/kg	<1.0 g/kg	*Without concurrent diabetes:* 0.55–0.6 g/kg *or* 0.28–0.43 g/kg with added keto acids to achieve 0.55–0.6 g/kg *With concurrent diabetes:* 0.6–0.8 g/kg
Sodium	1500 mg	3536 mg (U.S. Department of Agriculture [USDA], Agricultural Research Service [ARS], 2018)	<4000 mg (<3000 mg in clients with hypertension)	<2300 mg
Phosphorus	700 mg	1385 mg (USDA & ARS, 2018)	<1000 mg (limit phosphorus intake from preservatives and processed foods)	<800 mg (limit phosphorus intake from preservatives and processed foods; encourage more plant-based foods)
Potassium	Women: 2600 mg Men: 3400 mg	2323 mg/day (USDA & ARS, 2018)	Same as general population	≤2000–3000 mg

Source: Kalantar-Zadeh, K., & Fouque, D. (2017). Nutritional management of chronic kidney disease. *The New England Journal of Medicine*, *377*, 1765–1776; Ikizler, T. A., Burrowes, J. D., Byham-Gray, L. D., Campbell, K. L., Carrero, J.-J., Chan, W., Fougue, D., Friedman, A. N., Ghadder, S., Goldstein-Fuchs, D. J., Kaysen, G. A., Kopple, J. D., Teta, D., Wang, A. Y.-M., & Cuppari, L. (2020). KDOQI Nutrition in CKD Guideline Work Group. KDOQI clinical practice guideline for nutrition in CKD: 2020 update. *American Journal of Kidney Diseases*, *76*(3)(suppl 1), S1–S107. https://www.ajkd.org/article/S0272-6386(20)30726-5/pdf; U.S. Department of Agriculture & Agricultural Research Service. (2018). Nutrient intakes from food and beverages: Mean amounts consumed per individual, by gender and age, What We Eat in America, NHANES 2015–2016. https://www.ars.usda.gov/ARSUserFiles/80400530/pdf/1516/Table_1_NIN_GEN_15.pdf

BOX 23.3 Eating Tips for People with Chronic Kidney Disease

These recommendations are intended for all people with CKD.

- Choose heart-healthy options.
  - Grill, broil, bake, roast, or stir-fry instead of deep-fat frying.
  - Use nonstick cooking spray or olive oil instead of butter.
  - Trim fat from meat and remove poultry skin before eating.
  - Choose lean protein sources: loin or round cuts of meat, skinless white-meat poultry, fish, legumes, and low-fat milk, yogurt, and cheese.
  - Limit alcohol to moderate intake: no more than 1 drink/day for women and no more than 2 drinks/day for men.
- Control the type and amount of protein chosen.
  - Eat small portions of protein.
  - Use a mix of animal proteins (chicken, fish, meat, eggs, dairy) and plant proteins (legumes, nuts).
- Choose foods with less sodium to help control blood pressure.
  - Avoid salting food during cooking or at the table.
  - Buy fresh food more often.
  - Use spices, herbs, and sodium-free seasonings instead of salt.
  - Check the Nutrition Facts label to comparison shop. A Daily Value of ≥20% means the food is high in sodium.
  - Look for foods that are labeled sodium free, salt free, very low sodium, low sodium, reduced or less sodium.
  - Rinse canned vegetables, beans, and meats before eating.
  - Avoid processed meats and salted snacks and crackers.
  - Avoid high-sodium condiments, such as soy sauce, teriyaki sauce, and bottled salad dressings.

Additionally, these recommendations may be appropriate as kidney function deteriorates.

- Choose foods with less phosphorous.
  - Many packaged foods have added phosphorus. Look for phosphorus or words beginning with "phos" on ingredient lists.
  - Foods higher in phosphorus include
    - meat, poultry, and fish;
    - bran cereals and oatmeal;
    - chocolate, hot chocolate, and cocoa;
    - some whole grains;
    - dairy foods: milk, cheese, ice cream, milk, pudding, and yogurt;
    - lentils;
    - nuts, peanut butter, and seeds; and
    - cola and beer.
  - Foods lower in phosphorus include
    - fresh fruit and vegetables;
    - breads, pasta, rice;
    - corn and rice cereals;
    - non-enriched rice milk; and
    - light-colored soft drinks.
- Choose foods that have the appropriate amount of potassium.
  - Avoid salt substitutes unless approved by the health care provider.
  - Drain canned fruits and vegetables before eating.
  - Foods higher in potassium include
    - oranges, orange juice, avocado, banana, kiwifruit, prunes, prune juice, dried fruit, mango, nectarine, papaya, and pumpkin;
    - artichokes, avocado, brussels sprouts, okra, winter squash, potatoes, greens (except kale), tomatoes, and vegetable juice;
    - brown and wild rice, bran cereals;
    - milk and yogurt;
    - whole-wheat bread and pasta; and
    - legumes and nuts.
  - Foods lower in potassium include
    - apples, black berries, blueberries, cherries, grapes, grape juice, pears, pineapple, raspberries, and strawberries;
    - carrots, green beans, cabbage, celery, corn, cucumber, eggplant, kale, lettuce, green peas, and zucchini squash;
    - white bread, pasta, and rice;
    - cooked rice and wheat cereals; grits; and
    - unenriched rice milk.

Adapted from National Institute of Diabetes and Digestive and Kidney Diseases. (2016, October). *Eating right for chronic kidney disease*. https://www.niddk.nih.gov/health-information/kidney-disease/chronic-kidney-disease-ckd/eating-nutrition

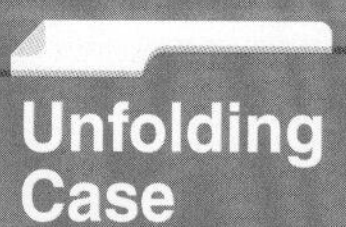

Consider Sonja. A diet history revealed she uses soy protein–based entrees, which she recently realized are high in sodium. Her typical pattern also includes 1 serving of yogurt per day, 1 serving of vegetables, 1 to 2 servings of fruit, and occasionally whole-wheat bread. She dislikes milk and gave up sugar-sweetened beverages. She drinks two "large" glasses of wine 3 to 4 days/week and admitted a weakness for white bread and potatoes. When she is stressed, she goes to the vending machine and buys two candy bars and hides them in her clothes so her coworkers won't know she is eating. Does her usual intake qualify as a healthy eating pattern? What are the positive features of her current pattern? What specific changes can she make in her intake to improve her diet quality? Is her alcohol intake considered moderate? What options would you suggest in place of high-sodium soy entrees?

Heart-Healthy Eating Pattern: Mediterranean Style

The Mediterranean diet has recently been suggested for adults with CKD Stages 1 to 5 not on dialysis or posttransplantation, with or without altered lipid levels, to improve lipid profiles (Ikizler et al., 2020).

- Emerging evidence in clients with CKD suggests that eating patterns rich in fruits and vegetables, such as the Mediterranean-Style Eating Pattern, may help delay the progression of CKD and prevent complications (Kelly et al., 2017).
- Better adherence to the Mediterranean-Style Eating Pattern has been consistently associated with a lower risk of ESRD in community-dwelling adults aged 51 to 70 years (Smyth et al., 2016).
- The potential mechanisms by which the Mediterranean-Style Eating Pattern may benefit clients with CKD are summarized in Box 23.4.

BOX 23.4 Selected Potential Mechanisms by Which the Mediterranean-Style Eating Pattern May Benefit Clients with Chronic Kidney Disease

- The amount of protein is similar to a controlled protein diet for CKD, supplying approximately 0.8 g/kg/day; but it mostly comes from heart-healthy vegetables, fish, and white meat.
- Red and processed meats are limited, which limits saturated fat, sodium, and phosphate intake.
- Half of the relatively high fat content is from monounsaturated fat due to the use of extra virgin olive oil; its polyphenols and vitamin E exert anti-inflammatory and antioxidant properties.
- Most of the carbohydrates are from high-quality, nutrient-dense sources, such as fruit, vegetables, whole grains, and nuts, which results in a low-glycemic index intake that may improve glucose control, hyperinsulinemia, insulin resistance, and blood lipid levels.
- Moderate intake of wine is included, which has anti-inflammatory and antioxidant properties due to the content of polyphenols (e.g., resveratrol) in red wine and phenols in white wine.
- Unrefined, minimally processed foods, which are lower in phosphorus and sodium than highly processed foods, are emphasized.
- Thirty to 50 g of fiber/day is provided, which positively affects the microbiome, constipation, uremic toxins, inflammation, and the risk of diabetes and heart disease.
- Its high content of fruits and vegetables is controversial.
  - On the plus side, they provide potassium which may help control blood pressure and have a low dietary acid load which may slow the decline in kidney function.
  - However, their high potassium content may increase the risk of CKD progression.

Source: Chauveau, P., Aparicio, M., Bellizzi, V., Campbell, K., Hong, X., Johansson, L., Kolko, A., Molina, P., Sezer, S., Wanner, C., ter Wee, P. M., Teta, D., Fouque, D., Carrero, J. J., & European Renal Nutrition (ERN) Working Group of the European Renal Association-European Dialysis Transplant Association (ERA-EDTA). (2018). Mediterranean diet as the diet of choice for patients with chronic kidney disease. *Nephrology Dialysis Transplantation*, *33*, 725–735. https://doi.org/10.1093/ndt/gfx085

Protein

A high-protein diet, usually defined as >1.2 g protein/kg body weight/day, is known to cause significant alterations in the function and health of kidneys (Ko et al., 2017). Conversely, low-protein diets can slow the progression of CKD but contribute to the state of malnutrition usually seen in CKD clients (Noce et al., 2016).

- Although it is agreed upon that excesses and deficiencies of protein should be avoided, the ideal intake of protein for clients with CKD is not known.
- Clients with CKD and diabetes may be allowed slightly higher amounts of protein than clients without diabetes to improve glycemic control.
- Where keto acid analogs are available, a very-low-protein diet supplemented with essential amino acids and keto acid mixtures may be considered for adults without diabetes, not on dialysis, and with an eGFR <20 mL/min/1.73 m^2.
    - Keto acid analogs are widely used for managing CKD in Europe, Asia, and other areas of the world. Their use in the United States is limited because of lack of availability.
    - These supplements ensure a sufficient balance of essential amino acids.
    - Crucial to the success of this type of regimen is a high level of client motivation, intensive education and support, and ongoing nutrition counseling.
- Low-protein diets (0.6–0.8 g protein/kg body weight/day) are not always prescribed in the United States as a means of slowing the progression of CKD, in part because of the risk of malnutrition and difficulty with compliance (Kalantar-Zadeh et al., 2016).
    - Most clients on a low-protein diet consume more protein than prescribed (Cupisti et al., 2018).

Sodium

Sodium restriction is recommended to control fluid retention and hypertension and to improve cardiovascular risk profile, even though it is not clear that it slows disease progression (Kalantar-Zadeh & Fouque, 2017).

- Generally, <2300 mg/day is recommended (Ikizler et al., 2020).
- For reference, the Chronic Disease Risk Reduction Intake for sodium for healthy Americans aged 14 and older is 2300 mg/day—meaning that all people should reduce their intake of sodium if it is >2300 mg (National Academies of Sciences, Engineering, and Medicine, 2019).
- Evidence supporting a sodium intake of <1500 mg for clients with renal insufficiency is lacking, given the risk of hyponatremia and adverse outcomes.

Phosphorus

Elevated parathyroid hormone highlights the importance of managing phosphorus intake even in clients who do not have hyperphosphatemia (Kalantar-Zadeh & Fouque, 2017).

- Phosphorus and protein share many sources, so a low-protein diet is lower in phosphorus than the typical American diet.
- Phosphorus absorption is higher from animal sources than from plants.
- Phosphate additives, widely used as food preservatives, are commonly found in frozen, convenience, and prepackaged foods. Because inorganic phosphate additives are better absorbed than naturally occurring phosphorus in foods, processed food intake should be minimized.
- "Nutrition Facts" labels are not required to list phosphorus content, making it difficult for clients to estimate phosphorus intake.
- Because serum phosphate levels are difficult to control through dietary restriction alone, ample use of phosphate binders may be prescribed with meals and snacks to avoid excessively stringent protein restriction to control hyperphosphatemia (Kalantar-Zadeh & Fouque, 2017).

Potassium

Clients with CKD are at risk of hyperkalemia due to reduced urinary excretion. Other contributing factors include metabolic acidosis, catabolism, and the use of ACEIs or ARBs to control blood pressure.

- Potassium restriction is often recommended for clients with hyperkalemia, especially clients in advanced stages of kidney disease. However, excessive potassium restriction may translate to less heart-healthy/more atherogenic eating patterns (e.g., fewer fruits, vegetables, and whole grains) and worsen constipation, which may result in higher gastrointestinal (GI) absorption of potassium (Kalantar-Zadeh & Fouque, 2017).
- In clients with hyperkalemia, limiting potassium intake to <3 g/day is recommended with the caveat that fruit, vegetable, and high-fiber intake not be compromised (Kalantar-Zadeh & Fouque, 2017).

Other Dietary Concerns

Calories, calcium, fiber, fat, and micronutrient supplements are other dietary concerns for clients with CKD.

Calories

Generally, 25 to 35 cal/kg/day are suggested depending on BMI, sex, level of physical activity, CKD stage, concurrent illness, and age.

- Adequate calories are needed to ensure that dietary protein is used for repair rather than being metabolized as a source of energy.
- Calorie intake is often inadequate due to anorexia, nausea, depression, and taste and smell abnormalities related to uremic toxicity (Cupisti et al., 2018).
- Specially formulated low-protein foods made from carbohydrates are available to boost calorie intake while providing negligible amounts of protein, potassium, sodium, and phosphorus. However, they tend to be expensive and lack palatability.
- Fats and simple sugars are considered "free" foods because they provide protein-free calories with only small amounts of potassium, sodium, and phosphorus when used in recommended amounts. Suggestions include the following:
  - Adding honey or sugar to cereals or beverages.
  - Adding oils or trans fat–free margarine to cooked rice, pasta, cereals, or vegetables.
  - Using jam or jelly on toast or crackers
  - Snacking on hard candy, gummies, lollipops, jelly beans, and marshmallows.

Calcium

Kidney disease alters calcium metabolism in several ways. The decrease in vitamin D activation in the kidneys decreases calcium absorption from the GI tract, although passive diffusion of calcium ion absorption continues. Urinary calcium excretion decreases, but calcium is released from the bone secondary to hyperparathyroidism.

- It is recommended that calcium intake from all sources be 800 to 1000 mg/day in clients with moderate-to-advanced CKD, a recommendation not too different than the normal RDA.
- Milk products, a rich source of calcium, are generally restricted because they are also high in phosphorus.

Dysbiosis
an imbalance in the natural microflora of the gut, a condition thought to contribute to the cause or persistence of diseases.

Fiber

Advanced CKD is characterized by **dysbiosis** of intestinal microbiota, which contributes to uremic toxicity and cardiovascular damage (Cupisti et al., 2018).

- Adequate fiber intake could reduce dysbiosis and circulating uremic toxins (Cupisti et al., 2018).

- High-fiber grains may promote a more favorable microbiome and help prevent constipation, but most are higher in phosphorus and potassium than refined grains. Some low-phosphorus grains that provide fiber include
    - bulgur,
    - high-fiber white bread,
    - unsalted popcorn, and
    - Grape Nut Flakes.

Fat

A low-protein diet results in a higher proportion of calories from carbohydrates and fat (Kalantar-Zadeh & Fouque, 2017).

- Pure fats are a concentrated source of calories and do not provide protein, phosphorus, and potassium. Like simple sugars; they are considered "free" foods.
- Because people with CKD are at high risk of CVD, heart-healthy unsaturated fats (e.g., olive oil, soy oil, or canola oil) are preferred over saturated fats (e.g., butter and stick margarine). Soy oil and canola oil also provide omega-3 fatty acids.

Micronutrient Supplements

Micronutrient imbalances may occur in clients with CKD from inadequate intake, impaired GI absorption, or altered metabolism.

- Iron is the most problematic mineral deficiency (Kalantar-Zadeh & Fouque, 2017).
- When assessment of micronutrient intake is determined to be inadequate, daily multivitamin supplements may be prescribed (Ikizler et al., 2020).
- Clients at any stage of CKD may be prescribed vitamin D supplements to correct impaired vitamin D metabolism resulting from decreased kidney function.
- At any stage of CKD, routine supplementation of selenium or zinc is not suggested because there is little evidence of benefit (Ikizler et al., 2020).

Renal Meal Plan

In contrast to the general guide for food selection outlined in Box 23.3, a renal meal plan is a more restrictive approach to managing the intake of specific nutrients. This detailed approach is particularly useful for CKD clients with diabetes who require a consistent carbohydrate intake. The meal plan varies with the stage of CKD and the client's calorie needs. Keep in mind that these generalizations listed as follows may differ from guidelines from other sources.

- Food lists and a meal plan are used to achieve relative consistency in the intake of nutrients of concern: protein, sodium, phosphorus, and potassium.
- Subgroups exist based on nutrient content.
- Box 23.5 outlines food choice lists for diabetes and CKD Stages 1 to 4, with examples of representative foods.
- An individualized meal plan specifies how many servings from each list or sublist should be consumed at each meal and snack.
- An example of the total daily amount of food from each food group allowed for someone with Stage 4 CKD is as follows:
    - 4 oz of meat
    - ½ c of milk
    - 2 servings of fruit (1 low potassium, 1 high potassium)

  - 3 servings of vegetables (1 each of low, medium, and high potassium)
  - 5 servings of bread, cereal, and grains
  - 6 servings of fats
  - 2 desserts/sweets
- Client adherence to traditional nutrition therapy for CKD is estimated to be approximately 31% (Cupisti et al., 2018). Strategies to help promote dietary adherence are listed in Box 23.6.

BOX 23.5 Food Choice Lists for Diabetes and Chronic Kidney Disease Stages 1–4: Examples of Representative Foods

Protein choice categories

- Meat, poultry, and fish
- Meat alternatives: eggs, nuts, and tofu
- Legumes: prepared from dried beans; not canned varieties
- Protein foods with higher amounts of sodium and phosphorus: bacon, sausage, canned fish, processed cheese, canned legumes, deli meats, and vegetarian meat alternatives

Dairy choice categories

- Dairy foods: low-fat or fat-free milk, low-fat or fat-free yogurt
- Dairy foods with higher amounts of calories, carbohydrates, and fat: eggnog, ice cream, whole milk, sweetened pudding, and regular sweetened or frozen yogurt
- Dairy alternatives: unenriched, unsweetened almond milk, rice milk, and soy milk; nondairy creamer

Bread, cereal, and grain choice categories

- Bread, cereal, or grain food: bread, many cooked cereals, crackers, pasta, popcorn, rice, and tortilla
- Additional grain choices: biscuits, muffins, oatmeal, dry cereal, pancake, waffle, and sandwich cookie
- Desserts and sweets: hard candies, jellybeans, sugar cookies, and low-fat vanilla wafers

Fruit choice categories

- Low-potassium fruits: apple, apple juice, applesauce, blackberries, blueberries, grapes, papaya nectar, pear, and strawberries
- Medium-potassium fruits: cantaloupe cherries, fig, grapefruit, mango, and fresh papaya
- High-potassium fruits: apricot, avocado, bananas, dates, kiwifruit, orange, orange juice, prune juice, and raisins

Vegetable choice categories

- Low-potassium vegetables: canned beets, cabbage, carrots, cauliflower, corn, eggplant, green beans, mushrooms, and onions
- Medium-potassium vegetables: asparagus, broccoli, celery, kale, green peas, summer squash, and zucchini
- High-potassium vegetables: artichokes, brussels sprouts, okra, potatoes, spinach, sweet potatoes, tomatoes, and winter squash

Fat choice categories

- Healthier, unsaturated fats: trans fat–free margarine, low-fat or nonfat mayonnaise, and oils (canola, corn, olive, peanut, soybean, sunflower)
- Saturated fats—limit use: bacon fat, butter, half and half, cream cheese, whipped cream, lard, sour cream, and whipped cream topping

Note. Lists are not complete or universally agreed upon

Source: Academy of Nutrition and Dietetics. (n.d.). *Diabetes and chronic kidney disease stages 1–4: nutrition guidelines.* https://www.nutritioncaremanual.org/

BOX 23.6 Strategies to Promote Dietary Adherence to Chronic Kidney Disease Diet

- Provide positive messages about what to eat rather than emphasizing food restrictions.
- Encourage social support from family and friends.
- Foster the client's perception as successfully adhering to the plan; people who are more confident in their ability to adhere to the eating plan make better choices.
- Provide feedback on self-monitoring and laboratory data; correlation of records with laboratory data enables the client to see cause and effect, reinforces the importance of nutrition therapy, and opens the door for problem-solving.
- Encourage clients to
  - eat a good breakfast if appetite decreases as the day progresses, which may occur secondary to uremia;
  - try highly seasoned or strongly flavored foods if uremia has caused a change in the sense of taste;
  - eat a consistent intake of carbohydrate with regularly timed meals to control blood glucose levels, if appropriate; and
  - seek physician approval before using any vitamin, mineral, or supplement.
- Provide pointers to help clients limit their intake of protein, which may be less than 5 to 6 oz/day for most men and less than 4 oz/day for most women.
  - Urge clients to think of meat as a side dish, not the main entrée.
  - Because too little or too much protein can cause uremic symptoms to return, encourage clients to initially, and periodically thereafter, weigh or measure protein portion sizes for accuracy.
  - Encourage the use of low-protein breads, cereals, cookies, and pastas. Acceptability varies greatly among low-protein products, so if a client does not like one brand, it does not mean they will not like another.
  - Urge clients to spread protein allowance over the whole day instead of saving it all for one meal.

Nutrition Therapy during Dialysis

Clients undergoing dialysis are at considerable increased risk of morbidity and mortality related to persistent inflammation, malnutrition, and metabolic abnormalities (Huang et al., 2013a). The goal of nutrition therapy is to match dietary intake with renal replacement therapy (RRT) while preventing nutrition deficiencies (Beto et al., 2014). The diet is complex and dynamic. Nutrient recommendations are used as a guideline; the client's actual needs are based on individual assessment.

In general, clients undergoing dialysis have the same nutrient recommendations as those listed for advanced CKD (Table 23.1) with the following exceptions:

Dialysate
the dialysis solution used to extract wastes and fluid from the blood.

- Protein recommendation increases to 1.0 to 1.2 g/kg/day or higher to account for the loss of serum proteins and amino acids in the **dialysate** (Ikizler et al., 2020).
  - Achieving a high protein intake within the confines of other restrictions, especially phosphorus restrictions, can be challenging.
- Total calcium intake should be <800 mg/day.
- For people on hemodialysis, fluid allowance equals the volume of any urine produced plus 1000 mL (Kalantar-Zadeh & Fouque, 2017).
  - Fluid intake is monitored by weight gain: Anuric hemodialysis clients should not gain more than approximately 2 pounds/day between treatments.
  - For many clients on hemodialysis, limiting fluid intake is the biggest challenge. Teaching *how* to control their intake and thirst is vital.
  - Strategies to relieve thirst are listed in Box 23.7.
  - Peritoneal dialysis clients usually have fewer problems with fluid retention.

BOX 23.7 Strategies to Relieve Thirst

- Very cold items are better at relieving thirst.
  - Use ice or popsicles within the fluid allowance.
  - Rinse your mouth without swallowing using refrigerated water.
  - Rinse your mouth occasionally with refrigerated mouthwash.
  - Try frozen low-potassium fruit, such as grapes.
- Suck on the following:
  - Hard candy
  - Mints
  - Lemon wedge
- Chew gum.
- Eat bread with applesauce or jelly and margarine.
- Control blood glucose levels, as appropriate.
- Use small drinking glasses instead of large ones.
- Apply petroleum jelly to the lips.

Kidney Transplantation

Kidney failure poses a significant challenge to maintaining adequate nutritional status and muscle mass. In fact, up to 20% of people have protein–calorie malnutrition and loss of muscle mass at the time of kidney transplant (Nolte Fong & Moore, 2018). After transplantation, the use of immunosuppressive drugs requires ongoing nutrition therapy to reduce the risks of obesity, hyperlipidemia, hypertension, diabetes, and osteoporosis (Hong et al., 2019). Arterial sclerosis, such as ischemic heart disease and stroke, is the leading cause of death in kidney transplant clients; therefore, a heart-healthy eating pattern is indicated. Unfortunately, nutrition practice guidelines for posttransplant clients are scarce (Nolte Fong & Moore, 2018).

- In the immediate postoperative period, calorie and protein needs are increased due to the stress and catabolism related to surgery. During the first 1 to 2 months of posttransplant, the need for protein may be 1.3 to 2.0 g/kg of body weight (Hong et al., 2019).
- Protein and calorie needs gradually decrease after the initial postoperative period. Table 23.2 outlines nutrient recommendations after transplant.
  - Relaxation of dietary restrictions and an increase in appetite secondary to steroids increase the likelihood of posttransplant weight gain, particularly visceral fat gain.
  - Visceral fat gain increases the risk of developing new-onset diabetes, dyslipidemia, and CVD (Nolte Fong & Moore, 2018).
  - Calorie intake should be adjusted to maintain desirable weight.
- Ongoing nutrition assessment and counseling are needed to maintain adequate nutritional status and adjust the diet as needed to prevent or alleviate side effects caused by the use of immunosuppressive drugs (Hong et al., 2019).
- The DASH diet and Mediterranean-Style Eating Patterns are suitable for posttransplant clients; however, longitudinal studies have not been conducted in this population (Nolte Fong & Moore, 2018). Both patterns are heart healthy, which is important to decrease the risk of obesity, hypertension, diabetes, and hyperlipidemia.

ACUTE KIDNEY INJURY

Acute kidney injury (AKI) is characterized by a sudden decrease (up to 48 hours) in kidney function. Common life-threatening complications include volume overload, hyperkalemia, acidosis, and uremia. AKI seldom exists as an isolated organ failure but rather is often a complication of sepsis, critical illness, burns, cardiac surgery, trauma, and multiple-organ failure.

Table 23.2 Nutrient Recommendations for Adults after Transplantation

Nutrient	Posttransplantation
Protein	0.8–1.0 g/kg of BW/day with 50% high biological value Limit protein with chronic graft dysfunction
Energy	Initially 30–35 cal/kg Thereafter, 25–35 kcal/kg of BW/day to achieve or maintain desirable body weight
Carbohydrate	Emphasize complex carbohydrate intake
Fat	Emphasize unsaturated fat intake
Sodium	Initial restriction if blood pressure/fluid status dictates After acute period, allowance based on blood pressure and/or edema
Potassium	No restriction unless hyperkalemia is present and then individualized
Calcium	1200–1500 mg (prolonged use of steroids increases the risk of osteoporosis)
Phosphorus	Initial supplementation may be needed to restore normal blood levels Thereafter, DRI level
Fiber	Same as general population: 25–35 g/day
Fluid	No restriction; matched to urine output if appropriate

Source: Beto, J. A., Ramirez, W. E., & Bansal, V. K. (2014). Medical nutrition therapy in adults with chronic kidney disease: Integrating evidence and consensus into practice for the generalist registered dietitian nutritionist. *Journal of the Academy of Nutrition and Dietetics*, *114*(7), 1077–1087; Hong, S., Kim, E., & Rha, M. (2019). Nutritional intervention process for a patient with kidney transplantation: A case report. *Clinical Nutrition Research*, *8*(1), 74–78. https://doi.org/10.7762/cnr.2019.8.1.74

PEW may affect up to 40% of AKI clients in the intensive care unit (ICU) and represents a major negative prognostic factor (Fiaccadori et al., 2013). The pathogenesis of PEW in AKI is complex and involves many factors, including a systemic inflammatory response, loss of kidney homeostatic function, insulin resistance, and oxidative stress (Fiaccadori et al., 2013). Dialysis may contribute to nutrient losses.

Nutrition Therapy

There is a consensus that nutritional support should be individualized according to the severity of hypercatabolism and the underlying disease, comorbidities, the use of dialysis, and the client's preexisting nutritional status (Ostermann et al., 2019). However, evidence-based guidelines are limited and high-quality trials have not been performed. Still, studies on general ICU populations regarding the type and timing of nutrition are likely to be applicable to critically ill clients with AKI (Ostermann et al., 2019). The following recommendations are based on expert opinion, the lowest grade of evidence (Ostermann et al., 2019).

- Calorie recommendation are generally 20 to 30 cal/kg.
  - Hypocaloric feedings (not greater than 70% of energy expenditure) progressing gradually to 80% to 100% of estimated need by day 3 are recommended for general ICU clients and may also be appropriate for clients with AKI.
  - Protein recommendations vary depending on whether dialysis is used in these critically ill clients; without dialysis: gradually increase to 1.3 g/kg/day or possibly 1.7 g/kg/day.
- On intermittent RRT: 1.0 to 1.5 g/kg/day.
- On continuous RRT: up to 1.7 g/kg/day.
- An oral diet is the preferred route; enteral nutrition within 24 to 48 hours is recommended if oral intake is inadequate.

KIDNEY STONES

Kidney stones form when insoluble crystals precipitate out of urine. They vary in size from sand-like "gravel" to large, branching stones. Although they form most often in the kidney, they can occur anywhere in the urinary system. Dehydration or low urine volume, urinary tract obstruction, gout, chronic inflammation of the bowel, and intestinal bypass or ostomy surgery are medical conditions that increase the risk for kidney stone formation.

Kidney stones are common, with an estimated prevalence in the United States of approximately 7.1% in women and 10.6% in men (Scales et al., 2012). The prevalence of stones has consistently increased over the last 50 years and that trend is expected to continue based on the rising prevalence of obesity, diabetes, and metabolic syndrome, which are considered risk factors for stone formation (Khan et al., 2016). A twin study estimated that 56% of the risk of stones is hereditary, implying that approximately 50% of stones could be prevented by modifiable risk factors (Ferraro et al., 2017).

Stone Composition

Oxalate
a salt of oxalic acid. Oxalate has no known function in the body and is normally excreted in urine. Excess oxalate can bind with calcium in the urine to form calcium oxalate kidney stones.

Approximately 80% to 85% of kidney stones contain calcium, and most calcium stones are composed primarily of calcium **oxalate** (Noori et al., 2014). Because dietary calcium favorably binds with dietary oxalate in the intestines to form an insoluble compound that the body cannot absorb, an adequate calcium intake helps reduce the risk of calcium oxalate stones.

Nutrition Therapy

Nutrition therapy cannot dissolve a kidney stone, although increasing fluid intake may help promote its excretion. However, nutrition and lifestyle may help prevent stones from forming. A study of 3 large prospective cohort studies found that the following actions were associated with a more than a 50% decrease in the incidence of kidney stones (Ferraro et al., 2017).

- Maintain a normal BMI
  - Obesity and weight gain increase the risk of stone formation, and the magnitude of the increased risk may be greater in women than in men (Taylor et al., 2005).
- Drink an adequate amount of fluid—at least 2 L/day
  - A well-accepted strategy for reducing the recurrence of stones is to increase fluid intake to dilute the urine, thereby reducing the risk of stone formation regardless of the composition (Ferraro et al., 2013).
- Consume a DASH-style eating pattern that is high in fruits, vegetables, and low-fat dairy products.
  - In a randomized controlled trial, the DASH diet, despite its high oxalate content, decreased the risk of stone formation by 35% (Noori et al., 2014).
  - The effectiveness of the DASH diet may be due to its ample content of calcium, magnesium, and potassium. The result is more calcium to bind with oxalate in the intestine and a favorable increase in urinary pH.
  - The study data do not support the common practice of restricting dietary oxalate (a single component), particularly if that means a lower intake of fruits, vegetables, and whole grains (a healthy eating pattern).
- Consume adequate calcium
  - Consuming 1200 mg calcium/day combined with a low intake of animal protein and lower sodium intake has been associated with a 51% decrease in stone recurrence compared to a low calcium intake (about 400 mg/day) in people affected with idiopathic calcium stones (Borghi et al., 2002).
- Avoid frequent intake of sugar-sweetened beverages
  - Frequent consumption of sugar-sweetened beverages (soft drinks and punch) has been reported to increase the risk of kidney stones by 30% to 40% (Ferraro et al., 2013).

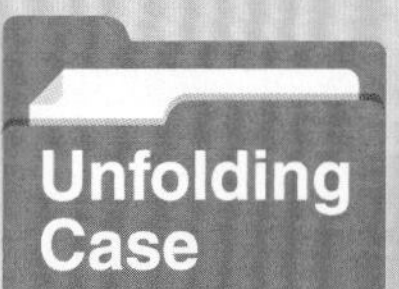

Recall Sonja. An increase in her stress level has caused her to give up on her lacto-ovo vegetarian eating pattern. Her blood pressure is increasing, and her weight loss has stalled. To make matters worse, she recently went to an ambulatory care center with excruciating back pain and was diagnosed with kidney stones, which she passed hours after receiving IV fluids. She is worried she will have more kidney stones that may eventually damage her only kidney. What would you tell her about reducing her risk of stone recurrence? What should her nutritional priorities be to maintain kidney health? What other lifestyle interventions would you recommend?

NURSING PROCESS Chronic Kidney Disease

Carlos is 66 years old and has had type 2 diabetes for 20 years. He is 5 ft 7 in. tall and weighs 172 pounds. His hemoglobin A1c is 8.2; he takes insulin twice daily. He has a history of hypertension and mild anemia and complains of sudden weight gain and "swelling." His blood urea nitrogen (BUN) and creatinine have been steadily increasing over the last several years, and his GFR is currently 63. During his last appointment, the doctor told Carlos to watch his sugar intake and avoid salt. At this visit, Carlos states he has never followed a "diet" before and does not want to start now. The doctor has asked you to talk to Carlos about his diet.

Assessment

Medical–Psychosocial History

- Medical history including cardiovascular disease, hypertension, diabetes, and renal disease
- Medications that affect nutrition such as diuretics, insulin, and lipid-lowering medications
- Physical complaints such as fatigue, taste changes, anorexia, and nausea
- Psychosocial and economic issues such as living situation, cooking facilities, financial status, employment, and education
- Understanding of the relationship between diet and diabetes, hypertension, renal function

Anthropometric Assessment

- Current height, weight, and BMI
- Recent weight history

Biochemical and Physical Assessment

- Blood values of the following:
  - BUN and creatinine
  - Sodium, potassium, and other electrolytes
  - Glucose
  - Lipid profile
  - Hemoglobin and hematocrit
- eGFR
- Blood pressure

Dietary Assessment

- What kind of nutrition counseling have you had in the past?
- How many meals and snacks do you usually eat?
- What is a typical day's intake for you?
- What gives you the most difficulty in changing your eating habits to limit sugar and salt?
- Do you have any eating issues, such as difficulty chewing or swallowing?
- What kind of protein do you eat most often? What is a typical serving size? Is it spread out over the day?
- How often do you eat sweets and sugar-sweetened beverages?
- How often do you eat high-sodium foods, such as cold cuts, bacon, frankfurters, smoked meats, sausage, canned meats, chipped or corned beef, buttermilk, cheese, crackers, canned soups and vegetables, convenience products, pickles, and condiments?
- Do you use a salt substitute?

NURSING PROCESS

Chronic Kidney Disease (continued)

- Do you regularly eat fruits and vegetables? How many servings of each do you consume in an average day?
- How much fluid do you drink daily? What is your favorite beverage?
- Do you have any cultural, religious, and ethnic food preferences?
- Do you have any food allergies or intolerances?
- Do you use vitamins, minerals, or nutritional supplements? If so, what, how much, and why do you use them?
- Do you drink alcohol?
- How often do you eat out?

Analysis

Possible Nursing Analysis

Food- and nutrition-related knowledge deficit related to lack of interest in making dietary changes as evidenced by his denial for the need to change his eating habits

Planning

Client Outcomes

The client will do the following:

- Understand the rationale for reducing sugar and salt intake.
- Implement the appropriate dietary strategies to achieve a lower intake of sugar and salt.
- Achieve adequate glucose control.
- Achieve and maintain normal blood pressure.
- Delay or prevent further kidney damage.

Nursing Interventions

Nutrition Therapy

Provide a 2000-calorie carbohydrate-controlled diet with 2300 mg sodium, as ordered.

Client Teaching

Instruct the client on the following:

- The role of nutrition therapy in the treatment of CKD.
- Eating plan essentials including the following:
  - The rationale for consuming a heart-healthy eating pattern.
  - Maintaining a consistent carbohydrate intake that is adequate in calories.
  - Limiting high-sodium foods, not adding salt during cooking or at the table.
- Behavioral matters including the following:
  - How to estimate portion sizes to improve accuracy.
  - Weighing oneself at approximately the same time every day with the same scale while wearing the same amount of clothing. Unexpected weight gain or loss should be reported to the physician.
- That heart-healthy cookbooks and cookbooks for diabetes may help increase variety and interest in eating.
- Changing eating attitudes.
  - Learn to view the diet as an integral component of treatment and a means of life support.
  - Adhering to the diet can improve the quality of life and decrease the workload on the kidneys.

Evaluation

Evaluate and Monitor

- Monitor food intake or records (if available) for compliance to limiting sugar and salt.
- Monitor weight.
- Monitor lab values, blood glucose, blood pressure, and urine output.
- Provide periodic feedback and reinforcement.

How Do You Respond?

Does cranberry juice prevent urinary tract infections? Cranberry, particularly in the form of cranberry juice, has long been associated with preventing and treating of urinary tract infections (UTIs) (Dong et al., 2018). Proanthocyanidins, one of the active phytonutrients in cranberry, have been shown to inhibit the adhesion of certain strains of *Escherichia coli* (the primary bacteria associated with UTIs) to the lining of the urinary tract. Unfortunately, study results are often conflicting, and standardization of doses, form (tablets, capsules), length of trial, and the amount of active ingredient used are not always reported (Dong et al., 2018). Given that the use of cranberry is without adverse effects and that it may be beneficial, clients who are prone to urinary tract infections and like cranberry juice should be encouraged to consume it regularly.

Are omega-3 fish oil supplements beneficial for people on hemodialysis? Omega-3 fatty acids in fish and fish oil can modify abnormal lipid levels, decrease platelet aggregation, and improve blood pressure, heart rate, oxidative stress, and inflammation (Saglimbene et al., 2020). Given these effects, their use is recommended for secondary cardiovascular prevention in the general population (Siscovick et al., 2017).

The potential benefits linked to omega-3 fatty acids, namely, improved lipid levels, less inflammation, and reduced blood pressure, suggest they may be beneficial for clients with CKD. However, study results using omega-3 fatty acids in clients with CKD are often conflicting (Svensson & Carrero, 2017). For instance, results from a recent meta-analysis of randomized controlled trials indicate that supplements of omega-3 fatty acids may decrease cardiovascular mortality in clients treated with hemodialysis but were uncertain whether they reduce the progression to ESRD in clients with CKD not yet receiving RRT (Saglimbene et al., 2020). More high-quality studies are needed.

REVIEW CASE STUDY

Dorothea is a 72-year-old Black woman who is 5 ft 5 in. tall and weighs 149 pounds. She has coronary heart disease and a long-standing history of hypertension with progressive loss of kidney function. She recently started receiving hemodialysis and is gaining about 4 pounds/day between treatments. She has convinced herself that because she is on dialysis, she can eat and drink whatever she wants and "the machine will take care of it."

Yesterday, she ate the following as shown on the right.

- What risk factors does Dorothea have for CKD?
- Based on her treatment with hemodialysis, what nutrients may she need to restrict or increase?
- Why is she gaining 4 pounds/day between treatments? What is a more reasonable goal? What would you suggest she do to achieve the goal?
- Evaluate her protein intake and recommend changes she could make to achieve her protein goals.
- What foods is she eating that are not heart healthy? What substitutions would you recommend?
- Evaluate her sodium intake and recommend changes she could make to limit her sodium intake.
- What foods is she eating that are high in potassium? What alternatives would you suggest?
- What would you tell Dorothea about the use of dialysis and her theory about eating anything she wants?
- Which is the lesser risk: getting enough calories and protein by eating non-heart-healthy foods or adhering to the sodium and other restrictions but not getting enough calories and protein?

Breakfast: Grits with cheese, bacon, biscuit with butter, and coffee
Lunch: Hamburger on bun with ketchup and mustard, potato chips, banana, and sweetened tea
Dinner: Fried chicken, macaroni and cheese, collard greens, pound cake, and sweetened tea

STUDY QUESTIONS

1 Which statement indicates the client understands the instructions about nutrition therapy for nephrotic syndrome?
   a. "I know I need to eat a high-protein diet to replace the protein lost in urine."
   b. "I need to limit my intake of fruit and vegetables that are high in potassium."
   c. "I should limit my sodium intake by not using salt in cooking or at the table and avoiding foods high in sodium such as processed foods, fast foods, and convenience foods."
   d. "I should lose weight to decrease the workload on my kidneys."

2 A healthy client with a family history of CKD asks how they can decrease their risk of developing kidney disease. Which of the following would be the nurse's best response?
   a. "If you have a positive family history, there is no way for you to lower your risk of CKD."
   b. "We don't know how to lower the risk of CKD so the best thing you can do is to have your kidney function monitored regularly."
   c. "Limit your intake of plants because they are high in potassium and phosphorus, 2 nutrients that make your kidneys work harder."
   d. "Eat a heart-healthy eating pattern; CVD and CKD share the same lifestyle risks.

3 When developing a teaching plan for a client who must restrict potassium, which fruits and vegetables would the nurse recommend for their low potassium content?
   a. Avocado, tomatoes, and potatoes
   b. Kiwifruit, prune juice, and acorn squash
   c. Apple, blueberries, and green beans
   d. Mango, spinach, and raisins

4 The nurse knows their instructions about preventing future kidney stones have been effective when the client verbalizes he should
   a. avoid milk, cheese, and other sources of calcium.
   b. limit fruit and vegetables.
   c. lose weight to maintain healthy body weight.
   d. eat a high-protein diet.

5 How do the protein recommendations for adults with CKD without diabetes differ from those who have diabetes?
   a. Protein is more restricted for people who do not have diabetes.
   b. Protein is more restricted for people who have diabetes.
   c. The protein recommendations do not differ for people with diabetes or without diabetes.
   d. There are no specific protein recommendations for people with diabetes because carbohydrates and fat are the priority concerns.

6 A client on hemodialysis asks if they can use popsicles to help relieve their thirst. Which of the following is the nurse's best response?
   a. "That's a great idea as long as you deduct the equivalent amount of fluid from your total daily fluid allowance."
   b. "Popsicles are empty calories. You are better off drinking just plain water."
   c. Popsicles are great at relieving thirst, and because they are solid, they do not count as fluid, so you can eat them as desired."
   d. "Hot things are better at relieving thirst than cold things. Try small amounts of hot tea or coffee to relieve your thirst."

7 What characteristics of a Mediterranean-Style Eating Pattern may be beneficial to clients with CKD? Select all that apply.
   a. It is low in red and processed meats, which limits saturated fat, sodium, and phosphate intake.
   b. It includes a moderate intake of wine, which has anti inflammatory and antioxidant properties.
   c. It is low in fat, which helps protect against CVD.
   d. Its protein content is similar to a controlled protein diet recommended for people with CKD.

8 The client asks if they will need to follow a diet after they recover from a kidney transplant. Which of the following is the nurse's best response?
   a. "You will always have to limit protein and phosphorus intake to help preserve the health of the new kidney."
   b. "After recovery, all restrictions are lifted and you can eat anything you want."
   c. "You may need to modify some aspects of your diet because of side effects from the medications you will be taking, and you should continue to eat a heart-healthy diet to decrease the risks of diabetes, hypertension, heart disease, and obesity."
   d. "All the restrictions you followed before dialysis will resume after you recover from the transplant."

CHAPTER SUMMARY NUTRITION FOR CLIENTS WITH KIDNEY DISORDERS

The kidneys are vital for maintaining overall health; impairments in kidney function can cause widespread disruptions in metabolism, bone health, fluid balance, nutritional status, and nutrient requirements.

Nutrition in Maintaining Kidney Health

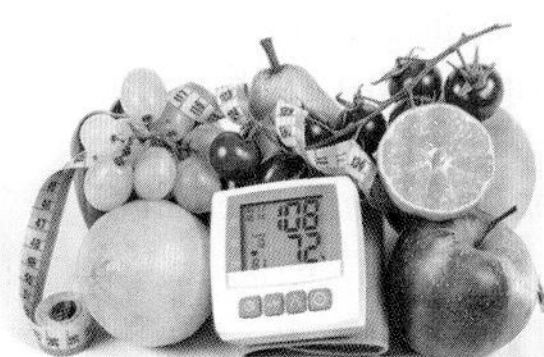

The typical American diet increases the risk of obesity, diabetes, hypertension, and CVD; each of these chronic diseases increases the risk of kidney disease. Heart-healthy nutrition and lifestyle interventions are likely also kidney healthy.

Healthy Eating Pattern. Certain eating patterns have been shown to reduce the incidence of CKD disease.

The DASH Diet. Benefits may be attributed to its effect on lowering blood pressure and reducing inflammation.

Mediterranean-Style Eating Pattern. May help preserve kidney function through favorable effects on endothelial function, inflammation, lipid levels, and blood pressure.

Nephrotic Syndrome

Hypoalbuminemia, proteinuria, hyperlipidemia, and edema are major features of nephrotic syndrome.

Nutrition Therapy. The primary objective of nutrition therapy is to reduce proteinuria. Protein intake should be adequate but not excessive. Sodium may be restricted. It is not known if restricting cholesterol and fat improves prognosis. Calories should be adequate and vitamin D supplements may be necessary.

Chronic Kidney Disease

CKD is a progressive, irreversible loss of kidney function.

Risk Factors for CKD. Diabetes and hypertension are the major risk factors. Others include CVD, obesity, advancing age, family history, and certain ethnic backgrounds.

Disease Progression. Loss of kidney function leads to impaired excretion of nitrogenous wastes, sodium, fluid, potassium, phosphorus, and hydrogen ions. Interrelated and multifactorial metabolic and clinical complications develop.

Nutrition Therapy. Varies in complexity according to the stage of CKD, comorbidities, and the client's nutritional status. Control of blood glucose and blood pressure is primary. Limiting sodium and protein and eating heart healthy are encouraged for all stages of CKD; additional restrictions for phosphorus and potassium are added as necessary. Actual nutrient recommendations vary among experts.

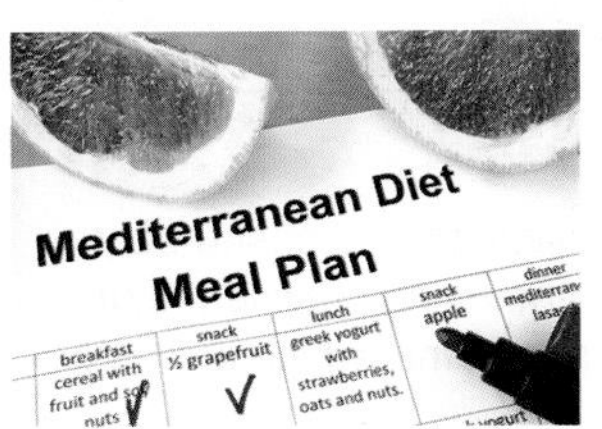

Mediterranean-Style Eating Pattern. Recommended for adults at all stages of CKD (but not on dialysis or posttransplant); may improve lipid levels and posttransplant may help delay the progression of CKD and prevent complications.

Protein. Low-protein diets can slow the progression of CKD but may contribute to the malnutrition.

Sodium. Restricted to control of blood pressure and edema.

Phosphorus. Restricted due to elevated parathyroid hormone, even when serum phosphorus is not high. Dietary control is difficult; phosphate binders allow for greater phosphorus intake.

Potassium. Serum levels become elevated due to impaired excretion, metabolic acidosis, catabolism, and certain antihypertensive medications. Many healthy foods, such as fruits, vegetables, whole grains, and legumes, are high in potassium.

Calories. Must be adequate to promote protein sparing.

Calcium. Restricted due to abnormal metabolism. Milk is restricted because it is also a rich source of phosphorus.

Fiber. Adequate intake is encouraged to improve intestinal dysbiosis, which contributes to uremic toxicity and cardiovascular damage.

Fat. Unsaturated fats are emphasized over saturated fats due to the high risk of CVD.

Micronutrient Supplements. Micronutrient imbalances may occur in clients from inadequate intake, impaired GI absorption, or altered metabolism. Daily supplements may be prescribed.

Renal Meal Plan. Food lists based on nutrient content are used to create a daily meal pattern. The diet is complex and multiple sublists are common.

Nutrition Therapy during Dialysis. With the exception of protein and fluid, dietary recommendations remain similar during dialysis. Protein intake is liberalized to account for losses in the dialysate and fluid is restricted.

Kidney Transplantation. The use of immunosuppressive drugs requires ongoing nutrition therapy to reduce the risks of obesity, hyperlipidemia, hypertension, diabetes, and osteoporosis.

(continued)

CHAPTER SUMMARY NUTRITION FOR CLIENTS WITH KIDNEY DISORDERS (continued)

Acute Kidney Injury. Usually occurs in combination with critical illness. Nutrient recommendations for critical illness are probably appropriate. Protein recommendations vary depending on whether dialysis is used.

Kidney Stones

The prevalence of stones has consistently increased over the last 50 years and is related to the rising prevalence of obesity, diabetes, and metabolic syndrome, which are risk factors for stone formation.

Stone Composition. Eighty to eighty-five percent of stones contain calcium. Adequate calcium is needed to bind with oxalate in the intestines so it is not absorbed and filtered through the kidneys.

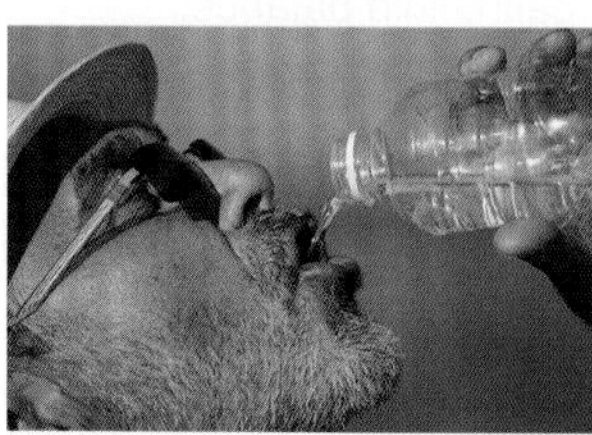

Nutrition Therapy for Kidney Stones. Many stones can be prevented by maintaining healthy body weight, drinking adequate fluid, eating a healthy eating pattern such as the DASH diet, consuming adequate calcium, and avoiding frequent consumption of sugar-sweetened beverages.

Figure sources: *shutterstock.com/ratmaner, shutterstock.com/Vitalii Vodolazskyi, and shutterstock.com/VILevi*

Student Resources on thePoint®
For additional learning materials, activate the code in the front of this book at https://thePoint.lww.com/activate

Websites

American Association of Kidney Patients at www.aakp.org
American Kidney Fund at www.kidneyfund.org
National Institute of Diabetes and Digestive and Kidney Diseases at www.niddk.nih.gov
National Kidney and Urologic Diseases Information Clearinghouse (NKUDIC) at http://kidney.niddk.nih.gov
National Kidney Disease Education Program (NKDEP) at www.nkdep.nih.gov
National Kidney Foundation at www.kidney.org
Oxalosis and Hyperoxaluria Foundation at www.ohf.org

References

Academy of Nutrition and Dietetics. (2020). *Nutrition care manual.* https://nutritioncaremanual.org

Agrawal, S., Zaritsky, J., Fornoni, A., & Smoyer, W. (2018). Dyslipidaemia in nephrotic syndrome: Mechanisms and treatment. *Nature Reviews Nephrology, 14*(1), 57–70. https://doi.org/10.1038/nrneph.2017.155

Beto, J., Ramirez, W., & Bansal, V. (2014). Medical nutrition therapy in adults with chronic kidney disease: Integrating evidence and consensus into practice for the generalist registered dietitian nutritionist. *Journal of the Academy of Nutrition and Dietetics, 114*(7), 1077–1087. https://doi.org/10.1016/j.jand.2013.12.009

Borghi, L., Schianchi, T., Meschi, T., Guerra, A., Allegri, F., Maggiore, U., & Novarini, A. (2002). Comparison of two diets for the prevention of recurrent stones in idiopathic hypercalciuria. *The New England Journal of Medicine, 346,* 77–84. https://doi.org/10.1056/NEJMoa010369

Cadnapaphornchai, M., Tkachenko, O., Shehekochikhin, D., & Schrier, R. (2014). The nephrotic syndrome: Pathogenesis and treatment of edema formation and secondary complications. *Pediatric Nephrology, 29,* 1159–1167. https://doi.org/10.1007/s00467-013-2567-8

Campbell, K. L., & Carrero, J. J. (2016). Diet for the management of patients with chronic kidney disease; it is not the quantity, but the quality that matters. *Journal of Renal Nutrition, 26*(5), 270–281. https://doi.org/10.1053/j.jrn.2016.07.004

Carrero, J. J., Biostat, F. T., Nagy, K., Arongundade, F., Avesani, C. M., Chan, M., Chmielewski, M., Cordeiro, A. C., Espinosa-Cuevas, A., Fiaccadori, E., Guebre-Egziabher, F., Hand, R. K., Hung, A. M., Ikizler, T. A., Johansson, L. R., Kalantar-Zadeh, K., Karupaiah, T., Lindholm, B., Marckmann, P., … Kovesdy, C. P. (2018). Global prevalence of protein energy wasting in kidney disease: A meta-analysis of contemporary observational studies from the International Society of Renal Nutrition and Metabolism. *Journal of Renal Nutrition, 28*(6), 380–392. https://doi.org/10.1053/j.jrn.2018.08.006

Centers for Disease Control and Prevention. (2017). *Chronic kidney disease initiative: Prevention and risk management.* https://www.cdc.gov/kidneydisease/prevention-risk.html

Centers for Disease Control and Prevention. (2019). Chronic kidney disease in the United States, 2019. US Department of Health and Human Services, Centers for Disease Control and Prevention.

Centers for Disease Control and Prevention. (2020). *Chronic kidney disease basics.* https://www.cdc.gov/kidneydisease/basics.html

Chauveau, P., Aparicio, M., Bellizzi, V., Campbell, K., Hong, X., Johansson, L., Kolko, A., Molina, P., Sezer, S., Wanner, C., ter Wee, P. M., Teta, D., Fouque, D., Carrero, J. J., & European Renal Nutrition (ERN) Working Group of the European Renal Association-European Dialysis Transplant Association (ERA-EDTA). (2018). Mediterranean diet as the diet of choice for patients with chronic kidney disease. *Nephrology Dialysis Transplantation, 33*(5), 725–735. https://doi.org/10.1093/ndt/gfx085

Cupisti, A., Brunori, G., Di Iorio, B. R., D'Alessandro, C., Pasticci, F., Cosola, C., Bellizzi, V., Bolasco, P., Capitanini, A., Fantuzzi, A. L., Gennari, A., Piccoli, G. B., Quintaliani, G., Salomone, M., Sandrini, M., Santoro, D., Babini, P., Fiaccadori, E., Gambaro, G., … Gesualdo, L. (2018). Nutritional treatment of advanced CKD: Twenty consensus statements. *Journal of Nephrology, 31*(4), 457–473. https://doi.org/10.1007/s40620-018-0497-z

de Boer, I., & Utzschneider, K. (2017). The kidney's role in systemic metabolism—still much to learn. *Nephrology Dialysis Transplantation, 32*(4), 588–590. https://doi.org/10.1093/ndt/gfx027

Dong, B., Zimmerman, R., Dang, L., & Pillai, G. (2018). Cranberry for the prevention and treatment of non-complicated urinary tract infections. *Symbiosis Open Access Journals Pharmacy and Pharmaceutical Sciences, 6*(1), 1–9. https://symbiosisonlinepublishing.com/pharmacy-pharmaceuticalsciences/pharmacy-pharmaceuticalsciences93.pdf

Estruch, R., Ros, E., Salas-Salvadó, J., Covas, M.-I., Corella, D., Arós, F., Gómez-Gracia, E., Ruiz-Gutiérrez, V., Fiol, M., Lapetra, J., Lamuela-Raventos, R. M., Serra-Majem, L., Pintó, X., Basora, J., Muñoz, M. A., Sorlí, J. V., Martínez, J. A., Fitó, M., Gea, A., … Hernán, M. A., PREDIMED Study Investigators. (2018). Primary prevention of cardiovascular disease with a Mediterranean diet supplemented with extra-virgin olive oil or nuts. *The New England Journal of Medicine, 378*(25), e34. https://doi.org/10.1056/NEJMoa1800389

Ferraro, P. M., Taylor, E. N., Gambaro, G., & Curhan, G. C. (2013). Soda and other beverages and the risk of kidney stones. *Clinical Journal of the American Society of Nephrology, 8*(8), 1389–1395. https://doi.org/10.2215/CJN.11661112

Ferraro, P. M., Taylor, E. N., Gambaro, G., & Curhan, G. C. (2017). Dietary and lifestyle risk factors associated with incident kidney stones in men and women. *The Journal of Urology, 198*(4), 858–863. https://doi.org/10.1016/j.juro.2017.03.124

Fiaccadori, E., Regolisti, G., & Maggiore, U. (2013). Specialized nutritional support interventions in critically ill patients on renal replacement therapy. *Current Opinion in Clinical Nutrition and Metabolic Care, 16*(2), 217–224. https://doi.org/10.1097/MCO.0b013e32835c20b0

Hong, S., Kim, E., & Rha, M. (2019). Nutritional intervention process for a patient with kidney transplantation: A case report. *Clinical Nutrition Research, 8*(1), 74–78. https://doi.org/10.7762/cnr.2019.8.1.74

Huang, X., Lindholm, B., Stenvinkel, P., & Carrero, J. J. (2013a). Dietary fat modification in patients with chronic kidney disease: n-3 fatty acids and beyond. *Journal of Nephrology, 26*(6), 960–974. https://doi.org/10.5301/jn.5000284

Huang, X., Jimenez-Moleon, J. J., Lindholm, B., Cederholm, T., Amlov, J., Riserus, U., Sjogren, P., & Carrero, J. J. (2013b). Mediterranean diet, kidney function, and mortality in men with CKD. *Clinical Journal of the American Society of Nephrology, 8*(9), 1548–1555. https://doi.org/10.2215/CJN.01780213

Ikizler, T. A., Burrowes, J. D., Byham-Gray, L. D., Campbell, K. L., Carrero, J.-J., Chan, W., Fougue, D., Friedman, A. N., Ghadder, S., Goldstein-Fuchs, D. J., Kaysen, G. A., Kopple, J. D., Teta, D., Wang, A. Y.-M., & Cuppari, L. (2020). KDOQI Nutrition in CKD Guideline Work Group. KDOQI clinical practice guideline for nutrition in CKD: 2020 update. *American Journal of Kidney Diseases, 76*(3)(suppl 1), S1–S107. https://www.ajkd.org/article/S0272-6386(20)30726-5/pdf

Kalantar-Zadeh, K., & Fouque, D. (2017). Nutritional management of chronic kidney disease. *The New England Journal of Medicine, 377*, 1765–1776. https://doi.org/10.1056/NEJMra1700312

Kalantar-Zadeh, K., Moore, L. W., Tortorici, A. R., Chou, J. A., St-Jules, D. E., Aoun, A., Rojas-Bautista, V., Tschida, A. K., Rhee, C. M., Shah, A. A., Crowley, S., Vassalotti, J. A., & Kovesdy, C. P. (2016). North American experience with Low protein diet for non-dialysis-dependent chronic kidney disease. *BMC Nephrology, 17*(1), 90. https://doi.org/10.1186/s12882-016-0304-9

Kelly, J. T., Palmer, S. C., Wai, S. N., Ruospo, M., Carrero, J. J., Campbell, K. L., & Strippoli, G. F. M. (2017). Healthy dietary patterns and risk of mortality and ESRD in CKD: A meta-analysis of cohort studies. *Clinical Journal of the American Society of Nephrology, 12*(2), 272–279. https://doi.org/10.2215/CJN.06190616

Khan, S. R., Pearle, M. S., Robertson, W. G., Gambaro, G., Canales, B. K., Doizi, S., Traxer, O., & Tiselius, H.-G. (2016). Kidney stones. *Nature Reviews Disease Primers, 2*, 16008. https://doi.org/10.1038/nrdp.2016.8

Ko, G. J., Obi, Y., Tortorici, A. R., & Kalantar-Zadeh, K. (2017). Dietary protein intake and chronic kidney disease. *Current Opinion in Clinical Nutrition and Metabolic Care, 20*(1), 77–85. https://doi.org/10.1097/MCO.0000000000000342

Kochanek, K., Murphy, S., Xu, J., & Arias, E. (2019). Deaths: Final data for 2017. *National Vital Statistics Reports, 68*(9). National Center for Health Statistics.

Koppe, L., Fouque, D., & Kalantar-Zadeh, K. (2019). Kidney cachexia or protein-energy wasting in chronic kidney disease: Facts and numbers. *Journal of Cachexia, Sarcopenia and Muscle, 10*(3), 479–484. https://doi.org/10.1002/jcsm.12421

Ku, E., Kopple, J., Johansen, K., McCulloch, C., Go, A., Xie, D., Lin, F., Hamm, L., He, J., Kusek, J., Navaneethan, S., Ricardo, A., Rincon-Choles, H., Smogorzewski, M., Hsu, C., & CRIC Study Investigators. (2018). Longitudinal weight change during CKD progression and its association with subsequent mortality. *American Journal of Kidney Diseases: The Official Journal of the National Kidney Foundation, 71*(5), 657–665. https://doi.org/10.1053/j.ajkd.2017.09.015

Lin, J., Fung, T. T., Hu, F. B., & Curhan, G. C. (2011). Association of dietary patterns with albuminuria and kidney function decline in older white women: A subgroup analysis from the Nurses' Health Study. *American Journal of Kidney Diseases, 57*(2), 245–254. https://doi.org/10.1053/j.ajkd.2010.09.027

National Academies of Sciences, Engineering, and Medicine. (2019). Consensus study report highlights. Dietary reference intakes for sodium and potassium. https://www.nap.edu/resource/25353/030519DRI-SodiumPotassium.pdf

Nishi, S., Ubara, Y., Utsunomiya, Y., Okada, K., Obata, Y., Kai, H., Kiyomoto, H., Goto, S., Konta, T., Sasatomi, Y., Sato, Y., Nishino, T., Tsuruya, K., Furuichi, K., Hoshino, J., Watanabe, Y., Kimura, K., & Matsuo, S. (2016). Evidence-based clinical practice guidelines for nephrotic syndrome 2014. *Clinical and Experimental Nephrology, 20*, 342–370. https://doi.org/10.1007/s10157-015-1216-x

Noce, A., Vidiri, M., Marrone, G., Moriconi, E., Bocedi, A., Capria, A., Rovella, V., Ricci, G., DeLorenzo, A., & Daniele, N. C. (2016). Is low-protein diet a possible risk factor of malnutrition in chronic kidney disease patients? *Cell Death Discovery, 2*, 16026. https://doi.org/10.1038/cddiscovery.2016.26

Nolte Fong, J. V., & Moore, L. W. (2018). Nutrition trends in kidney transplant recipients: The importance of dietary monitoring and need for evidence-based recommendations. *Frontiers in Medicine, 5*, 302. https://doi.org/10.3389/fmed.2018.00302

Noori, N., Honarkar, E., Goldfarb, D., Kalantar-Zadeh, K., Taheri, M., Shakhssalim, N., Parvin, M., & Basiri, A. (2014). Urinary lithogenic risk profile in recurrent stone formers with hyperoxaluria: A randomized controlled trial comparing DASH (Dietary Approaches to Stop Hypertension)-style and low-oxalate diets. *American Journal of Kidney Diseases, 63*(3), 456–463. https://doi.org/10.1053/j.ajkd.2013.11.022

Ostermann, M., Macedo, E., & Oudemans-van Straaten, H. (2019). How to feed a patient with acute kidney injury. *Intensive Care Medicine, 45*, 1006–1008. https://doi.org/10.1007/s00134-019-05615-z

Pluta, A., Strozecki, P., Kesy, J., Lis, K., Sulikowska, B., Odrowza-Sypniewska, G., & Manitium, J. (2017). Beneficial effects of 6-month supplementation with omega-3 acids on selected inflammatory markers in patients with chronic kidney disease stages 1–3. *BioMed Research International, 2017*, Article ID 1680985, https://doi.org/10.1155/2017/1680985

Rebholz, C., Crews, D., Grams, M., Steffen, L. M., Levey, A. S., Miller, E. R., III, Appel, L. J., & Coresh, J. (2016). DASH (Dietary Approaches to Stop Hypertension) diet and risk of subsequent kidney disease. *American Journal of Kidney Diseases, 68*(6), 853–861. https://doi.org/10.1053/j.ajkd.2016.05.019

Saglimbene, V. M., Wong, G., van Zwieten, A., Palmer, S. C., Ruospo, M., Natale, P., Campbell, K., Teixeira-Pinto, A., Craig, J. C., & Strippoli, G. F. M. (2020). Effects of omega-3 polyunsaturated fatty acid intake in patients with chronic kidney disease: Systematic review and meta-analysis of randomized controlled trials. *Clinical Nutrition, 39*(2), 358–368. https://doi.org/10.1016/j.clnu.2019.02.041

Salas-Salvado, J., Guasch-Ferre, M., Lee, C.-H., Estruch, R., Clish, C. B., & Ros, E. (2016). Protective effects of the Mediterranean diet on type 2 diabetes and metabolic syndrome. *Journal of Nutrition, 146*(4), 920S–927S. https://doi.org/10.3945/jn.115.218487

Scales, C. Jr., Smith, A., Hanley, J. M., & Saigal, C. (2012). Prevalence of kidney stones in the United States. *European Urology, 62*(1), 160–165. https://doi.org/10.1016/j.eururo.2012.03.052

Siscovick, D., Barringer, T., Fretts, A., Wu, J. H. Y., Lichtenstein, A. H., Costell, R. B., Kris-Etherton, P. M., Jacobson, T. A., Engler, M. B., Alger, H. M., Appel, L. J., Mozaffarian, D. and on behalf of the American Heart Association Nutrition Committee of the Council on Lifestyle and Cardiometabolic Health; Council on Epidemiology and Prevention; Council on Cardiovascular Disease in the Young; Council on Cardiovascular and Stroke Nursing; and Council on Clinical Cardiology. (2017). Omega-3 polyunsaturated fatty acid (fish oil) supplementation and the prevention of clinical cardiovascular disease. *Circulation, 135*, e867–e884. https://doi.org/10.1161/CIR.0000000000000482

Smyth, A., Griffin, M., Yusuf, S., Mann, J. F. E., Reddan, M., Canavan, M., Newell, J., & O'Donnell, M. (2016). Diet and major renal outcomes: A prospective cohort study. The NIH-AARP Diet and Health Study. *Journal of Renal Nutrition, 26*(5), 288–298. https://doi.org/10.1053/j.jrn.2016.01.016

Svensson, M., & Carrero, J. J. (2017). n-3 polyunsaturated fatty acids for the management of patients with chronic kidney disease. *Journal of Renal Nutrition, 27*(3), 147–150. https://doi.org/10.1053/j.jrn.2017.02.003

Taylor, E. N., Stampfer, M. J., & Curhan, G. C. (2005). Obesity, weight gain, and the risk of kidney stones. *The Journal of the American Medical Association, 293*(4), 455–462. https://doi.org/10.1001/jama.293.4.455

U.S. Department of Agriculture & Agricultural Research Service. (2018). Nutrient intakes from food and beverages: Mean amounts consumed per individual, by gender and age, What We Eat in America, NHANES 2015–2016. https://www.ars.usda.gov/ARSUserFiles/80400530/pdf/1516/Table_1_NIN_GEN_15.pdf

Valdivielso, J., Rodriguez-Puyol, D., Pascual, J., Barrios, C., Bermudez-Lopez, M., Sanchez-Nino, M. D., Perez-Fernandez, M., & Ortiz, A. (2019). Atherosclerosis in chronic kidney disease: More, less, or just different? *Atherosclerosis, Thrombosis, and Vascular Biology, 39*(1), 1938–1966. https://doi.org/10.1161/ATVBAHA.119.312705

Chapter 24

Nutrition for Clients with Cancer or HIV/AIDS

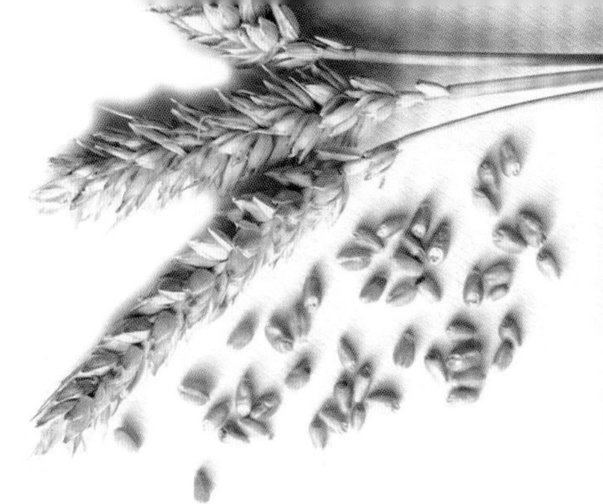

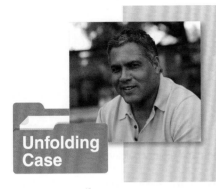

Unfolding Case

Patrick Hannon

Patrick is 50 years old, is 6 ft tall, and considers himself healthy. His normal adult weight is 258 pounds. He is a "meat-and-potatoes" kind of guy and admits to being sedentary. His beverage of choice is sweetened tea, which he prefers over water. His wife convinced him to have a routine colonoscopy—since it is recommended at age 50 years—which led to a diagnosis of stage 3 colon cancer. He had a partial colectomy and lymph node removal. He is undergoing adjuvant chemotherapy.

Learning Objectives

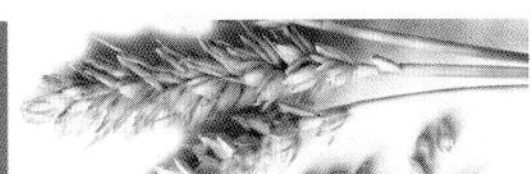

Upon completion of this chapter, you will be able to:

1 Evaluate a person's usual intake according to nutrition guidelines for cancer prevention.
2 Summarize how cancer and cancer therapies can affect nutritional status.
3 Give examples of ways to modify the diet to alleviate side effects of anorexia, nausea, fatigue, taste changes, mouth sores, dry mouth, and diarrhea.
4 Discuss ways to increase a client's calorie and protein intake.
5 Explain how HIV/AIDS affects nutritional status.
6 List food safety practices.
7 Teach a person living with HIV/AIDS guidelines for a healthy eating pattern.

Cancer and HIV/AIDS are combined in this chapter because they can have similar effects on nutritional status, whether from the disease itself or from disease treatments. Although nutrition therapy cannot cure either disease, it has the potential to maximize the effectiveness of drug therapy, alleviate the side effects of the disease and its treatments, and improve overall quality of life.

This chapter presents nutrition recommendations for cancer prevention, the effects of cancer and cancer treatments on nutrition, and nutrition therapy for clients being treated for cancer, for those with advanced cancer, and for cancer survivors. Also presented are the nutritional consequences of HIV and AIDS and nutrition therapy recommendations.

CANCER

Cancer is a group name for more than 100 different types of malignancies characterized by the uncontrolled growth of cells. Individual cancers differ in where they develop, how quickly they grow, the type of treatment they respond to, and how much they affect nutritional status. In the United States, 40 out of 100 men and 39 out of 100 women will develop cancer during their lifetime (American Cancer Society [ACS], 2020). Cancer was responsible for 21.3% of all deaths in 2016 and 2017, making it the second leading cause of death in the United States (Heron, 2019).

Nutrition in Cancer Prevention

In 2014, an estimated 42% of incident cancers and almost 50% of all cancer deaths were attributed to potentially modifiable risk factors (Islami et al., 2018). Tobacco cessation is inarguably the leading behavioral strategy for reducing the risk of cancer (Box 24.1). For nontobacco users, the most important modifiable determinants of cancer risk are body weight, dietary choices, and levels of physical activity.

Figure 24.1 depicts cancer prevention recommendations by the American Institute for Cancer Research (AICR). These recommendations are similar to those published by the American

BOX 24.1 Percent of Cancer Deaths Attributed to Various Lifestyle Factors

Risk Factor	% Cancer Deaths
Cigarette smoking	29%
Excess body weight	7%–8%
Alcohol intake	4%–6%
Poor diet (e.g., low intake of fruit, vegetables, fiber, and dietary calcium and consumption of red and processed meat)	4%–5%
Physical inactivity	2%–3%

Source: Islami, F., Sauer, A., Miller, K., Siegel, R., Fedewa, S. A., Jacobs, E. J., McCullough, M. L., Patel, A. V., Ma, J., Soerjomataram, I., Flanders, W. D., Brawley, O. W., Gapstur, S. M., & Jemal, A. (2018). Proportion and number of cancer cases and deaths attributable to potentially modifiable risk factors in the US. *CA: A Cancer Journal for Clinicians*, *68*(1), 31–54. https://doi.org/10.3322/caac.21440

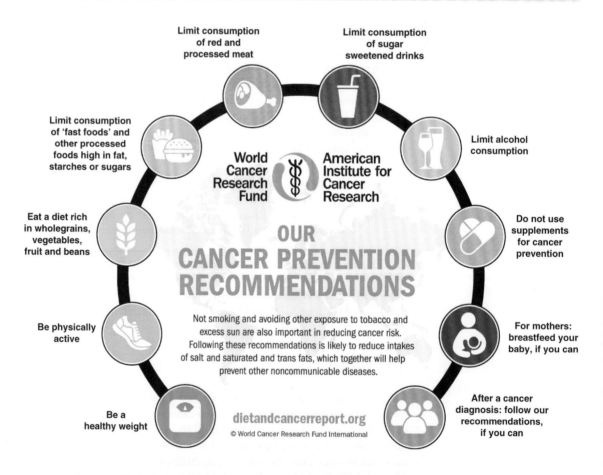

Figure 24.1 ▲ **10 Cancer prevention recommendations as an overarching "package."** (*Source:* Reproduced from World Cancer Research Fund/American Institute for Cancer Research. Diet, Nutrition, Physical Activity and Cancer: A Global Perspective. Continuous Update Project Expert Report 2018. Available at dietandcancerreport.org.)

Cancer Society and the American Heart Association (Chapter 2, Table 2.3). A large systematic review of 10 large prospective studies showed that high versus low adherence to ACS or AICR nutrition and physical activity cancer prevention guidelines consistently and significantly reduced the overall risk of cancer incidence and mortality (Kohler et al., 2016). Risk reduction ranged from 10% to 45% for cancer incidence and 14% to 61% for cancer mortality. For people who most closely adhered to cancer prevention recommendations, consistent reductions in incidence were shown for breast cancer (19%–60%), endometrial cancer (23%–60%), and colorectal cancer in both men and women (27%–52%).

Despite evidence showing nutrition and physical activity guidelines consistently and significantly lower cancer risk, the role of diet in cancer prevention is difficult to study. For instance, the human diet is complex and the food supply is ever changing (Kushi et al., 2012). Lifelong eating patterns may be important but cannot be detected by relatively short-term, randomized clinical trials (PDQ® Supportive and Palliative Care Editorial Board, 2020). In addition, cancer takes years to develop, making randomized controlled trials of dietary interventions to prevent cancer impractical (Kushi et al., 2012). Although not all studies on the role of diet as a cause of cancer reach the same conclusions, evidence that certain dietary factors and patterns are associated with a lower risk of cancer is consistent and serves as the foundation of the ACS and AICR nutrition and lifestyle guidelines. Table 24.1 lists potential mechanisms by which nutrition-related guidelines may help reduce the risk of cancer.

Although following nutrition and lifestyle recommendations has been shown to lower cancer incidence and mortality, there is insufficient evidence to recommend one particular eating pattern (e.g., Mediterranean-style or DASH diet) to reduce the risk of *all* cancers. It may be that the effectiveness of an eating pattern on cancer risk depends on the type of cancer or on other risk factors, such as family history, gender, age, other lifestyle factors, comorbidities, or gut microbiota profiles (Steck & Murphy, 2020).

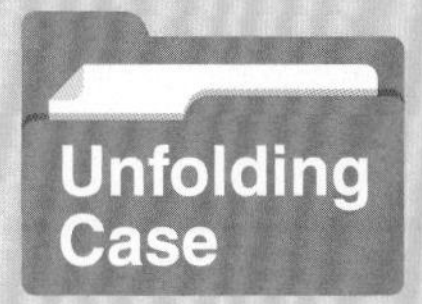

Think of Patrick. What lifestyle factors may have increased his risk for cancer? Is it appropriate for him to adopt healthy lifestyle behaviors while he is undergoing chemotherapy?

Table 24.1 Potential Mechanisms by Which Nutrition-Related Guidelines May Help Reduce the Risk of Cancer

Recommendation	Rationale
Maintain a healthy weight	Excess body fat can promote chronic inflammation, causing a favorable environment for cancer growth; can cause excess estrogen production which can increase the risk of breast and endometrial cancer; and causes high levels of insulin and other hormones that may stimulate cancer cell growth.
Choose a healthy diet with an emphasis on plants	It is not known which components of plants may be protective; therefore, eating a variety is important. Supplements cannot duplicate the myriad of naturally occurring substances in plants. A plant-based eating pattern can also help manage weight.
Limit calorie-dense, nutrient-poor, refined, and processed foods	These foods can displace the intake of nutrient-dense, minimally processed foods. These foods can be high in calories, making weight management more difficult.
Limit consumption of red and processed meat	High meat intake can displace the intake of nutrient-dense foods and regular intake of processed meat can lead to weight gain. Red and processed meat are associated with an increased risk of colorectal cancer.
Limit consumption of sugar-sweetened drinks	Sugar-sweetened beverages are generally a source of empty calories that can make weight management difficult.
Limit alcohol consumption	The metabolism of ethanol may damage DNA which can alter cell growth and function. Alcohol is associated with an increased risk of oral, esophageal, breast, and colorectal cancer (in men) and may also increase the risk of liver cancer and colorectal cancer in women.

Source: American Institute for Cancer Research. (n.d.). *10 cancer prevention recommendations*. https://www.aicr.org/cancer-prevention/; National Cancer Institute. (2020). *Cancer prevention overview (PDQ)-Health professional version*. https://www.cancer.gov/about-cancer/causes-prevention/hp-prevention-overview-pdq

Nutrition Complications Related to Cancer

The effect of cancer on nutritional status and intake varies with baseline nutrition status, disease site, stage of disease, and treatment approach (PDQ® Supportive and Palliative Care Editorial Board, 2020). For a number of reasons, cancer clients are among the most malnourished of all client groups (Ryan et al., 2016), with a reported malnutrition prevalence ranging from 25% to over 70% (Muscaritoli et al., 2017). Malnutrition in cancer clients differs dramatically from malnutrition caused by simple starvation in that the negative calorie balance and loss of skeletal muscle are powered by a combination of inadequate food intake and alterations in metabolism (Arends et al., 2017). However, there is not a universally agreed-upon standard definition of malnutrition (PDQ® Supportive and Palliative Care Editorial Board, 2020).

Local Tumor Effects

Local tumor effects occur when the tumor impinges on surrounding tissue, impairing its ability to function. Nutrition complications vary with the site and size of the tumor and are usually most severe with gastrointestinal (GI) or head and neck tumors (Table 24.2).

Tumor-Induced Changes in Metabolism

Cancer metabolism has intrigued cancer researchers for almost a century (Nelson, 2017).

- Tumor-induced alterations in metabolism can directly impair nutritional status.
- Tumor-induced weight loss occurs frequently in clients with solid tumors of the lung, pancreas, and upper GI tract.
- Although altered metabolism is universally accepted as one of the hallmarks of cancer, many questions remain as to how reprogrammed metabolism is related to cancer (Wu & Zhao, 2013).

Table 24.2 Common Side Effects Based on Tumor Site

Site	Potential Effects
Brain/CNS	Eating disabilities Chewing and swallowing difficulties
Head and neck	Dysphagia/odynophagia Xerostomia Taste alterations
Esophagus, stomach	Dysphagia, odynophagia Early satiety Nausea/vomiting Abdominal pain Diarrhea/malabsorption Anorexia/weight loss Obstruction, which may necessitate enteral or parenteral nutrition
Pancreas, liver, small intestine	Early satiety Nausea/vomiting Abdominal pain Diarrhea/malabsorption Constipation/obstruction Anorexia/weight loss
Large intestine	Diarrhea/ malabsorption Constipation/obstruction, which may necessitate enteral or parenteral nutrition Anorexia/weight loss

Source: PDQ® Supportive and Palliative Care Editorial Board. (2020). PDQ Nutrition in Cancer Care. National Cancer Institute. https://www.cancer.gov/about-cancer/treatment/side-effects/appetite-loss/nutrition-hp-pdq.

Inadequate Intake

Inadequate intake has been determined to be present if a client cannot eat for more than a week or if the client consumes <60% of their estimated calorie requirement for >1 to 2 weeks (Arends et al., 2017). The causes of inadequate intake are complex and multifactorial.

- Anorexia is a major cause of inadequate intake. It may be present at the time of diagnosis or may occur as a side effect of treatments or the tumor.
- Other factors that may contribute to inadequate intake include mouth ulcers, poor dentition, dry mouth, taste alterations, intestinal obstruction, malabsorption, constipation, diarrhea, nausea, vomiting, decreased GI motility, uncontrolled pain, depression, anxiety, and side effects of medications (Arends et al., 2017).
- Inadequate intake can lead to weight loss, which has been correlated with adverse outcomes, including increased incidence and severity of treatment side effects and increased risk of infection, thereby reducing the chance of survival (PDQ® Supportive and Palliative Care Editorial Board, 2020).

Muscle Protein Depletion

Lean Body Mass
the weight of the body minus the weight of fat.

Sarcopenia is the condition of severe muscle depletion. The loss of **lean body mass**, with or without fat loss, is an independent risk factor for poorer outcomes (PDQ® Supportive and Palliative Care Editorial Board, 2020). It predicts risk of physical impairment, postoperative complications, chemotherapy toxicity, and mortality (Arends et al., 2017).

- Sarcopenia is present in 20% to 70% of cancer clients depending on the type of tumor (Ryan et al., 2016). However, a universal definition of sarcopenia does not exist (PDQ® Supportive and Palliative Care Editorial Board, 2020).
- Identifying muscle loss has become increasingly difficult as 40% to 60% of cancer clients are overweight or obese, even in the setting of metastatic disease (Ryan et al., 2016). Sarcopenic obesity is an independent risk factor for poor prognosis (PDQ® Supportive and Palliative Care Editorial Board, 2020).
- Impaired physical activity may also contribute to loss of muscle mass.

Systemic Inflammation Syndrome

Systemic inflammation syndrome (SIS) is frequently activated in clients with cancer; it is associated with the development of fatigue, impaired physical activity, anorexia, and weight loss (Arends et al., 2017). SIS impacts all relevant metabolic pathways, although the degree of impact varies.

- **Protein metabolism:** Altered protein turnover, loss of fat and muscle mass, and increase in acute phase proteins.
- **Carbohydrate metabolism:** Insulin resistance and impaired glucose tolerance.
- **Fat metabolism:** Fat oxidation is maintained or increased, especially in the presence of weight loss.

Interactions and Outcomes

Weight loss, impaired physical performance, and SIS in cancer clients are all independently associated with an unfavorable prognosis (Arends et al., 2017).

- Consequences include increased toxicity of anticancer treatments leading to an interruption of treatment and reduced quality of life (Arends et al., 2017).
- Interactions between weight loss, impaired physical performance, and SIS lead to a continuous deterioration of the client's well-being.

Cancer Cachexia

Cancer cachexia is an incompletely understood, multifactorial syndrome characterized by unstoppable muscle wasting that cannot be fully reversed by conventional nutrition support and leads to progressive impairment (Fearon et al., 2011).

- Altered metabolism of carbohydrates, protein, and fat is evident.
- Weight loss can occur from poor intake and/or an increase in metabolism (PDQ® Supportive and Palliative Care Editorial Board, 2020).
- Cachexia can increase toxicity related to treatment, aggravate symptoms, worsen quality of life, and shorten survival (Zhou et al., 2018).

Stages of cancer cachexia are as follows (Fearon et al., 2011):

- Precachexia, characterized by loss of appetite and altered glucose intolerance that precede substantial weight loss.
- Cachexia, characterized by significant weight loss or sarcopenia in the absence of simple starvation and defined as
  - weight loss >5% in the past 6 months or
  - body mass index (BMI) <20 and degree of weight loss >2% or
  - Sarcopenia and any degree of weight loss >2%.
- Refractory cachexia is cachexia that usually associated with advanced stage cancer or rapid progression of disease that is unresponsive to treatment.

Nutrition Complications Related to Cancer Treatments

Cancer treatments include surgery, chemotherapy, radiation, biotherapy, hemopoietic cell transplantation, or a combination of therapies. Each treatment modality can contribute to progressive nutritional deterioration related to localized or systemic side effects that interfere with intake, increase nutrient losses, or alter metabolism. Comorbidities may complicate treatment and nutritional status. The success of treatment is influenced by the client's ability to tolerate therapy, which is affected by nutritional status.

Surgery

Surgery is often the primary treatment for cancer. People who are malnourished prior to surgery are at higher risk of postoperative morbidity and mortality.

- If time allows, nutritional deficiencies are corrected before surgery and may require the use of oral nutrition supplements (ONS), enteral or parenteral nutrition, and/or use of medications to stimulate appetite.
- Postsurgical nutritional requirements increase for protein, calories, vitamin C, B vitamins, and iron to replenish losses and promote healing.
- Physiological or mechanical barriers to good nutrition can occur depending on the type of surgery, with the greatest likelihood of complications arising from GI surgeries.
- Table 24.3 outlines potential side effects and complications incurred for various types of surgery.

Chemotherapy

Given alone or in combination, chemotherapy drugs damage the reproductive ability of both malignant and normal cells, especially rapidly dividing cells such as well-nourished cancer cells and normal cells of the GI tract, respiratory system, bone marrow, skin, and gonadal tissue.

- The side effects of chemotherapy vary with the type of drug or combination of drugs used, dose, rate of excretion, duration of treatment, and individual tolerance.
- Chemotherapy side effects are systemic and, therefore, potentially more numerous than the localized effects seen with surgery or radiation.
- The most commonly experienced nutrition-related side effects are anorexia, taste alterations, early satiety, nausea, vomiting, mucositis/esophagitis, diarrhea, and constipation (PDQ® Supportive and Palliative Care Editorial Board, 2020).
- Side effects increase the risk of malnutrition and weight loss, which may prolong recovery time between treatments. When subsequent chemotherapy treatments are delayed, successful treatment outcome is potentially threatened.

Table 24.3 Potential Complications of Surgery

Type	Potential Complications
Head and neck resection	Impaired ability to speak, chew, salivate, swallow, smell, taste, and/or see Enteral nutrition support dependency Negative impact on nutritional status can be profound
Esophagectomy or esophageal resection	Early satiety Regurgitation Fistula formation Stenosis Vagotomy → decreased stomach motility, decreased gastric acid production, diarrhea, steatorrhea
Gastric resection	Dumping syndrome: crampy diarrhea that develops quickly after eating, accompanied by flushing, dizziness, weakness, pain, distention, and vomiting Hypoglycemia Esophagitis Decreased gastric motility Fat malabsorption and diarrhea Deficiencies in iron, calcium, and fat-soluble vitamins Vitamin B_{12} malabsorption related to lack of intrinsic factor
Intestinal resection	Malnutrition related to generalized malabsorption Fluid and electrolyte imbalance Diarrhea Increased risk of renal oxalate stone formation Metabolic acidosis
Massive bowel resection	Steatorrhea Malnutrition related to severe generalized malabsorption Metabolic acidosis Dehydration
Ileostomy or colostomy	Fluid and electrolyte imbalance
Pancreatic resection	Generalized malabsorption Diabetes mellitus

Source: PDQ® Supportive and Palliative Care Editorial Board. (2020). PDQ Nutrition in Cancer Care. National Cancer Institute. https://www.cancer.gov/about-cancer/treatment/side-effects/appetite-loss/nutrition-hp-pdq

Radiation

Radiation causes cell death; particles of radioactive energy break chemical bonds, disrupting reproductive ability. Although radiation injures all rapidly dividing cells, it is most lethal for the poorly differentiated and rapidly proliferating cells of cancer tissue. Side effects are localized. Recovery from sublethal doses of radiation occurs in the interval between the first dose and subsequent doses. Normal tissue appears to recover more quickly from radiation damage than does cancerous tissue.

- The type and intensity of radiation side effects depend on the type of radiation used, the site, the volume of tissue irradiated, the dose of radiation, the duration of therapy, and individual tolerance.
- Clients most at risk for nutrition-related side effects are those who have cancers of the head and neck, lower neck and mid chest, abdomen and pelvis, and brain (Table 24.4).
- Side effects usually develop around the second or third week of treatment and then diminish 2 or 3 weeks after radiation therapy is completed. Some side effects may be chronic.

Biotherapy

Biotherapy is treatment to enhance the body's immune system to boost the body's own response against cancer or to help repair normal cells damaged as a side effect of treatment (PDQ® Supportive and Palliative Care Editorial Board, 2020).

Table 24.4 Potential Complications of Radiation

Area	Potential Complications
Head and neck	Altered or loss of taste (mouth blindness) Xerostomia (dry mouth) Thick salivary secretions Difficulty swallowing and chewing Loss of teeth Mucositis Stomatitis Esophagitis
Chest	Acute: esophagitis with dysphagia Delayed: fibrosis, esophageal stricture, dysphagia Nausea/vomiting Edema Anorexia
Abdomen and pelvis	Acute or chronic bowel damage can cause diarrhea, nausea, vomiting, enteritis, and malabsorption Bowel constriction, obstruction, or fistula formation
Brain	Anorexia Nausea/vomiting Dysphagia/odynophagia

- The side effects most likely to impact nutrition status are fatigue, fever, nausea, vomiting, and diarrhea (PDQ® Supportive and Palliative Care Editorial Board, 2020).
- Actual side effects depend on the type of biotherapy used, such as growth factors, monoclonal antibodies, and vaccines.

Hemopoietic Cell Transplantation

Hemopoietic cell transplants are preceded by high-dose chemotherapy and possibly total-body irradiation to suppress immune function and destroy cancer cells.

- Treatments frequently result in nutrition-related side effects, such as mucositis and significant diarrhea (PDQ® Supportive and Palliative Care Editorial Board, 2020).
- Acute or chronic graft-versus-host disease may also occur, impairing intake and the body's ability to process adequate protein and calories (PDQ® Supportive and Palliative Care Editorial Board, 2020).
- Parenteral or enteral nutrition support may be necessary for clients who are malnourished and not expected to eat or absorb adequate calories for >7 to 14 days (PDQ® Supportive and Palliative Care Editorial Board, 2020).
- **Neutropenia** leaves the client susceptible to infection, so precautionary measures must be taken to prevent foodborne illness (Box 24.2): A **neutropenic diet** may be recommended, although they have not been found to be superior to a regular diet in neutropenic cancer clients (PDQ® Supportive and Palliative Care Editorial Board, 2020).

Neutropenia
abnormally low number of neutrophils in the blood, which increases the risk of infection.

Neutropenic Diet
a diet intended to protect people with low neutrophil counts from bacteria and other organisms in some food and drinks; eliminates fresh fruits, vegetables, raw nuts, yogurt, and other products with live active cultures.

Nutrition Therapy during Cancer Treatment

The goals of nutrition therapy are to maintain or improve intake, maintain skeletal muscle mass and physical performance, reduce the risk of reductions or interruptions of scheduled anticancer treatments, and improve quality of life (Arends et al., 2017). Goals are individualized according to the client's nutrition status, type and stage of disease, comorbid conditions, and overall medical treatment plan (PDQ® Supportive and Palliative Care Editorial Board, 2020). Early and regular nutrition screening is recommended to identify nutritional problems at an early stage; however, there is no agreement on which screening/assessment tools are most accurate for assessing malnutrition in cancer clients (Muscaritoli et al., 2017).

BOX 24.2 Strategies to Reduce the Risk of Foodborne Illness

Storage

- Refrigerate perishable and prepared foods immediately after purchase.
- Refrigerate leftovers immediately after eating; thoroughly reheat before eating.
- Discard leftovers after 24 hours.
- Keep hot foods >140°F and cold foods <40°F.
- Use expiration dates on food packaging to discard foods that may be unsafe to eat.

Food Preparation

- Wash hands before and after handling food and eating and after using the restroom.
- Wash fruits and vegetables thoroughly in clean water.
- Avoid cross-contamination by using separate cutting boards and work surfaces for raw meats and poultry; keep work surfaces clean.

Thawing

- Thaw food in the refrigerator, never at room temperature.
- If the microwave is used to thaw frozen meat, cook the meat immediately after it is defrosted.

Cooking

- Cook all meat, fish, and poultry to the well-done stage.

Foods to Avoid

- Raw or undercooked meat and poultry
- Raw or undercooked fish, such as sushi, ceviche, or refrigerated smoked fish
- Unpasteurized milk and fruit juices
- Soft cheeses made from unpasteurized milk such as feta, brie, camembert, Queso fresco
- Foods that contain raw or undercooked eggs, such as homemade Caesar salad dressing, raw cookie dough, and eggnog
- Raw sprouts (alfalfa, bean, and others), unwashed fresh vegetables, and any moldy or damaged fruits and vegetables
- Hot dogs, deli meats, and luncheon meats that have not been reheated
- Unpasteurized, refrigerated pates or meat spreads
- Salad bars and buffets when eating out

Calories

Adequate calories are needed to maintain healthy weight and help maintain lean body mass. Unfortunately, few studies have assessed total calorie requirements of cancer clients (Arends et al., 2017).

- If indirect calorimetry is not available, calorie needs can be estimated with the same general formula applied to healthy adults, which is 25 to 30 cal/kg/day.
- Body weight and muscle mass are monitored to assess the adequacy of calorie intake.

Protein

The optimal amount of protein for cancer clients has not been determined; however, studies have shown that a high protein intake promotes muscle protein anabolism in cancer clients (Arends et al., 2017).

- Recommendations state that protein intake should not be less than 1 g/kg/day and should be up to 1.5 g/kg/day if possible.
- In people with normal kidney function, protein intake up to and above 2 g/kg/day is safe and may promote a positive protein balance in clients with cancer.

Promoting an Oral Intake

The best way to maintain or increase calorie and protein intake is through normal food (Arends et al., 2017).

- For clients who have difficulty consuming an adequate amount of food, modifications to increase the calorie or protein density can improve overall intake without increasing the volume of food needed (Box 24.3).
- Interventions to mitigate side effects or complications of cancer or its treatments can improve oral intake (Box 24.4).

BOX 24.3 Ways to Increase the Protein and Calorie Density of Foods

To Increase Protein and Calories

- Add skim milk powder to milk to make double-strength milk; chill well before serving.
- Use double-strength milk on hot or cold cereals and in scrambled eggs, soups, gravies, casseroles, milk shakes, and milk-based desserts.
- Substitute whole milk for water in recipes.
- Add grated cheese to soups, casseroles, vegetable dishes, rice, and noodles.
- Use peanut butter as a spread on slices of apple, banana, pear, crackers, or waffles; use as a filling for celery.
- Add finely chopped, hard-cooked eggs to sauces; add cream to soups and casseroles.
- Choose desserts made with eggs or milk such as sponge cake, angel food cake, custard, and puddings.
- Dip meat, poultry, and fish in eggs or milk and coat with bread or cereal crumbs before baking, broiling, or pan frying.
- Use yogurt, especially Greek yogurt, as a topping for fruit, plain cakes, or other desserts; use in gravies and dips.

To Increase Calories

- Mix cream cheese with butter and spread on hot bread and rolls.
- Whenever possible, add butter to hot foods: breads, pancakes, waffles, soups, vegetables, potatoes, cooked cereal, rice, and pasta.
- Substitute mayonnaise for salad dressing in salads, eggs, casseroles, and sandwiches.
- Add dried fruit, nuts, or granola to desserts and cereal.
- Use whipped cream on pies, fruit pudding, gelatin, ice cream, and other desserts and in coffee, tea, and hot chocolate.
- Use marshmallows in hot chocolate, on fruits, and in desserts.
- Top-baked potatoes, vegetables, and fruits with sour cream.
- Snack frequently on nuts, dried fruit, candy, buttered popcorn, cheese, granola, and ice cream.
- Use honey on toast, cereal, and fruit and in coffee and tea.

BOX 24.4 Recommendations for Managing Side Effects or Complications That Affect Nutrition

Anorexia

- Plan a daily menu in advance.
- Overeat during "good" days.
- Eat a high-protein, high-calorie, nutrient-dense breakfast if appetite is best in the morning.
- Eat a small high-calorie meals every 2 hours.
- Seek help preparing meals.
- Add extra protein and calories to food.
- Eat high-protein foods first, such as meat, fish, poultry, eggs, legumes, and yogurt.
- Limit liquids with meals to avoid early satiety and bloating at mealtime.
- Use ONS (instant breakfast mixes, milk shakes, commercial supplements) in place of meals when appetite deteriorates or the client is too tired to eat.
- Make eating a pleasant experience by eating in a bright, cheerful environment, playing soft music, and enjoying the company of friends or family.
- Avoid strong food odors if they contribute to anorexia. Cook outdoors on a grill, serve cold foods rather than hot foods, or use takeout meals that do not need to be prepared at home. In the hospital, the tray cover should be removed before the tray is placed in front of the client so that food odors can dissipate.
- Try different foods.
- Perform frequent mouth care to reduce aftertastes.
- Be as active as possible to stimulate appetite.

Nausea

- Rinse mouth before and after eating.
- Eat 5 or 6 small meals daily instead of 3 large ones.
- Do not skip meals.
- Some people feel better by eating dry toast, crackers, or breadsticks throughout the day.
- Slowly sip fluids throughout the day.
- Drink ginger ale or ginger tea.
- Eat foods served cold, such as chicken salad, instead of hot baked chicken or deli roast beef instead of pot roast.
- Eat high-carbohydrate, low-fat, easy-to-digest foods such as toast, crackers, pretzels, yogurt, sherbet, cooked cereal, soft or canned fruits, watermelon, bananas, fruit juices, and angel food cake.
- Avoid fatty, greasy, fried, spicy, or foods with a strong odor.
- Sit up for 1 hour after eating.
- Keep track of and avoid foods that cause nausea.
- Avoid eating 1–2 hours before chemotherapy or radiotherapy.
- Take antiemetics as prescribed even when symptoms are absent.

Fatigue

- Eat a hearty breakfast because fatigue may worsen as the day progresses.
- Engage in regular exercise if possible.
- Consume easy-to-eat foods that can be prepared with a minimal amount of effort, such as frozen dinners, takeout foods,

BOX 24.4 Recommendations for Managing Side Effects or Complications That Affect Nutrition (continued)

sandwiches, instant breakfast mixes and liquid formulas, cheese and crackers, peanut butter on crackers, yogurt, and pudding.
- If weight loss isn't a problem, avoid overeating for energy. Excess weight worsens fatigue.
- Enlist the help of friends and family to provide meals.

Taste Changes

- Eat cold or frozen foods.
- Use sugar-free lemon drops, gum, or mints to counter a metallic or bitter taste in the mouth.
- Brush your teeth or rinse with a mouthwash before eating.
- Eat small frequent meals.
- Use plastic utensils if food has a metallic taste.
- Drink tart juice before eating, such as cranberry or orange juice, to mask a metallic taste.
- Experiment with tart foods such as pickles, vinegar, or relishes to help overcome metallic taste.
- Eat meat with something sweet, such as pork with applesauce or turkey with cranberry sauce.
- Substitute poultry, eggs, cheese, and mild fish for beef and pork if they have a "bad," "rotten," or "fecal" taste.
- Avoid foods that are offensive; stick to those that taste good.
- Try new foods, such as lemon yogurt in place of strawberry.

Sore Mouth (Stomatitis)

- Practice good oral hygiene (thorough cleaning with a soft-bristle toothbrush or cotton swabs plus frequent mouth rinses with normal saline and water or baking soda and water). Commercial mouthwashes containing alcohol may irritate and burn the oral mucosa.
- Eat cold or room-temperature foods.
- Eat soft, nonirritating foods that are easy to chew and swallow, such as bananas, applesauce, watermelon, canned fruit, cottage cheese, yogurt, mashed potatoes, macaroni and cheese, puddings, milk shakes, ONS, scrambled eggs, oatmeal, and other cooked cereals.
- Add gravy, broth, or sauces to increase the fluid content of foods, as appropriate.
- Cook food until soft and tender.
- Cut food into small pieces or puree in a blender.
- Numb the mouth with frozen bananas, ice chips, ice cream, or popsicles.
- Avoid spices, acidic foods, coarse foods, salty foods, alcohol, and smoking that can aggravate an already irritated oral mucosa.
- Consume high-calorie, high-protein drinks in place of traditional meals.
- Use a straw to drink liquids.
- Avoid wearing ill-fitting dentures.
- Glutamine swishes may reduce the duration and severity of mucositis.

Xerostomia (Dry Mouth)

- Use an alcohol-free mouth rinse before eating.
- Drink fluids with meals and all day long.
- Eat moist foods softened with gravies or sauces. Casseroles and stews are easier to eat than baked or roasted meats.
- Avoid dry, coarse foods and very spicy or salty foods.
- Avoid foods that stick to the roof of the mouth such as peanut butter.
- Avoid sugary food and beverages that promote dental decay.
- Drink high-calorie, high-protein liquids between meals.
- Stimulate saliva production with citrus fruits if tolerated, such as lemons, oranges, limes, and grapefruit.
- Consume frozen desserts, such as ice cream and frozen yogurt.
- Eating papaya may help break up "ropy" saliva.
- Use ice chips and sugar-free hard candies and gum between meals to relieve dryness.
- Use a straw to drink liquids.
- Apply a moisturizer to the lips to help prevent drying.
- Brush after every meal and snack.
- Avoid tobacco and alcohol because they dry the mouth.

Diarrhea

- Replace fluid and electrolytes with broth, soups, sports drinks, and canned fruit.
- Drink at least 1 cup of liquid after each loose bowel movement.
- Limit caffeine, hot or cold liquids, and high-fat foods because they aggravate diarrhea.
- Avoid gassy foods and liquids such as dried peas and beans, cruciferous vegetables, carbonated beverages, and chewing gum.
- Try foods high in pectin and other soluble fibers to slow transit time, such as oatmeal, cooked carrots, bananas, peeled apples, and applesauce.
- Avoid sugar-free candy or gum containing sorbitol because it can contribute to osmotic diarrhea.
- Unless tolerance to lactose has been confirmed, limit or avoid milk.

Constipation

- Increase fiber gradually by eating more fruits, vegetables, and legumes. Replace refined grains with whole-grain bread and cereals.
- Consume 2 tbsp wheat bran, which can be sprinkled on cooked or ready-to-eat cereal, salad, applesauce, or yogurt. After 3 days, increase by 1 tbsp daily until constipation is resolved. Bran intake should not exceed 6 tbsp/day.
- Eat dried fruit, such as raisins, dates, or prunes.
- Eat high-fiber foods throughout the day.
- Drink 8–10 cups of fluid/day.
- Take walks and exercise regularly.

Table 24.5 Drugs Commonly Used for Anorexia-Cachexia Syndrome

Drug Category	Common Drugs Used	Effectiveness
Progesterone analogs	Megestrol acetate	Improved weight gain Shown to improve appetite for clients with advanced cancer
	Medroxyprogesterone	Improved appetite and stimulated weight gain
Corticosteroids	Dexamethasone	Similar efficacy to megestrol acetate in improving appetite
	Methylprednisolone	Increased appetite but negligible weight change
	Prednisolone	Short-term appetite improvement but no weight gain
Cannabinoids	Dronabinol	Inconsistent evidence of effectiveness; is inferior to megestrol acetate for appetite improvement and weight gain
Antihistamines	Cyproheptadine	Increases appetite but may not decrease weight loss in adults
Anti-inflammatory agents	Melatonin	Several systemic literature reviews have failed to show conclusive evidence of efficacy No improvement in weight or appetite vs. megestrol or placebo
	Omega-3 fatty acids (EPA)	Poor compliance with high doses but results suggest improved lean body mass Low doses had no effect on weight gain or appetite
	Pentoxifylline	No effect on weight gain or improvement in appetite
	Thalidomide	Shown to reduce weight loss compared to placebo at 200 mg daily

Source: PDQ® Supportive and Palliative Care Editorial Board. (2020). PDQ Nutrition in Cancer Care. National Cancer Institute. https://www.cancer.gov/about-cancer/treatment/side-effects/appetite-loss/nutrition-hp-pdq; Childs, D., & Jatoi, A. (2019). A hunger for hunger: A review of palliative therapies for cancer-associated anorexia. *Annals of Palliative Medicine*, *8*(1), 50–58. https://doi.org/10.21037/apm.2018.05.08

- ONS, which may be nutritionally complete, can be used to supplement or replace oral meals and snacks.
  - Most ONS provide between 230 to 360 calories and 10 to 20 g protein per 8 oz serving.
  - ONS may be the easiest and most consistent way to achieve a high-calorie, high-protein intake.
- Appetite stimulants are helpful for a subgroup of cancer clients who struggle with loss of appetite (Table 24.5) (Childs & Jatoi, 2019).
  - Although they may improve appetite, they do not appear to improve quality of life or survival.

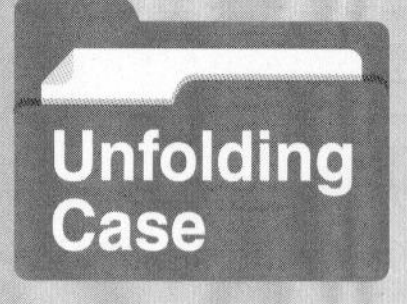

Recall Patrick. He is experiencing anorexia, nausea, vomiting, and mouth sores from chemotherapy and now weighs 236 pounds. What percentage of his usual weight has he lost? Is that significant? What strategies would you suggest he try to maintain an adequate oral intake?

Nutrition Support

For both physiological and psychological reasons, an oral diet is preferred whenever possible. When oral intake is inadequate or contraindicated, enteral or parenteral nutrition can provide supplemental or complete nutrition.

- Nutrition support is not used routinely but is indicated in clients who are malnourished and are expected to not be able to consume adequate oral nutrition for an extended period (PDQ® Supportive and Palliative Care Editorial Board, 2020).
- Enteral nutrition is preferred over parenteral nutrition whenever the GI tract is functional.
- Parenteral nutrition support is an option when the GI tract is nonfunctional, such as in the case of a complete bowel obstruction or failure.

Additional Considerations

Additional considerations as put forth in the European Society for Clinical Nutrition and Metabolism (ESPEN) guidelines on nutrition in cancer clients are as follows (Arends et al., 2017):

- Cancer clients who are losing weight and have insulin resistance may benefit from lowering the percentage of calories from carbohydrate and increasing calories from fat. This change decreases the glycemic load and increases calorie density.
- The use of a multivitamin and mineral that provides RDA levels of nutrients is useful and safe. In general, single, high doses of micronutrients should be avoided.
- The use of any diet that is not based on clinical evidence is not recommended.
  - Fad diets have the potential to cause micronutrient deficiencies and exacerbate malnutrition.
  - No diets have been proven to cure or prevent the recurrence of cancer.
- Maintaining or increasing physical activity, including resistance exercise, is recommended to support muscle mass, physical function, and health-related quality of life.

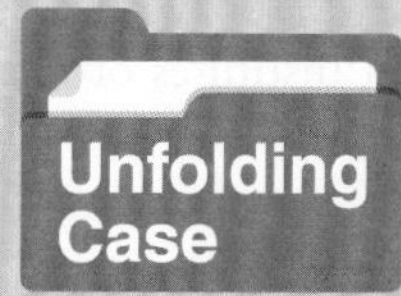

Recall Patrick. His weight loss continues and he is having difficulty staying hydrated due to mouth sores and vomiting. Are there additional diet modifications you would recommend that may enable him to consume adequate fluids and calories? Is he a candidate for EN? What are the potential risks and benefits?

Nutrition in Advanced Cancer

Refractory cachexia develops as a result of very advanced cancer or rapidly progressive disease (PDQ® Supportive and Palliative Care Editorial Board, 2020). It is associated with active catabolism and weight loss that are not responsive to nutrition therapy. At the end of life, clients often severely restrict their intake of food and fluids as part of the normal dying process (PDQ® Supportive and Palliative Care Editorial Board, 2020).

- The goals of nutrition intervention in clients with advanced cancer are to promote the best possible quality of life and manage nutrition-related symptoms that cause distress (Box 24.3) (PDQ® Supportive and Palliative Care Editorial Board, 2020).
- Eating is encouraged as a source of pleasure, not as an adjunct to treatment, and the client's preferences are the primary consideration.
- Studies on the last week of life do not support the use of artificial nutrition, and studies on artificial hydration had mixed results (PDQ® Supportive and Palliative Care Editorial Board, 2020).

Nutrition for Cancer Survivors

Cancer survivors are urged to follow nutrition and physical activity recommendations for cancer prevention—namely, maintain a healthy weight, be physically active, and eat a mostly plant-based diet (Fig. 24.1). Several reviews indicate that obesity and metabolic syndrome might be independent risk factors for recurrence and reduced survival in breast and gastric cancer clients (Arends et al., 2017). Cancer survivors are at a significantly higher risk of developing second primary cancers and other chronic diseases such as coronary heart disease, diabetes, and osteoporosis (Ng & Travis, 2008), emphasizing the importance of a healthy lifestyle.

Consider Patrick. He completed the recommended course of chemotherapy and will be closely followed to ensure the treatment was effective. He has high anxiety and fear that the cancer will return and wants to do everything he can to reduce the risk. What would you say to Patrick to help manage his fear? What weight, intake, and exercise goals would you recommend Patrick set?

HIV AND AIDS

HIV is a chronic infectious disease that attacks the immune system, specifically CD4 cells. It is diagnosed with an enzyme-linked immunosorbent assay test (ELISA) and confirmed with a Western blot test. HIV progresses to AIDS when CD4 cell count is <200 cell/mL and/or an AIDS-defining illness is diagnosed. Poor nutrition can impact the course of HIV; untreated HIV can have significant effects on nutritional status (Box 24.5). The chronicity of HIV infection intensifies the challenge to nutrition.

Antiretroviral Therapy (ART) a combination of ART medications that are typically used to control and reduce viral load.

When the HIV/AIDS pandemic began in the 1980s, people often died from opportunistic infections within years or even months of diagnosis. Since the introduction of potent **antiretroviral therapy (ART)** in the mid-1990s, HIV has been transformed from a fatal illness to a manageable chronic condition (Harris et al., 2018). Today, successfully treated HIV-positive clients have a near-normal life expectancy (National Institutes of Health, National Institute of Allergy and Infectious Diseases, 2019).

Nutrition-Related Complications

Although people living with HIV/AIDS (PLWH) are still at risk for undernutrition and wasting, the use of ART has reduced many of the acute malnutrition-related concerns associated with HIV (Tate et al., 2012). With increased life expectancy, PLWH are facing the challenges of chronic disease (Thuppal et al., 2017).

- Researchers have found that even when HIV is well controlled with ART, immune cells undergo persistent activation that causes chronic inflammation in organs and body systems (National Institutes of Health, National Institute of Allergy and Infectious Diseases, 2019).
- Because inflammation is a key driver of many chronic diseases, PLWH have higher risks of obesity, metabolic syndrome, cardiovascular disease (CVD), and type 2 diabetes as they age.
- Public health concerns over nutrition and HIV have shifted from acute malnutrition to providing optimal nutrition to improve quality of life and overall health (Thuppal et al., 2017).
- Selected nutrition-related complications and comorbidities are outlined in Box 24.6.

BOX 24.5 Effect of HIV on Nutritional Status

- Inflammatory, hormonal, and immune responses to HIV can increase metabolic rate and nutrient requirements, promote loss of lean body tissue, cause anorexia, and alter nutrient storage and availability.
- Infections in the intestines can lead to diarrhea, malabsorption of nutrients, blood loss, and damage to the intestinal lining.
- Opportunistic infections and cancers often result in weight loss.
- Severe infection increases the risk of malnutrition.
- ART medications have multiple adverse side effects that may affect overall intake, metabolism, or nutrient utilization.

BOX 24.6 Nutrition-Related Complications and Comorbidities of HIV/AIDS

Undernutrition

Both malnutrition and HIV impair immune system functioning; when malnutrition and HIV are combined, the effects on the immune system are magnified (Willig et al., 2018).

- Death rates are higher in PLWH who have malnutrition, even those receiving ART.
- HIV and ART may cause a dysregulation of metabolism that negatively affects nutritional status and alters nutrient needs. Protein-energy malnutrition, anemias, and micronutrient deficiencies are common.

HIV-Associated Wasting

HIV-associated wasting was defined in 1987 as an AIDS-defining condition (CDC, 1987). Before the advent of ART, the prevalence of wasting was estimated to be as high as 37%. Some studies suggest the current prevalence may be 20% to 34%, but the degree of wasting is less severe (Myhre & Sifris, 2019).

- It is defined as an involuntary weight loss of >10% with either diarrhea, or weakness and fever for ≥30 days with no other concurrent illness or condition other than HIV infection that could explain the findings (e.g., cancer, tuberculosis, etc.) (CDC, 1987).
- Losses of both fat and lean body mass occur.
- Causes may include HIV, opportunistic infections, or inflammatory changes that increase calorie expenditure and protein breakdown.
- Although ART improves weight loss and malnutrition in PLWH, it may not necessarily prevent the loss of muscle mass or replace it once body weight is restored (Myhre & Sifris, 2019).

Overweight and Obesity

As with the general population in the United States, the prevalence of overweight and obesity in PLWH has been rising.

- More than 60% of PLWH are overweight or obese (Hernandez et al., 2017).
- Some people are obese at the time of HIV diagnosis, and others experience significant weight gain after initiation of ART (Willig et al., 2018).

Lipodystrophy

Lipodystrophy syndrome is characterized changes in body fat distribution and metabolic disturbances.

- Peripheral fat wasting may occur with loss of subcutaneous fat in the face, arms, legs, and buttocks.
- Abnormal fat accumulation may occur in the abdomen (visceral), back of the neck, and breast (gynecomastia).
- Some clients have only fat gain, some have only fat loss, and some have both.
- Metabolic disturbances of HIV lipodystrophy include impaired glucose tolerance, insulin resistance, and hyperlipidemia, which increase the risk of diabetes and atherosclerotic CVD.
- Factors associated with the development of lipodystrophy include ART's protease inhibitor, HIV clinical stage, age at the start of ART, race, and exercise level (dos Santos et al., 2018).
- Body changes due to lipodystrophy may stigmatize clients, causing low self-esteem, problems in social and sexual relations, anxiety, and depression (Shenoy et al., 2014).

Chronic Disease

HIV infection is associated with CVD, hypertension, diabetes, osteoporosis, frailty, and cognitive impairment (Willig et al., 2018).

- PLWH are 50% to 100% more likely to develop CVD than people without HIV, in part due to the chronic inflammatory nature of HIV (NIH, 2019).
- The age-adjusted and body mass index–adjusted rate of diabetes is over 4 times greater in HIV-infected men compared to noninfected men (Brown et al., 2005).

Nutrition Therapy for HIV/AIDS

Viral Load
the level of virus or viral markers measured in the blood.

Nutrition therapy has the potential to promote optimal nutritional status; prevent foodborne illnesses; improve quality of life by managing symptoms of HIV or side effects of medications that affect food intake; and manage or reduce the risk of comorbidities. A well-nourished PLWH who has a controlled **viral load** is more likely to withstand the effects of HIV infection and delay disease progression (Willig et al., 2018). General healthy eating recommendations are the same for PLWH as they are for non-HIV individuals (Box 24.7)

- Because nutrition-related alterations can occur early in HIV infection, nutrition intervention should begin soon after diagnosis (Willig et al., 2018).
- There is not a one-size-fits-all diet for HIV/AIDS nor are there unanimously agreed-upon recommendations for calories or nutrients despite the universal goals of maintaining body weight and lean body mass.
- Recommended intake ranges for macronutrients are the same Dietary Reference Intakes (DRI) levels as those set for the general public: 45% to 65% calories from carbohydrate, 10% to 35% calories from protein, and 20% to 35% calories from fat (Willig et al., 2018).

BOX 24.7 General Healthy Eating Recommendations for Clients with HIV

Overall

- Eat a calorie-appropriate, balanced eating pattern rich in a variety of fruit, vegetables, and whole grains.
- Eat some carbohydrate, protein, and fat at each meal and snack.
- Drink adequate fluid.
- Practice food safety guidelines.
- Manage side effects or symptoms that affect nutrition, such as anorexia, nausea, vomiting, and diarrhea.

Protein

- Choose lean sources such as skinless poultry, lean cuts of beef and pork, fish and seafood, and legumes.
- Eat fish and seafood for healthy omega-3 fats.

Dairy

- Choose low-fat or nonfat milk or yogurt.

Fats

- Eat healthy fats in moderation, such as olive and canola oils, seeds, nuts, nut butters, and avocados.
- Limit saturated and trans fats such as butter, margarine, and shortenings and foods made with solid fats.

Added sugars

- Limit sugar-sweetened beverages and foods with added sugar such as candy, cookies, cakes, and ice cream.

Calories

Calorie needs may be higher or lower than normal depending on the client's current weight and clinical status. Resting energy expenditure (REE) is higher in PLWH than in HIV-negative people and is higher in clients with lipodystrophy than in those with no lipodystrophy (Willig et al., 2018).

To maintain weight, calorie needs may be 10% higher in asymptomatic PLWH and 20% to 30% higher during symptomatic HIV and AIDS (World Health Organization, 2003).

- Calorie reduction for prevention of weight gain may be the primary focus in clients who are overweight or obese (Willig et al., 2018).

Protein

No recent studies of protein need for PLWH have been conducted (Willig et al., 2018)

- An individualized diet with the 10% to 35% of calories from protein (the DRI) is recommended (Willig et al., 2018).

Micronutrients

Recent studies on micronutrients in well-controlled HIV infection are lacking (Willig et al., 2018).

- Supplements of vitamin D and calcium may reduce the loss of bone density that occurs with ART (Overton et al., 2015).
- Clients who do not consume adequate amounts of micronutrients should be counseled on how to improve their intake of micronutrients through better food choices.
- Micronutrient supplements should be used only in the case of deficiencies (Willig et al., 2018).

Manage Symptoms

Clients with HIV/AIDS may experience problems with appetite and intake similar to those of cancer clients. Diet modifications recommended for side effects or complications of cancer are also appropriate for people infected with HIV (see Box 24.4).

Nutrition for Comorbidities

The management of comorbidities and HIV has largely been extrapolated from non-HIV–infected populations (Willig et al., 2018).

- It is not known if nutrition guidelines for hypertension and diabetes in the general public also apply to PLWH (Willig et al., 2018).

- The following are among the modifiable risk factors associated with reducing bone loss in PLWH: Maintain optimal weight; avoid smoking, alcohol, and caffeine; and consume foods rich in calcium and vitamin D (Overton et al., 2015).
- The primary interventions for clients with ART-related dyslipidemia are nutrition and lifestyle (Calza et al., 2016).
  - Recommendations include reducing the intake of saturated fat and cholesterol and increasing the intake of vegetables and fiber.
  - The general healthy eating guidelines outlined in Box 24.7 are appropriate.
  - Increasing physical activity and maintaining healthy body weight usually produce a significant improvement in lipid profile (Calza et al., 2016).

Food and Drug Interactions

ART involves taking a combination of HIV drugs with the goal of reducing viral load to an undetectable level. Although ART does not cure HIV, it enables PLWH to live longer, healthier lives and reduces the risk of HIV transmission (USDHHS, 2020). ART is recommended for all people beginning at the time of HIV diagnosis. The actual drugs included in a person's treatment regimen vary with the individual's needs. The bioavailability of some medications depends on the medication being taken with food (Table 24.6).

Table 24.6 Single HIV/AIDS Medications and Timing of Food Intake

Generic Name (Brand Name)	Take with Food	Take on Empty Stomach	Take with or without food
Nucleoside reverse transcriptase inhibitors (NRTIs)			
Abacavir (Ziagen)			✓
Emtricitabine (Emtriva)			✓
Lamivudine (Epivir)			✓
Tenofovir (Viread)			✓
Zidovudine (Retrovir)			✓
Nonnucleoside reverse transcriptase inhibitors (NNRTIs)			
Doravirine (Pifeltro)			✓
Efavirenz (Sustiva)		✓ Preferably at bedtime	
Etravirine (Intelence)	✓ After eating		
Nevirapine (Viramune)			✓
Rilpivirine (Edurant)	✓		
Protease inhibitors			
Atazanavir (Reyataz)	✓		
Darunavir (Prezista)	✓		
Fosamprenavir (Lexiva)	✓ (Liquid)		✓ (Tablets)
Ritonavir (Norvir)	✓		
Saquinavir (Invirase)	✓		
Tipranavir (Aptivus)	Take within 2 hours after a meal.		
Fusion inhibitors			
Enfuvirtide (Fuzeon)			✓
CCR5 Antagonists			
Maraviroc (Selzentry)			✓
Integrase inhibitors			
Dolutegravir (Tivicay)			✓
Raltegravir (Isentress)			✓
Pharmacokinetic enhancers			
Cobicistat (Tybost)	✓		

Source: USDHHS, AIDSinfo. (2020). FDA-Approved HIV Medicines. https://aidsinfo.nih.gov/understanding-hiv-aids/fact-sheets/21/58/fda-approved-hiv-medicines

Food Safety

Because clients infected with HIV have compromised immune systems, steps should be taken to reduce the risk of foodborne illness. Food safety strategies are listed in Box 24.2 (see Chapter 10 for more on foodborne illness).

NURSING PROCESS Cancer

Karen is a 59-year-old former smoker who now calls herself a "health nut." She was recently diagnosed with lung cancer. She had surgery to remove her right lung and is receiving chemotherapy for cancerous "spots" on the left lung and stomach. She has lost 28 pounds and complains of nausea, vomiting, and a bad taste in her mouth. Because she has followed a healthy diet to prevent cancer for years, she is reluctant to now change her eating habits and eat more protein, fat, and calories. Right now, she is eating mostly fruit, sherbet, and skim milk.

Assessment

Medical–Psychosocial History

- Medical history such as diabetes, heart disease, or hypertension.
- Types of drugs the client is receiving through chemotherapy; other prescribed medications that affect nutrition.
- Physician's goals and plan of treatment.
- Pattern of nausea and vomiting.
- Client's understanding of increased nutritional needs related to cancer and cancer therapies.
- Willingness to change her attitudes toward food and nutrition.
- Psychosocial and economic issues such as financial status, employment, and outside support system.
- Usual activity patterns.

Anthropometric Assessment

- Height, current weight, usual weight.
- Rate of weight loss; percentage of usual body weight lost.
- BMI.

Biochemical and Physical Assessment

- Laboratory data: prealbumin, serum electrolytes, any abnormal values.
- General appearance/evidence of muscle wasting.

Dietary Assessment

- How many daily meals and snacks are you eating?
- What is a typical day's intake for you?
- When is your appetite the best?
- What do you do to alleviate nausea?
- How has your sense of taste changed? What do you do to cope with the changes?
- Do you have any food allergies or intolerances?
- Do you have any cultural, religious, or ethnic food preferences?
- Do you use vitamins, minerals, or nutrition supplements?
- Do you use liquid formulas, such as instant breakfast mixes or commercial products?
- How much liquid do you consume in a day?
- Do you use alcohol?

Analysis

Possible Nursing Analysis

Malnutrition risk related to nausea, vomiting, and taste changes secondary to cancer/cancer therapy as evidenced by 28-pound weight loss.

Planning

Client Outcomes

The client will do the following:

- Eat six times daily.
- Increase the protein and calorie density of foods she eats.
- Drink at least 16 oz of a high-calorie, high-protein ONS daily.
- Switch from skim milk to whole milk, as tolerated.

NURSING PROCESS

Cancer (continued)

- Verbalize interventions she will try to help alleviate nausea and taste alterations.
- Verbalize the importance of consuming adequate protein and calories and the role of fat in providing calories.
- Maintain present weight until chemotherapy is completed.

Nursing Interventions

Nutrition Therapy Client Teaching

Provide regular diet as ordered with high-protein, high-calorie, in-between meal supplements.

Instruct the client on the following:

- An adequate nutritional status reduces the side effects of treatment, may make cancer cells more receptive to treatment, and may improve quality of life; poor nutritional status may potentiate chemotherapeutic drug toxicity.
- A preventive eating style is no longer appropriate; consuming adequate protein and calories (even fat calories) is the major priority.

Instruct the client on eating plan essentials, including the following:

- Protein sources the client may tolerate despite nausea and taste changes such as eggs, cheese, nuts, dried peas and beans, yogurt, milk shakes, eggnogs, puddings, ice cream, instant breakfast mixes, and commercial supplements.
- How to increase the protein and calorie density of foods eaten (see Box 24.4).
- To eat small, frequent "meals" to help maximize intake but to avoid eating 12 hours before chemotherapy.
- To drink ample fluids 1–2 days before and after chemotherapy to enhance excretion of the drugs and to decrease the risk of renal toxicity.

Instruct the client on interventions to minimize nausea, as follows:

- Eating foods served cold or at room temperature.
- Eating high-carbohydrate, low-fat foods such as toast, crackers, yogurt, sherbet, cooked cereal, soft or canned fruits, watermelon, bananas, fruit juices, and angel food cake.
- Avoiding fatty, greasy, fried, and strongly seasoned foods.

Instruct the client on behavior to help maximize intake, including the following:

- Viewing food as a medicine, rather than a social pleasure, that must be "taken" even when the desire to eat is lacking.
- Keeping track of and avoiding foods that cause nausea.
- Taking antiemetics as prescribed even when symptoms are absent.
- Sucking on sugarless hard candy during chemotherapy and using plastic utensils and dishes to mitigate the "bad taste" in her mouth.
- Avoiding anything that tastes unpleasant.

Evaluation

Evaluate and Monitor

- Monitor weight.
- Monitor food intake records.
- Monitor management of side effects; suggest additional interventions as needed.

How Do You Respond?

Why do cancer prevention guidelines suggest red meat intake be limited? According to the World Cancer Research Fund/American Institute for Cancer Research Continuous Update Project (2018), there is strong evidence that the intake of red meat is a probable cause of colorectal cancer and convincing evidence that processed meat is a cause of colorectal cancer. The risk may be related to substances that occur naturally in red meat (e.g., heme iron, fat content) and substances that are produced when red meat is processed (e.g., nitrites that can become carcinogenic compounds) or cooked (e.g., heterocyclic amines formed at high heat). Other hypotheses are that processed meats are high in fat, contributing to an excess calorie intake and an increase in bile acids and that people who have a high red meat intake tend to eat less plant-based foods and thus miss out on their cancer-protective substances. It is recommended that red meat consumption be limited to no more than 3 portions per week, or about 12 to 18 ounces of cooked weight. Very little, if any, processed meat should be eaten based on data that show no level of intake can confidently be associated with a lack of risk.

Doesn't canola oil cause cancer? The rumor that canola oil causes cancer stems from the fact that canola is derived from rapeseed. Rapeseed is naturally high in erucic acid, a fatty acid shown to be harmful to animals. However, in the 1970s, traditional plant breeding methods led to the creation of a low–erucic acid rapeseed, which is used to make canola oil. Other objections about hexane used to extract the oil and trans fats created during the process of deodorizing the oil are not significant enough to cause concern (Crosby, 2015). Canola oil is a safe and healthy form of fat.

REVIEW CASE STUDY

Steve is a 39-year-old male who has been HIV positive for 6 years. His waistline is expanding, and he blames that for his recent onset of heartburn. Based on a physical examination and insulin resistance, his doctor diagnosed lipodystrophy syndrome. Steve is 6 ft tall and weighs 190 pounds. His weight has been stable for the last several years, although he feels "fatter." He is on ART but is thinking of discontinuing the medication if it is the cause of his change in shape. He is willing to exercise but wants maximum benefit from minimum effort. He is also willing to change his eating habits but relies heavily on eating out. A typical day's intake is shown on the right:

- Evaluate Steve's current weight. Would you recommend weight loss?
- How does Steve's weight affect heartburn and insulin resistance?
- How does his usual intake affect heartburn and insulin resistance?
- What are Steve's nutrition-related problems? What nutrition therapy recommendations would you make?
- What would you tell Steve about exercise?
- What criteria would you monitor to evaluate the effectiveness of nutrition therapy?

Breakfast: A fast-food egg, bacon, and cheese sandwich on an English muffin; hash browns; and large black coffee
Lunch: Double hamburger, french fries, and cola
Dinner: Grilled steak, baked potato with sour cream, and water
Snacks: Chips

STUDY QUESTIONS

1 The nurse knows their instructions about healthy eating to reduce the risk of cancer have been understood when the client states,
   a. "If I follow those healthy eating guidelines, I will not get cancer."
   b. "To reduce the risk of cancer, I have to eat a vegetarian diet."
   c. "There is not enough known about diet and cancer to make informed choices about what to eat to reduce the risk of cancer."
   d. "A mostly plant-based diet may reduce the risk of cancer."

2 The nurse knows their instructions on how to reduce the risk of foodborne illness have been understood when the client states,
   a. "It is okay to thaw food at room temperature as long as I cook it immediately after it is defrosted."
   b. "Leftovers are not safe to eat."
   c. "Fruits and vegetables do not need to be washed if I peel them or eat them after they are cooked."
   d. "Hot dogs, deli meats, and luncheon meats should be reheated before being eaten."

3 Which of the following strategies would the nurse suggest to help the client increase the protein density of their diet?
   a. Top-baked potatoes with sour cream.
   b. Mix cream cheese with butter and spread on hot bread.
   c. Substitute milk for water in recipes.
   d. Add whipped cream to coffee.

4 Which of the following meals would be most appropriate for a client who has nausea?
   a. Cottage cheese and fresh fruit plate
   b. Fried chicken and coleslaw
   c. Hamburger and french fries
   d. Spaghetti with marinara sauce and salad

5 The client asks what foods they can eat for protein because meat tastes "rotten." Which of the following would be the nurse's best response?
   a. Cheese omelet, cold chicken sandwich, and shrimp salad
   b. Vegetable soup, pulled-pork sandwich, and chili
   c. Pasta salad, beef taco salad, peanut butter, and jelly sandwich
   d. Hot dogs, hamburgers, and vegetable pizza

6 A client asks if it is okay to drink nutrition supplements in place of eating solid food because it seems to be the only thing they tolerate. Which of the following is the nurse's best response?
   a. "Oral nutrition supplements are okay to use as a supplement in your diet, but they do not provide enough nutrition to use them in place of a meal."
   b. "Oral nutrition supplements are rich in nutrients and can be used in place of meals if they are what you are able to tolerate best."
   c. "It is fine to rely on oral nutrition supplements but vary the brand to ensure you are getting adequate nutrition."
   d. "Oral nutrition supplements generally are too high in calories and protein to use in place of meals."

7 Which statement indicates the client with HIV understands instruction about healthy eating?
   a. "Eating fat increases my chances of getting fat around my middle, so I am trying to choose all nonfat or low-fat food."
   b. "Because I have HIV, it is too late for healthy eating to be beneficial."
   c. "Protein is the most important nutrient, so I am eating extra red meat at every meal."
   d. "Unsaturated fats in olive oil, canola oil, nuts, and avocado are healthiest. I am eating those in place of solid fats."

8 When should nutrition therapy become part of the care plan for a client with HIV?
   a. Soon after diagnosis
   b. When the client begins to lose weight
   c. After the first acute episode of illness
   d. When weight loss is >5% of initial weight

CHAPTER SUMMARY NUTRITION FOR CLIENTS WITH CANCER OR HIV/AIDS

Cancer is a group name for different types of malignancies characterized by the uncontrolled growth of cells. Thirty-nine to forty percent of Americans will develop cancer in their lifetime

Nutrition in Cancer Prevention

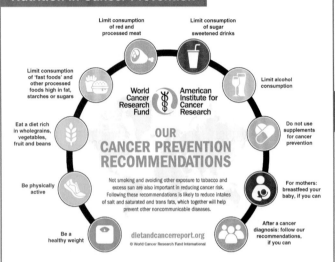

- Potentially modifiable risk factors are estimated to be responsible for more than 40% of incident cancers and almost 50% of all cancer deaths.
- The two largest modifiable risk factors are tobacco use and overweight/obesity.
- Nutrition-related recommendations for cancer prevention include a plant-based diet with limited consumption of fast foods, processed foods, red and processed meat, sugar-sweetened beverages, and alcohol.

Nutrition Complications Related to Cancer

Cancer clients are among the most malnourished of all client groups. Malnutrition differs from starvation-related malnutrition in that inadequate food intake is accompanied by an alteration in metabolism.

- **Local tumor effects:** Occur when the tumor impinges on surrounding tissue and are most severe with GI and head and neck cancers.
- **Tumor-induced changes in metabolism:** Considered a hallmark of cancer but exact mechanisms are not fully understood.
- **Inadequate intake:** The causes are complex and multifactorial and may occur prior to diagnosis or be the result of cancer or cancer treatments.
- **Muscle protein depletion:** Loss of lean body mass is an independent risk factor for poorer outcomes. Sarcopenia can be difficult to identify in clients who are obese.
- **Systemic inflammation Syndrome:** Alters the metabolism of carbohydrates, protein, and fat and is associated with fatigue, impaired physical activity, anorexia, and weight loss.
- **Interactions and Outcomes:** Weight loss, impaired physical functioning, and systemic inflammation in cancer clients are all independently associated with unfavorable outcomes and interact to diminish client well-being.
- **Cancer cachexia:** Multifactorial syndrome characterized by unstoppable muscle wasting that cannot be fully reversed by conventional nutrition support.

Nutrition Complications Related to Cancer Treatments

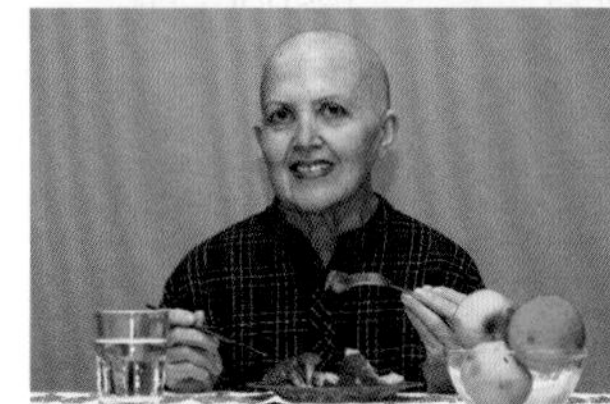

Treatments can contribute to progressive nutritional deterioration due to localized or systemic side effects. The success of treatment is influenced by the client's ability to tolerate therapy.

- **Surgery:** Healing from surgery increases the requirement for protein, calories, vitamin C, B vitamins, and iron. GI surgeries have the greatest likelihood of nutrition complications.
- **Chemotherapy:** Cancer cells and healthy cells of the GI tract, respiratory system, bone marrow, skin, and gonadal tissue are most vulnerable. Side effects are systemic; anorexia, taste changes, early satiety, nausea, vomiting, mucositis, diarrhea, and constipation are most common.
- **Radiation:** Side effects are localized; some may be chronic. Nutrition-related side effects are most common from radiation to the head and neck, lower neck and mid-chest, abdomen and pelvis, and brain.
- **Biotherapy:** Most common nutrition-related side effects are fatigue, fever, nausea, vomiting, and diarrhea.
- **Hemopoietic cell transplantation:** Mucositis and significant diarrhea are frequent side effects. Enteral or parenteral support may be indicated.

Nutrition Therapy during Cancer Treatment

Goals of nutrition therapy are individualized according to the client's nutrition status, type and stage of disease, comorbid conditions, and treatment plan.

- **Calories:** Can be estimated at 25 to 30 cal/kg/day and adjusted as needed.
- **Protein:** Optimum intake is unknown; ≥1.0 to 2.0 g/kg/day may be needed to promote positive protein balance.

CHAPTER SUMMARY NUTRITION FOR CLIENTS WITH CANCER OR HIV/AIDS (continued)

- **Promoting an oral intake:** Ideally clients meet their need orally through food. Calorie and protein density can be increased in food. ONS can be used to supplement or replace meals as needed.
- **Nutrition support:** May be necessary if oral diet is inadequate or contraindicated.
- **Additional considerations:** A low-carbohydrate diet may benefit cancer clients with insulin resistance; a multivitamin and mineral supplement at 100% of the DRI is useful; fad diets are not recommended; and physical activity is recommended.

Nutrition in Advanced Cancer

Refractory cachexia develops in clients with very advanced cancer or rapidly progressive cancer. It is not responsive to nutrition therapy. Clients often self-restrict food and fluid intake at the end of life. Nutrition-related symptoms that cause distress should be managed.

Nutrition for Survivors of Cancer

Cancer prevention guidelines—eat a plant-based diet, maintain healthy weight, and be physically active—should be followed to potentially decrease the risk of recurrence, second primary cancers, and other chronic diseases.

HIV and AIDS

Poor nutrition impacts the course of HIV; HIV can have significant effects on nutrition status. PLWH/AIDS now have a life expectancy near normal.

Nutrition-Related Complications. PLWH have higher risks of obesity, metabolic syndrome, CVD, and type 2 diabetes as they age related to the inflammatory nature of HIV. Focus has shifted from acute malnutrition to managing chronic diseases.

Nutrition Therapy for HIV/AIDS. A PLWH who has a controlled viral load is more likely to withstand the effects of HIV infection and delay disease progression. General healthy eating recommendations for the general public are appropriate for PLWH: Eat a plant-based diet that provides a variety of fruit, vegetables, whole grains, and lean protein and limit the intake of saturated fat, trans fat, and added sugar.

- **Calories:** PLWH may have a higher REE than noninfected people. Calorie needs may be 10% higher in the absence of symptoms and 20% to 30% higher during symptomatic HIV/AIDS. Prevention of weight gain may be appropriate for PLWH who are overweight or obese.
- **Protein:** Exact requirements are unknown. Protein should provide 10% to 35% of total calories (normal DRI).
- **Micronutrients:** Preferable source is food. Vitamin D and calcium supplements may reduce loss of bone density with ART. Other supplements should be used only in the case of documented deficiencies.
- **Manage symptoms:** Nutrition interventions may help relieve problems with appetite and intake.
- **Comorbidities:** It is not known if nutrition guidelines for hypertension and diabetes are the same for PLWH as they are for the general public. Bone loss may be reduced with dietary and lifestyle interventions. A heart-healthy eating pattern may improve dyslipidemia.

Food and Drug Interactions. The bioavailability of some drugs is influenced by the presence of food.

Food Safety. Food safety is especially important for PLWH because of their compromised immune system.

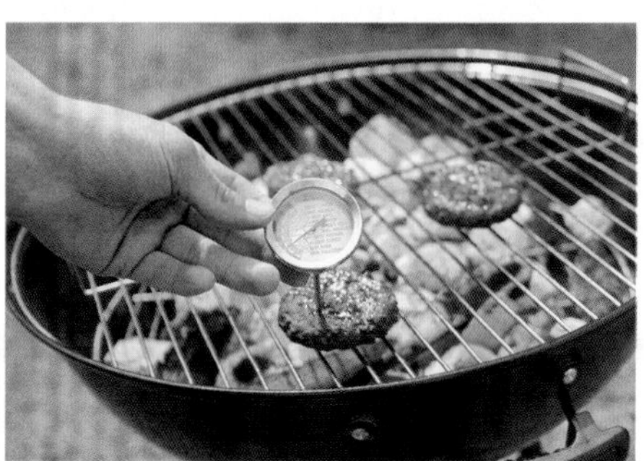

Figure sources: *shutterstock.com/OKcamera and shutterstock.com/ESB Professional*

Student Resources on thePoint®
For additional learning materials, activate the code in the front of this book at https://thePoint.lww.com/activate

Websites

Websites related to cancer

American Cancer Society at www.cancer.org
American Institute for Cancer Research at www.aicr.org
National Cancer Institute at www.cancer.gov
National Center for Complementary and Alternative Medicine (NCCAM) at www.nccam.nih.gov
Oncology Nursing Society at www.ons.org

Websites related to HIV/AIDS

AIDSinfo (A Service of the U.S. Department of Health and Human Services) at www.aidsinfo.nih.gov
Center for HIV Information from the University of California San Francisco School of Medicine at www.hivinsite.org

References

American Cancer Society. (2020). *Cancer facts & figures 2020.* American Cancer Society; 2020. https://www.cancer.org/content/dam/cancer-org/research/cancer-facts-and-statistics/annual-cancer-facts-and-figures/2020/cancer-facts-and-figures-2020.pdf

Arends, J., Bachmann, P., Baracos, V., Barthelemy, N., Bertz, H., Bozzetti, F., Fearon, K., Hutterer, E., Isenring, E., Kaasa, S., Krznaric, Z., Laird, B., Larsson, M., Laviano, A., Muhlebach, S., Muscaritoli, M., Oldervoll, L., Ravasco, P., Solheim, T., Strasser, F., van der Schueren, M., & Preiser, J.-C. (2017). ESPEN guidelines on nutrition in cancer clients. *Clinical Nutrition, 36*(1), 11–48. https://doi.org/10.1016/j.clnu.2016.07.015

Brown, T. T., Cole, S. R., Li, X., Kingsley, L. A., Palella, F. J., Riddler, S. A., Visscher, B. R., Margolick, J. B., & Dobs, A. S. (2005). Antiretroviral therapy and the prevalence and incidence of diabetes mellitus in the multicenter AIDS cohort study. *Archives of Internal Medicine, 165*(10), 1179–1184. https://doi.org/10.1001/archinte.165.10.1179

Calza, L., Golangeli, V., Manfredi, R., Bon, I., Carla Re, M., & Viale, P. (2016). Clinical management of dyslipidaemia associated with combination antiretroviral therapy in HIV-infected patients. *Journal of Antimicrobial Chemotherapy, 71*(6), 1451–1465. https://doi.org/10.1093/jac/dkv494

Centers for Disease Control and Prevention. (1987). Revision of the CDC surveillance case definition for acquired immunodeficiency syndrome. Council of State and Territorial Epidemiologists; AIDS Program. *Center for Infectious Diseases MMWR Morbidity and Mortality Weekly Report, 36*(suppl 1), 1S–15S.

Childs, D., & Jatoi, A. (2019). A hunger for hunger: a review of palliative therapies for cancer-associated anorexia. *Annals of Palliative Medicine, 8*(1), 50–58. https://doi.org/10.21037/apm.2018.05.08

Crosby, G. (2015). Ask the expert: concerns about canola oil. The Nutrition Source, Harvard School of Public Health. https://www.hsph.harvard.edu/nutritionsource/2015/04/13/ask-the-expert-concerns-about-canola-oil/

dos Santos, A., Navarro, A., Schwingel, A., Alves, T. C., Abdalla, P. P., Venturini, A. C. R., de Santana, R. C., & Machado, D. R. L. (2018). Lipodystrophy diagnosis in people living with HIV/AIDS: Prediction and validation of sex-specific anthropometric models. *BMC Public Health, 18*, 806. https://doi.org/10.1186/s12889-018-5707-z

Fearon, K., Strasser, F., Anker, S., Bosaeus, I., Bruera, E., Fainsinger, R., Jatoi, A., Loprinzi, C., MacDonald, N., Mantovani, G., Cavis, M., Muscaritoli, M., Ottery, F., Radbruch, L., Ravasco, P., Walsh, D., Wilcock, A., Kaasa, S., & Baracos, V. (2011). Definition and classification of cancer cachexia: An international consensus. *Lancet Oncology, 12*(5), 489–495. https://doi.org/10.1016/S1470-2045(10)70218-7

Harris, T., Rabkin, M., & El-Sadr, W. (2018). Achieving the fourth 90: Healthy aging for people living with HIV. *AIDS (London, England), 32*(12), 1563–1569. https://doi.org/10.1097/QAD.0000000000001870

Hernandez, D., Kalichman, S., Cherry, C., Kalichman, M., Washington, C., & Grebler, T. (2017). Dietary intake and overweight and obesity among persons living with HIV in Atlanta Georgia. *AIDS Care, 29*(6), 767–771. https://doi.org/10.1080/09540121.2016.1238441

Heron, M. (2019). Deaths: Leading causes for 2017. *National Vital Statistics Reports, 68*(6), 9. Hyattsville, MD: National Center for Health Statistic.

Islami, F., Sauer, A., Miller, K., Siegel, R., Fedewa, S. A., Jacobs, E. J., McCullough, M. L., Patel, A. V., Ma, J., Soerjomataram, I., Flanders, W. D., Brawley, O. W., Gapstur, S. M., & Jemal, A. (2018). Proportion and number of cancer cases and deaths attributable to potentially modifiable risk factors in the US. *CA: A Cancer Journal for Clinicians, 68*(1), 31–54. https://doi.org/10.3322/caac.21440

Kohler, L., Garcia, D., Harris, R., Oren, E., Roe, D. J., & Jacobs, E. T. (2016). Adherence to diet and physical activity cancer prevention guidelines and cancer outcomes: A systematic review. *Cancer Epidemiology, Biomarkers & Prevention, 25*(7), 1018–1028. https://doi.org/10.1158/1055-9965.EPI-16-0121

Kushi, L., Doyle, C., McCullough, M., Rock, C. L., Demark-Wahnefried, W., Bandera, E. V., Gapstur, S., Patel, A. V., Andrews, K., Gansler, T., The American Cancer Society 2010 Nutrition and Physical Activity Guidelines Advisory Committee. (2012). American Cancer Society guidelines on nutrition and physical activity for cancer prevention. *CA: A Cancer Journal for Clinicians, 62*(1), 30–67. https://doi.org/10.3322/caac.20140

Muscaritoli, M., Lucia, S., Farcomeni, A., Lorusso, V., Saracino, V., Barone, C., Plastino, F., Gori, S., Magarotto, R., Carteni, G., Chiurazzi, B., Pavese, I., Marchetti, L., Zagonel, V., Bergo, E., Tonini, G., Imperatori, M., Iacono, C., Maiorana, L., Pinto, C., … and on behalf of the PreMiO Study Group. (2017). Prevalence of malnutrition in patients at first medical oncology visit: The PreMiO study. *Oncotarget, 8*(45), 79884–79896. https://doi.org/10.18632/oncotarget.20168

Myhre, J., & Sifris, D. (2019). *Understanding HIV wasting syndrome.* https://www.verywellhealth.com/hiv-wasting-syndrome-aids-defining-condition-48955

National Institutes of Health, National Institute of Allergy and Infectious Diseases. (2019). *Treatment for HIV coinfections and complications.* https://www.niaid.nih.gov/diseases-conditions/treatment-hiv-complications

Nelson, W. (2017). Metabolism and cancer. *Cancer Today.* https://www.cancertodaymag.org/Pages/Fall2017/Metabolism-and-Cancer-William-G-Nelson.aspx

Ng, A., & Travis, L. (2008). Second primary cancers: An overview. *Hematology/Oncology Clinics of North America, 22*(2), 271–289. https://doi.org/10.1016/j.hoc.2008.01.007

Overton, E., Chan, E., Brown, T., Tebas, P., McComsey, G. A., Melbourne, K. M., Napoli, A., Hardin, W. R., Ribaudo, H. J., & Yin, M. (2015). Vitamin D and calcium attenuate bone loss with antiretroviral therapy initiation: A randomized trial. *Annals of Internal Medicine, 162*(12), 815–824. https://doi.org/10.7326/M14-1409

PDQ® Supportive and Palliative Care Editorial Board. (2020). PDQ Nutrition in Cancer Care. National Cancer Institute. https://www.cancer.gov/about-cancer/treatment/side-effects/appetite-loss/nutrition-hp-pdq

Ryan, A., Power, D., Daly, L., Cushen, S. J., Bhuachalla, E. N., & Prado, C. M. (2016). Cancer-associated malnutrition, cachexia and sarcopenia: The skeleton in the hospital closet 40 years later. *Proceedings of the Nutrition Society, 75*(2), 199–211. https://doi.org/10.1017/S002966511500419X

Shenoy, A., Ramapuram, J. T., Unnikrishan, B., Achappa, B., Madi, D., Rao, S., & Mahalingam, S. (2014). Effect of Lipodystrophy on the quality of life among people living with HIV (PLHIV) on highly active antiretroviral therapy. *Journal of the International Association of Providers of AIDS Care, 13*(5), 471–475. https://doi.org/10.1177/2325957413488205

Steck, S., & Murphy, E. (2020). Dietary patterns and cancer risk. *Nature Reviews Cancer, 20,* 125–138. https://doi.org/10.1038/s41568-019-0227-4

Tate, T., Willig, A., Willing, J., Raper, J. L., Moneyham, L., Kempf, M. C., Saag, M. S., & Mugavero, M. J. (2012). HIV infection and obesity: Where did all the wasting go? *Antiviral Therapy, 17*(7), 1281–1289. https://doi.org/10.3851/IMP2348

Thuppal, S., Jun, S., Cowan, A., & Bailey, R. L. (2017). The nutritional status of HIV-infected US Adults. *Current Developments in Nutrition, 1*(10), e001636. https://doi.org/10.3945/cdn.117.001636

USDHHS, AIDSinfo. (2020). *HIV treatment: The basics.* https://aidsinfo.nih.gov/understanding-hiv-aids/fact-sheets/21/51/hiv-treatment--the-basics

Willig, A., Wright, L., & Galvin, T. (2018). Practice paper of the Academy of Nutrition and Dietetics: Nutrition intervention and human immunodeficiency virus infection. *Journal of the Academy of Nutrition and Dietetics, 118*(3), 486–498. https://doi.org/10.1016/j.jand.2017.12.007

World Cancer Research Fund/American Institute for Cancer Research. Continuous Update Project. (2018). Diet, nutrition, physical activity and cancer: A global perspective. The Third Expert Report. https://wcrf.org/dietandcancer

World Health Organization. (2003). Nutrient requirements for people living with HIV/AIDS: Report of a technical consultation. www.who.int/nutrition/publications/Content_nutrient_requirements.pdf

Wu, W., & Zhao, S. (2013). Metabolic changes in cancer: Beyond the Warburg effect. *Acta Biochimica et Biophysica Sinica, 45*(1), 18–26. https://doi.org/10.1093/abbs/gms104

Zhou, T., Wang, B., Liu, H., Yang, K., Thapa, S., Zhang, H., Li, L., & Yu, S. (2018). Development and validation of a clinically applicable score to classify cachexia stages in advanced cancer patients. *Journal of Cachexia, Sarcopenia and Muscle, 9*(2), 306–314. https://doi.org/10.1002/jcsm.12275

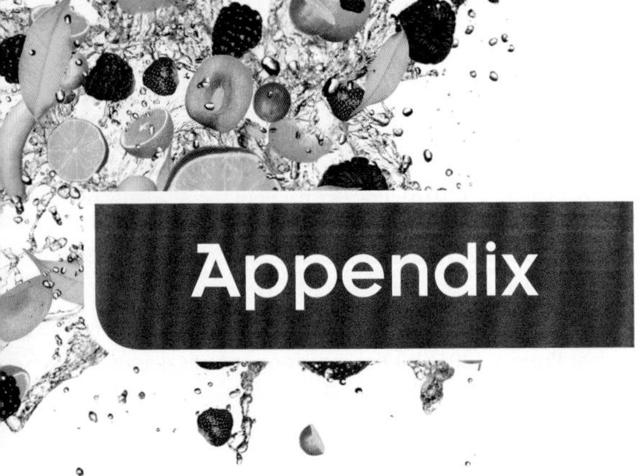

Appendix

Answers to Study Questions

Chapter 1
1. a
2. b
3. c
4. b
5. a

Chapter 2
1. a
2. c
3. c
4. a
5. c
6. a
7. a
8. b

Chapter 3
1. c
2. a
3. d
4. d
5. c
6. a
7. c
8. a

Chapter 4
1. b
2. d
3. b
4. b
5. a
6. c
7. d
8. a

Chapter 5
1. b
2. d
3. b
4. b
5. a
6. a
7. d
8. c

Chapter 6
1. b
2. c
3. c
4. c
5. d
6. b
7. c
8. a

Chapter 7
1. b
2. a
3. c
4. b
5. c
6. a
7. d
8. c

Chapter 8
1. c
2. b
3. c
4. b
5. c
6. b
7. a
8. b

Chapter 9
1. b
2. c
3. b
4. c
5. d
6. c
7. c
8. d

Chapter 10
1. c
2. d
3. c
4. a
5. a, c, d
6. c
7. a
8. a

Chapter 11
1. b
2. c
3. b, c, d
4. a, b, c, d
5. a, b, d
6. d
7. b
8. a

Chapter 12
1. b
2. a
3. d
4. c
5. b
6. a
7. a
8. c

Chapter 13
1. d
2. a
3. b
4. b
5. a, b, c
6. c
7. a
8. d

Chapter 14
1. d
2. c
3. a
4. b
5. b
6. a, b, c
7. a
8. d

Chapter 15
1. a
2. b
3. a
4. b
5. b, c, d
6. d
7. b
8. c

Chapter 16
1. c
2. b
3. c
4. a, c, d
5. b
6. a
7. a, b
8. a

Chapter 17
1. b
2. a, b, c
3. a
4. c
5. b
6. a
7. c
8. b

Chapter 18
1. b
2. c
3. d
4. c
5. c
6. c
7. d
8. b

Chapter 19
1. a
2. a
3. c
4. b
5. b
6. b
7. d
8. d

Chapter 20
1. b
2. a
3. b
4. b
5. b
6. a
7. a
8. d

Chapter 21
1. c
2. d
3. d
4. d
5. a
6. b
7. c
8. a, b, c

Chapter 22
1. b
2. c
3. a
4. a
5. a, b, c, d
6. d
7. c
8. b

Chapter 23
1. c
2. d
3. c
4. c
5. a
6. a
7. a, b, d
8. c

Chapter 24
1. d
2. d
3. c
4. a
5. a
6. b
7. d
8. a

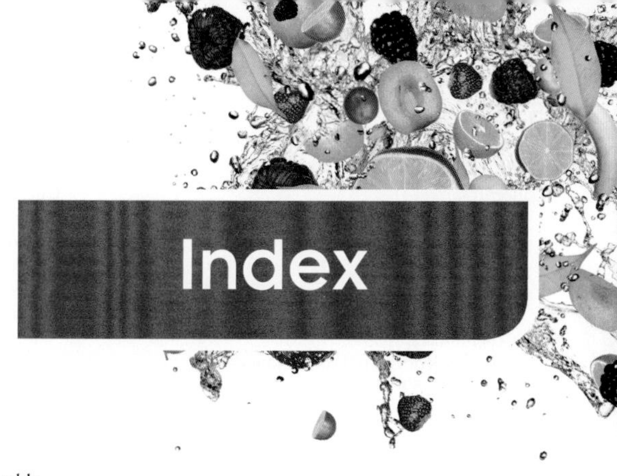

Index

Note: Page numbers followed by *b* indicate a box; those followed by *f*, an illustration; and those followed by *t*, a table.

D

E

F

CCS0521